ORAL MEDICINE AND RADIOLOGY

TOTAL SOLUTIONS

EXAM PREPARATORY MANUAL FOR UNDERGRADUATES

ORAL MEDICINE AND RADIOLOGY

TOTAL SOLUTIONS

EXAM PREPARATORY MANUAL FOR UNDERGRADUATES

Dr. Sunita Prashant Kulkarni, B.D.S, M.D.S
Professor and Head
Department of Oral Medicine and Radiology
Swargiya Dadasaheb Kalmegh Smruti Dental College and Hospital,
Nagpur (Maharashtra)

ARYA MEDI PUBLISHING HOUSE PVT. LTD.
4806, Bharat Ram Road, 24 Darya Ganj
New Delhi - 110 002 (India)

Oral Medicine and Radiology

First Edition : 2018

ISBN: 81-86809-65-1

Published by:
Mr. Sudhir Kumar Arya
For **ARYA MEDI PUBLISHING HOUSE PVT. LTD.**
4806 Bharat Ram Road, 24 Darya Ganj,
New Delhi-110 002
Email: mail@aryamedipublishing.com
www.aryamedipublishing.com

Foreword

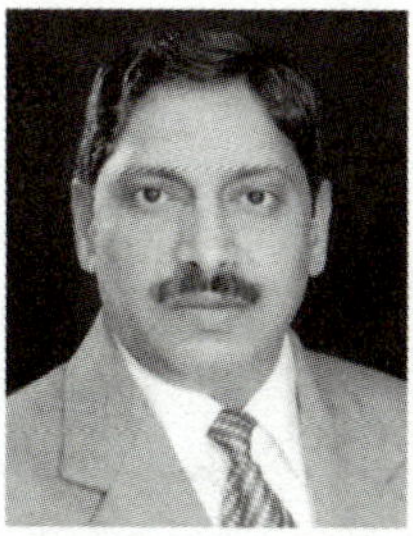

Dr. R. S. Sathawane
MDS (OMR), MA (Public Admn)
*Ex-Professor & HoD, Govt. Dental College, Nagpur
*Ex-Dean, Maitri College of Dentistry, Durg
*President, Indian Academy of Oral Medicine & Radiolgy-2011
*Ex-Member, Academic Council, Board of Studies and Faculty of Dentistry
*President, Indian Dental Association, Nagpur Br -2004-05
*Consultant Oral Physician & Maxillofacial Radiologist

It is indeed a privilege and pleasure in writing this Foreword to this book "Oral Medicine And Radiology including Forensic Odontology – Total Solutions" authored by Dr. Sunita P. Kulkarni, Professor & Head, Dept. of Oral Medicine and Radiology, Swargiya Dadasaheb Kalmegh Smruti Dental College and Hospital, Nagpur.

The initiative and well orchestrated efforts precisely articulated by her in bringing out this book is exemplary & praiseworthy. It is indeed a diligent effort to compile all intellectual inputs covering the vast subject in to a simple, easy and understandable question – answer format. I am sure this book fulfills the need of UG/PG students as a quick reference and help for the examination.

Dr. Sunita P. Kulkarni with her vast experience as a teacher has brought out this book that would be useful not only to undergraduate students but also to postgraduate aspirants/ students and teachers in the speciality of Oral Medicine & Radiology including Forensic Odontology. I congratulate her and strongly recommend this book to all, especially UG/ PG Students.

Dr. R. S. Sathawane

Dedicated to

My husband
Mr Prashant Kulkarni,

my daughter and son-in-law
Ms. Shweta Kulkarni and *Lt. Col Mihir Ghooi*

my parents
Mr. Vijay Puranik and *Mrs. Nalini Puranik,*

my sisters
Anjali and *Jayashree*

Preface

Oral medicine and Radiology is an interesting but vast subject with two components,Oral Medicine and Oral Radiology.Forensic Odontology has also been included in the syllabus since recent times.Its a tough subject to study and internalise.Especially the universities following the semester system there is hardly any time to prepare this subject properly.It was my long desired wish to make things a little easier for the students and prepare them from the exam point of view.I noticed that students who solved and read the question papers fared well in the exams.I hence came up with the idea of giving the students solved questions according to the marks allotted.I have included actual questions asked by various universities and have tried my best to give well researched answers to them.I have also quoted references for further reading by the students.It is thus my humble wish that this book should come in handy for the undergraduate students of Final Year B.D.S.

Dr. Sunita Kulkarni

Acknowledgements

I wish to express my gratitude to Honourable Mr. Sharad Kalmegh, Founder President and Chairman, Local Management Committee, Swargiya Dadasaheb Kalmegh Smruti Dental College and Hospital, Nagpur,for motivating me to come up with this idea of writing solved questions,due to his passion for students to acquire honours and gold medals in exams. Heartfelt gratitude to Dr. Sharath Bontha for his encouragement and motivation.

I wish to thank my colleagues Dr. Rakhi Chandak, Dr. Ashish Lanjekar and Dr. Romita Gaikwad for their support and encouragement.

I also would like to thank my friend Dr. Deepti Gattani for her encouragement and motivation.

A great appreciation for my P.G students, Dr. Sonali Akhade, Dr. Sonal Sonule, Dr. Rashmi Wasekar, Dr. Farheen Khan, Dr. Shubhangi Badole, Dr. Usha Rathod, Dr. Rucha Pandhripande, Dr. Vaishali Agrawal and Dr. Gunjan Moon for their help and support.

I thank all my family members for their constant encouragement and support.

Dr. Sunita Kulkarni

Contents

Foreword v
Preface vii
Acknowledgements ix

Short Answer Questions

Oral Medicine including Forensic Odontology

Sr No	Topic	Page No
1	Case History	3-8
2	Investigations in Dentistry	9-38
3	Drugs in Dentistry	39-49
4	Developmental Disorders of Teeth	50-55
5	Developmental Disorders of Craniofacial Structures	56-60
6	Red And White Lesions of Oral Mucosa	61-78
7	Benign Tumours of Orofacial Region	79-91
8	Oral Cancer	92-97
9	Malignant Tumours of Orofacial Region	98-103
10	Ulcerative and Vesiculobullous Lesions	104-127
11	Orofacial Pain	128-145
12	Oral Pigmented Lesions	146-155
13	Diseases of Tongue	156-164
14	Gingival and Periodontal Diseases	165-171
15	Granulomatous Diseases	172-178
16	Temporomandibular Joint Disorders	179-187
17	Salivary Gland Disorders	188-206

18	Disorders of Maxillary Sinus	207-208
19	Infections of Oral Cavity	209-215
20	Bacterial Infections	216-219
21	Viral Infections	220-225
22	Diseases of Cardiovascular System	226-234
23	Acquired Immunodeficiency Syndrome	235-243
24	Endocrine Disorders	244-248
25	Blood Disorders	249-269
26	Metabolic Disorders	270-272
27	Neuromuscular Disorders	273-275
28	Miscellaneous	276-302
29	Forensic Odontology	303-323

Short Answer Questions:

Oral and Maxillofacial Radiology

Sr No	Topic	Page No
1	Radiation Physics	327-336
2	Radiation Biology	337-339
3	Production of X Rays	340-347
4	Properties of X Rays	348-350
5	Radiation Protection	351-363
6	Projection Geometry	364-366
7	Imaging Principles	367
8	X Ray Films and Accessories	368-378
9	Processing of X Ray Film	379-387
10	Intraoral Radiographic Techniques	388-398
11	Radiographic Anatomy	399-402
12	Faulty Radiographs	403-408
13	Panoramic Radiography	409-413
14	Extraoral Radiographic Techniques	414-423
15	Specialized Imaging Techniques	424-440
16	Dental Caries	441-448
17	Infections and Inflammatory Lesions of the Jaws	449-459
18	Cysts of Jaws	460-462

19	Benign Tumors of Jaws	463-469
20	Malignant Tumors of Orofacial Region	470-473
21	Fibro-Osseous Lesions	474-478
22	Radiopaque Lesions of Jaws	479-482
23	Radiolucent Lesions of Jaws	483-486
24	Miscellaneous	487-492

Long Answer Questions:

Oral Medicine

Sr No	Topic	Page No
1	Ulcerative, Vesicular and Bullous Lesions	495-519
2	Red and White Lesions of Oral Mucosa	520-560
3	Pigmented Lesions of Oral Mucosa	561-565
4	Oral Cancer	566-575
5	Salivary Gland Diseases	576-589
6	Temporomandibular Joint Disorders	590-594
7	Orofacial Pain	595-612
8	Gingival and Periodontal Diseases	613-616
9	Diseases of Maxillary Sinus	617-621
10	Immunologic Diseases	622-626
11	Hematologic Diseases	627-632
12	Miscellaneous	633-654

Long Answer Questions

Oral and Maxillofacial Radiology

Sr No	Topic	Page No
1	Radiation Biology	657-662
2	Radiation Protection	663-667
3	Processing of X Ray Films	668-678
4	Intraoral Radiographic Examination	679-683
5	Panoramic Imaging	684-687
6	Periodontal Diseases	688-693
7	Inflammatory Lesions of Jaws	694-702
8	Cysts of Jaws	703-713
9	Benign Tumors of Jaws	714-722

10	Fibro-Osseous Lesions	723-726
11	Diagnostic Imaging of Temporomandibular Joint	727-732
12	Trauma to Teeth and Facial Structures	733-736
13	Salivary Gland Radiology	737-740
14	Periapical Radiolucencies and Radiopacities	741-745
15	Miscellaneous	746-767

ORAL MEDICINE INCLUDING FORENSIC ODONTOLOGY

SHORT ANSWERS

CHAPTER 1

Case History

INTRODUCTION

Case history can be considered as a planned, professional conversation that enables the patient to communicate his symptoms, feelings and fears, to the clinician, so that the nature of the patient's real and suspected illness and attitudes can be determined.

To establish a good rapport with the patient, the dentist should show interest, warmth and compassion so that a detailed clinical history can be obtained.

It should be taken in a pleasant environment with nice decor and furniture and the atmosphere should be different from the dental operatory.

Diagnosis is made by history, physical examination and investigations.

Q 1) Significance of medical history

TNMGRU APRIL 2001 (5 Marks)

Obtaining a medical history is a process for gathering information and getting a complete assessment of the health status of the patient.

The medical case history consists of a detailed information of the patient's chief complaint, a complete history of the chief complaint, information about past and present medical conditions, social and family history, and a systematic review of symptoms organ wise. It also includes detailed history about where the patient resides and what kind of conditions he is living in and complete address so that it can be used to identify the patient.

Obtaining patients medical history is of high importance as it can give information about the health status of the patient and can facilitate better diagnosis of the oro-facial complaint of the patient.

A proper interpretation of all the information gathered during the medical history can give us three important objectives:

1. it helps to understand and monitor the medical conditions and evaluate the systemic symptoms that the patient may be unaware about.
2. it provides information about the fact as to whether the dental treatment carried out may affect the overall health of the patient.

3. it also gives an initial information about whether the systemic conditions can influence the patient's oral health and dental treatment required.

Components of Medical History:

(i) **Details of patient's residential address:** Writing the patients name, detailed address and land line or mobile numbers, any proof of identity, recording age and sex, race and ethnic origin, and also obtaining any contact information of the patients kith and kin or close friend, phone numbers of the referring dentist or clinician and also the same of patients family dentist or physician.

(ii) **Recording of the chief complaint and the history of present illness:** The chief complaint is obtained by taking a detailed history of the problems that the patient is troubled with the most and is seeking treatment for the same. It is recorded as much as possible in patient's own words and should not be written in any technical terms unless the patient uses it.

(iii) **Past Dental History:** It is a very important part of the patient's history. (PDH)

It is especially important in cases where patient presents with restorative and periodontal conditions along with medical complications like Diabetes. Certain important points to be recorded are the past dental visits, any restorative, periodontal or endodontic and oral surgical procedures, reasons for loss of teeth if any, history of any complications during previous treatment.

Fluoride history, source of water for drinking, any previous orthodontic treatment or dental prosthesis and radiation therapy for oro-facial lesions.

(iv) **Past Medical History:** (PMH) consists of information about any previous illnesses either in childhood or as adult.

The PMH can be categorised as: 1) Any serious illness. 2) History of previous hospitalisation. 3) Blood transfusions. 4) Allergies. 5) Medications. 6) Pregnancy.

(v) **Social History:** This includes details of marital status, area of residence, educational qualification, occupation, religion, use of tobacco, alcohol, in both cases the frequency and amount of each, any history of drug abuse.

(vi) **Thorough review of systems (ROS):** It comprises of complete review of subjective symptoms affecting different parts of the body. The ROS and physical examination in combination helps to get a systematic patient history.

Both the negative and positive responses have to be recorded.

More questions can be asked to collect additional data to either confirm or rule out certain diseases that have been noted by the clinician as a likely explanation for the patient's symptoms.

This will help the clinician to become alert about the underlying systemic conditions that were not mentioned in the PMH. The ROS will help to monitor the changes in medical conditions.

Different pieces of information makes up the patient's medical history that gives a complete picture about that individual's current and past health. It can provide information about the following:

1. **Assess in the diagnosis of oral disease:** Several systemic disorders have oral manifestations. Hence medical history would help for eg. in herpes virus infection, negative history of RHL and positive history of contact with primary or recurrent herpes patient would help in diagnosis.
2. By taking medical history any systemic condition that the patient is not aware of can be detected.
3. **Management of patient:** The general health status can be ascertained which would help in proper treatment planning.Presence of quite a few systemic disorders can alter the line of treatment of dental complaints of a patient and may need modifications.
4. Consultations with other professionals: Proper medical history would determine whether any additional information is needed to assess the medical status and may be required to communicate with a medical professional in following instances:
   (i) **Known medical problems:** Consultation with a medical professional may be required before a stressful dental procedure if the patient has a medical problem that can complicate a dental procedure.
   (ii) **Unknown medical problem:** In some patients certain medical abnormalities can be detected during recording of history, physical examination or laboratory procedures which would require consultation with a medical professional.
   (iii) **High risk patients:** Some patients may have high risk for development of certain problems. Eg. obese patients may have a risk of hypertension.

   Patients with diabetes may be at risk for developing complications during dental surgical procedures and consultation with concerned physician and his consent may be vital.
5. Medical history can give indication of presence of medical conditions like retardation, depression, hypertension, cerebral palsy or other mental health conditions which may have effect on dental procedures.

   Anesthetics containing epinephrine may be contraindicated in hypertensive patients. Prophylactic antibiotics may be indicated in patients with prosthetic valves and joints, a history of rheumatic fever, congenital heart murmurs, etc.
6. History of known allergies : Medical history would give information on presence of allergies to certain food stuff or drugs.
7. Past or present illnesses: Information on previous serious or chronic illnesses like tuberculosis, asthma, or diabetes is very important as it may have effect on the dental procedures.

8. History of taking medications like immunosuppresants are very important prior to going in for dental surgical procedure. Antibiotics may decrease the effectiveness of birth control pills .
    1. Information about patient's medical consultants: Medical history can give information about the names and phone numbers of the patient's health care providers that include, doctors, or psychiatrists.
    2. Names and phone numbers of family and friends, in case of emergency can be obtained during medical history.
    3. History of any previous surgeries the patient has had.
    4. Previous hospitalisation and their dates and reason.
    5. History of any medical history in the family like cancer, mental illness or heart disease and diabetes. Certain diseases are hereditary and family medical history might help in diagnosis eg.Recurrent aphthous stomatitis, has a family history that is positive in about 60-70% cases.
    6. Records and dates of immunisation done in the past.
    7. Medical questionnaire:During medical history a complete questionnaire on various systems evaluation is filled out from the patient which can have direct or indirect effect on the dental treatment procedures.In this procedure general information, and information on various systems like cardiovascular, respiratory, haematologic, and nervous system, metabolic and endocrine, gastrointestinal, hepatic, biliary tracts and genitourinary systems.Particular importance must be given to disorders like diabetes, bleeding disorders, asthma, hypertension, hepatitis B, myocardial infarction, diphtheria, rheumatoid heart disease, tuberculosis, gonorrhoea etc.
    8. History of taking medications like immunosuppresants are very important prior to going in for dental surgical procedure. Antibiotics may decrease the effectiveness of birth control pills.

Suggested reading:

1. Anil Govind Rao Ghom, Text Book of Oral Medicine, Third edition, page 29-31.
2. Burket's, Oral Medicine Diagnosis and Treatment 10th edi. Pg no. 9-12.

Q 2) Percussion test

BFU 2009 MAY (5 Marks)

Percussion test is done during a patients history taking and helps to evaluate the status of the periodontium surrounding the tooth.

- Percussion test is done to find out the offending tooth and determining the peri-radicular diagnosis.
- This is done by using the metal handle of a mouth mirror and the tooth is gently tapped occlusally and then buccally to elicit a response.

- The intensity of tapping should be minimal but can be repeated several times and the intensity of tapping becoming slightly pronounced with repetition.
- A painful response is suggestive of periradicular inflammation and the intensity of pain can be compared with the other teeth by increase in the severity of the symptoms of the affected tooth when it is repeatedly percussed.
- Teeth adjacent to the symptomatic tooth can be sensitive but the intensity of pain does not progress like the problematic tooth after being tapped repeatedly.
- In case the pain and discomfort does not increase with repeated tapping, it can be termed as a sensitive tooth that can be evaluated in the next appointment to ascertain whether the symptoms have disappeared.

There are two types of percussion tests that are carried out:

(i) Vertical percussion test.
(ii) Horizontal percussion test.

(i) **Vertical percussion test:**
   - In case the vertical percussion test is positive it indicates the presence of periapical pathology.
   - To carry out this test, the tooth is struck a quick, moderate blow initially with low intensity by the finger and then with increasing intensity by using the handle of the instrument, to determine whether the tooth is tender.
   - The adjacent tooth is tapped first and then the affected one is tapped in a vertical direction.
   - The response to tapping is judged by patient's body language and movement and the reflex of the eyes. If the tooth is tender, the patient will blink the eyes due to pain.

(ii) **Horizontal percussion test:**
   - Positive horizontal percussion test indicates periodontium associated problems. The procedure is same as that of vertical percussion but the direction of blow is in horizontal direction.

Categories for Percussion:

1. **None (-):** Tapping on the incisal edge of a tooth with the tip of the fingernail or with the end of a mirror causes no discomfort at all. The patient is likely to not respond at all, or may respond with phrases like "no problem" or "it feels like the other teeth".
2. **Mild (+):** Tapping on the incisal edge of a tooth with the tip of the fingernail or with the end of a mirror causes little discomfort, but may be noticeable by the patient. The patient is likely to respond with phrases like "that feels different from the other teeth".
3. **Moderate (++):** Tapping on the incisal edge of a tooth with the tip of the fingernail or with the end of a mirror causes some noticeable discomfort. The patient is likely to respond with phrases like "I

feel that", and there may be non-verbal communication such as frowning or squinting of the eyes.

4. **Severe (+++):** Tapping on the incisal edge of a tooth with the tip of the fingernail or use of the end of a mirror many times to excessive causes definitive discomfort. The patient is likely to respond with phrases like "Ouch" or "Please do not do that again", and there will likely be non-verbal communication such as frowning or squinting of the eyes.

Suggested reading:

1. Anil Govindrao Ghom, Textbook of oral medicine, chapter 4 page no 44.
2. Manish Garala, BDS, MS. Contemporary Endodontic Evaluation and Diagnosis: Implications for Evidence-Based Endodontic Care, A Peer-Reviewed Publication.

CHAPTER 2

Investigations in Dentistry

INTRODUCTION

There are various diagnostic tests that are required to diagnose, and treat successfully several oral disorders.Laboratory studies include examination in which tissue, blood, urine, or other specimens are obtained from patients and subjected to histological or immunological examination. The information thus obtained can help in final diagnosis of the disease.

Q 1) Exfoliative Cytology

TNMGRU APRIL 2001 (5 Marks)
RGUHS APRIL1998 (5 Marks)

It is a fast and rapid, non-invasive procedure to assess dysplastic changes in the oral epithelium. It involves removal of surface cells.

Cytology indicates study of cells

It is of great importance when a clinician or dentist decides it best not to perform biopsy. It aids in the differential diagnosis of an unidentified lesion of the oral mucosa or benign lesion and also helps in detecting carcinoma-in situ and other premalignant lesions or velvety red, granular patches and in cases of confirming a lesion suggestive of oral cancer where the patient is not ready for biopsy.

1. It's a quick and simple procedure which is painless and no anesthesia is required.
2. It is low cost and rapid procedure and is safe with almost no complications.
3. It acts as a screening procedure for lesions whose gross appearance is such that the biopsy is not warranted.
4. Diagnosis is fast.
5. As a check against false negative biopsies.
6. Follow up detection of recurrent carcinoma.
7. Should not be done on pigmented and vascular lesions.

Indications:

(i) As a preferred procedure when patient refuses biopsy.
(ii) Follow up for recurrence in patients who had radiation therapy for

lesion that was superficial or adjacent to bone.

(iii) In debilitated and very old patients where it is difficult to localise a proper biopsy site.

(iv) Periodic review of lesions like leukoplakia, lichen planus.

(v) As an aid to diagnose some diseases like candidiasis, pemphigus, white sponge nevus, oral premalignant and malignant lesions.

(vi) For population screening for detection of oral cancer.

Procedure:

(a) Tissue is obtained by rubbing the lesion with wet wooden spatula & transferring some of the cells on the slide for H/P examination.

(b) A tongue blade may be used as it is or split into longitudinal halves so that there is a smooth and sharp edge for scraping the lesion. It is made certain that the working tips of the tongue blade are soaked in tap water before use.

(c) As the tissue is stretched the square edge of the instrument is positioned at the back of the lesion and is firmly held and brought forward and pressure is then applied until some material that is visible is collected.Vigorous scraping of the surface of the lesion may be done with a metal cement spatula or a moistened tongue blade.

(d) The slide is prepared by gently smearing the cells on it and then spraying with a fixative while the slide is still wet or immersed in the jar containing fixative.

(e) Fixing is done by dipping it in 95 percent ethyl alcohol or in equal quantities of 95 percent ethyl alcohol and ether or spraying it with commercial fixative.

(f) After the slides are air dried they are sent to the pathologist for processing and evaluation.

(g) They are usually stained with papinicolaou.

(h) The slides are carefully screened by a cytotechnologist, who marks the cells that are suspicious and can be considered as malignant.

(i) The slides that are marked are then reviewed by the pathologist who makes the final evaluation.

(j) The final report generally contains a description of the types of cells present (epithelial, inflammatory etc.) and also assessment of malignancy.

(k) The evaluation may reveal a)negative for cancer, b)suspicion of cancer, c)positive for cancer.

Interpretation:

1. **Class I (Normal):** only normal cells observed.
2. **Class II (Atypia):** Presence of atypia but no evidence of malignant changes.
3. **Class III:** It is an intermediate stage between class I and class IV where the smear may be suggestive of cancer but there is no clarity and may represent precancerous lesion or carcinoma in situ and a biopsy is recommended in such cases.

4. **Class IV (suggestive of cancer):** There may be few cells with malignant characteristics or many cells with border line features. Biopsy is mandatory in such cases.
5. **Class V (positive of cancer):** Cells that show obvious malignancy. Biopsy is compulsory in such cases.

Suggested reading:

1. Anil Govindrao Ghom Text book of Oral Medicine Third Edition page 64-66.
2. Sugerman PB, Savage NW. Aust Dent J. 1996 Apr;41(2): 71-4. Exfoliative cytology in clinical oral pathology.

Q 2) Toulidine Blue Staining

TNMGRU FEBRUARY 2011 (6 Marks)

William Henry Perkin discovered Toulidine Blue in 1856 and is being used in various medical applications. It is a acidophilic metachromatic dye which is also called as tolonium chloride, that stains selectively the acidic components of tissues like sulfates, carboxylates and phosphate radicals. It has affinity for nucleic acid and hence binds with the tissue's nuclear material having a high content of DNA and RNA.

This dye is currently being used extensively as an aid in diagnosis of oral premalignant disorders and oral cancers. It is used as a mouth wash or topical application. It has a good sensitivity and very low chances of false negative results. It can very effectively demonstrate dysplasia and early malignant lesions which are not clinically recognisable.

It is also known as methlananine or aminotoulene. It has three isoforms that are ortho/para/and metatoulidine. It has been used extensively as a vital stain for mucosal lesions and in tissue sections to stain certain components due to its metachromatic properties. This dye reacts with tissues based on the principle of metachromasia to produce a colour different from the original dye and the rest of the tissues.

- Vital staining with this dye on the oral epithelium has been used as a means for screening patients who have high risk for oral cancer development.
- This stain has been used for high-lighting the oral potentially malignant lesions and has the ability to identify early lesions that can be easily missed out on clinical examination.
- It can outline the entire extent of the dysplastic lesion or carcinoma before it can be excised and can detect multicentric or second tumours and in patients with oral cancer helps in follow up.
- It is of great help in selecting sample site for biopsy in premalignant lesions and marginal control of carcinoma can be obtained.
- In toulidine blue-stained lesions loss of heterozygosity can be detected.
- Toulidine blue staining of tissues appear dark or pale royal blue in colour.
- **Mechanism:**

- **Binding with DNA:** Belongs to the thiazine group and is an acidophilic metachromatic nuclear dye which is soluble partially in both water and alcohol and stains selectively acidic components of tissues especially the DNA and RNA. Dysplastic and anaplastic areas contain more DNA than normal cells and hence retain the dye.
- **Intracellular canals:** Malignant epithelium contains intra-cellular canals that are wider than the normal epithelium, and hence helps in penetration of the dye.
- **Effect on the normal epithelium:** The normal epithelium stains blue after application of 1% toulidine blue dye, but the staining is removed after application of 1% acetic acid solution. But the stain is retained in the dysplastic epithelium.
- **Effect on benign lesions:** There is a well defined uptake of the dye at the margins, but the dysplastic or malignant ulcers show diffuse marginal uptake patterns.

Method

The toulidine blue, staining kit is easily available and contains three components. The first kit contains 1% toulidine blue 10ml solution. Second and third kit contains 1% acetic acid as pre and post rinse solutions.

The kit contains:

- 1gm Toulidine blue.
- 10ml 1% Acetic acid.
- 4.19cc absolute alcohol.
- 86cc distilled water.
- pH adjusted to 4.5.

(i) Patient is asked to rinse the mouth first with plain water twice for 20 second each. After rinsing with water, the patient is again made to rinse for 20 seconds with 1% acetic acid.

(ii) The suspected area is then gently dried with gauze, taking care not to abrade the tissue while drying.

(iii) The 1% toulidine blue stain is applied to the lesion with a cotton swab.

(iv) The patient is again asked to rinse with acetic acid for about a minute.This is followed by rinsing with water.

(v) If the mucosa is stained positive then the procedure is repeated in one to two weeks. Biopsy of the sites that stain positive on two successive visits is advised.

Suggested reading:

1. Anil Govindrao Ghom, Text book of oral medicine, third edition, page 60.
2. Epstein JB, Scully C, Spinelli J, Toluidine blue and Lugol's iodine application in the assessment of oral malignant disease and lesions at risk of malignancy. J. Oral Pathol Med. 1992 Apr; 21(4):160-3.
3. Gokul Sridharan and Akhil A Shankar, Toluidine blue: A review of its chemistry and clinical utility, J Oral Maxillofac Pathol. 2012 May-Aug; 16(2): 251–255.

Q 3) Immune Fluorescence Test

TNMGRU FEBRUARY 2011 (6 Marks)

It is an antigen-antibody reaction where the antibodies are labeled with a fluorescent dye and the antigen-antibody complex is visualised using a ultraviolet microscope.

The fluorochromes are dyes that absorb ultra-violet rays and emit visible light and this process is called fluorescence.

Commonly used fluorochromes are Acridine Orange, Rhodamine, Lissamine and Calcofluor white.

However, these fluorochromes are used for general fluorescence.

When fluorescein (FITC) is excited by a blue (wavelength 488nm) light, it will emit a green (520nm) colour.

Phycoerythrin (PE) emits an orange (570nm) colour.

The fluorochromes commonly used are fluorescin isothiocyanate (green) and tetramethyl rhodamine isothiocyanate (red).

Types

- Direct.
- Indirect.
- Microimmunofluorescence.
- Sandwich technique of immunofluorescence.

Direct Immunofluorescence

In this technique antigen in clinical specimens are detected using specific fluorochrome labeled antibody.

It consists of following steps.

(i) Fixing of the smear on the slide.
(ii) Treating with labeled antibody.
(iii) Incubation at 37°C to allow the antigen and labeled antibody to react.
(iv) Washing with buffered normal saline so as to remove the unbound excess labeled antibody and visualising under a fluorescent microscope. On doing so the field is dark and areas with bound antibody fluoresce green.

This technique can be used to detect viral. parasitic, tumour antigens from patient specimens or monolayer of cells. Another application is identification of anatomic distribution of an antigen within a tissue or compartments of a cell.

Indirect Immunofluorescence

This technique is used to detect antibodies in patient serum.

(i) The antigen on the smear is made to react with specific unlabelled antibody and is washed.
(ii) The unbound antibody gets washed off.
(iii) The presence of specific mouse antibody bound to the antigen on the smear is detected by adding another antibody.
(iv) The second antibody is labeled with anti-gammaglobulin antibodies. This binds to the fragment crystallisable (Fc) region

of first antibody and persists despite washing. The presence of second antibody is detected by observing under fluorescent microscope.

(v) It is often used to detect autoantibodies.

(vi) It is commonly used in detection of antinuclear antibodies (ANA) in the serum of patients with SLE.

Advantages

- Brighter fluorescence because several fluorescent anti-globulin molecules bind onto each of the antibody molecules in the specific antiserum.
- There is considerable cost saving and versatility to the indirect technique, which requires only one labeled antiserum.
- Staining of more than one tissue component per slide can also be accomplished.

Microimmunofluorescence

It is a serological technique used to detect antibodies in patient serum. The principle is the same as that of indirect immunofluorescence but is performed on Teflon slides with many wells dotted with antigens. It is used in the serodiagnosis of Qf fever, Mediterranean spotted fever. Detection of Ig G, IgA and IgM Antibodies to Chlamydia, toxoplasmosis, epidemic typhus etc.

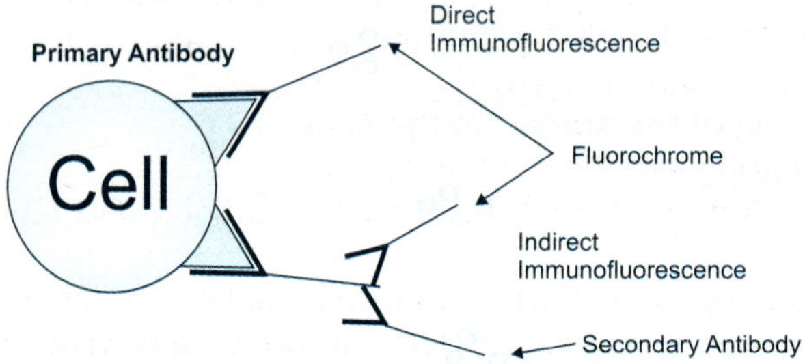

Fig. Direct and Indirect immunofluorescence.

Sandwich technique of immunofluorescence:

(i) In this technique antigen is sandwiched between two layers of the same specific antibody, one labeled and one not.

(ii) **Reaction of solution of antigen with antibody:** Appropriately fixed tissue sections are reacted with a solution of the antigen for which specific antibody is to be identified in the section.

(iii) **Application of fluorescein isothiocyanate (FITC)s labeled antiserum:** Following incubation and washing, FITC labeled antiserum with the same specificity as that to be identified in the section, is applied to the section. The labeled antiserum again identifies the location of the tissue component.

Suggested reading:

1. Anil Govindrao Ghom, Text book of oral medicine, third edition, page 67.

Q 4) Immunofluorescent test and their application in oral diseases

TNMGRU APRIL 1998 (5 Marks)

It is a powerful technique that uses fluorescent-labeled antibodies to detect specific target antigens. It is used widely in both scientific research and clinical laboratories. It is technique based on microscope used clinically to diagnose certain cutaneous diseases by detection of autoantibody-antigen complexes.

The techniques include:

- **Direct immunofluorescence:** It is performed on patient's skin using fluorophore-labeled antibodies that directly bind to the pathogenic autoantibody-antigen complexes in the skin.
- **Indirect immunofluorescence:** Its used in dermatological disorders to detect circulating pathogenic autoantibodies.
- Salt -split skin technique: Certain diseases cannot be distinguished using direct immunofluorescence techniques. Eg. Bullous pemphigoid with autoantibodies against BP 180 and BP 230 antigens and Epidermolysis bullosa aquisita with autoantibodies against collagen VII, both create a linear band of IgG and complement at the dermal-epidermal junction. Splitting the skin prior to evaluation allows these target antigens to be more accurately localised.
- These techniques are used depending on the clinical scenario.
- **Applications in various oral diseases:** The cutaneous diseases have oral manifestations and the immunofluorescent techniques are helpful in their diagnosis.

A) Pemphigus vulgaris:

The intercellular space fluorescent pattern results from binding of antibodies to the desmosomal proteins around the keratinocytes cell surface and is characteristic of the pemphigus group of disorders. In Pemphigus vulgaris the pattern of fluorescence is the deposition of IgG around epidermal cells.

B) Paraneoplastic pemphigus:

In paraneoplastic pemphigus there is deposition of IgG in the intercellular space and basement membrane zone.

C) Bullous pemphigoid:

In bullous pemphigoid deposition of IgG, C3 or both is seen at the basement membrane zone.

D) Epidermolysis bullosa Aquisita:

In Epidermolysis bullosa aquisita multiple deposits at the basement membrane zone is the pattern seen. Intense IgG deposition is consistently present.

E) Linear IgA Disease:

Deposition of IgA in linear pattern at the basement membrane zone is characteristic of this disease.

F) Dermatitis Herpetiformis:

In the papillary dermis and along the basement membrane zone granular deposition of IgA and C3 is characteristic of this disease.

G) Lupus Erythematosus:

Since the frequency of deposition, its morphology and site of deposition vary among various subsets of lupus erythematosus, direct immunofluorescence could be quite helpful in distinguishing between different subsets.

H) Lichen Planus:

Mucosal Lichen Planus can be differentiated from other mucosal erosive and bullous diseases such as mucosal pemphigoid by direct immunofluorescence. Within the cytoid bodies immune deposits are present in the superficial dermis and also along the dermo-epidermal junction. IgM and fibrinogen are the most frequently present immune deposits.

Suggested reading:

1. Ian D Odell and Deborah Cook Immunofluorescence Techniques Journal of Investigative Dermatology (2013) 133, e4.
2. Wojnarowska F, Eady RA, Burge SM. Bullous eruptions. In: Champion RH, Burton JL, Burns DA, Breathnach SM, eds. Textbook of Dermatology.6th edn. Oxford: Blackwell Science; 1998. p. 1817-98.

Q 5) Capillary fragility test

TNMGRU FEBRUARY 2014 (5 Marks)

It is also called as tourniquet test and Rumpel Leede test which determines the patient's hemorrhagic tendency by clinical diagnostic method. There is assessment of fragility of capillary walls and is used to identify thrombocytopenia.

This test is defined by WHO as one of the necessary requisites for diagnosis of Dengue fever.

It is the test of the ability of superficial capillaries of the skin of the forearm and hand to withstand an increased intraluminal pressure and a certain degree of hypoxia. It is done by occluding veins of the upper arm with a blood pressure cuff for five minutes.

A circle of diameter 2.5 cms, the upper edge of which is 4 cms below the crease of the elbow, is drawn on the inner aspect of the forearm. and pressure is applied midway between systolic and diastolic blood pressure using a sphygmomanometer above the elbow for 15 minutes and the petechiae count within the circle is made. Count of 10 is considered normal, 10-20 is marginal and above 20 is abnormal.

Indications:

1. **Bleeding abnormalities:** It is used to screen for bleeding abnormalities, especially where there is suspicion of platelet disorder.
2. **Petechiae in oral cavity:** The discovery of petechiae in the oral cavity or on the skin is the most common indication for capillary

Fragility Test, especially where the petechiae are confined to the oral cavity and could also conceivably have resulted from local trauma or denture irritation.

3. **Scurvy:** in dental practice, it is used as a screening test for scurvy, which is an etiological factor in periodontal disease.

Technique:

(a) **Equipment:** sphygmomanometer and cuff, microscope slide.

(b) **Patient position:** the patient is seated with one arm supported on the chair or thigh.

(c) **Instruction to patient:** the dentist should explain the patient that his blood pressure will be taken and cuff will be left on a little longer than the patient may be used to and also the procedure may make the patients arm a little numb and even painful, but that discomfort will quickly disappear once the cuff is removed.

(d) **Examination of hand of patient:** during this time, the dentist examines the patients forearms and hands for any petechiae and record their location with an ink spot. The blood in a petechial hemorrhage lies extravascularly and should not disappear upon pressure with the surface of a glass microscope slide.

(e) **Application of sphygmomanometer:** the sphygmomanometer is applied customarily and the patients systolic and diastolic arterial blood pressure is recorded.

(f) **Inflation of cuff**: the pressure in the cuff is reduced to zero and the cuff is reinflated to a point halfway between systolic and diastolic pressure. The pressure is maintained for 5 minutes during which the forearm and the hands are examined for development of new petechiae. The patient should not be moved vigorously while the cuff is in place because movement will increase anaerobic muscular glycolysis, lactate accumulation and thus result in pain.

(g) **Result:** after 5 minutes, the cuff is removed and the patient is allowed to exercise his arm to resolve the circulation in the arm. The blood vessels of normal individual will withstand these conditions and petechial haemorrhages will not appear on the forearm and hand from rupture of superficial capillaries.

(h) **Positive test:** if any unequivocal petechiae develops distal to the cuff after cuff has been applied, the test is recorded as positive.

(i) **Negative test:** if only one or two petechiae are seen or if those seen are not convincing in their appearance, a negative test is recorded, retesting is done if required by investigating dentist.

Suggested reading:

1. Anil Govindrao Ghom, Textbook of oral medicine, Investigations in dentistry, 2nd ed, pg no. 73-74.
2. Eric S. Halsey, Stalin Vilcarromero, Brett M. Forshey, Claudio Rocha, Isabel Bazan, Steven T. Stoddard, Tadeusz J. Kochel, Martin Casapia, Thomas W. Scott, and Amy C. Morrison, Performance of the Tourniquet Test for Diagnosing Dengue in Peru, Am J Trop Med Hyg. 2013 Jul 10; 89(1): 99–104.

Q 6) Glucose Tolerance Test

TNMGRU AUGUST 2014 (5 Marks)

Glucose tolerance test is a diagnostic test for diabetes mellitus. Diabetes mellitus is a metabolic disease characterized by dysregulation of carbohydrate, protein, and lipid metabolism. The most common forms of Diabetes are Type 1 and Type 2.

Type 1 diabetes was previously called insulin-dependent diabetes in which autoimmune destruction of pancreatic beta cells occurs following which the patient develops an absolute insulin deficiency and can no longer produce insulin .Type 2 diabetes used to be known as non-insulin dependent diabetes or adult onset diabetes.

Glucose tolerance can be defined as 'the capacity to dispose off administered glucose under standard conditions'.

There are two types of Glucose tolerance test:

1. Oral Glucose tolerance test.
2. Intravenous Glucose tolerance test. This test is also called fasting blood sugar test (FBS).

1) Oral Glucose Tolerance Test:

The diagnosis of diabetes can be made on the basis of individuals response to the oral glucose load, commonly known as oral glucose tolerance test.

A. Preparation of subject for GTT:

The person should have been taking carbohydrate rich diet for at least 3 days prior to the test. All drugs known to influence carbohydrate metabolism should be discontinued for at least 2 days. The subjects should avoid strenuous exercise on the previous day of the test. He should be in an overnight (at least 10 hrs) fasting state. During the course of GTT, the person should be comfortably seated and should refrain from smoking and exercise.

B. Procedure for GTT:

Glucose tolerance test should be conducted preferably in the morning (ideal 9 to 11 AM). A fasting blood sample is drawn and urine is collected. The subject is given 75g glucose orally, dissolved in about 300ml of water, to be drunk in about 5minutes. Blood and urine samples are collected at 30 minute intervals for at least 2 hours. All blood samples are subjected to glucose estimation while urine samples are qualitatively tested for glucose.

C. Interpretation of GTT:

The fasting plasma glucose level is 75-110mg/dl in normal persons. On oral glucose load, the concentration increases and the peak value (140 mg/dl) is reached in less than an hour which returns to normal by 2 hours. Glucose is not detected on any of the urine samples.

In individuals with impaired glucose tolerance, the fasting (110-126mg/dl) as well as 2 hour plasma glucose level (140-200mg/dl) are elevated. These subjects slowly develop frank diabetes at an estimation rate of 2%

per year. Dietary restriction and exercise are advocated for the treatment of impaired glucose tolerance.

A person is said to be suffering from Diabetes Mellitus if his/her fasting glucose exceeds 7.0 mmol/l (126mg/dl) and, at 2 hrs 11.1 mmol/l (200mg/dl).

2) Intravenous Glucose Tolerance Test:

There are two methods which are commonly employed for intravenous glucose tolerance test:

(a) The continuous infusion of a weak solution of glucose.
(b) The rapid injection of more concentrated solutions.

The continuous infusion of a weak solution of glucose method is cumbersome for routine clinical practice compared to rapid injection of more concentrated solutions method which has been used by the majority of workers.

Preparation of subjects:

(a) The person should have been taking at least 250 g of carbohydrate rich diet for at least 4 days prior to the test. The subject, who had fasted for 15 hours, should be kept completely at rest during the test and for half an hour prior to it.
(b) The solution used for intravenous administration should contain 50 g of glucose per 100 ml sterile distilled water.
(c) Syringes of 50 ml capacity is used and in every instance the injection into an arm vein should be completed within 3 minutes.
(d) Capillary blood was used for glucose analysis, 0-2 ml of blood was drawn up into a pipette from a stab puncture made with a scalpel blade in the thumb.
(e) The samples should be drawn at an interval of 30 seconds each.
(f) After three fasting blood samples had been taken over a period of 15 minutes, the glucose was injected again.
(g) Exactly 4 minutes after the completion of the injection another sample was obtained and this time was regarded as zero. Thereafter at intervals of 5 or 10 minutes for a total period of 60 to 90 minutes, further samples were taken. Analysis is carried out and graphs are plotted according to the readings.

Technically, the intravenous glucose tolerance test is difficult for a routine hospital laboratory procedure, hence, not performed as routine test to check glucose tolerance when compared to oral glucose tolerance test which is easy, less time consuming and causes less harm to the patients.

Suggested reading:

1. L J Duncan, The Intravenous Glucose Tolerance Test. Quarterly Journal Of Experimental Physiology and Cognate Medical Science. s1956; 41(1): 85-96.
2. U Satyanarayana, Biochemistry, Insulin Glucose Homeostatsis and Diabetes Mellitus, 3rd ed, pg no. 679-681.

Q 7) Biopsy

RGUHS OCTOBER 1997 (5 Marks)

Biopsy is a procedure of removal of a piece of tissue or a sample of cells from the body so as to analyse in a laboratory. It is the removal of cells or tissue for examination by a pathologist. He may observe the tissue under a microscope or perform other tests on the cells or tissues. A proper biopsy contains tissue which is representative of the lesion and depend mainly on three factors: Selection of biopsy site, the type of biopsy and adequate submisssion of the specimen to the laboratory.

The region that is selected for biopsy, especially in the larger lesions, must be representative of overall pathology that is present in the lesion. In such cases, multiple smaller biopsies may be needed of the lesion so as to provide tissue that is representative of the lesion to give the pathologist to examine.

Indications:

- **Undiagnosed clinical condition:** If a case is being difficult to be diagnosed confirmation with a biopsy is advised.
- **Nature of the lesion:** To determine the exact histologic nature of the lesion.
- **Screening:** To test and diagnose the abnormal tissues removed from the oral cavity, like a granuloma or cyst.
- **Confirmation of malignancy:** When a clinically diagnosed malignant lesion needs to be confirmed by histologic test so that treatment can be started urgently.
- **Diagnostic tests:** For evaluation of non-neoplastic lesions such as mucosal nodules, papilloma, erosive lichen planus, erythema multiforme, lupus erythematosus, pemhigus, pemphigoid, and desquamative gingivitis.

Uses:

(i) **Diagnosis:** Biopsy is useful for the diagnosis of lesions. It helps in differentiating between benign and malignant lesions.
(ii) **Grading of tumours:** It aids in determining the grading of tumours.
(iii) **Metatstatic lesions:** Helpful in diagnosis of metastatic lesions.
(iv) **Recurrence:** For evaluation of recurrence of lesions.
(v) **Assessment:** Useful for therapeutic assessment of the lesion by differentiating between benign and malignant lesions.

Instrument and materials:

- **Excisional and incisional biopsy:** Local anesthesia, scalpel, pointed surgical scissors, tissue forceps, and surgical haemostat. Sterile sponge, curved needles and sutures, needle holder and wide mouthed bottle containing 10% formalin.
- **Intraosseous biopsy:** Periosteal elevator, bone burr, curette.
- **Aspiration biopsy:** Syringe 10-20cc with a fine long needle.

When a biopsy specimen is taken from the oral cavity, immediate immersion into a fixative is important. If not adequately fixed the tissue may degenerate and the interpretation may become difficult. The most commonly used fixative is 10% neutral buffered formalin.

Types of biopsy:

The commonly used biopsy techniques are incisional, excisional, fine needle aspiration cytology, punch, scrape, and trephine as some techniques like bite, cone, core, endoscopic, irrigation, pressure, shave and sponge are less commonly used.

(i) **Excisional biopsy:** Total excision of a small lesion for microscopic examination is called excisional biopsy. It is a diagnostic and therapeutic procedure. Normal tissues on the margin of the lesion is also included in the specimen.
It is generally carried out in small lesions less than 1 cm, sessile or pedunculated lesions and movable lesions.

(ii) **Incisional biopsy:** It is performed by removing a wedge shaped tissue from the lesion which also includes surrounding normal zone.
It is done for larger and diffuse lesions which extend deeply in the surrounding tissues where total removal is not easy or possible by local anesthesia.
This type also helps to determine whether the treatment should be conservative or radical.

(iii) **Intraosseous biopsy:** Less frequently performed and in the form of exploratory curettage. It is done to determine the nature of large radiological alterations.

(iv) **Punch biopsy:** It is a less invasive procedure .No suturing is required as the surgical defect is small.
It is done with a sharpened hollow tube which is varying millimetres in diameter. It is rotated until the underlying muscle is reached.The tissue is then removed in the same way as that of incisional or excisional biopsy.

(v) **Frozen section biopsy:** It is performed when an immediate histologic report of a lesion is required. It is done to determine whether a lesion is malignant or not. Also to evaluate the margins of an excised malignancy to determine whether the entire lesion was removed during surgery.
The tissue is obtained from the lesion and kept in deep freezer and the frozen tissue is sectioned and stained to get a correct diagnosis. However the slides cannot be preserved for future reference.

(vi) **Exfoliative cytology:** The surface of the lesion is scraped and smeared on a slide, stained with papanicolaou and examined under microscope. It is the examination of cells shed from the epithelium. Some cancer cells have such peculiar features that they can be recognised individually and this has lead to the development of this technique and is called a pap smear.

(vii) **Fine needle aspiration cytology (FNAC):** The microscopic examination of the aspirate obtained by a fine needle from a lesion is called FNAC. It is a relatively painless and safe procedure for fast diagnosis. It was first discovered by Kun in 1847 and later reintroduced by Martin and Ellis in 1930.

The aspirate is put on the slides and later stained with either papanicolaou or hematoxyllin and eosin stain.

(viii) **Oral CDX Test:** It is a specialised computer assisted analysis of oral brush biopsy performed on oral tissue. It is very recently developed oral biopsy technique. This is a reliable technique for determining the need for scalpel biopsy in cases of benign appearing oral mucosal leukoplakia. This technique is especially designed to detect as few as just two abnormal cells among the thousands of cells in each biopsy specimen.

Suggested reading:

1. RM Logan, AN Goss, Biopsy of the oral mucosa and use of histopathology services, Volume 55, Issue s1 June 2010 Pages 9–13.
2. Molly S Rosebush, K. Mark Anderson, Swati Y .Rawal, Harry H Mincer, Yeshwant B. Rawal, The Oral Biopsy :Indications, Techniques, And Special Considerations, Journal Of Tenesse Dental Association, March 2010, 90-92.

Q 8) Rose Waaler Test

RGUHS OCTOBER 2004 (2 Marks)

The Rose Waaler test is a slide haemagglutination test for qualitative and semi-quantitative detection in human serum of the rheumatoid factor. Sheep erythrocytes that are stabilised and sensitised with rabbit IgG anti-sheep erythrocytes are agglutinated when mixed with samples that contain RF.

Dr. Erik Waaler, a Norwegian scientist in 1940 first described this test and it was then again described by Dr. H.M Rose and his colleagues in 1948.

When the red blood cells of sheep are coated with a concentration of anti-serum to red blood cells of sheep which is very low for causing agglutination, then the serum from a patient with rheumatoid arthritis when added will cause agglutination.

Rose Waaler test is positive in 70% of patients with rheumatoid arthritis. It is a rapid slide haemagglutination test that is used to detect rheumatoid factor in serum of humans. The RF is usually found in the serum of patients with rheumatoid arthritis and it is thought that they are IgM antibodies which are directed against the immunoglobulin G of the patients own. The RF also shows activity against the IgG in animals. Because there are a wide variety of the rheumatoid factors a single test that is unique doesnot exist to detect them all.

Suspension of stabilised sheep red blood cells with rabbit anti-sheep IgG is the reagent of the Rose Waaler test. Clear agglutination is seen when the RF is present in the sample.

The limit of detection is 8 IU/ml of RF in the serum of the patient and the calibration of the reagent is according to the WHO International Reference Preparation.

Clinical significance:

A group of antibodies that are directed to the determinants in the fractional crystallisation portion of the immunoglobulin G molecule are the Rheumatoid Factors. The rheumatoid factors are also found in another rheumatoid disorder like systemic lupus erythematosus, Sjogren's syndrome, and certain non-rheumatic conditions. Its most important role in the clinic is as an aid in the diagnosis of rheumatoid arthritis.

Limitations of the test:

A low or suspected positive result should be reassessed. Just based on one clinical assay, the diagnosis should not be made. While interpreting the test, its highly important to take in to consideration the entire clinical data. The RF tests are very important in distinguishing between Rheumatoid Arthritis, autoimmune and other inflammatory disorders. It should however be taken into consideration that with every case of clinically diagnosed rheumatoid arthritis every test will not give positive result for RF.

Suggested reading:

1. H. A. Otten and F. Westendorp Boerma, Significance of the Waaler-Rose Test, Streptococcal Agglutination, and Antistreptolysin Titre in the Prognosis of Rheumatoid Arthritis, Ann Rheum Dis. 1959 Mar; 18(1): 24–28.

Q 9) Glycosylated Hemoglobin Test

TNMGRU AUGUST 2012 (5 Marks)

Glycosylated Hemoglobin test is a diagnostic test for diabetes mellitus. Diabetes mellitus is a metabolic disorder that is characterised by faulty regulation of carbohydrate, protein and lipid metabolism. The most common forms of diabetes are Type 1 and type 2 where in type 1 was called insulin-dependent diabetes or juvenile and diabetes in which there occurred autoimmune destruction of beta cells of the pancreas. Due to the destruction the patient has an absolute insulin deficiency and the production of insulin is hampered. Type 2 diabetes was known as non-insulin dependent diabetes or adult-onset diabetes.

- It is often useful to assess the long-term control of glycemia, especially in known diabetic patients.
- The glycated (or glycosylated) hemoglobin assay (also called the glycohemoglobin test) allows the determination of blood glucose status over the 30 to 90 days prior to collection of the blood sample. As glucose circulates in the bloodstream, it becomes attached to a part of the hemoglobin molecule on red blood cells. The higher the plasma glucose levels are over time, the greater is the percentage of hemoglobin that becomes glycated.

There are two different glycated hemoglobin assays which measure two different portions of the hemoglobin molecule,

(a) Hemoglobin A1 (HbA1) test and
(b) Hemoglobin A1c (HbA1c) test.

- The normal HbA1 value is less than approximately 8% whereas the normal HbA1c value is less than 6.0 to 6.5%. These tests are not currently standardized across all laboratories therefore, glycated hemoglobin values must be interpreted in the context of normal ranges for the specific laboratory performing the test.

- The American Diabetes Association recommends that individuals with diabetes should have target HbA1c value of less than 7% whereas patients having HbA1c value of more than 8% suggests that a change in patient management may be needed to improve glycemic control.
- The glycated hemoglobin assay is not currently recommended as a screening tool or as an initial test for the diagnosis of diabetes. It is used to monitor glycemic control in patients with previously diagnosed diabetes.

Suggested reading:

1. Burket's, Oral Medicine, Diagnosis and Treatment, 10th ed, pg 566.

Q 10) Schilling's test

TNMGRU AUGUST 2013 (5 Marks)

Its a medical investigation to detect vitamin B12 deficiency. It is done to detect the presence of pernicious anemia. It is named after Robert. F Schilling.

There is defective absorption of vitamin B12 (cyanocobalamine)in pernicious anemia which is caused by the absence of intrinsic factor(IF) in the stomach. It was designed to reveal and differentiate causes of vitamin B12 deficiency.

Indication:

- This test is of value in establishing the diagnosis of pernicious anaemia (Addisonian anaemia), whether or not treatment with vitamin BI2 has already commenced.
- In addition, the test can provide contributory evidence for the diagnosis of generalised malabsorption.

Patient Preparation:

- The patient fasts overnight and for 2 hours following administration of the test dose.
- The patient should not have received other radioactive isotopes in the recent past. The test may be performed on in-patients or out-patients.

Procedure:

- Part I of the vitamin B12 absorption (Schilling)test involves administration of non-radioactive vitamin B12 (1000/tg) intramuscularly, followed immediately by vitamin B12 (0.5 /tg approximately; 18.5kBq, O.5/tCi) given orally in 50 ml of water; the rinsings from the container are also taken, in order to ensure that the dose is complete.
- Part II of the 'Schilling test' can be performed 72 hours later and consists of repeating Part I with, in addition, administration of one

capsule of IF.

- Immediately before commencing either part of the test, the bladder is emptied and the urine discarded; a 24 hour urine collection in a plain polythene bottle is started at this time.
- The 24 hour urine collection is sent to the laboratory for measurement of urine volume and radioactivity.
- Normally more than 10% of the administered dose should be excreted in the first 24 hour in Part 1 of the test, with no significant increase in Part II.
- In Part I of the test, excretion of less than 1.5% of the administered Cyanocobalamine is diagnostic of pernicious anaemia; this is assuming that the patient took the dose, that there was no vomiting and that urine collection was complete.
- Excretion of 4-8% is compatible with generalized intestinal malabsorption. Impaired glomerular filtration delays excretion and can produce very low result in the first 24 hour collection, but further collections over the next few days may permit summation of radioactivity excreted over that period; in these circumstances a total value of greater than 10% excretion of Co would indicate normal vitamin B12 absorption.
- Administration of other radioactive isotopes to the patient may produce very high values of radioactivity, though these may decay rapidly, unlike the radioactive cobalt isotopes used here. Repeat counting of the samples 1 week later could be informative.
- In Part II of the test, in patients with pernicious anaemia, there will be no effect on the intermediate values found in generalised malabsorption.
- Part III: Vitamin B12 and antibiotics.
  This stage is useful for identifying patients with bacterial overgrowth syndrome.
- Part IV: Vitamin B12 and pancreatic enzymes.

This stage where in pancreatic enzymes are administered can be helpful in identifying patients with pancreatitis.

Schilling test procedure is not being done very regularly, because of lack of production of the cobalt radioisotopes and labeled -B12 test substances.

More over replacement by injectable B12 has become relatively inexpensive and also can be administered by the patient himself and mega dose of oral B12 is also cheap and affordable.

Since the above mentioned treatment plans can be given for most cases of B12 malabsorption even if the exact cause is identified, the diagnostic test may be omitted without any harm to the patient.

Suggested reading:

1. Majid Moridani, PharmD, PhD, DClinChem, 1, 2 Shana Ben-Poorat, BS Laboratory Investigation of Vitamin B12 Deficiency. Labmedicine _ Volume 37 Number 3 _ March 2006.
2) Zuckier LS, Chervu LR (September 1984). "Schilling evaluation of pernicious anemia: current status".Journal of Nuclear Medicine 25 (9).

Q 11) Serological test for syphilis

RGUHS APRIL 2001 (5 Marks)

Treponema pallidum causes the sexually transmitted disease, syphillis in which case it penetrates the intact mucosa or enters the body through small defects in the epithelium.

Serological laboratory tests for syphilis:

Serological tests for syphilis is the most reliable laboratory diagnostic method, which ever stage of infection it is in.

Syphilis serological tests are divided into two categories.

- Non-treponemal assays measures during the treponemal infections antibodies against non-specific cardiolipin antigen. They are:
  - (a) VDRL(Venereal disease research laboratory)
  - (b) RPR- Rapid Plasma Reagin
- Treponemal assays measures antibodies that directly reacts with the syphilis-causing organism i.e. Treponema. Pallidum. The various types of treponemal assays are:
  - (i) FTA-ABS that is fluorescent treponemal antibody-absorbed test.
  - (ii) TPHA that is treponema pallidum hemagglutination assay.
  - (iii) TPPA that is treponema pallidum particle agglutination and EIA which is enzyme immunoassay.

1. **Nontreponemal Serologic Tests:** Syphilis may be confirmed either through blood tests or direct visualisation through a microscope. The diagnosis is through blood tests using treponemal/or non-treponemal tests. The non-treponemal tests used initially are the VDRL and the rapid plasma reagin test (RPR), occasionally give false positive results and confirmation with TPHA or FTA-ABS tests may be required.
   - (a) **VDRL tests:** This test is used as a confirmatory serlogical test which is a micro-flocculation test used for detection of antibodies to syphillis.
     - Qualitative testing: Results are interpreted as:
     - Reactive (medium to large clumps)
     - Weakly reactive (small clumps)
     - Non-reactive (No clumping or only slight roughness)
     - Quantitive testing is done on all serum samples to the end point that produce reactive results in the qualitative slide test.
   - b) **Rapid Plasma Reagin Test:** The Rapid Plasma Reagin is a non-treponemal test for serologic detection of syphilis. The RPR Card test detects the non-specific antilipid antibody. The antigen suspension of RPR reagin consists of lecithin, cholesterol, cardiolipin which are bound to the charcoal particles that help to make the reaction visible.

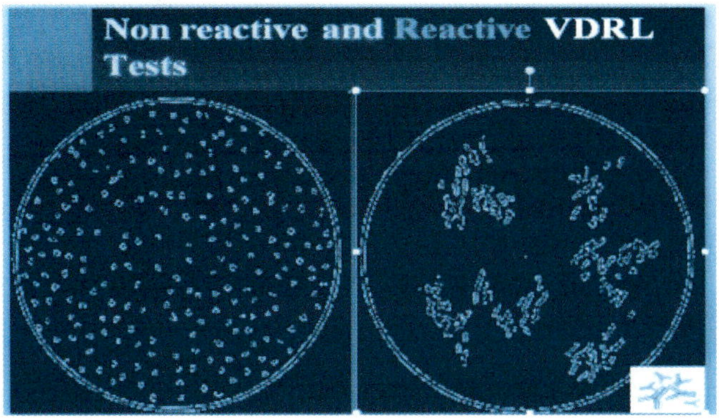

Fig. Results of VDRL test

2. **Treponemal tests:** These tests are based in antigens derived from T. pallidum, they allow specific anti-treponemal antibodies detection. These tests have a higher sensitivity and specificity than the non-treponemal tests. They are used to confirm the presence of syphillis after a reactive non-treponemal screening test.
   a) **FTA-ABS test:** This technique is an indirect fluorescent -antibody technique and the antigen that is used is pallidum subspecies (Nichol's strain).The serum of the patient is diluted to 1:5 in a sorbent so as to remove the group treponemal antibodies which are produced in some patients as a response to non-pathogenic treponemes. The absorbed serum is layered on a microscopic slide to which treponema pallidum has been fixed. In case the antibody is present in the patient's serum, it coats the treponeme. The test that is gold standard serological test for laboratory diagnosis of syphilis is FICT-labeled antihuman immunoglobulin which is added and it combines with the antibodies of the patient and results in FICT stained spirochetes that can be visible when they are examined by a fluoresence microscope.
   Treponemal specific tests should be used to confirm the results of serum RPR and the VDRL tests.
   (b) **TPHA and TPPA:** Its a test that detects reactive antibody that agglutinates red blood cells sensitised with Treponema pallidum antigen and is a simpler test. A formalised sheep erythrocytes are sensitised with ultrasonicated antigen from treponema pallidum Nichol's strain. The patient's serum is first mixed with adsorbing diluents made from non-pathogenic Reiter treponemes and other adsorbents and stabilisers.The reaction is performed in a microtitre plate. A smooth mat of agglutinated cells are formed when the serum containing antibody reacts with these cells in the microtitre plate. Unsensitised cells are used as a control for non-specific reactivity.

Suggested reading:

1. Neuza Satomi Sato, Laboratorial Diagnosis of Syphilis Center of Immunology, Institute Adolfo Lutz São Paulo, SP Brazil.

Q 12) Investigations for candidiasis

TNMGRU APRIL 1998 (5 Marks.)

Candidiasis is an opportunistic infection caused by yeast like fungus called candida. Various species of candida can cause oral or systemic candidiasis however the most common cause is candida albicans.

The investigations include:

Identification of risk factors:

In many cases, risk factors may be evident from history or examination, such as known HIV infection, hyposalivation/xerostomia, use of dentures, malnutrition, advanced malignancy, cancer chemotherapy or radiotherapy, pregnancy, or recent immunosuppressive or antibiotic therapy. In the absence of overt risk factors, the following investigations may be indicated in adults with oral candidiasis:

- Urinalysis, random or fasting blood glucose, or glucose tolerance test to exclude diabetes.
- HIV test.
- Sialometry.
- Electrolyte panel to exclude endocrinopathy (e.g., diabetes mellitus, hypoparathyroidism, pregnancy, hypoadrenalism).

Laboratory tests:

Diagnosis of oral candidiasis is done by the superficial smears of the lesions and observed by microcsope.

- In case of a wet mount, the scrapings or smears are taken from, nails, skin, vaginal or oral mucosa which are examined by a microscope for the presence of hyphae, pseudohyphae, or the budding yeast cells.
- Direct demonstration of the fungal cells can be done by a potassium hydroxide smear, Gram's stain or methylene blue.
- To identify the etiologic agent for onychomycosis, cultures from affected nails may help and can rule out other infectious agents.
- The smear sample may be sent to the laboratory, requesting a periodic acid-Schiff stain of fixed scrapings from the lesions, for microscopic visualisation of the Candida yeast form or hyphae.
- Superficial candida hyphae may be few in erythematous candidiasis, but in pseudomembranous forms they are numerous, and the smear test is more likely to be positive.
- If the smear sample is negative for Candida, this may be due to an inadequate smear sample or an infection that has invaded deep into the tissue. In this situation, a biopsy of a lesion may be performed.
- Histological examination of tissue samples demonstrate Candida

hyphae, extending into the spinous cell layer of the epithelium, with marked parakeratosis, acanthosis, and spongiosis, as well as a submucosal neutrophil response.

- Culture of a mouth rinse sample may be used for mycological surveillance, to determine the level of candidal carriage and risk of infection.
- Candida is present in the normal flora, so when culture is performed, moderate to heavy growth of yeast should be considered for intervention. This amounts to approximately greater than or equal to 400 colony-forming units/mL.

Identification of invasive disease:

Oropharyngeal candidiasis may be associated with oesophageal candidiasis, especially in the setting of HIV infection.

Therefore, patients who present with signs and symptoms such as dysphagia or odynophagia are investigated with an upper GI endoscopy for possible oesophageal involvement.

To establish the diagnosis of esophageal candidiasis, lesions are visualised and biopsies may be taken for histopathological demonstration of characteristic Candida yeast forms and culture confirmation of the presence of Candida species.

In cases of disseminated infections the blood cultures are helpful but may yield positive results only in 50-60% of cases.

Analysis of urine can be helpful and can show either colonisation or renal candidiasis.

Biopsy of lung is mandatory to certainly establish the diagnosis of candidiasis of the respiratory tract because of high frequency of colonisation of the respiratory tract by the yeast.

Identification of species:

- Species of candida like the c. albicans, c.stellatoidea, c. dubliniensis can be morphologically identified by germ tube formation or biochemical assays.
- Chrom agar candida can help in identification of various species by the use of colour reactions in the specialised media that can demonstrate the different colours of the colonies depending on the species of candida.
- Biochemical assays AP120C and AP132C help in the identification of different species of candida with greater precision. These assays help in evaluation of assimilation of several carbon substrates and help in generating profiles that help in identification of different fungal species.
- The candida albicans can be identified in 24-48 hours by the C. albicans peptide nucleic acid (PNA) fluorescence in situ hybridisation test when the probe is added to smears that are made directly from the blood culture bottle and is followed by hybridisation.
- Simultaneous identification of either C. albicans or C. glabrata can be done by the newer version of this test.

- Polymerase chain reaction and DNA probes molecular assays appear promising but are still under development and in early investigational phases.

Susceptibility testing of antifungals:

Candida species susceptibility testing in vitro is now standardised by using the Clinical Laboratory Standards Institute (CLSI) microbroth dilution.

Suggested reading:

1. Alexander BD, Pfaller MA. Contemporary tools for the diagnosis and management of invasive mycoses. Clin Infect Dis. 2006. 43:S15-S27.

Q 13) VandenBergh Test

TNMGRU FEBRUARY 2006 (5 Marks)

The Van den Bergh test is done to assess the levels of billirubin in blood.It determines the amount of conjugated bilirubin in the blood more specifically.

Van den Bergh reaction: Ehrlich in 1883 first made the observation that when diazonium salts was added to a solution of billirubin, a new compound azo-billirubin is formed. The solution becomes coloured and the colour depends upon the reaction of the solution.

It becomes red when neutral and blue when it is acidic. The practical importance of this reaction was brought to notice by the works of Himans van den Bergh and Snapper, when they applied it to clinical work.

Van den Bergh found the test to be more reliable than many of those tried earlier, both for the detection and quantitative estimation of billirubin.

Van den Bergh thus transferred the outlook on jaundice from the colour of skin to quantitive changes in blood.

The reaction is very delicate and may help to detect billirubin as great as 1:1, 500000.Normal blood serum contains between 0.1 and 0.25 mg of billirubin per 100 cc or 0.2-0.5 units.

Quantitative studies have shown that sera of normal individuals may contain excess quantities of billirubin in the absence of conditions with which jaundice is usually associated.

Vanden Bergh thus points out that the sallow complexion of apparently healthy individuals can thus be explained where in the serum may contain as much as 2-3 units of billirubin per 100cc.

Van den Bergh working with the diazo reaction, found that some specimens of bile gave a colour reaction when treated with the reagent directly, while others required the addition of alcohol before a change in colour could be seen.

He observed that a direct reaction was obtained when the reagent was added to the serum of obstructive jaundice, where as a negative reaction was obtained when the reagent was added to the serum of hemolytic jaundice.

Procedure:

Reagent No. 1: Dissolve 53.60 mg of malic acid, 0.25 mg of sodium nitrite, and 4.80 mg of disodium hydrogen phosphate (Na_2HPO_4) in 2.0 ml of distilled water.

Reagent No. 2: Dissolve 53.60 mg of malic acid, 75.00mg of Duponol, 1.20mg of sulfanilic acid, and 4.00 mg of disodium hydrogen phosphate (Na2HPO4) in 2.0 ml of distilled water.

To each 'test' and 'serum blank' tube, 2.0 ml of reagent No. 1, followed by 2.0 ml of reagent No. 2 to the "test" tube is added, and 2.0 ml of distilled water to the "serum blank" tube. The contents of both tubes are thoroughly mixed and allowed to stand 1 min. at ambient temperature (250 C). A 200 micro l2 aliquot of untreated serum or standard is added to both tubes, mixed, and incubated in a 37 ± 0.5°C water bath for 6 min. The "serum blank" is adjusted for zero absorbance and the "test" absorbance is read at 560 nm within 10 minutes of the end of the incubation.

Types of Van den Berg reactions:

- If a reddish violet colour reaction occurs immediately on adding the reagent to the serum and reaches a maximum within about 30 seconds, the reaction is known as immediate direct.
- When with the same technique the reddish colour is observed to develop only after some time about, 1-10 minutes and then deepens to a violet hue then the reaction is called as delayed direct.
- When a reddish colour appears immediately and only after some time deepens to a violet hue, the reaction is known as biphasic direct.
- When no colour reaction occurs, after the addition of the reagent to the blood directly but does occur after the blood proteins have been precipitated with alcohol and the reagent has been applied to the clear alcoholic filtrate, the reaction is known as indirect.
- Though the above reactions are the most frequently seen there are quite a few slight differences.
- Van den Bergh found out the explanation of these differences and it was the result of his hard work because of which a basis was formed for the use of this test in clinical medicine .

When used by itself the Van den Bergh reaction is of value only in detection of latent jaundice, and in doubtful cases of icteroid tints of the skin, and its quantative studies are of value in measuring progress in cases of definite jaundice when the colour of skin alone may be deceptive.

Van den Bergh test when used in conjunction with the urobilinogen reaction can provide very important laboratory diagnosis and estimation of progress in many cases of jaundice.

Limitations of the test:

At times the results that are obtained appear to be incompatible with known physiology, pathology and clinical experience. And in such situations it becomes the prerogative of the clinician to label the test as useful or not.

Suggested reading:

1. Frederick C. Peariman and Robert T. V. Lee, Detection and Measurement of Total BilirubininSerum, with Use of Surlactants as SolubilizingAgents, CLIN. CHEM. 20/4, 447-453 (1974)
2. I. M. Rabinowitch, Jaundice And The Application of The Van Den Bergh And Urobilinogen Tests, Can Med Assoc J. 1931 Sep; 25(3): 255–265.

Q 14) L.E cell test

TNMGRU OCTOBER 1997 (5 Marks)

Systemic lupus erythematosus is a recurrent, chronic, potentially multisystem involving inflammatory disorder that can be very difficult in diagnosing. This disorder has no single means of diagnostic marker but is identified through various combinations of clinical and laboratory criterion. Correct diagnosis of this disorder is essential because the right treatment can reduce the morbidity and mortality associated especially from lupus nephritis.

In 1948 Hargraves, Richmond and Morton reported the L.E cell phenomenon. These cells are usually polymorhonuclear leukocytes containing a round, homogenous, or more rarely reticular or granular body.

The L.E cell test was the first diagnostic laboratory test described for systemic lupus erythematosus(SLE)

The L.E cell reaction is positive in about 50-70% of patients with acute disseminated lupus.

LE Cell is a phagocytic leucocyte, commonly polymorphonuclear leukocytes which engulfs the denatured nucleus of injured cells. It is recognised as neutrophil polymorphonuclear leukocyte whose nuclear lobes are compressed to the periphery of the cell by inclusion of homogenous material which stains a reddish purple with the usual blood stains.

This test was at one time performed to diagnose SLE but has been replaced for this purpose by antinuclear antibody testing.

The production of L.E cells from bone marrow or blood of patients suffering from systemic lupus erythematosus is essential for a complete diagnosis.

Many methods have been developed for producing L.E cells from venous blood, but the one devised by Marten and Blackburn has been found to be reliable.

Three essential factors are involved in L.E cell formation:

(i) Plasma or serum from an S.L.E patient.
(ii) Nucleoprotein from nuclei of damaged cells, which form substrate.
(iii) Active phagocytic polymorphonuclears.

Lupus Erythematosus (L.E) cell testing is performed by using any of the following:

(i) Heparinised bone marrow.
(ii) Heparinized venous blood.
(iii) Oxalated venous blood.

(iv) Defibrinated venous blood.
(v) Clotted venous blood.
(vi) LE factor and donor cells.

Over the past few years many tests have been used for their detection.

The techniques using anticoagulants with or without bone marrow have been tedious.

A simple method that is used is as follows:

20 mls of venous blood is defibrinated by agitation in a universal container holding a bent paper clip. The defibrinated blood is transferred to a conical tube and centrifuged for 5 minutes at 1800 rpm. The upper cellular layer is transferred by a pipette to a Wintrobe tube, which is again centrifuged at 1800 rpm for 5 minutes. Smears are made from the buffy coat, and stained by Leishman's method. The number of L.E cells/500 leucocytes is then determined.

The inclusions show varying grades of density and of colour from deep blue to pink.

When approximately 2-30% of the cells seen on the slide in the neutrophil count are L.E cells, the L.E cell test is considered to be positive. The technical skill and observation of the test performer decides the integrity of the test.

Antinuclear antibody testing has replaced L.E cell testing in the diagnosis of systemic lupus erythematosus.

Antinuclear antibodies (ANA) cannot penetrate the intact cells and thus cell nuclei should be exposed to bind them with the ANAs.

Rheumatoid arthritis, chronic hepatitis, scleroderma, dermatomyositis, poly arteritis nodosa, acquired hemolytic anemia and Hodgkin's disease may also show positive reactions. In persons taking phenylbutazone and hydralazine the test might be positive.

Suggested reading:

1. H. Lempert and G. M. Berlyne Improved L.E. Cell Test Using Finger-prick Blood Br Med J. 1957 May 4; 1(5026): 1041–1043.
2. R. H. Marten and E. K. Blackburn A Simple Method for the Detection of L.E. Cells, J Clin Pathol. 1953 Feb; 6(1): 89–90.

Q 15) Fine needle aspiration cytology

TNMGRU AUGUST 2006, (5 Marks)

Fine needle aspiration cytology is a atraumatic, easy and inexpensive, simple procedure for diagnosis of disease sites.

Introduction:

- It is the microscopic examination of an aspirate obtained by inserting a fine needle into the lesion.
- First discovered by Kun in 1847.
- It was reintroduced in 1930 by Martin and Ellis.
- It is a painless and safe procedure for rapid diagnosis.

- It is a technique of obtaining cellular material for cytological examination and diagnosis.
- Performed by using a 21 gauge or smaller needle and using a 5, 10 or 20 ml syringe either freehand or by using special syringe holders.
- It is a minimally invasive, rapid diagnostic method applied to tissue samples but it does not preserve the histological architecture.

Indications:

- The technique can be: Diagnostic or Therapeutic e.g. evacuation of cysts.
- The major indication for FNAC relates to diagnosis of either primary malignancy or metastatic disease.
- As a chairside investigation to differentiate between a tumour or cyst. A cyst will yield cystic fluid.
- As a diagnostic tool for evaluating potentially malignant conditions FNAC has the following indications:
    (i) Initial evaluation before treatment and predicting prognosis.
    (ii) Evaluation of recurrence following therapy.
    (iii) Evaluation of metastasis.
- Salivary gland pathology: FNAC of salivary gland is a useful procedure for evaluation of salivary gland tumor.
- As a replacement of extensive biopsy: It is indicated in lesions in which open biopsy requires extensive procedures.
- Can be used to differentiate inflammatory, reactive, cystic and neoplastic processes.
- Suspicious lymph nodes: For examination of enlarged, clinically suspicious lymph nodes.
- Recurrence: To check against recurrence or local extension of lesions.
- Metastatic lesions: Detection of metastatic squamous cell carcinoma within cervical nodes.

Procedure:

- Plastic disposable syringe of 20 ml is most commonly used, coupled with 21, 23 or 25 gauge needle.
- The skin is cleaned with an antiseptic and the tumour is held firmly with one hand and needle is then inserted directly into it.
- The plunger of the syringe is pulled back so as to exert suction. This is maintained with the thumb and the needle is moved through the tumour three or four times in different directions.
- With the needle still in the tumour, the suction is slowly released. The needle is then removed from the tumour and the syringe from the needle.
- The syringe is then filled with air, reconnected to the needle and the contents of the needle blown on to the clean and dry slides, which are rapidly air dried.

- They can be then stained with Giemsa, Romanowsky or papinicollaou stain.
- Romanowsky stain is preferred because it is not possible to stain the air dried smears satisfactorily by Hematoxylin stain.

Advantages:

- This method is cheap and cost effective.
- Has much lesser risk than surgical biopsy.
- It is easily repeatable for multifocal lesions.
- There is minimal physical and psychological discomfort for the patient.
- The reporting and diagnosis of neoplastic, hyperplastic and inflammatory masses can be done rapidly.
- Can be used as chair side diagnostic tool:
- It can be a good therapeutic procedure for evacuation of a cystic lesion.
- It is a very fast way of confirming recurrence of previously treated malignancy without the need for surgery.

Limitations:

- The samples obtained are scanty and the histological architecture is lost. Hence there is possibility that the inflammatory, neoplastic or degenerative lesions may mimic malignancy.
- In certain cases such as follicular adenoma diagnosis may be indefinite.
- There could be difficulty in cytological diagnosis in certain conditions like lymphomas.

Suggested reading:

1. Jv Lever, P A Trott, and A J Webb, Review Article: Fine Needle Aspiration Cytology; J Clin Pathol 1985;38: 1-11.

Q 16) Laboratory investigations for bleeding disorders

TNMGRU FEBRUARY 2006 (5 Marks)

To detect bleeding disorders, laboratory tests are very important which could be the result of deficiencies or defects in the Von Willebrand's Factor (vwf). platelets, coagulation factors or fibrinolytic proteins.

In bleeding disorders, many of the common causes are mild conditions, with mucocutaneous bleeding symptoms, but in many cases the causes are due to defects that are presently undefined.

In order to investigate bleeding problems, the tests that are advised are influenced by number of factors, that include family history of bleeding problems and the clinical scenario, such as the nature of bleeding symptoms, and whether they are acute or chronic, immediate or delayed in onset with challenges, or whether they are associated with drug exposure, vitamin k deficiency and other coagulopathies.

Some of the tests that are carried out are:

1. **Platelet count:** Normal range is 1,50,000-4, 50,000/mm^3.
   - Surgical or traumatic hemorrhage can occur below 50,000/mm^3.
   - If the levels go down below 10,000-20,000/mm^3 then spontaneous hemorrhage can occur.
2. **Bleeding time**: It is the time interval between skin puncture and arrest of bleeding.

   Method:

   Patient is seated comfortably. The sphygmomanometer cuff is applied to the upper arm and inflated to 40mm of hg. A lancet is used to puncture the forearm midway between the wrist and the elbow. The lancet is removed and the time is noted. Every 30 seconds an edge of filter paper is touched against the drop of blood that wells up. The time required till the bleeding ceases is the bleeding time in minutes.
   - Normal bleeding time is 3-6 minutes.
   - It is a sensitive measure of platelet function.
   - It is increased in Thrombocytopenia, Von Willebrand's disease, and platelet dysfunction.
3. **Clotting time:** Time taken for the blood to clot after collection from the body. Normal values are 3-8 minutes.

   Method:

   Blood prick is made under sterile conditions and it is collected in a capillary tube. At the end of two minutes small portions of the tube end is snapped at intervals of 15 seconds and noting the formation of fibrin thread. The time is noted when the first thread is seen.
   - Clotting time is decreased in menstruation and before parturition.
   - Pathologic conditions where it is increased are:
     - (i) Hemophilia.
     - (ii) Liver damage.
     - (iii) Any clotting factor deficiency.
     - (iv) Vitamin K deficiency.
     - (v) Anticoagulant treatment.
     - (vi) Disseminated intravascular coagulation.
4. **Prothrombin time:**

   Blood is collected and oxalated so that prothrombin doesnot convert to thrombin. Then a large quantity of tissue thromboplastin and calcium ion is added to this blood. The time that is taken by blood to clot after the addition of tissue thromboplastin is called prorombin time.

   Normal values are 12-14 seconds. It is increased in:
   - Warfarin therapy.
   - Vitamin K deficiency.
   - Deficiency of factors V, VII, X, prothrombin and fibrinogen.

5. **Thrombin time:** It assesses the final step of coagulation, that is conversion of fibrinogen to fibrin in the presence of thrombin.
   Basic principle: Thrombin is added to plasma and the clotting time is measured which is affected by the concentration and reaction of fibrinogen and by the presence of inhibitory substances including fibrinogen/fibrin degradation products and heparin.
   Normal range: 15-19 seconds.
6. **Activated partial thromboplastin time (APTT):**
   - It is screening test for intrinsic limb and common pathway of coagulation system.
   - Blood samples are collected in tubes with oxalate or citrate to arrest coagulation.
   - In order to activate the intrinsic pathway, phospholipids and calcium are added to the plasma.
   - The time is measured until the clot forms.
   - The test is termed partial due to absence of tissue factor from the reaction mixture.
   - Normal range is below 45 seconds.
   - It is increased in haemophilia.
7. **INR: International normalised ratio:**
   - As prothrombin time estimated in different laboratories is different INR has been established to introduce standardisation.
   - INR=Prothrombin time of patient/prothrombin time of control.
   - Normal value is 1.
   - When INR is below 3.5 extraction of teeth can be carried out normally with out any change in anticoagulant therapy.
8. **Mixing test:** Unexplained prolongation of PT or (APTT) can be investigated with simple correction test by mixing the patient's plasma with normal plasma. Correction indicates a possible factor deficiency where as inability to correct indicates the presence of an inhibitor.
   It is done by performing PT and/or APTT on control, patient and a 50-50 mixture of the control and the patient's plasma.
9. **Fibrinogen assay**: Usually done by Clauss technique.
   The diluted plasma is clotted with a strong thrombin solution.
   The plasma must be diluted to give a low level of any inhibitor, for example FDPs (fibrin degradation factors) and Heparin.
   A strong thrombin solution must be used so that the clotting time over a range is independent of the thrombin concentration.
   Normal values: 1.8-3.6gm/l.
10. **Hess's capillary fragility test:** Cuff is wrapped on upper arm and pressure is maintained midway between systolic and diastolic blood pressure for 15 minutes. 4cms below the elbow joint, a circle of 2.5 cm diameter is drawn on the anterior aspect of forearm.
    Up to 10 new hemorrhagic spots are normal. But more than 20 new spots are considered pathological.

11. Second line of laboratory investigations are:
- Clot solubility test.
- Specific factor assay for suspected factor deficiency, especially factor VIII.
- PFA (platelet function analyser) 100.It is being increasingly used to detect bleeding disorders.

Suggested reading:

1. Catherine P.M. Hayward, Karen A. Moffat, Elizabeth Plumhoff, 3, 4 and Elizabeth M. Van Cott, Approaches to investigating common bleeding disorders: An evaluation of North American coagulation laboratory practices, American Journal of Hematology Volume 87, Issue S1, February 2012.
2. H.R Umarji, concise oral medicine, 140.
3. Palmer RL. Laboratory diagnosis of bleeding disorders. Basic screening tests, Postgrad Med. 1984 Dec; 76(8):137-42, 147-8.

CHAPTER 3

Drugs in Dentistry

INTRODUCTION

It is very important to have a complete and profound knowledge about the drugs used in dentistry. The drugs commonly used are antibiotics, analgesics and anti-inflammatory, anticancer drugs, antivirals, corticosteroids, anti-fungals, immunomodulators, emergency drugs, desesnsitising agents, mouthwashes and gum paints. The dentist should be well aware of its uses, dosage, modes of administration and their side effects.

Q 1) Corticosteroids In Dentistry

TNMGRU APRIL 2001 (5 Marks)

Adrenal cortex produces a class of steroid hormones called corticosteroids. They are involved in a wide range of physiologic systems like immune, stress response and regulation of inflammation, carbohydrate and protein metabolism, blood electrolyte levels and behavior.

They can be manufactured synthetically as drugs which can be available as tablets or fluid form to be used as injectables.

Steroids play an important role in dentistry and can be used as anti-inflammatory drugs to control pain, relieve stress and anxiety and also treatment of some oral diseases.

1) Use of corticosteroids in oral surgery:

For morning surgeries two 4mg dexamethasone tablets the night before surgery.

For the afternoon and evening surgeries four 4mg tablets of dexamethasone preoperative in the morning and four 4mg tablets of dexamethasone, three hours preoperatively and two tablets of dexamethasone at bed time followed by 4 tablets of the same drug the first preoperative morning.

2) Corticosteroids in temporomandiblar joint disorders:

In the treatment of TMDs various corticosteroids are used which have a dramatic effect in controlling hypomobility, pain, inflammation, especially associated with T.M.J problems.

Oral corticosteroids are mainly being used for acute TMJ discomforts.

Intra articular injections of corticosteroids are useful in reducing pain, swelling and dysfunction in inflammatory diseases of TMJ.

Hydrocortisone 20-240mg/day, prednisone 50 to 60 mg/day, dexamethasone 0.75-9.0mg/day, betamethasone 0.6-7.2 mg/day are being used.

3) Steroids in endodontics:

Ledermix, a combination of steroid and antibiotic are used as intracanal medication for management of root resorption with a fair amount of success.

Hydrocortisone is mixed with zinc oxide eugenol to be used root canal sealers.

4) Corticosteroids in ulcerative and vesiculobullous lesions:

a) Recurrent aphthous stomatitis:

Topical corticosteroids like 0.1% triamcinolone acetonide as gel or lotion suffice for minor ulcers but for major ulcers topical along with intralesional injections also need to be given.

Systemic corticosteroids generally of short course should be given for very severe cases.

b) Pemphigus vulgaris:

Corticosteroids are used for minor lesions but for severe lesions local and systemic corticosteroids along with immunosuppresives may be required.

Pemphigus vulgaris can be primarily treated with systemic administration of corticosteroids at doses of 1-2mg/kg/day which has been found to be effective.

In order to maintain remission, topical steroids can be given, also allowing reduction in systemic doses. Isolated lesions can be treated with injectable corticosteroids.

c) Behcet's syndrome:

This syndrome can be treated almost similar to severe or major recurrent aphthous stomatitis.

d) Mucous membrane pemphigoid:

Often the initial site of involvement is the oral mucosa. Fluocinomide (0.05%) and clobetasol propionate (0.05%) in an adhesive vehicle can be used three times a day for up to 6 months. Systemic therapy includes prednisone, usually given at a dose of 1-1.5 mg/kg/day, with appropriate monitoring for side effects.

e) Bullous pemphigoid:

The primary treatment of bullous pemphigoid is moderate dose of systemic prednisone.

Clobetasol propionate 20 mg to 40 mg/day is more effective for the treatment of bullous pemphigoid.

f) Erythema multiforme and Steven's johnson's syndrome:

If treated in high doses for a short time with proper tapering of doses corticosteroids can be very effective in these conditions. Early therapy of systemic predinisone of 0.5-1.0mg/kg/day or pulse methyl prednisolone 1mg/kg/day for 3 days, intravenous pulsed dose of methyl prednisolone, 3 consecutive daily infusions of 20-30 mg/kg to a maximum of 500 mg given over 2-3 hours and dexamethasone pulse therapy of 1.5mg/kg over 30-60 minutes on 3 consecutive days have been shown to be very effective.

5) Premalignant conditions:

(i) Oral lichen planus: The erosive, bullous or ulcerative lesions of lichen planus are treated with high potency topical steroids, such as 0.05% fluocinonide ointment.
A gingival tray can also be used to deliver 0.05% clobetasol propionate with 1,00,000 IU/ml of Nystatin in orabase.
Intralesional injection of triamcinolone acetonide of 10-20 mg or short-term regimens of 40 mg of prednisone daily for 5 days, followed by 10 to 20 mg daily for an additional 2 weeks, have also been used in most severe cases.

(ii) **Oral submucous fibrosis:** Local application of steroids like 0.1% triamcinolone acetonide or betnesol oral drops may show good response. Intralesional dexamethasone mixed with hyaluronidase is also used with varying results.

6) Central giant cell granuloma:

In case of non-surgical treatment intracellular corticosteroid injections are generally given and triamcinolone acetonide has been found to be effective which may act by suppressing the angiogenic component of the lesion.

7) Bell's Palsy

Treatment includes prednisone, about 60-80mg daily for the first 5 days and then taper over the next 5 days.

8) Mucocele:

The most common site of occurrence in oral cavity is the lower lip, whereas the less common sites include floor of the mouth, anterior ventral tongue, palate, buccal mucosa and retromolar pad.

Mucoceles have been treated successfully by intralesional injections of corticosteroids.

SUMMARY:

Aggressive treatment with 40-60 mg of oral prednisone daily should be considered when the severity of lesions affects the patient's concentration, diet and other functions.

When the lesions are few and accessible, localised or mild vesiculobullous conditions should be treated topically.

In cases of numerous and inaccessible lesions, which cannot be easily treated topically, dexamethasone elixir, 0.5mg/5ml may be used as a oral rinse. There should be vigourous rinsing 3-4 minutes qid after meals and then the patient should expectorate.

Direct injections of corticosteroids may be required around the margins of recalcitrant lesions. Injectable 0.5-1.0 ml dexamethasone phosphate, 4mg/ml or triamcinolone 10mg/ml can be given twice weekly until the lesions heal.

Suggested reading:

1. Vigneshwar Sambandam, Prasanna Neelakanta. Steroids in Dentistry - A Review Int. J. Pharm. Sci. Rev. Res., 22(2), Sep – Oct 2013; n° 44, 240-245 .

Q 2) Antifungal drugs

RGUHS 2000 (5 Marks)

Fungal infections are caused by organisms that can invade the epithelial tissue which includes yeasts, molds, rusts and mushrooms. Opportunistic fungal infections are likely to occur in patients on steroid, immunosuppressants or antimetabolite therapy, patients with aids, diabetes mellitus, tuberculosis, leukemia, lymphoma, burns etc.

Candida albicans is a normal resident in the oral cavity, it invades to cause infection when host defense is impaired or the oral flora is disturbed.

Antifungal are used topically or systemically. Superficial infections are treated by topical therapy and systemic therapy is reserved for chronic cases, resistant fungal infection, immunocompromised patients, deep fungal infections etc.

Classification of Antifungal agent:

Five classes of antifungal agents are used in the treatment of fungal infections.

- **Polyenes:** Amphotericin B, Nystatin. (broad spectrum, naturally occurring derived from fermentation of sterptomyces.)
- **Azoles:**
  - o Imidazol: Clotrimazole, Ketaconazole, Micoanozole, Econazol.
  - o Triazole:
  - o Fluconazole, Itraconazole, Voriconazole, Posaconazole.
- **Pyrimidine analogues** : Flucytosine
- **Allylamines:** Terbinafine
- **Echinocandins:** Caspofungin, Micafungin, Anidulafungin.

1. **Nystatin:** broad spectrum topical antifungal, parenteral administration causes systemic toxicity and side effects, available forms are pastille: 2 lac units, 1-2 pastilles QID.

   Trade names- mycostatin, nilstat, biostatin.

   For oral candidiasis 1 lac unit 4 times/day and continue for 48 hrs after the lesion have healed, dosage: 5-10 lac units 2-3 times daily.

Adverse effects: bitter taste, nausea. And should not be used in chlorhexidine gluconate as it inactivates both the drugs.

Contraindications: hypersensitivity.

2. **Amphotericin B:** broad spectrum microcyclic prolene, was considered as gold standard for antifungal therapy.Trade name-Fungizone, Amphocin as tablet and injections. Dosage: 50-100mg QID.
   - Topical is available as suspension & lozenge form, swish and swallow topical suspension 1 ml QID (100mg/ml).
   - Systemic available as powder to be diluted with glucose 0.3-0.7 mg/kg is slowly infused over 4-8 hours daily.

   Uses: candidiasis, cryptococcosis, aspergillosis, histoplamosis, zygomycosis, coccidiodomycosis, leishmaniasis etc.

   Contraindication: renal impairment, epilepsy.

   Adverse effects: fever, chills, rigors, malaise, nausea, vomiting, headache on parenteral infusion and long term use causes nephrotoxicity.
3. **Clotrimazole:** topical antifungal, having antistaphylococcal activity, 1st line of treatment for superficial oral candidiasis available as troche, lotion, gel or cream 1% 3 times a day. 10 mg Troche orally 5 times / day trade name: candid mouth paint, Mycelex troche. side effects: nausea, vomiting, unpleasant, itching and burning sensation and high sucrose content so use with caution if dental caries is a concern.
4. **Ketaconazole:** Trade name nizral, tocon, available as tablet, dose 200mg OD/BD Indication: systemic candidiasis, dermatomycosis.
   Contraindicated: children below 2 years.
   Adverse effects: hepatitis, rashes, GIT upset.
5. **Fluconazole:** trade name: F-zole, Fluzone; available as capsule tablet, infusion ; dose:200mg on 1st day followed by 100mg OD.
   Indication: Systemic vaginal and mucosal candidiasis.
   Contraindications: hypersensitivity.
   Adverse effects: nausea, headache, skin rashes and abdominal pain.
6. **Itraconazole:** trade name : itrole, canditral; available as capsule.
   Dose: 100-200mg OD for 6 months.
   Indication: Oropharyngeal candidiasis, systemic mycosis, chronic mucocutaneous endocrinopathy.
   Contraindication: Hypersensitivity.
   Adverse effect: Nausea, headache, skin rashes, and abdominal pain.
7. **Caspofungin:** trade name: cancidas; available as white lyophilized powder.
   Dose: 50-70 mg vials.
   Indication: refractory mucosal candidiasis.

Contraindications: Hypersensitivity.

Adverse effects: fever phlebitis at the site of infusion, headache & nausea.

Suggested reading:

1. Anil Govindrao Ghom, 'Textbook of oral medicine'. Ch:46 Pg : 977- 982

Q 3) Anti inflammatory drugs

RGUHS APRIL 2001 (5 Marks)

A drug that inhibits or suppresses most inflammatory responses of an allergic, bacterial, traumatic or anaphylactic origin, as well as being immunosuppressant are called anti-inflammmatory drugs.

Inflammation is a process caused by release of chemicals from tissues and migrating cells. Prostaglandins, leukotrienes, histamine, bradykinin, and platelet activating factor (PAF) and interleukin-1 are most strongly implicated in the process.

Classification:

A) Steroidal anti-inflammatory drugs: The steroidal anti-inflammatory drugs like corticosteroids prevent the formation of prostaglandins and leukotrienes by causing release of lipocortin, which by inhibition of phospholipase A2 reduces arachidonic acid release.

Classification:

Glucocorticoids:

1. **Natural (short acting):** a) Cortisone. b) Hydrocortisone.
2. **Synthetic (Intermediate acting):** Prednisone, prednisolone, methyl prednisolone acetate and triamcinolone.
3. **(Long acting):** a) Betamethasone. b) Dexamethasone. C) Fluocinolone.

B) **Non-steroidal anti-inflammatory drugs:**

- In short called as NSAIDS are a drug class that groups together drugs that provide analgesia and antipyretic effects and in higher doses also exerts anti-inflammatory effect.

Most NSAIDs, inhibit the activity of cyclooxygenase-1(COX-1) and cyclooxygenase-29COX-2) and thus the synthesis of prostaglandins and thromboxanes. Inhibition of COX-2 leads to anti-inflammatory, analgesic, and antipyretic effects and the NSAIDs that also inhibits COX-1, particularly aspirin, can cause gastrointestinal bleeding and ulcers.

Clasification:

A. **Non-selective COX inhibitors (conventional NSAIDs)**

1. Salicylates, Aspirin, Diflusinal.
2. Pyrazolone derivatives: Phenyl butazone, Oxyphenbutazone.
3. Indole derivatives: Indomethacin, Sulindac.
4. Propionic acid derivative:Ibuprofen, Naproxen, Ketoprofane, Flurbiprofen.

5. Anthranilic acid derivatives: Mephenamic acid.
6. Aryl-acetic derivatives: Diclofenac.
7. Oxicam derivatives: Piroxicam, Tenoxican
8. Pyrrolo-pyrrole derivatives: Ketorolac.

B. Preferential COX-2 inhibitors: Meloxicam, Nabumetone, Nimusulide.

C. Selective COX-2 inhibitors: Celecoxib, Rofecoxib, Valdecoxib,

D. Analgesics-antipyretics with poor anti-inflammatory action.

1. Para-aminophenol derivatives: Paracetamol(Acetaminophen)
2. Pyrazolone derivatives: Metamizol. Propiphenazone.
3. Benzoxazocine derivatives: Nefopam.

NSAIDs are usually used to bring about symptomatic relief of following conditions:

Osteoarthritis, Rheumatoid arthritis, mild to moderate pain due to inflammation and tissue injury, low back pain, ankylosing spondilytis, psoriatic arthritis, reactive arthritis, tennis elbow, headache, migrine, acute gout, dysmenorrhoea, metastatic bone pain, post-operative pain, muscle stiffness, and pain due to Parkinson's disease, pyrexia and renal colic.

They are also given to neonate infants whose ductus arteriosus is not closed within 24 hours of birth.

Anti-inflammatory drugs usage in dentistry:

- After extraction of third molar patients who have moderate to severe pain and who received a single dose of nimesulide, 300mg tablet showed very good pain control.
- A single dose of oral dipyrone 500mg showed very good results for dental post operative pain.
- Ibuprofen has been found to be highly effective for dental pain associated with oral surgery as well as periodontal surgery which includes elevation of surgical flap which is quite often of considerable size, and which includes reshaping of bone and implantation of material to replace the lost bone, and can last for 2-3 hours. 200-400mg of ibuprofen has been found to be quite superior in its effect as compared to various other drugs to control pain in such cases.
- Administering a single dose of ibuprofen 400mg has been found to be very effective in patients under going orthodontic treatment who can experience various degrees of discomfort especially during the first few days of treatment.
- Use of NSAIDs also plays a major role in managing endodontic pain. Patients seek urgent treatment in case of pulpal and periapical pain and the primary aim is to remove the necrotic material and inflammed tissue , but in such cases a variety of pro-inflammatory mediators are released and may contribute to post-operative pain and in such cases ibuprofen has been found to be effective.

- Flurbiprofane has been used widely for managing acute pain and discomfort associated with rheumatoid and osteoarthritis of the TMJ.
- Ketorolac is the first NSAID approved for intramuscular administration for short term management of moderate to severe pain associated with oral surgical as well as endodontic procedures.
- Selective COX-2 inhibitors like Rofecoxib has been found to be very effective to control acute dental pain.
- Orfenadrine –100 mg bid orally- anticholinergic drug to treat painful muscle spasms of the face.
- Diprospan suspension containing 5mg betamethasone as dipropionate and 2mg betamethasone as sodium phosphate in a sterile buffered vehicle can be given as intramuscular or intra-articular or even in soft tissues which has been found to be effective in rheumatoid arthritis and osteoarthritis of TMJ.
- Steroidal anti-inflammatory drugs are used in various conditions like aphthous ulcers, pemhigus, pemphigoid, erythema multiforme, lichen planus, oral submucous fibrosis. They produce anti-inflammatory as well as immunosuppressive effect.
- Intralesional steroids are also used for treatment of oral submucous fibrosis and lichen planus.

Side effects of NSAIDS:

NSAIDs when used for long term can cause gastric erosions which can become ulcers and in some extreme cases can cause hemorrhage resulting in death. In adults aged 16-45 the risk of death due to gastro-intestinal bleeding caused by use of NSAIDs is 1 in 12000. Above the age of 75 the risk increases twenty fold. Other risks of NSAIDs are exacerbation of asthma and kidney damage. Apart from aspirin, the risk of myocardial infarction and stroke risks are increased by prescription and over the counter NDAIDs. It is hence best to prescribe NSAIDs which would not cause gastric erosions or increase the risk of strokes and myocardial infarction.

Side effects of steroidal anti-inflammatory drugs:

Immunosupression, osteoporosis, redistribution of fat like moon face, buffalo hump, hyperglycemia, glaucoma.

Suggested reading:

1. K D Tripathi, Essentials Of Medical Pharmacology, 6th edition, 184

Q 4) Immunomodulators

TNMGRU APRIL 1995 (5 Marks)

Definition: Substances that modify the immune system's response to a threat upon it are called immunomodulators. They weaken or modulate the activity of immune system.

- Types:
  - Immunostimulants.
  - Immunosuppressants.

Immunostimulants:

- These agents are inherently non- specific in nature as they are seen to enhance body's resistance against infection.
- They can act through innate immune response and through adaptive immune response .
- In healthy individuals the immunostimulants are expected to serve as prophylactic and promoter agents i.e. as immunopotentiators by enhancing basic level of immune response, and in the individual with impairment of immune response as immunotherapeutic agents.

Immunosuppressants:

They suppress the activity of immune system.

Immunosuppressant Drugs:

These are a structurally and functionally heterogeneous group of drugs, which are often concomitantly administered in combination regimens to treat various types of organ transplant rejection and autoimmune diseases.

These drugs have major role in organ transplantation and auto immune diseases. The drugs are:

1. *Calcineurin inhibitors(specific-T cell inhibitors).*

Cyclosporin:

- It is a lipophillic cyclic polypeptide composed of 11 amino acids.
- The drug is extracted from a soil fungus. It profoundly and selectively inhibits T lymphocyte proliferation, IL2 and other cytokine production and response to inducer T-cells.
- Lymphocytes are arrested in G0 to G1 phase. KDT 837 cyclosporin is used in prevention of rejection of kidneys, liver and cardiac allogenic transplants.

Tacrolimus: (TAC)

- It is a newer immunosuppressant, macrolide.
- Tacrolimus is used in prevention of rejection of liver and kidney and is given with corticosteroids and antimetabolites.

2. Anti-proliferative drug (cyto-toxic drugs)

Azathioprine:

- It is a purine antimetabolite. Its selective uptake into immune cells and intracellular conversion to the active metabolite 6-mercaptopurine, which then undergoes further transformation to inhibit de novo purine synthesis and damage to DNA. It is approved for prevention of renal and other graft rejection.

Cyclophosphamide:

- This drug has more effect on B cells and humoral immunity compared to that on T cells and cell- mediated immunity. It is used in bone marrow transplant.

- Other drugs of this category are
- Methotrexate,
- Chlorambucil,
- Mycophenolate mofetil (MMF)

3. Glucocorticoids:

Prednisolone:

- The steroids are used to suppress acute rejection of solid allograft and in chronic graft versus host disease.
- Lymphocyte populations can be rapidly reduced by lysis or redistribution by the steroids. After entering the cells, they bind to the gluccocorticoid receptors and the complex passes in to the nucleus and regulates the translation of DNA.

4. Antibodies:

- **Muromonab CD3:** It is a murine monoclonal antibody against the CD3 glycoprotein which is located near to the T cell receptor on helper T cells.
- It is used for treatment of acute rejection of renal allografts as well as cardiac and hepatic transplantation.
- **Antithymocyte globin (ATG):** Is a polyclonal antibody purified from horse or rats immunized with human thymine lymphocytes. It binds to T-lymphocytes and depletes them.
- It is a potent immunosuppressant used for suppressing acute allograft reject episodes.
- **Other drugs of this category are:**
- Rho (D) immunoglobin.
- Efalizumab.

Immunostimulant drugs:

The immune system is stimulated by these drugs to fight against immunodeficiencies like AIDS, infections and cancers.

1. **Levamisole:** It is an antihelminthic drug which also restores the functions of B lymhocytes, T-lymphocytes, monocytes and macrophages. It is hence being used in cancer along with 5 FU.
2. **Thalidomide:** Different effects of this old drug has been utilised in conditions such as:
   Erythema nodosum: Anti inflammatory effect.
   Multiple myeloma: Anti-angiogenesis.
   Rheumatoid arthritis: Anti Tumour necrosis factor effect.
3. **BCG:** Used in carcinoma bladder.
4. **Recombinant cytokines:**
   Interferons: In tumours and chronic hepatitis B and C.
   Interleukin 2: It has been used in renal cell carcinoma and melanoma.

Suggested reading:

1. Priyanka Saroj et al, J Adv Scient Res, 2012, 3(1): 07-12

Q 5) Contraindications of corticosteroids

MUHS, NOVEMBER 2009, (2 Marks)

Corticosteroids are substances that are produced naturally in the body by adrenal glands and help in regulating fats, proteins and carbohydrate metabolism. They regulate the immune system and helps to maintain salt-water balance. They help to reduce inflammation.

Steroids in dentistry are usually used as anti-inflammatory drugs to control pain, relieve anxiety, and also for the treatment of various oral diseases.

It is important for dentists to know the contraindications.

Following are the conditions in which they are contraindicated:

1. **Cushings syndrome:** It occurs in patients who are given high dosages of corticosteroids of 100 mg/day for longer than 2 weeks and is characterized by rounded face appearance, narrow mouth, supraclavicular hump, obesity of trunk with relatively thin limbs. Its essential to recognise the condition and not prescribe steroids.
2. **Patients with active or incompletely treated tuberculosis:** latent tuberculosis reactivated after initiation of gluccocorticoid therapy.
3. **Active viral or fungal infections:** It is contraindicated in cases of primary herpetic gingivostomatitis and candidiasis. Especially contraindicated in cases of ocular herpes as it can cause suppression of host response and dissemination of herpes.
4. **Ocular Disease:** It is contraindicated in ocular diseases as it increases intraocular pressure.
5. Patients with a history of acute psychoses or psychotic tendencies.
6. In patients with primary bacterial infections and hypersensitivity topical corticosteroids are contraindicated.
7. **Hypertension:** As it increases intracranial hypertension due to hypokalemia and hypochloremic alkalosis.
8. **Diabetes mellitus:** As it precipitates hyperglycaemia and glycosuria.
9. **Osteoporosis:** It decreases calcium absorption from intestine, increases renal excretion of calcium, and increases bone resorption.
10. **Myasthenia gravis:** Corticosteroids causes muscle wasting.
11. Acute or long standing infections.
12. **Active or latent peptic ulcer:** Increases the risk of bleeding and silent perforation of the ulcers.
13. **Pregnancy and lactation:** It is best to avoid in 1st trimester of pregnancy due to risk of cleft palate and intrauterine growth retardation of the fetus.
14. **Renal insufficiency**.
15. **Heart diseases like coronary heart disease:** Sodium retention may precipitate risk of congestive heart failure.

Suggested reading:

1. Anil Ghom, text book of oral medicine, 3rd edition, chapter 42, pg no.957.
2. KD Tripathi, Essential of pharmacology for Dentistry, 1st edition, chapter 14, pg no-227-228.

CHAPTER 4

Developmental Disorders of Teeth

Q 1) Regional odontodysplasia

RGUHS APRIL 1997 (5 Marks)

Definition:

- Its a rare developmental anomaly involving both mesodermal and ectodermal dental components in a group of contiguous teeth. It is also called as ghost teeth.
- In this condition all elements of teeth are hypocalcified and hypoplastic.

Introduction:

- The condition probably was first described by Hitchin in 1934 but many authors give credit to McCall and Wald as reporting first but only showing radiographic features.
- As this condition affects only one quadrant, the term regional odontodysplasia was thought to be the best to describe it.
- It has also been known as odontogenic dysplasia, localised arrested tooth development, ghost teeth, odontogenesis imperfecta, unilateral dental malformation, familial amelodentinal dysplasia etc.

Etiology:

- The etiology is uncertain, but several factors such as trauma, infection, teratogenic drugs, local circulatory disorders, Rh incompatibility, hyperpyrexia, metabolic and nutritional disorders, irradiation, neural damage, and vitamin deficiency have been quoted as contributing factors.
- It seems to be non-inherited condition.
- It also seems to be associated with the activation of latent viruses in the odontogenic epithelium, and with the presence of nevi, hemangiomas and hydrocephaly.
- This condition is primarily diagnosed by clinical and radiographic criteria.

Clinical features:

- Both primary and permanent dentitions can be affected by regional odontodysplasia.
- Though it affects only one arch it may in some cases cross the midline.
- It affects the maxilla twice as much as the mandible and the maxillary left quadrant is most commonly affected.
- The anterior teeth that is the central and lateral incisors are more commonly affected than the posterior teeth.
- It is more common in women than in men.
- The mediolateral expansion of the maxillary posterior alveolar process, which extends from the canine to the maxillary tuberosity and its associated gingiva along with abnormal spacing, absence of premolars and/or molars occurs in the affected quadrant.
- The teeth that are affected have an abnormal morphology, irregular surface contour, and there may be pitting and grooves on the surface.
- There is discolouration, hypoplasia and hypocalcification of the affected teeth.
- The enamel is thin and soft on probing and the teeth are discoloured, yellow or yellowish brown.
- Some teeth may show no alterations in the affected quadrant.
- The teeth that are affected are very friable, fracturing at slightest trauma and more susceptible to caries.
- There is delay in tooth eruption or may not erupt at all.
- After the teeth erupt, the most common clinical findings are gingival swelling, periapical infection, and abscess formation in the absence of caries.
- The range of severity varies in this condition. In some mild cases the roots might develop well and may not have any infections or complicatons.
- This condition may be associated with vascular nevi, hemangioma, hydrocephalus and epidermal nevus syndrome.

Radiographic features:

- Ghost like appearance due to reduced thickness and radiodensity of enamel and dentin, is seen in the affected teeth.
- Demarcation between hypomineralised dentin and enamel is not visible.
- The teeth are generally shorter, with short roots, wide open apices, and abnormally wide pulp chambers and canals.
- Sometimes only the shell of enamel remain on the teeth, and this appearance is called shell teeth.
- The affected bone is dense and sclerotic, and has coarse, irregular and vertically oriented trabeculae.
- Histological features:
- The affected teeth, histologically show fibrous enlargement of the

pulp and an irregular pulp/dentin interface with pseudo inclusions and pulp stones. Tubular defects are found in the coronal part of dentin from the level of pulp horn to the tip of the cusp. Tubular structure is seen in the circumpulpal dentin of the apical half and there is focally deficient odontoblastic layer and also presence of wide spread external resorption.

- Gingiva may show dense collagenous fibrous tissue, focal aggregations of calcified bodies, and several islands of odontogenic epithelium.

Diagnosis:

- **Clinical diagnosis:** Irregular shaped teeth with brown discoloration.
- **Radiological diagnosis:** Shell teeth appearance seen radiologically.

Differential diagnosis:

(i) Shell teeth in case of dentinogenesis imperfecta: There is familial involvement which is not the case in regional odontodysplasia. Enamel is not hypoplastic in shell teeth as compared to ghost teeth.

Treatment:

- Conservative approach such as use of restorations to protect the permanent teeth or just long term follow up is done.
- Some experts favor immediate extraction and replacement with prosthesis.

Suggested reading:

1. Rafaela Scariot, Regional odontodysplasia: A case report. Rev Odonto Cienc 2012; 27(3):246-250.

Q 2) What is taurodontism and fusion?

MUHS DECEMBER- 2005 2 Marks

a) Taurodontism:

- It is one of the tooth anomaly in which tooth is enlarged at the expense of root. It was first described in 1913 by Sir Arthur Keith.
- The clinical and anatomical crown is of normal shape and size, an elongated body, short roots and longitudinally enlarged pulp chambers.
- Involved tooth are generally rectangular in shape.
- **Etiology:**
  - (i) Hereditary-Cause is due to genetically determined trait.
  - (ii) Developmental-It usually occurs as a result of failure of Hertwig's epithelial root sheath to invaginate at proper horizontal level.
  - (iii) Mutation-As a result of odontoblastic deficiency during dentinogenesis of the root.

Classification:

(a) **Hypotaurodont:** It is mild form of taurodontism and there is slight apical displacement of pulpal floor.

(b) **Mesotaurodont:** There is a moderate pulpal floor displacement which is at about midline of the root of the teeth.

(c) **Hypertaurodont:** A severe form with apical displacement of pulpal floor which is present at the apex.

- **Associated syndrome**-Klinfelter syndrome, Rapp hodkins, Down's syndrome & dento-osseous syndrome.
- **Radiographically:** The pulp chamber is unusually large with much greater apico-occlusal height than normal pulp and lack the usual constriction at the cervix of tooth.

  Roots and the root canals are very short. The dimension between the CEJ and furcation is also increased.

Treatment: No specific treatment is needed as it does not cause any clinical problem.

b. Fusion:

It is also called as 'synodontia'. It represents the embryonic union of normally separated tooth germs. Two separate tooth germs initially close together, as they grow and expand, they contact with each other and the germ fuse to varying degree.

- **Etiology:**
  - **Genetic:** It is transmitted as autosomal dominant trait with reduced penetration.
  - **Physical:** Physical force or pressure generated during development causes contact of tooth germ.
- **Clinical features:**
  - More commonly in anterior teeth region.
  - Deciduous dentition more affected than Permanent dentition.
  - Size of the tooth is twice in size than normal, with separate or fused root canals.
  - It results in reduced number of teeth in the jaw.
  - Large tooth with missing adjacent tooth will help in diagnosis.
- **Radiographic features:**
  - True nature and extent of the union will be more evident on radiograph.
- **Management:**
  - **Endodontic treatment:** Morphology of teeth should be determined radiographically for endodontic treatment.
  - **Reshaping of tooth:** After endodontic treatment, tooth may be reshaped with a restoration that will mimic independent crown.
  - Extraction and extraoral separation of teeth followed by immediate replantation can also be done.

Suggested reading:

1. Anil Govindrao Ghom, Text book of Oral Medicine, 3rd edition, chapter 6, pg no-85.91.

Q 3) Dentinogenesis Imperfecta

TNMGRU AUGUST 2004 (5 Marks)

It is also known as hereditary opalescent dentin and is a dentin development disorder with autosomal dominant transmission that affects both the primary and permanent dentition.

DGI is a genetic disorder that involves tooth development. It is a type of dentin dysplasia that causes tooth discolouration, quite often blue-gray or yellowish-brown colour giving an opalscent sheen. The teeth tend to be weaker than normal and they undergo rapid wear, breakage and loss. It can affect both the primary and permanent teeth.

Dentinogenesis Imperfecta type I:

Persons having DGI-I also suffer from osteogenesis imperfecta. The teeth involving both dentitions appear amber and translucent and reveal substantial attrition. Radiographs show teeth having short, constricted roots and dentin hypertrophy causing pulpal obliteration before or just after eruption. Some teeth may show total pulpal obliteration while in others the dentin may appear normal.

Dentinogenesis Imperfecta type II:

The dental features are similar to that of DGI-I but penetrance is almost complete and osteogenesis imperfecta is not present. The crowns are bulbous with accentuated constriction at the cervical region.

Dentinogenesis Imperfecta type-III:

This form is found in a tri-racial population from Maryland and Washington DC known as the Brandywine isolate. The clinical features are variable and similar to those seen in DGI-I and DGI-II but the primary teeth show multiple pulp exposures and radiographically they show shell teeth due to hypotrophy of dentin.

Clinical features:

They are variable, however, the teeth usually involved and seriously affected are the primary teeth in DGI-I but in type DGI-II both dentitions are equally affected.

The teeth appear gray-yellowish brown. They exhibit translucent or opalescent hue. Enamel is lost early but the teeth are not more susceptible to caries than the normal teeth.

The enamel frequently separates easily from underlying dentin due to which the crown erodes easily.

The usually exposed dentin becomes stained and teeth may appear dark brown or even black. Most of the times though the pulp is obliterated with excess dentin production, some teeth show normal sized pulp or pulpal enlargement giving the typical appearance of shell teeth.

Certain patients with DGI may suffer from multiple periapical abscesses apparently resulting from pulp strangulation secondary to pulp obliteration or pulp exposure because of extensive crown wear. Apical surgery may be required to save the teeth.

Radiographic features:

The teeth have bulbous crowns and there may be attrition of the occlusal surface. Type I and Type II show partial or complete obliteration of pulp chambers. Root canals may be absent or if present may appear thread like. This occurs due to obliteration of pulp by the dentine.

The pulp chambers and canals may be normal, or contain pulp stones or often may be partially or totally obliterated. Roots may often be short but could be of normal length and sometimes may be absent.

Sometimes periapical radiolucencies are seen associated with a sound tooth without any pulpal involvement.

Differential diagnosis:

Dentinal dysplasia:

Radiographic appearance of dentinogenesis imperfecta may simulate that of dentinal dysplasia. But teeth with dentinogenesis imperfecta have typical bulbous crowns with constriction at the cervical area as compared to normal shape, size and proportions of the crowns in dentinal dysplasia.

Periapical rarefying osteitis associated with non-carious teeth are more commonly seen in dentinal dysplasia.

Hypocalcified form of amelogenesis imperfecta: As opposed to DGI the teeth are usually sensitive and on radiographs enamel is less radio-dense than dentine. Pulp chamber and root canals are usually not sclerosed.

Intrinsic discoloration:

Congenital erythropoietic porphyria:

The discolouration of teeth range from yellow to green, brown and grey to black is usually found at the necks of teeth and enamel hypoplasias are usually located in the coronal third of teeth.

Tetracycline stains: can cause permanent discolouration which ranges from yellow to grey to brown depending on the dose or type of the drug received in relation to body weight. However the normal shape and size of teeth and pulp chambers can differentiate from dentinogenesis imperfecta.

Treatment:

Prevention and restoration are important as well as esthetics is a major consideration. In most cases full-coverage crowns are needed for esthetic appearance, as well as to prevent further attrition. Another treatment option is bonding or putting lighter enamel on the weakened enamel of teeth and with several such treatments the teeth appear whiter outwardly but inside the colour is the same. Due to the weak teeth, treatments like bridges and orthodontic braces are not advisable as they can cause damage than the conditions they were meant to correct.

Dental bleaching is contraindicated as it may lighten the colour of DGI affected teeth but with only some success.

Suggested reading:

1. Martin J Barron, Sinead T McDonnell, Iain MacKie and Michael J Dixon, Hereditary dentine disorders: dentinogenesis imperfecta and dentine dysplasia Orphanet Journal of Rare Diseases2008 3:31.

CHAPTER 5

Developmental Disorders of Craniofacial Structures

Introduction

Several developmental disorders of the craniofacial structure have oral and dental manifestations and several syndromes associated with it can be recognised by an expert dental clinician. It is therefore important to know and understand and recognise these disorders.

Q 1) Ectodermal Dysplasia

TNMGRU OCTOBER 1996 (5 Marks)

This condition is an inherited X-linked recessive disorder which is characterised by defective formation of ectodermal structures like skin, teeth, nails, sweat glands, sebaceous glands and hair follicles etc.

The disease appears in two forms hydrotic and hypohydrotic or anhydrotic.

Features of Hydrotic form:

(i) Most often autosomal dominant.
(ii) Scalp hair is soft, and darker in colour.
(iii) Teeth show anodontia or hyodontia.
(iv) Lips show no abnormality.
(v) Sweat glands are active.
(vi) Nasal bridge shows no flattening.
(vii) Nails show dystrophic nails.
(viii) Eyebrows are frequently absent.
(ix) Eye lashes/pubic hair/axillary hair are scanty or absent.

Features of Hypohydrotic form:

(i) Most often autosomal recessive.
(ii) Scalp hair are fine in texture, fair and short.
(iii) Teeth show andontia or hypodontia.
(iv) Lips are protruding type.
(v) Sweat glands are almost absent.

(vi) Nasal bridge shows underdevelopment.
(vii) Nails show no abnormality.
(viii) Eyebrows are absent.
(ix) Eyelashes/pubic hair/axillary hair are affected with variability.

Clinical features:

The three most outstanding features are:

1. Hypohydrosis(lack of sweating)
2. Hypotrichosis(absence of hair)and
3. Hypodontia(absence of teeth)

Affects males more than females.

Soft, dry and smooth skin with little or no tendency for sweating.

There may be unexplained fever and patients cannot endure warm temperature.

The hair on the scalp and eyebrows are fine and scanty and blonde and the sebaceous glands are absent.

The patient may suffer from rhinitis, sinusitis, and pharyngitis etc. with dysphagia and hoarseness of voice.

The patient frequently exhibits "pili tori" (kinky hair) & cleft Palate.

Treatment:

For patients with anhydrosis and hypohydrosis airconditioned atmosphere is advised for home, school and work.

Frequent consumption of cool liquids to maintain adequate hydration and thermoregulation.

Patients are advised to wear cool and comfortable clothing like cottons.

In patients with dental defects, early evaluation and interventional treatment is helpful and routine dental hygiene should be encouraged.

Dental implants could be advised for missing teeth.

Orthodontic treatment is advised for cosmetic reasons.

Adequate nutritional intake is advisable.

Denture prosthesis with soft liners are given and changed from time to time to accommodate the growth of jaws and artificial saliva given to keep the mouth moist.

Artificial tears in case of reduced lacrimation.

Wigs for alopecia so that the patient feels confident and not subconscious.

Suggested reading:

1. Anil Govindrao Ghom, Textbook of Oral Medicine. Edition 3rd chapter 7; page. No.136.
2. Hickey AJ, Vergo TJ. Prosthetic treatments for patients with ectodermal dysplasia. J Prosthet Dent. 2001 Oct. 86(4):364-8.
3. Jyothi Sharma, GP Mamatha, Hereditary Ectodermal Dysplasia: diagnostic dilemmas, Rev. Clín. Pesq. Odontol. Curitiba, v. 4, n. 1, p. 35-40, jan./abr. 2008

Q 2) Gardner's Syndrome

MUHS NOVEMBER 2014 (3 Marks)

It is also called as familial multiple polyposis.

It is an inherited autosomal dominant disorder. Typically one parent tends to have this syndrome.

It is recently known to be caused by mutation in the APC gene located in the chromosome 5q21.

This syndrome was described by Gardner which consists of hereditary intestinal polyposis with osteomas and multiple cutaneous and subcutaneous lesions in the year 1953.It has been since then modified by the addition of other features such as osteomas, supernumerary teeth, dental abnormalities, fibrous dysplasia of the skull, fibromas, desmoid tumours, epidermoid cysts and number of malignant tumours.

Clinical features:

- Occurs usually in 2nd decade of life with male predilection.
- The most important feature of this syndrome is the association of multiple colonic polyps, with sebaceous cysts and jaw osteomas.
- The significance of this dominantly inherited condition for the dentist is that the colonic polyps usually undergo malignant change by the fourth decade and the extra-intestinal lesions may be apparent before those in the intestine.
- Osteomas are very commonly seen on the mandible, especially in angle region, maxilla, frontal and sphenoid bone.
- The osteomas may be either exostoses, often called as peripheral osteomas, or endostoses which are detectable only radiographically.
- These osteomas lead to facial deformity.
- A large osteoma involving the mandible may interfere with mouth opening.
- Some patients may suffer from epidermoid cyst, thyroid carcinoma, and desmoid tumour.
- The main cutaneous lesions in this syndrome are multiple epidermoid cysts, present in about 50-65% of cases. The cysts arise before puberty and occur mostly on the face, scalp and extremeties.
- Dental abnormalities are present in about 30% of cases with this syndrome and may include supernumerary teeth, compound odontomas, hypodontia, abnormal tooth morphology and impacted or unerupted teeth.
- The highest incidence of dental abnormalities is found in patients with multiple osteomas, but dental changes may be determined in the absence of skeletal lesions, and the dental anomalies are not secondary to bony changes.

Diagnosis: Presence of multiple osteomas and unerupted supernumerary teeth will favor diagnosis of gardner's syndrome.

Management: Prophylactic colectomy to prevent malignancy is suggested. Jaw osteomas can be removed surgically to improve esthetic value.

Suggested reading:

1. Guvenc Basaran and Mustafa Erkan, One of the Rarest Syndromes in Dentistry: Gardner Syndrome, Eur J Dent. 2008 Jul; 2: 208–212.

Q 3) Cleidocranial Dysostosis

RGUHS APRIL 2005 4 Marks

Introduction:

Cleido-cranial dysostosis is also known as Marie-Sainton syndrome, Sheuthauer-Marie Sainton syndrome and Mutational Dysostosis.

Its a syndrome characterised by defective development of cranial bones and by complete or fibular bones, absence of pubic bone, partial absence of the clavicles.

There is delayed ossification of midline structures.

Etiology:

- Though not completely clear, is thought to be due to core binding factor activity1(CBFA1), gene defect on the short arm of chromosome 6p21.
- CBFA1 is necessary for differentiation of stem cells into osteoblasts, and hence any defect in this gene can cause defects in the membranous and endochondral bone formation.

Clinical features:

- The disease affect men and women with equal frequency.
- People with CCD have a characteristic facial appearance.
  - They tend to have brachycephaly and frontal bossing.
  - There is delayed closure of fontanels and in some cases the fontanels are open.
  - The eyes are widely spaced and the nasal bridge is often flat. The neck appears long and the shoulders are narrow and sloping downwards.
  - The deciduous teeth are over-retained and there is delayed eruption of permanent teeth.
- Adults affected with this syndrome have mixed dentition.
- There are great numbers of supernumerary teeth.
- The maxilla is under developed and the paranasal sinuses may be ill-formed.
- There is skeletal class III tendency, that is the mandible is prognathic.
- The classic characteristic is that, one or both the clavicles are frequently partially or in about 10% of cases completely absent.
- Rudimentary sternal and acromial stubs are present and the mid-clavicular portion is absent.
- Clavicular deformity along with the dysplastic muscle attachments give rise to elongated neck, narrow dropping and hypermobility of the shoulders along with the tendency to approximate the shoulders anteriorly.
- There is under development of bones and joints and patients are shorter and their body frames are smaller than their siblings who donot have this condition.

- Vertebral abnormalities.
- Other features are: parietal bossing, abnormal ear structures with hearing loss, supernumerary ribs, hemivertebrae with spondylosis, small and high scapulae, hypoplasia of iliac bone, short/absent fibular and radial bones and hypoplastic terminal phalanges.

Radiological findings:

- Panoramic radiographs show multiple unerupted abnormal teeth.
- Narrow ascending ramus, slender and pointed coronoid process, thin zygomatic arch, small or absent maxillary sinuses, coarse trabeculation of mandibular bone, cyst formation with supernumerary teeth especially in the premolar region.
- Increased density of alveolar bone over unerupted teeth.
- Skull radiographs show brachycephaly, a persistently open anterior fontanel, multiple wormian bones, open skull sutures, small sphenoid bones, and calvarial thickening over the occiput and wormian bones.
- Narrow thorax, oblique ribs, and absence of clavicles.

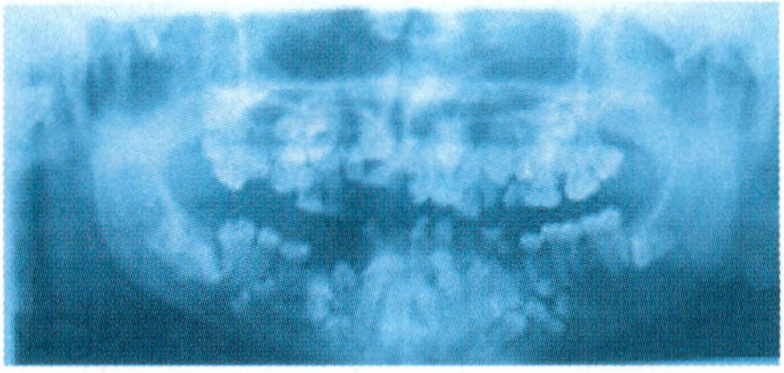

Fig. Panoramic view of jaws with multiple unerupted supernumerary teeth, missing gonial angles, underdeveloped sinuses, in a case of cleidocranial dysostosis.

Differential Diagnosis:

Includes Crane-Heise syndrome, mandibulo-acral dysplasia, pycnodysostosis, Yunis-Varon syndrome, hypophosphatasia.

Management:

- Cranio-facial surgery may be necessary to correct skull defects.
- In case of open fontanelle, appropriate head gear may be advised for protection from injury.
- Skull and clavicle anomalies- there is no treatment required for this anomaly. Patient can live normal life.
- Dental care as the patient may be having supernumerary teeth, they should be extracted.
- Prosthetic replacement of teeth should be carried out.
- Unerupted teeth should be extruded orthodontically.

Suggested reading:

1. Anil Govindrao Ghom Textbook of Oral Medicine, 129.

CHAPTER 6

Red and White Lesions of the Oral Mucosa

Introduction

Red and white lesions are quite a common occurrence in the oral cavity and a thorough knowledge about their diagnosis and treatment plan is essential for dentists.

A white lesion is described as an abnormal area of the oral mucosa that appears whiter than the surrounding tissue and are usually slightly raised, roughened, or different texture from adjacent normal tissue. The white lesion may be smooth, folded, shaggy, elevated, lacy or annular. They could also be fissured, ulcerated, eroded or inflammed. They can be solitary, multiple, focal or diffuse.

Q 1) Treatment of oral submucous fibrosis

MUHS SUMMER 2013 (3 Marks)

Medical management of oral submucous fibrosis:

TNMGRU AUGUST 2012 (3 Marks)

A) Patient Education:

- Advising the patient to discontinue the habit of betelnut and kharra chewing.
- Avoidance of spicy food.
- Balanced and healthy diet to avoid malnutrition.
- Proper oral hygiene maintenance education.
- Scheduling regular oral examination.

B) Medical Management:

Supportive therapy:

- Prescribing vitamin A rich diet .
- Iodine-B complex preparation subscription.

1) Mouth opening more than 35 mm:

(i) Systemic:

- Capsule vitamin Bcomplex, Dose-200mg BDx3 months.
- Iodine +B complex preparation: Injection Ranodine 2ml ampule daily intramuscularly-5 injections.
- Tablet lycopene–Dose-2000 micrograms BDx 3 months. (SM Fibro)
- Iron supplements (Dexorange syrup or Haemup syrup)

(ii) Topical applications:

- Triamcinolone acetonide 0.13% (kenalog/Tess) xTDS. or
- Crushed dexamethasone tablets in 20 ml of water to be used as mouth rinse.

(iii) Newer drugs for systemic use:

- Tablet pentoxyphyllin 400 mg BDx 3 months. (Trental/Flexital) or
- Interferon gamma injections 0.01-10U/ml TDS × 6 months. In patients with OSMF this plays an important role due to its immunomodulatory effects. IFN-gamma is a known antifibrinolytic cytokine. It alters collagen synthesis and appears to be a key factor in the treatment of this condition. or
- Tablet levamisole 50mg TDS for 3 consecutive days /week x 4-6 weeks.

2) Mouth opening : 30-35 mm:

Combination of treatment protocols for mouth opening of more than 35 mm along with following:

(i) **Intralesional injection:** Combination of dexamethasone (4mg/ml)+Hyaluronidase 1500 IU+2ml of 2% lignocaine, as 0.2ml/site twice a week for 3 months. or

(ii) **Injection of placental extract:** Placentrex 2ml once a week for 1 month. or

(iii) Combination of i+ii/once a week for 3 months. or

(iv) Immune milk powder 45 ml BDx 3 months.

3) Mouth opening 20-30mm:

(i) Combination of treatment protocols of 1+2 as follows:

- Steroid + vitamins + minerals
- Steroids + Hyaluronidase + Vitamins
- Steroids + Placental extracts.
- Steroids or pentoxyphyllin + vitamins + minerals.
- Levamisole + Vitamin A.
- Steroids + Hyaluronidase + Immune milk.

(ii) **Ayurvedic treatments:**

- Tulsi extract powder+glycerineTDSx 3 months.
- Turmeric tablets TDS x 3 months.
- Aloe vera gel TDS x 3 months.

B) Surgical management of OSMF:

Surgical management is the treatment of choice in case where the mouth opening is less than 20mm. Biopsy in such cases reveals marked degree of dysplasia and there is trismus and symptoms of dysphagia.

Surgical modalities include:

- Excision of the fibrous bands followed by tongue flap.
- Excision of fibrous bands followed by reconstruction using bilateral full thickness nasolabial flap.
- Bilateral palatal flap along with bilateral temporalis myotomy and coronoidectomy.
- After excision of fibrous bands implantation of bits of fresh human placenta is giving good results.
- **Oral stent:** An appliance made up of acrylic having bilateral posterior vertical stops is made and is placed after surgery to allow tissues to heal upto a new height.
- CO2 lasers are used to excise the fibrous bands to reduce restricted mouth opening.
- Cryosurgery which is method of local tissue destruction by freezing. Available as liquid sprays and better suited for mucosal lesions.
- Short wave diathermy is used in some early and moderately advanced cases. Low current of (20watts × 2450 cycles) is used. It acts by physiofibrolysis of bands. It can be used in combination with other treatment modalities.

C) Oral physiotherapy:

- Oral exercises are advised in early and moderate cases of OSMF where in ballooning of mouth is advised.
- Bunch of icecream sticks held together with rubber bands are placed in the anterior teeth for 10 minutes for 4-5 times daily to facilitate mouth opening.
- Forceful mouth opening by gags or acrylic screws.
- Warm saline gargles 3-4 times/day to increase the blood supply to the tissues.

Suggested reading:

1. Haque MF, Meghji S, Nazir R, Harris M. Interferon gamma (IFN-gamma) may reverse oral submucous fibrosis. J Oral Pathol Med. 2001 Jan. 30(1):12-21.

Q 2) Management of oral lichen planus

MUHS MAY 2007 (2 Marks)

TNMGRU OCTOBER 1999 (5 Marks)

It is a chronic inflammatory disorder that affects the mucous membrane of oral cavity.

It is a T-cell mediated autoimmune disorder in which CD8+T-cells trigger the process of apoptosis of the basal cells of the oral epithelium.

Pharmacologic management:

1) Corticosteroids:

This group of drugs is most commonly used for treatment of this condition.

The reason of usage is the ability of these drugs to modulate inflammation and immune response. They act by reducing the lymphocytic exudates and stabilising the lysosomal membrane.

- Topical mild potency drugs like Triamcinolone acetonide is given as 0.1% TID/day for I month.
- High potent fluorinated corticosteroids such as fluocinonide acetonide is given as 0.025% TID for two months. Tapering frequency of local application is advised.
- Super potent halogenated corticosteroids like clobetasol is given 0.05% local application cream BID for two months for symptomatic cases.
- Clobetasone 17-butyrate is given as 0.05% BID x 1 month and then OD x 1 month.
- Betamethasone valerate as 0.05% cream for mild to moderate lesions.
- Small and accessible erosive lesions located on palate and gingiva can be treated with corticosteroid cream or lotion mixed with denture adhesive paste in custom made trays for close contact and gives excellent reduction of pain and burning.
- Soluble prednisolone tablets, 5 mg dissolved in 15 ml water can be used as mouth rinse 3-4 times a day for atrophic and erosive lichen planus.
- Systemic steroids like tablet prednisolone for short duration of 40-80mg for 5-7 days.
- This regimen can be followed for severe or recalcitrant cases and erosive or erythematous lichen planus cases not responding to topical application.
- Intra lesional steroids like injection triamcinolone 0.5 ml OD/week for 4 weeks can be given for recalcitrant cases.

2) Other immunomodulatory and immunosuppressant agents:

(i) **Calcineurin Inhibitors:**

- **Cyclosporin**: Its used as a mouth rinse or topically with adhesive bases in oral lichen planus. However the solution is very expensive and should be reserved for highly recalcitrant cases of OL. Its systemic absorption is very low and it is known to cause gingival hyperplasia which reduces when the drug is withdrawn.
- Azathioprine is given in resistant cases and can be used in combination with corticosteroids and cyclosporine. It is given as 50-150mg for 1 month.
- **Tacrolimus:** It is 10-100 times as potent as cyclosporin and has greater percutaneous absorption. It is very effective in cases of recalcitrant OLP.

  Given as 0.1-0.3% (tacroz forte) topical ointment.
- **Pimecrolimus: 1**% topical cream of pimecrolimus has been used successfully in OLP. It has significant anti-inflammatory

activity and immunomodulatory capabilities but with low systemic immunosuppressive potential.

2. **Retinoids:** such as tretinoin and fenretinide with their immunomodulatory properties have been reported to be very effective in OLP. White striae can be reversed with topical retinoids, although effects may be temporary.
    - Retinol palmitate (chewable vitamin A) 50000 IU.
    - Tretinoin 0-1% in an adhesive gel 4 times/day for 2 months.
    - Isotretinoin 0.1% 2 times/day for 2 months.

      Systemic retinoids have been used in cases of severe lichen planus with variable degrees of success.
    - Etretinate 1-6 mg/kg/day for 2 months followed by maintenance dose of 0.3 mg/kg/day.
    - Isotretinoin can be used in dosage of 10-60mg/day for 2 months.
3. **Dapsone:** It probably acts as an anti-inflammatory agent by inhibiting the release of chemotactic factors for mast cells and are used in treatment of OLP.
    - Given as doses of 50mg TDS for 3 consecutive days/week for 4-6 weeks.
4. **Mycophenolates:** Originally used for treatment of psoriasis, is now being used to treat severe case of oral lichen planus.
5. **Low dose low molecular weight heparin:** This promises to be simple, effective and safe treatment for OLP when injected subcutaneously as it has no side effects.

Non-Pharmacologic management of oral lichen planus:

1. **PUVA Therapy:**

   It is a non-pharmacologic approach which uses photochemotherapy with 8-methoxypsoralen and long wave ultraviolet light (PUVA).

   Methoxypsoralen is given orally, followed by administration of 2 hours of UV radiation, intraorally at the affected site.
2. **Photodynamic therapy:**

   It is a technique which uses a photosensitising compound like methylene blue, activated at a specific wavelength of laser light so as to destroy the targeted cells by strong oxidisers which cause cellular damage, membrane lysis, and protein inactivation.

   May help in reversing the hyperproliferation and inflammation of lichen planus.
3. **Laser therapy:**

   In severe and painful cases of erosive lichen planus which are unresponsive to even the topical superpotent corticosteroids, surgical management using cryosurgery and different types of lasers have been tried.

   A 980nm Diode laser, CO2 laser evaporation, biostimulation with a pulsed diode laser using 904-nm pulsed infra-red rays and low -dose excimer 308-nm laser with UV-rays have been tried.

- **Natural alternative therapy:**
  - Lycopene 4mg BD for 1 month.
  - Curcumin-tablet turmix (curcumin300mg+piperine 5 mg) TDS for 1 month.
  - Green tea extract.
  - Aloe vera-5mg TDS topically for 3 months.

Suggested reading:

1. N Lavanya, P Jayanthi, Umadevi K Rao, and K Ranganathan, Oral lichen planus: An update on pathogenesis and treatment, J Oral Maxillofac Pathol. 2011 May-Aug; 15(2): 127–132.

Q 3) White Sponge Nevus

RGUHS APRIL 1997 (5 Marks)

It is an autosomal dominant disorder and is rare. It is a oral genodermatosis which was described by Cannon in 1935.

It predominantly affects nonkeratinised stratified squamous epithelium.

The lesions of WSN may be present since birth or may first manifest and become more intense towards puberty.

Etiopathogenesis:

It is an inherited disorder exhibiting autosomal-dominant transmission with no sex predilection for mutations. The mutations affecting keratin protein interfere with immediate filament assembly. Thus according to a putative pathogenic mechanism, the intermediate filament can be easily damaged as a result of mild mechanical trauma, inducing cytokine flooding of underlying basal cells, and, as a consequence, excessive basal cell proliferation leading to mucosal hyperkeratosis. Suprabasal keratinocytes of the buccal, nasal, esophageal and anogenital epithelia specifically express K4 and K13 and mutations in K4 and K13 genes have been associated with white sponge nevus. Hence, the lesions are restricted to mucosal epithelia.

Clinical Features:

- No particular sex predilection and children are more commonly affected.
- The most common sites are cheeks, palate, gingiva, floor of the mouth, and portions of tongue. Generally present as bilateral, symmetric white, soft, spongy or velvety thick plaques on the buccal mucosa.
- It may also involve the mucous membrane of nose, esophagus, genitalia and rectum.
- Mucosa appears as thickened, folded, or corrugated with soft spongy texture and a white opalescent line. It may have a furrowed, wrinkled appearance.
- May vary from a small patch to involving large areas of the mucosa.
- The condition is usually asymptomatic and doesnot show tendency towards malignant change.

- Friction may cause the superficial keratotic area to strip off and may leave behind normal looking epithelium or raw area.

Diagnosis:

- **Clinical diagnosis:** The thickened white folded appearance which doesnot disappear after stretching is typical of white sponge nevus.
- **Laboratory diagnosis:** The typical histopathological features are epithelial thickening, parakeratosis, a peculiar perinuclear condensation of the cytoplasm, and vacuolisation of the suprabasal layer of keratinocytes.
- Electron microscopy of exfoliated cells show numerous cellular granules composed of disordered aggregates of tonofilaments.

Differential Diagnosis:

(i) **Leukedema:** They have white folded appearance like white sponge nevus but they disappear on stretching.

(ii) **Leukoplakia:** Is generally seen in older individuals.

(iii) **Hereditary benign intraepithelial dyskeratosis or pachyonichia congenita.**

(iv) **Pseudomembranous candidiasis:** Appearance is curdy white and there may be associated systemic symptoms .Scraping the lesions will leave raw erosive areas.

(v) **Habitual cheek biting:** There will be history of cheek biting and are seen only on the buccal mucosa.

(vi) **Chemical burns:** History will help in diagnosis and the lesions will be painful.

(vii) **Lichen planus:** Lesions will generally show wickham's striae and are present especially in elderly persons with female predilection.

(viii) **Lupus erythematosus:** Other system involvement will help in differentiating.

(ix) **Darriers disease and dyskeratosis congenita:** Presence of extra oral lesions associated with them will help in diagnosis.

Treatment:

No treatment is indicated for this benign and asymptomatic condition. Some cases may require palliative treatment if the condition is symptomatic.

Although the patients suffer from no pain, they do complain of altered texture of the mucosa or that the lesions are unaesthetic.

Reassurance is all that is required, although numerous therapy models have been tried. None are likely to be effective unless they take into account the genetic nature of the lesions.

Vitamins, antihistaminics, and mouthrinses have been suggested but with almost no success.

In some cases of white sponge nevus, penicillin has been used with some success.

Suggested reading:

1. Anil Govindrao Ghom, Text Book Of Oral Medicine, Third Edition, 163.

Q 4) Management of chronic atrophic candidiasis

RGUHS OCTOBER 2005 (5 Marks)

Chronic atrophic candidiasis, also known denture stomatitis or denture sore mouth and is a common form of oral candidiasis which manifests as a diffuse inflammation of the denture bearing area of the maxillary arch.

DSM exhibits three progressive clinical stages:

- Petechiae.
- Diffuse erythema involving almost the entire maxillary denture bearing area.
- Palatal papillary hyperplasia.

In mild cases topical antifungal therapy is the first line of treatment. The use of clotrimazole or nystatin lozengez and/or pastilles after the denture is removed from the mouth is recommended. The application of antifungal agents, on the tissue- contacting surface of the denture is also recommended.

I) *Topical Therapy:*

1. **Clotrimazole:** 10 mg /tablet to be dissolved in mouth 5 times daily.
2. 1% gentian violet locally.
3. **Nystatin:** One tablet, 100000 units to be dissolved in mouth 3 times a day.
4. Nystatin oral suspension 100000 units/cc, 1 tsp with 1/4 cup of water as oral rinse.
5. Topical creams and ointment containing nystatin, ketoconazole, or clotrimazole.
6. **Idoquinol:** it has antifungal and antibacterial properties.
7. Amycostatin B (0.1 mg/ml) mouth rinse is given for 7-10 days 3-4 times/day. With 0.2 -1% chlorhexidine mouth wash for rinsing 7-10 days 2 times/day.
    - Proper denture wearing habits and mechanical plaque control are very important measures in the treatment of DSM. Denture cleansing and sanitisation is of utmost importance.
    - Daily thorough brushing and scrupulous denture hygiene is very important. The denture has to be soaked in antiseptic solution like chlorhexidine or dilute sodium hypochlorite. However if the denture base contains metal component then soaking in hypochlorite solution should be avoided because it can cause tarnishing of the metal. Another advantage of soaking dentures overnight is the removal of dentures for a long time providing relief. Removal of the denture provides minimisation of additional irritation and is important aspect of treatment.
    - Palatal papillary hyperplasia usually needs to be surgically removed before the denture is emplaced or relined. In mild

cases antifungal treatment without surgery might be an alternative before dentures are relined or replaced.

II) Systemic Therapy:

Systemic antifungal agents should be reserved for candidal infections in debilitated or immunocompromised patients.

1. Nystatin is given in a dose of 250 mg TDS –2 weeks followed by 1 troche /day for 3rd week.
2. Ketoconazole is given in a dose of 200 mg tablet with food once / day. It can cause hepatotoxicity. Careful monitoring of liver function on long term use is important.
3. Fluconazole is given as 100mg tab once a day for 2 weeks.
4. Itraconazole is given as 100mg capsule in a dose of 200mg /day orally for 14 days.

Suggested reading:

1. Burket's, Oral Medicine Diagnosis and Treatment 10th edi. 96-98.

Q 5) Angular Cheilitis

TNMGRU FEBRUARY 2009 6 Marks

Definition:

It is an inflammatory condition that affects one or both angles of the mouth. It typically presents with erythema, cracking, scaling, bleeding and ulcerations at the corner of the mouth. Though it can occur spontaneously it often develops in persons wearing oral dentures and appliances, in those required to wear masks as part of occupation, and in small children who slobber and use pacifiers.

Also known as Perleche. It is a clinical diagnosis for majority of lesions affecting the lip commissures, when other specific lesions such as recurrent herpes labialis, ulceration due to known trauma, environmental exposure or syphilis is excluded.

Etiology:

(i) Candida albicans mainly but also there can be role of staphylococci and streptococci.

(ii) Over closure of jaws as in edentulous patients or patients with artificial dentures, with reduced vertical dimensions. Saliva gets collected in the folds at the corner of the mouth and the skin gets masserated, fissured and secondarily infected. Riboflavin, folate and iron deficiency with a superimposed bacterial and fungal infection.

(iii) General protein deficiency can also cause this condition.

(iv) Atopic dermatitis involving the face is frequently associated with angular cheilitis.

(v) Hypersalivation, Down's syndrome, large tongue where in constant dribbling of saliva could be a causative factor.

(vi) Rarely it could be associated with diabetes, AIDS, and neutropenia.
(vii) Excessive use of mouth washes and very aggressive dental flossing can also lead to this condition.
(viii) Use of orthodontic braces can lead to nickel-induced angular cheilitis.
(ix) In children who frequently lick their lips and indulge in thumb sucking are also prone to develop this condition.

Clinical Features:

(i) Can occur in children as well as in adults.
(ii) There is feeling of dryness and burning sensation at the corner of the mouth.
(iii) There is triangular area of erythema and edema at one or more commonly both the corners of the mouth.
(iv) Wrinkling, fissuring and ulceration with mild bloody crust in some cases may be seen.
(v) In denture wearers and in certain severe cases linear furrows or fissures radiating from the angle of the mouth.
(vi) Spontaneous remissions may occur.

Diagnosis:

Erythematous, furrowed, wrinkled, maserated appearing lesions at the corner of the mouth are highly suggestive of angular cheilitis.

A detailed history including the patient's dental status, oral hygiene practices and occupation should be taken.

It is important to find out about the patient's medical illnesses such as anemias, and diseases causing immunodeficiency, smoking, use of tobacco, alcohol consumption, cutaneous disorders, (psoriasis, lichen planus, atopic dermatitis), allergic disorders (asthma, eczema) and use of any oral medications.

Swabbing both angles of the mouth for microbiological investigation can be done.

Management:

(i) The underlying primary cause should be removed.
(ii) When the cause is not clear simple treatment like applying petroleum jelly to the lesions could be effective.
(iii) Vitamin B complex, folic acid and iron supplements should be given.
(iv) In staphylococcal infections, the lesions are swabbed and cleaned, and fusidic acid ointment or cream is applied four times a day.
(v) If causative agent is candida, miconazole ointment is applied locally.
(vi) This could also be applied to the affected areas as well as to the surface of the dentures if infected.
(vii) Gentian violet application is useful in some cases.

(viii) In old patients having dentures and other prosthesis, it is important that they be of appropriate size and shape and well fitting.

(ix) Maintenance of good oral hygiene is essential to prevent recurrences.

Suggested reading:

1. Burket's Oral Medicine Diagnosis and Treatment, 9th edition, 66-67.
2. Warnakulasuriya KA, Samaranayake LP, Peiris JS Angular cheilitis in a group of Sri Lankan adults: a clinical and microbiologic study. J Oral Pathol Med. 1991 Apr; 20(4):172-5.

Q 6) Thermal and chemical burns and their treatment

BFU NOVEMBER 2009 (7½ Marks)

Thermal burns:

Causes:

- Very hot food and beverages, like tea and coffee, melted cheese in pizza.
- Co2 burns (snow, dry ice).
- Popsicles, icecream.
- Iatrogenic; Sudden removal of cotton roll placed in the mouth to keep the area dry.

Clinical features:

- Common sites are anterior tongue and palate.
- White lesions that can be scraped off are formed due to superficial coagulation necrosis and may leave ulcerated areas on scarring.
- Pizza burns cause whitish, grayish or ulcerated lesions on the middle third of palate.Superficial necrosis and ulceration due to hot cheese sticking to the palate.
- Dry ice, popsicles or icecream can cause burns on the tongue and lips and it can cause persistent redness, swelling, and the epithelium becomes dry and rough than the surrounding tissues.

Management:

Treatment consists of pain control, mainly by local anesthetics, systemic analgesics and topical Hydrocarbon in emollient base.

To prevent secondary infection antibiotics can be given.

Chemical burns:

- **Aspirin burns:** Common cause of burns as the patients may hold it in the mucobuccal fold for long time to relieve pain and causes tissue damage.
- Silver nitrate is used often as a chemical cautery and its use can destroy the tissues around the area where its used and may cause severe necrosis.

- Hydrogen peroxide mouth rinses are used commonly to treat periodontal lesions and in concentrations more than 3% can cause epithelial necrosis.
- Mouth washes and dentifrices can cause chemical burns in the oral cavity. The cinnamon aldehyde in dentifrices can cause allergy type reaction causing severe ulcerations and sloughing of mucosa. Caustic burns on the lips, tongue and mouth can occur in patients using mouth washes containing alcohol and chlorhexidine.
- Tooth ache drops containing creosote and guiacol can cause chemical burns.
- Sodium hypochlorite is used as an irrigant of root canal and can lead to severe burns and ulcerations.
- Acid used to etch teeth can also lead to chemical burns.
- Accidental or suicidal ingestion of certain household chemicals can lead to burns in the mouth.

Clinical features:

The typical lesions are located on the mucobuccal fold region and gingiva. The lesion is irregular in shape and whitish with pseudomembrane covering. These can be very painful. Prolonged contact with aspirin, phenol, sodium hypochlorite, paraformaldehyde can lead to severe damage and sloughing of the necrotic mucosa.

In case of brief contact it can cause superficial white, wrinkled appearing lesions without necrosis.

Treatment:

- The best treatment is prevention.
- In children aspirin and other caustic agents should be given under supervision.
- Proper use of rubber dams during endodontic and other procedures can reduce risk of iatrogenic chemical burns.
- Careful debridement of the necrotic tissue, followed by antibiotic coverage should be done.
- A protective emollient film of methyl cellulose may give relief.
- Pain control can be achieved by local anesthetics like lidocaine and diclonine hydrochloride. Protective coat of emollient paste or hydroxypropyl cellulose can give relief.
- Ingestion of caustic chemicals or accidental exposure to severely corrosive agents can cause extensive scarring that may need surgery/and /or/ prosthetic rehabilitation.

Suggested reading:

1. Burket's Oral Medicine Diagnosis And Treatment, 10th edition, 88-89.

Q 7) Describe the clinical features of stomatitis nicotina palatine

MUHS DECEMBER 2012 (3 Marks)

Stomatitis nicotina palatine or smokers palate is a condition which occurs on the hard and soft palate of persons who are heavy smokers, pipe and cigar users, and is caused due to the reaction of the palatal mucosa to chronic heat.

Clinical features:

1. **Age and sex distribution:** usually seen in men who are pipe smokers and in reverse smoking. Common in middle aged and elderly people.
2. **The condition is painless.**
3. If the person wears a denture which is proper fitting and is a chronic smoker the mucosa underneath is unaffected by this condition.
4. **Site:** As the name suggests it affects the palate. In fact these lesions are found only on the palatal mucosa. They have a whitish cobblestone appearance, usually with red dots in the centre of the cobble stones like lesions. These lesions cannot be scraped off. This lesion usually affects the posterior part of the hard palate and the adjacent soft palate.
5. **Onset:** In the initial stages there is redness and inflammation of the palate.
6. In early stages mucosa is reddened. It then changes to grayish, white, thickened and fissured.
   - Fissures and cracks could appear giving a wrinkled irregular, cracked mud like appearance.
   - In some cases there may be papular or multinodular appearance.
   - Tonsillar pillars are erythematous.
7. **Dried mud appearance**: In certain cases the palatal keratin becomes very thickened imparting fissured or dried mud appearance.
8. **Salivary gland opening:** There is distribution of red spots all over the lesion that represents opening of the minor salivary gland ducts. Discoloration is homogenous. It represents focal thickening surrounding the orifice of the salivary gland which appears as a white umbilicated nodule having a red center that may stain brown due to deposition of tar.

Suggested reading:

1. Anil Govindrao Ghom, textbook of oral medicine, 3rd edition,
2. Treister NS, Bruch JM(2010), Clinical oral medicine and pathology, New York: Humana Press, page 46.

Q 8) Erosive Lichen planus

RGUHS APRIL 2005 (4 Marks)

Erosive lichen planus: It is a type of lichen planus that affects the oral mucosa, esophagus and the anogenital systems. It is an autoimmune disorder and is more painful than the other types of lichen planus. It also has a high malignant potential.

Etiology:

- **Drug therapy:** NSAID's, hydrochlorothiazide, penicillamine. Its partial response to antifungals and antibiotics suggests that there could be an abnormal response to the local microflora especially candida albicans.
- Chronic hepatitis.
- Dental restoration.
- Graft versus host disease.
- Stress and anxiety.
- Increased levels of IL 17, interleukins and IL23 by cytokine profiling has been found.

Clinical manifestations:

- Age: average 50 years.
- Sex: female to male ratio 2:1
- Site: Buccal mucosa, lingual mucosa commonly.
- Symptoms: Burning sensation and pain.
- The lesions appear as eroded and frankly ulcerated lesions. Lacy white pattern may be present at the periphery.
- The lesions are irregular and appears as raw and painful area.
- The surface of the lesion appears granular and brightly erythematous and bleed on slight pressure.
- Due to severe pain and burning it may interfere with eating leading to weight loss, nutritional deficiencies, and may also cause depression.
- Malignant potential: 1 to 25%.
- Healing: heal in period of 10 days to weeks. Some cases may take long to heal and may become recalcitrant cases.

Diagnosis:

- Clinical diagnosis: ulcerative lesions with white lacy pattern.

Lab diagnosis: The epithelium may show saw tooth like reteridges and, liquefaction degradation of basal cell layer with juxtaepithelial inflammatory cell infiltrate.

- Immunofluorescent staining will help in diagnosis.

Differential diagnosis:

- Speckled leukoplakia.
- Lichenoid drug reaction.
- Electrogalvanic muscosal reaction.
- Psoriasis.
- Cicatricial pemphigoid.
- Erythema multiforme.
- Squamous cell carcinoma.

Management:

- Removal of cause.

- **Steroids:** Steroid spray, Steroid coating in soft custom tray, intralesional steroid injection (0.5-1.5ml) for 3 weeks.
- **Systemic steroid:** Prednisolone 5 mg tablet size can be given in doses of maximum 40-80mg/day, maximum for 5-7 days.
- **Topical application:** Flucinolone acitonide, 0.1% Triamcinolone acetonide, and 0.025% clobetasol propionate give relief.
- Combination of prednisolone and levamisol is also used.
- Topical application of antifungal agent.
- Vitamin A analog as local application.
- Cyclosporine as topical application.
- Local application of tacrolimus and pimecrolimus 0.1% as local application is used in severe cases.
- Local application of Aloe Vera gel has shown significant reduction of burning sensation in several cases.
- Dapsone, mycophenolate, efalizumab, enoxaparine are used for anti-inflammatory and immunosuppressive effects.
- Methotrexate in doses of 10-20 mg once weekly is given. To reduce the chance of adverse effects folic acid is added. This combination may be very effective in treatment of erosive lichen planus and may improve the healing process in one to three months.
- PUVA, Photodynamic and laser therapy also are being used as treatment modalities.
- **Surgery:** If solitary lesion and well defined borders.

Suggested reading:

1. Eisen D, Carrozzo M, Bagan Sebastian JV, Thongprasom K Number V Oral lichen planus: clinical features and management. Oral Dis. 2005 Nov; 11(6):338-49.
2. N Lavanya, P Jayanthi, Umadevi K Rao, and K Ranganathan Oral lichen planus: An update on pathogenesis and treatment, J Oral Maxillofac Pathol. 2011 May-Aug; 15(2): 127–132.

Q 9) Differential diagnosis of non-scrapable white patch on tongue

TNMGRU AUGUST 2010 (6 Marks)

Non scrapable white patch on tongue can be:

1) Leukoplakia:

It can be defined as a white patch that cannot be scraped or rubbed off and cannot be characterised clinically or histopathologically as any other disease.

It can involve the tongue and it can be classified as:

Homogenous: Generally a well defined white patch, which can be localised or extensive and is slightly elevated, fissured or wrinkled with a corrugated surface. When palpated they have a leathery feel and have typical cracked mud like appearance and hence can be differentiated from other white patches.

Nodular or speckled leukoplakia: It can occur as a white patch but has interspersed red component which cannot be scraped off. The typical white plus red specks help in diagnosis.

Verrucous or papillary leukoplakia: These are thick white lesions with papillary projections and the typical appearance can help in diagnosis. These are heavily keratinised and seen in older people in the 7th to 8th decades of life.

2) Lichen planus:

This is a white iesion that can be seen as white patch on tongue. It is keratotic and cannot be scraped off. These can be differentiated from other white patches as it has a typical lacy pattern that is reticular lichen planus and can be seen in annular, papular, hypertrophic type of patterns. The peculiarity of the lesions is the presence of Wickham's striae that are present at the periphery. Tiny white elevated dots at the intersection of white radiating white or grayish velvety striae also help in differentiating from other white non-scrapable white patches.

3) Hyperplastic candidiasis or candidal leukoplakia:

It is so called because of firm and adherent white patch that cannot be easily scraped off.

It occurs commonly in middle or older men and especially in chronic smokers. It is a very chronic form of candidiasis and occurs as firm leathery patch quite often involving the tongue. It cannot be scraped or rubbed off on lateral pressure. They can range from slightly white to densely white patch with cracks and fissure occasionally present and can be confused with leukoplakia. But scraping of the lesion will show candidal hyphae in large numbers and can thus be differentiated.

Lichen planus can be differentiated by the concurrent presence of skin lesions and presence of wickham's striae at the periphery of the lesion and hairy leukoplakia generally occurs on the lateral borders of the tongue and has folded appearance.

4) Oral hairy leukoplakia:

It might be the first sign of HIV infection in some patients. The virus indicated in its causation is the Epstein-Barr Virus.

This lesion most commonly involves the lateral border of the tongue but may extend to the ventral or dorsal surfaces. These lesions are usually corrugated and may have a shaggy or frayed appearance and may mimic lesions caused by tongue chewing. They cannot be scraped off.

The lesions may appear plaque like and are often bilateral.

Oral hairy leukoplakic patches usually donot cause any discomfort and have no effect on the taste of food or liquids.

In some cases, however, some times can cause mild pain and may cause alterations in taste and heightened sensitivity to food temperatures.

Clinically the mostly bilateral folded or corrugated white lesion and history of AIDS will help in diagnosis.

Histopathologically it shows the presence of homogenous viral nuclear inclusions with a residual rim of normal chromatin which is characteristic. Definitive diagnosis can be achieved by showing the presence of Epstein Barr Virus by in situ hybridisation, electron microscopy or polymerase chain reaction (PCR).

5) Pachyonichia Congenita:

Its a genetic disorder which is rare and is characterised by hypertrophy of the nails and hyperkeratosis of the skin and mucosae.

In this condition about 50% of cases have oral leukokeratosis which can be painful, white lesions which are in the form of irregular plaques which are sensitive to touch. Focal or generalised white thickening of the mucosa of the tongue could be present.

The clinical features along with the oral lesions can help in diagnosis. There is palmoplantar keratosis which can be painful and cause difficulty in walking. There is excessive sweating, sparse hair and there is thickening and brownish discoloration of nails.

6) Hereditary benign intraepithelial dyskeratosis:

Also known as Witkop-Von Sallman syndrome.

These lesions appear as white, spongy, macerated lesions with or without folds and can be seen on the ventral and lateral borders of the tongue. They vary from delicate opalscent white membranous areas to rough and shaggy lesions.

The typical macerated and spongy lesions of the oral cavity along with the eye lesions which appear as superficial, foamy, gelatinous white plaque overlying the cornea which can cause blindness can help in differentiating from other nonscrapable white patches on the tongue.

7) Dicoid lupus erythematosus:

Occurs in the 3rd or 4th decades and common in women.

Common sites are skin, oral mucosa, chest, back and extremeties.

Skin lesions are red or purple macules covered by grey or yellow adherent scales.

Oral discoid lesions are characterised clinically by the presence of white papules, central erythema, typically a border zone of irradiating white striae and peripheral telangiectasia. Buccal mucosa, lips and palate are commonly involved but may also involve the tongue.

The typical rounded lesions with peripheral radiating striae and presence of skin lesions will help in diagnosis.

8) Syphilitic leukoplakia:

It is a term used to describe a white lesion associated with syphilis especially in the tertiary stage of syphilis. It is not considered to be type of idiopathic leukoplakia as the causative agent Treponema pallidum is known. Though now-a-days it is rarely seen, when syphilis was a more common phenomenon, this patch usually was seen on the dorsal surface of tongue and had a high risk of malignant transformation.

9) Systemic lupus erythematosus:

This is a disorder that leads to multiorgan damage is an immunologically mediated inflammatory condition. The oral lesions consist of keratotic plaques, white striae or papules and tongue may be rarely involved.

10) Geographic tongue:

Geographic tongue, which is also called as erythema migrans, benign migratory glossitis is a common benign condition affecting mainly the dorsal surface of the tongue.

Though the lesions have atrophic centers the periphery has raised white borders that cannot be scraped off.

The typical circinate lesions with migratory characteristic will help in diagnosis.

Suggested reading:

1. Alexander BD, Pfaller MA. Contemporary tools for the diagnosis and management of invasive mycoses.Clin Infect Dis. 2006. 43:S15-S27.
2. Burket's, Oral Medicine Diagnosis and Treatment 10th edi., 93-118.

CHAPTER 7

Benign Tumours of Orofacial Region

Introduction:

Tumours are growth representing the tissue of origin. The study of tumours of orofacial region and adjacent structures is of importance in dentistry because a dentist plays an important role in diagnosing and treating the disease.

Characteristics of benign tumours:

- Insidious onset.
- Usually painless.
- Well defined mass.
- They are smaller and grow slowly than the malignant tumours.
- They cause displacement of adjacent structures.

Q 1) Clinical features of Sturge Weber Syndrome

MUHS MAY2005 (2 Marks)

Sturge Weber Syndrome also known as encephalo-trigeminal angiomatosis is a sporadically occurring neuro-cutaneous syndrome which is characterised by malformation of vascular tissue, with capillary venous angiomas involving the face, choroid of the eyes and leptomeninges which results in the neurological and orbital manifestations and rarely internal organ involvement.

Clinical Features:

1. Shows variable clinical course with some children experiencing mental retardation, seizures and recurrent episodes of which are like strokes.
2. Nevus flammeus that is angiomatosis of the face, with variable distribution that sometimes matches the dermatomes of one or more trigeminal nerve divisions.
3. Leptomeningeal angiomas, particularly of the parietal and occipital lobes of the brain.
4. Characteristic intracranial calcifications.
5. Contralateral hemiplegia; and one or more of the neurologic symptoms.

6. In cutaneous manifestation port wine stains are seen.
7. Leptomeningeal angiomatosis is most often on the same side as of the facial nevus.
8. Ocular features such as glaucoma, enlargement of the eye balls.
9. The oral changes in this syndrome occur in 40% of the cases and may include severe gingival enlargement, haemangiomatous lesions, labial angiomas, asymmetric jaw growth and tooth eruption sequence, due to differential blood flow to the affected area.
10) Unilateral port-wine nevus involving the upper eyelid and the forehead region which is supplied by the first branch of trigeminal nerve and varies in colour from pink to red to purple in colour.
11) Maxillary midline diastema, maxillary anterior teeth spacing and proclination and increased overjet between maxillary and mandibular anterior teeth are some of the inter-arch discrepancies observed in the patient which could possibly have contributed to the macroglossia.

The diagnosis of Sturge Weber Syndrome is usually made when an infant or child with port wine stains develops neurological complications, and the magnetic resonance imaging of the brain with contrast studies demonstrate the presence of leptomeningeal angiomatosis and accompanying cortical abnormalities.

Laser treatments have become the standard modality of care for port wine stains and should be done early to prevent thickening and nodularity of skin.

Suggested reading:

1. Chaudhary SC, Sonkar SK, Kumar V, Golchha S, Sturge Weber syndrome: J Assoc Physicians India. 2011 May; 59:327-9.

Q 2) Hemangioma

TNMGRU FEBRUARY 2013 (5 Marks)

Hemangioma, tumour like malformations is composed of disorganised endothelial lined vessel masses which are filled with blood and are connected to the main blood vascular system.

They are present all over in and around the oral cavity and face and facial bones, salivary glands, temporomandibular joints, and also on the mucosa and skin surface.

They can occur as:

- Single or isolated lesions in the oral cavity.
- Multiple lesions that can affect different parts of the body.
- May also occur in association with other developmental anomalies as part of various angiomatous syndromes.

Classification:

- Capillary hemangioma.
- Cavernous hemangioma.

- Angioblastic or hypertrophic hemangioma.
- Racemose type.
- Diffuse systemic hemangioma.
- Metastasising hemangioma.
- Nevus vinosus or portwine stain.
- Hereditary hemorrhagic telangiectasis.

Clinical features:

- May occur as simple flat red patches(port wine stain), or birth marks that do not raise above the surface on the mucosa or skin.
- May become large fungating masses, which may bury the teeth and cause severe deformity and disfigurement.
- Small lesions may look like pyogenic granuloma and venous varicosities.
- Most commonly there are two types: Capillary and cavernous type.
- The cavernous type consists of relatively large blood filled lakes.
- Capillary type contains masses of proliferating vessels of capillary dimension.
- Both the types have a simple endothelial lining of the vascular channels and very little connective tissue stroma.
- The lesions bleed profusely when traumatised.
- Many hemangiomas are evident at birth and may increase in size along with the general body growth.
- Large lesions may be warm and even pulsatile.
- Hemangiomas may occur centrally within the bone also.

Oral manifestations:

- Occur in infants, children, and more common in females.
- Hemangiomas of oral soft tissues appear as flat or raised lesions of mucosa and are deep red or bluish red and rarely well circumscribed.
- They are readily compressible and fills very slowly when it is released. The more common sites are the tongue, lips, buccal mucosa and the palate.
- Central hemangiomas of maxilla and mandible occur occasionally. Central hemangiomas appear as honeycomb, spokes of a wheel or sunburst appearance.

Diagnosis:

(i) **Diascopy:** It shows blanching on pressure. This procedure is done by pressing gently on the lesion with a glass slide or glass test tube. Blanching of the lesion indicates positive result indicating that the blood is within the vascular spaces and is displaced out of the lesion by pressure.

(ii) **For bony lesions:** Computed tomography, Doppler and conventional ultrasound, scintigraphic scanning, super selective microangiography are used to define the extent of the lesion.

These tests will reveal bony defects as well as the presence of phleboliths in the cheek and salivary glands that mark the location of abnormal vessels.

Differential diagnosis:

- **Mucocele, ranula, superficial cysts:** Hemangioma will blanch on pressure where as the other lesions are soft fluctuant and non-emptiable.
- **Varicosity:** These are elongated enlargement of superficial vein rather than flat, nodular or dome shaped lesions.
- **Arteriovenous shunt or aneurysm:** In these cases pulse will be detected, which will not be so in hemangioma. Arteriovenous shunt and aneurysm will occur as dome shaped, rubbery, non-fluctuant lesions and throbbing will be obvious.

Management:

Treatment of hemangiomas can be very difficult and there is danger of severe, uncontrollable hemorrhage.

Conventional techniques of surgery are replaced by cryosurgery and laser often preceded by the injection of sclerosing agents.

Intravascular embolisation with plastic spheres is also used successfully.

Intralesional injections of corticosteroids are used to treat some cases in infants.

Radiation can be used to sclerose these lesions but there is danger of inducing neoplastic and other degenerative changes in the future and hence is contraindicated, especially in children.

Suggested reading:

1. Burket's Oral Medicine Diagnosis And Treatment, 9th edition, 145-147.

Q 3) Pyogenic Granuloma

BFU MAY 2008 (5 Marks)

It is a reactive hyperplastic lesion of connective tissue that occurs in response to local irritants. A tumour like growth of the oral cavity, which is frequently located surrounding the anterior teeth.

The pyogenic granuloma does not contain pus and is actually not a granuloma, hence the term is misnomer.

Poncet and Dor, two french surgeons described it in 1897.

It is thought to be a capillary hemangioma of the lobular type by some and hence very often quite prone to bleeding.

Etiology:

(i) **Microorganisms:** Botryomycotic infection, staphylococci and streptococci.

(ii) May occur due to trauma which creates a pathway for entry of microorganisms.

(iii) Low grade irritation and traumatic injury could be the stimuli.

(iv) **Hormonal imbalance:** Contributing factor in some cases of pyogenic granuloma. It is believed that female sex hormones may play important role.

(v) Certain drugs are implicated in its pathogenesis.

Clinical Features:

(i) Females are more commonly affected than males and occurs between 11-40 years of age.

(ii) Commonly occurs on gingiva. alveolar mucosa, vestibules, lips and tongue, buccal mucosa.

(iii) Its a asymptomatic papular, nodular or polypoid mass.

(iv) Lesions can be either pedunculated or sessile and smooth lobulated or warty surface.

(v) Surface is vulnerable to ulceration, bleeding, on slightest trauma or pressure.

(vi) Colour is red to purple depending on vascularity, and is soft in consistency, though it could some times be fibrous and pink in colour.

Size may range from few milimeters to centimeters and average size is 1.5 cms.It may grow rapidly and then the size may remain constant for a long time.

Diagnosis:

Clinical diagnosis is on the basis of reddish, purple colour, and soft consistency, which bleeds quite easily.

Biopsy shows granulation tissue which is exuberant and usually localised. Overlying epithelium may be thin and atrophic. Though it could be hyperplastic.

Differential diagnosis:

(i) **Small benign and malignant mesenchymal tumors:** These are less common than pyogenic granulomas.

(ii) **Capillary hemangioma:** These blanch on pressure but the pyogenic granulomas donot.

(iii) **Peripheral giant cell granuloma:** The lesions are more bluish in colour. It also causes radiological changes like superficial cuffing of alveolar bone.

(iv) **Peripheral fibroma with calcifications:** In some peripheral fibromas the radiographs will show foci of calcification as radiopacities.

Management:

(i) **Surgical excision:** It is a treatment of choice and it is important to remove the calculus of adjacent teeth so that the chances of recurrence are minimised.

(ii) As it is a benign growth, it is treated with excisional therapy which is the treatment of choice although some alternative therapies like cryosurgery, excision, by Nd YAG laser, flash lamp pulsed dye laser, injection of corticosteroid or ethanol, and sodium tetradecyl sulfate sclerotherapy are thought to be effective.

(ii) Elimination of causative agent is important.

Suggested reading:

1. Bhaskar SN, Jacoway JR Pyogenic granuloma--clinical features, incidence,

histology, and result of treatment: report of 242 cases. J Oral Surg. 1966 Sep; 24(5): 391-8.
2. Pushpendra Kumar Verma, Ruchi Srivastava, HC Baranwal, TP Chaturvedi, Anju Gautam, and Amit Singh, "Pyogenic Granuloma - Hyperplastic Lesion of the Gingiva: Case Reports" Open Dent J. 2012; 6: 153–156.

Q 4) Peripheral giant cell granuloma

BFU MAY 2007 (5 Marks)

Also known as peripheral giant cell reparative granuloma.It occurs much more commonly than the central type.

It seems to originate from either periodontal ligament or mucoperiosteum.

It is the most common giant cell lesion of the oral cavity which appears as a soft tissue, extraosseous, purplish red nodule which consists of multinucleated giant cells against a background of mononuclear stromal cells and extravasated red blood cells.

It is not present as a true neoplasm but as a reactive lesion. Though the exact cause is not known, it is thought to be due to local irritation or trauma.

It has a close resemblance microscopically to central giant cell granuloma, and according to some pathologists it represents the soft tissue counterpart of the central bony lesion.

Etiology:

- It is an unusual response to injury. The trauma could be caused due to tooth extraction or dental irritation.
- Chronic oral infections can lead to this condition.
- It can also occur due to primary or secondary hyperparathyroidism.

Clinical Features:

- Occurs above 20 years of age, with average age of 45 years. Females more commonly affected and more common in whites.
- Mandible is more commonly affected and in the anterior region to molars.
- It appears commonly as a soft tissue extraosseous reddish purple or bluish purple lump with smooth and shiny or papillomatous surface. It is a well defined exophytic lesion.
- It may be pedunculated or sessile and may not show ulceration.
- In the early stages appears as discolouration and slight swelling of the buccal gingiva. In the later stages it may increase in size, become rounded and pedunculated.
- It may develop an hour glass shape with the centre between two teeth and the extreme ends projecting buccally and lingually.
- May be red or bluish in colour. The more fibrous lesions are pale in colour.
- Consistency may be soft to hard.
- The lesions may vary from 0.5-1.5 cms in size.
- It is generally vascular and hemorrhagic and ulceration may be present. It could be tender on palpation.

- In edentulous patients it may appear as ovoid or fusiform vascular region on the crest of the ridge and may be 1-2 cms in diameter. A granular mass may occur on the ridge.

Histopathologic features:

It consists of nodules of multinucleated giant cells against a background of plump ovoid and spindle shaped mesenchymal cells, and extravasated red blood cells. The giant cells may contain only a few nuclei or several dozens of them. Some are large vesicular nuclei and some have pyknotic nuclei.

Radiological features:

- In edentulous areas there is erosion of the bone with peripheral cupping of the bone.
- In dentulous areas there could be superficial resorption of the alveolar margins or crest of the interdental bone.

Diagnosis:

Clinically red coloured lesion on the gingiva, soft to hard in consistency often having hourglass shape can help in clinically diagnosing this condition.

Laboratory diagnosis may reveal multinucleated giant cells and young connective tissue spindle shaped cells are scattered through out the granulation tissue in delicate reticular and fibrillar connective tissue stroma.

Differential diagnosis:

- The differential diagnosis of this lesion includes central giant cell lesion, pyogenic granuloma, peripheral ossifying fibroma, fibrous hyperplasia, irritation fibroma, hemangioma, lymphangioma, and amelanotic melanoma which all may have similar clinical and histopathologic features.
- Hemangioma: Present at birth and seldom occurs on the gingiva.
- Lymphangioma: It is rare on the gingiva and the colour is the same as the tissue.
- Metastatic carcinoma: There will be presence of primary tumour.
- Oral nevi and nodular melanoma: will be darker in colour.

Management:

- Excision with borders of normal tissue with the entire base of the lesion is done to avoid recurrence.
- Elimination of chronic irritation.

Suggested reading:

1. Padam Narayan Tandon, S.K Gupta, D.S Gupta, S.K. Jurel, Abhishek Saraswat, Periheral Giant Cell Granuloma: Contemporary clinical dentistry, April 2012, vol 3, supplement 1, 118-120.
2. Rodrigo Gadelha Vasconcelos1; Marcelo Gadelha Vasconcelos2; Lélia Maria Guedes Queiroz, Peripheral and central giant cell lesions: etiology, origin of giant cells, diagnosis and treatment, J Bras Patol Med Lab, v. 49, n. 6, p. 446-452, December 2013.

Q 5) Fibroma

TNMGRU FERUARY 2005 (5 Marks)

Fibromas are benign tumors that are composed of fibrous connective tissue.They can occur in all organs which arise from mesenchymal tissue.

It is a benign soft tissue tumor found in the oral cavity.

It is also referred to as a traumatic fibroma, focal fibrous hyperplasia, oral polyp or fibrous nodule.

While the term fibroma indicates that it is a benign lesion, most of them represent reactive focal fibrous hyperplasia due to trauma or local irritation.

Etiology:

Chronic irritation like cheek or lip biting, rubbing of mucosa against a rough tooth or dentures and other oral prosthesis.

Clinical manifestations:

Common in 3rd or 4th decades, it can occur at any age and has no sex perdilection.

Although any oral site may be involved it is commonly observed most often on the buccal mucosa along the plane of occlusion of the maxillary and mandibular teeth, gingiva, tongue and palate.

In case it develops under a denture it will be flat with the shape of a leaf.

It is a round or ovoid or dome shaped, asymptomatic, with a smooth surface and sessile or pedunculated mass. Lesions on lips and tongue present as circumscribed nodules.

It may vary in size of about 1-2 cms. The surface of the lesion is of similar colour of the surrounding mucosa but could be hyperkeratotic or ulcerated due to repeated trauma.

It is usually a solitary lesion.In case there are several lesions present, diagnosis to be considered are tuberous sclerosis, cowden syndrome, familial fibromatosis and fibrotic papillary hyperplasia of the palate. They donot develop into oral cancer.

They are usually painless, but if frequently traumatized can become inflamed and painful and cause discomfort.

Consistency ranges from soft and myxomatous to firm and elastic. According to consistency the tumor is termed as hard fibroma and soft fibroma.

Histological features:

Histopathologically, a fibroma shows encapsulation, and solid, nodular mass of dense and sometimes, hyalinised fibrous connective tissue, which is often arranged in haphazard fascicles. A mild chronic inflammatory infiltration may be present. The surface of the lesion could be hyperkeratotic, hyperplastic, or atrophic and ulcerated.

Differential diagnosis:

Neurofibroma, giant cell fibroma, peripheral giant cell granuloma, schwannoma, mucocele, benign and malignant salivary gland tumours.

Management:

Various treatment modalities are used for treatment of fibromas like surgical excision with scalpel, ablation with carbon dioxide (CO2) and erbium-doped yttrium aluminum garnet (Er:YAG) lasers, and cryosurgery.

Surgical excision is the most common modality used and it is combined with removal of local causes of irritation so as to prevent recurrence.

The Light Scalpel 10.6 μm CO2 dental surgical laser with light scalpel angled tipless handpiece which is an invaluable tool for the dentist especially for treatment of fibromas which has been found to be very comfortable and less painless than surgical excision with very good healing.

Suggested reading

1. Barker DS, Lucas RB. Localised fibrous overgrowths of the oral mucosa. Br J Oral Surg. 1967 Nov. 5(2):86-92.
2. De Santana Santos T, Martins-Filho PR, Piva MR, de Souza Andrade ES. Focal fibrous hyperplasia: A review of 193 cases. J Oral Maxillofac Pathol. 2014 Sep. 8 (Suppl 1).

Q 6) Papilloma

TNMGRU FEBRUARY 2009 (6 Marks)

A papilloma is benign epithelial tumour which grows exophytically in often finger-like projections.

The oral squamous papilloma is a benign proliferation of the stratified squamous epithelium that results in a papillary or verrucous exophytic mass.

Oral squamous papillomas are proliferative epithelial lesions generally considered to be caused due to HPV of sub types 6 and 11 being commonly implicated.

Isolated reports of an association with subtypes 2 and 16 have not been confirmed.

Classification:

- Squamous cell papilloma: Which may arise in the tongue, cheeks, lips and esophagus.
  - Can be congenital and may be present since birth.
  - Infective types can occur due to viruses.
  - A soft variety of papilloma can be seen on the eyelids of elderly.
  - Keratin horns that are formed due to excessive keratin formation can be seen in older people.
- Basal cell papilloma:
  - Also known as seborrhoeic or senile wart and occurs on trunk, face and armpits.

Clinical features:

- Squamous papillomas usually occur in the third to the fifth decades, most commonly as isolated palatal lesions. Other areas involved are, lips, and labial commisures.

- When they occur on lips they do pose an esthetic problem and can be removed by laser.
- More common in females and in the 4th and 5th decades.
- Very few cases, about 20% occur below 20 years of age.
- Rounded shape followed by cauliflower shape is common.
- Lesions are whitish in colour and often pedunculated. Colour may also be grayish pink.
- When these lesions occur on the keratinized surface of the lips, alveolar gingivae, or palate, they are well keratinized and wart like, often with a narrow pedicle.
- On the nonkeratinized mucosal surface, they may appear soft and redder and may be hard to differentiate from the lesions of fibrous hyperplasia described earlier.
- Size is generally from 2mm to few centimetres but most commonly less than 2cms.
- Although these lesions are probably infectious, a history of direct contact with another infected person is unusual.
- It is firm in consistency when keratinised and softer when less keratinised.
- Papillomas can be associated with certain syndromes like the focal dermal hyperplasia syndrome where in there are multiple oral papillomas, dermal hyperplasia and syndactyly, fatty herniation, coloboma and strabismus.
- Other syndromes with multiple papillomas are Cowden's and Down's syndrome.

Diagnosis:

- **Clinical:** Typical cauliflower like growth with finger like projections and usually pedunculated, in the oral cavity can help in easy clinical diagnosis.
- **Histopathology:** The typical appearance for oral squamous papilloma is squamous epithelium arranged in finger like projections, normal maturation patterns, and the presence of hyperparakeratosis of the epithelium, koilocytosis due to perinuclear cytoplasmic vacuolisation of cells of the spinous layer of the epithelium, which produces perinuclear pale halos, and pyknosis and the presence of basilar hyperplasia.

Differential diagnosis:

- Intraoral verruca vulgaris: Commonly occurs on skin and has a sessile base.
- Papillary squamous cell carcinoma: It is rapidly growing and more than a centimetre in size with a sessile base.
- Verrucous carcinoma: Generally occurs in the 6th -7th decades and is associated with habits of tobacco chewing and snuff dipping. These are bigger lesions and the base is as wide as the lesion. The finger like projections are lesser than the papilloma.

- Condyloma acuminata: They are less common and history of oral sex will be positive.
- Pseudoepitheliomatous hyperplasia: Lesions have a sessile base.
- Verruciform xanthoma: It is rare in the oral cavity and has a sessile base and vertical projections as in papilloma are absent.

Management:

- **Surgical excision:** Common modality of treating papilloma. The incision is given at the base of mucosa where the pedicle is inserted. If properly excised, recurrence is rare. Surgical removal using laser, cryotherapy or cautery is also done.
- **Other modalities:**
  - Salicylic acid: It is often first line of therapy chosen by patients as it is available over the counter. It is a keratolytic therapy.
  - Chemical cautery: Silver nitrate is most commonly used.
  - Occlusal duct tape therapy was introduced by Dr. Jeremy Litt in 1978.
  - Components of garlic have been shown to possess antiviral activity and also to inhibit cellular proliferation of virally infected cells.

Suggested reading:

1. Burket's, Oral Medicine Diagnosis and Treatment 10th edi., 166.
2. Michelle M. Lipke, An Armamentarium of Wart Treatments, Clin Med Res. 2006 Dec; 4(4): 273–293.
3. Thallasa E, Carneiro, Sandra A. Marinho, Flaviana D. Verli, Ana T.M. Mesquita, Nadia L. Lima and Joao L. Miranda, Oral squamous papilloma: clinical, histologic and immunohistochemical analyses, Journal oral science, Vol.51, No.3, 367-372, 2009.

Q 7) Ossifying Fibroma:

TNMGRU APRIL 1998 (5 Marks)

It is a benign, slow growing, well circumscribed tumour of the bone. It is often included in the classification of a benign fibro-osseous lesion.

They probably arise from cells of the periodontal ligament.

Clinical features:

- It is benign tumour which is relatively rare and affects the mandible and maxilla.
- Usually occurs as a single lesion but multiple lesions have also been reported.
- Occurs commonly in the third to fourth decades of age.
- Females are affected more than males.
- Mandible is affected more than the maxilla.
- In more than 50% of cases the posterior part of the mandible is involved.
- In OF, swelling is the most common clinical sign seen in the affected region.

- As they are usually painless they are ultimately identified when routine radiographs are taken.
- Some cases of OF may cause displacement of tooth and resorption of roots in adjacent teeth.
- A variant of ossifying fibroma is termed as juvenile OF and appears in younger individuals.
  - This tumour exhibits more aggressive behavior and a greater propensity for recurrence.

Histopathological features:

- Microscopically, OF consists of cellular fibrous connective tissue which shows mineralised material, and osteoblastic rimming is usually observed on the surface of that mineralised material.
- Consists of varying amounts of osteoid and bone.
- The other histological variants of OF are the juvenile trabecular OF(JTOF) and juvenile psammomatoid OF (JPOF).
- The JTOF and JPOF involve most commonly the maxilla and bony walls of the paranasal sinuses respectively in contrast to the conventional OF. The JTOF and JPOF show predilection for occurence in the second decade of life and the JTOFs tend to have aggressive and rapid growth pattern.

Radiographic Findings:

- The radiographic appearance depends on the amount of mineralised tissue within the tumour. They usually appear as unilocular, well defined or circumscribed lesions and may show variable amount of radiopaque foci within the lesion.
- It typically shows mixed radiopaque/radiolucent appearance.
- When the mandible is involved, in large number of cases there is buccolingual expansion and in several cases there is downward displacement of lower border of mandible.
- When maxilla is involved most of the case can be seen involving the maxillary antrum.
- The lesions may be completely evaluated with computerised tomography.
- Several image examinations like panoramic radiography, cone beam computerised tomography and CT scans are important to correctly assess the diagnosis of the intraosseous lesions.

Differential diagnosis:

- The most important lesion in the D/D of this lesion includes fibrous dysplasia which appears as a diffuse, homogenous ground glass, radio-dense region where as the OF appears as a well demarcated mixed radiolucent/radiopaque appearance.
- The other lesion to be considered in D/D of OF is the focal osseous dysplasia(FOD)in its early, intermediate and late stages. FOD affects

patients in the 4th -5th decades of life and usually has a ill defined radiographic borders. More over the FOD lesions are smaller than the OF and frequently affect the periapical region.

- When OF appears as a radiolucent lesion, lesions like ameloblastoma, odontogenic cysts, central giant cell lesions, chronic apical periodontitis and idiopathic bone cavity should be considered in the differential diagnosis.
- In the mixed lesions of OF calcifying epithelial odontogenic cysts, calcifying epithelial odontogenic tumour, osteoblastoma, should be considered in the DD.
- In cases of radiopaque OF, idiopathic osteosclerosis and complex odontoma should be considered in the DD.
- It may resemble a cementoblastoma in case it is placed around the root of a tooth, but cementoblastoma is fused with the root and OF is not.
- Osteosarcomas should be considered in the DD in case of large OFs since they affect the jaws of patients in almost the same age range as that of the OFs.

Management:

The most usual way of treating the OFs is the complete removal by excision or curettage.

Conservative surgical excision of the OFs seems to be a secure, satisfactory and versatile mode of treatment.

In case of larger lesions, in order to minimise or avoid the chances of recurrence, a partial or enbloc resection of the jaw is preferred.

After treatment the patients should be followed up carefully because though the recurrence rates of OFs is very low, this tumour has sometimes displayed aggressiveness and a tendency to recur after conservative surgical excision.

Suggested reading:

1. Burket's, Oral Medicine Diagnosis and Treatment, 11th edition, 143-144.
2. MacDonald-Jankowski DS, Ossifying fibroma: a systematic review, Dentomaxillofac Radiol. 2009 Dec; 38(8): 495-513.
3. Márcia de Andrade, Yara Teresinha Corrêa Silva-Sousa, Maria Fernanda Teiga Marques, Maria Luiza dos Anjos Pontual, Flávia Maria de Moraes Ramos-Perez, Danyel Elias da Cruz Perez, Ossifying Fibroma of the Jaws: A Clinicopathological Case Series Study, Braz. Dent. J. vol.24 no.6 Ribeirão Preto Nov./Dec. 2013.

CHAPTER 8

Oral Cancer

Q 1) Types of Radiotherapy

TNMGRU AUGUST 2012 (5 Marks)

Accurately targeted x-rays to destroy the cancer cells is called Radiotherapy. It utilises high energy x-rays, gamma rays and electrons to deliver ionizing radiation to patients with malignant diseases.

The principal treatment for primary tumors remains surgery and radiotherapy. The basic decision to be made is between radical radiotherapy and elective surgery. If the former is chosen salvage surgery should be done. If surgery is chosen, radiotherapy may be used in an adjuvant manner, either pre or post operatively.

Types of Radiotherapy:

1. External Beam Therapy – Using machine such as linear accelerator, cobalt machine.
2. Brachytherapy – Using a localized radioisotope implant.
3. Internal or systemic irradiation: (Radionuclide therapy) : Using a systemic radioisotope preparation.

1) Teletherapy/External beam radiation:

Teletherapy is the most commonly used modality accounting for 90% of radiation therapy & in this modality, there is delivery of electromagnetic radiation(eg. x-rays, gamma rays) or particulate radiation (eg.protons, electrons) from a linear accelerator or radionucleide source, such as 60cobalt kept at a distance away from the patient. It is of two types depending on energy of rays, which are used for this purpose.

Kilovoltage Therapy:

(i) Superficial X-rays (50-150 kV)
(ii) Orthovoltage X-rays (150-300 kV).

Megavoltage Therapy:

(i) Cobalt gamma rays (1.17-1.33 mV)
(ii) Linear accelerators (4-25 mV) (1 mV = 1000 kV).

2. Brachytherapy:

(a) The term brachytherapy was first proposed by Dr G Forsell in 1931. The prefix 'brachy' simply mean a short range delivery of radiation.

(b) The National Council on Radiation Protection (1972) defined the term brachytherapy as a method of radiation therapy in which an encapsulated source or a group of such sources is utilized to deliver gamma or beta radiation at a distance of up to a few centimeters, either by surface, intracavitary or interstitial application.

(c) Sources suitable for brachytherapy use consist of small amounts of radionuclide which are totally encapsulated by a non toxic and inert material, such as stainless steel or platinum.

(d) The radioactive sources come in the form of small needles, wires, rods or spheres. The commonly used isotopes are Radium226, Cesium137, Iridium192 and Iodine.125 Generally a dose of 65 Gray over 6-7 days is given when it is used as the sole treatment.

Types of Brachytherapy:

(a) Interstitial Brachytherapy: In this, radioactive sources are inserted into the tumor via surgical intervention. For example, in carcinoma of tongue and buccal mucosa.

(b) Mold Therapy: The radiation source is placed into a plastic mold on the patient's skin or mucous membrane. The radiation dose from a mold falls off rapidly and is therefore ideal for treating superficial tumors. For example, carcinoma of hard palate and skin cancer.

(c) Intracavitary Brachytherapy: Radioactive isotopes are kept inside a body cavity. For example, carcinoma of nasopharynx and cervix, oesophageal and lung tumors.

Advantages

(i) A high dose of radiation can be delivered directly to the tumor sparing surrounding normal tissue.

(ii) Treatment time is short.

Disadvantages

(i) It can be used only in selected cases especially in the early stage of disease at accessible sites.

(ii) It requires anesthesia and excel.

3) Internal Or Systemic Irradiation:

Radioisotope is either administered intravenously or parenterally. Commonly used isotopes are Iodine-131, Phosphorous-32, Yittrium-90.

Other types of radiotherapy:

(a) Radiotherapy to different parts of the treatment area with different doses of radiotherapy can be given by Intensity modulated radiation therapy (IMRT) which actually shapes the radiotherapy beam making it possible. Hence the treatment of cancers that are close to the important organs and structures can be done very precisely and with minimum damage to other structures.

(b) Images taken using an x-ray or CT scan machine, to show the shape, size and location of the tumour just before treatment is the principle behind Image Guided Radiotherapy(IGRT).

Suggested reading:

1. Vikrant Kasat, Sunil Sahuji, Manjiri Joshi . Radiotherapy: An Update. JIAOMR 2010; 22(4):S26-30.

Q 2) Staging of oral cancer:

TNMGRU FEBRUARY 2011 6 Marks

Staging of oral cancer is the extent of spread of tumor within patients.

Assessment:

It is assessed by following ways:

- Clinical examination: staging can be assessed clinically by the size and extent of primary lesion.
- Investigations: investigations like radiology, sonography can lead to staging of disease.
- Pathological examination: this is very important part while staging of neoplastic process is done. Mainly biopsy, cytology are used.
- Infiltration: Degrees of infiltration of primary lesion should be carried out.
- Metastasis: it includes presence or absence of metastasis to regional lymphnodes, presence or absence of distant metastasis, involvement of contralateral or ipsilateral node and whether nodes are fixed or not.

Objectives:

- Treatment planning: it aids the clinician in the planning of treatment.
- Prognosis: to give some indication of prognosis.
- Evaluation of treatment: to assist in evaluation of the result of treatment.
- Exchange of information so as to make easy the exchange of information between treatment centers.
- Investigations: to contribute to the continuing investigations of human cancer.

1) TNM staging:

TNM tumour-node-metastasis staging system was first reported by Pierre Denoix in the 1940s. it is universally accepted system which is developed by UICC (union international centre of cancer).

(a) Primary tumor (T): local extent is major factor contributing to prognosis

Tx-Inability to assess the primary tumour.

To-There is no evidence of primary tumour.

Tis-Carcinoma-in-situ.

T1-Tumour that is 2cms or less in diameter.

T2 - Tumor 2cm to 4cm in diameter.

T3 - Tumor more than 4cm in greatest diameter.

T4a-(lip) Tumour which invades through the cortical bone, inferior alveolar nerve, floor of the mouth, skin of the face.

T4a (Oral cavity) -Tumour which invades through the cortical bone, into deep extrinsic muscles of the tongue, maxillary sinus , or skin of the face.

T4b-(lip and oral cavity)- Tumour invades the masticator space, pterygoid plates or skull base or encases the internal carotid artery.

(b) N-Regional lymph nodes.

NX-Regional lymph nodes cannot be assessed.

NO-There is no evidence of regional lymph node metastasis.

N1-There is presence of metastasis in a single ipsilateral lymph node that is 3 cms or less in greatest dimension.

N2-There is metastasis in a single ipsilateral lymph node which is 3cms but not more than 6 cms in the greatest dimension, or in multiple ipsilateral lymph nodes more than 6 cms in greatest dimension, or in bilateral or contralateral lymph nodes, none more than 6 cms in greatest dimension.

N2a-There is metastasis in single ipsilateral lymph node more than 3 cms but not more than 6 cms.

N2b-There is metastasis in multiple ipsilateral lymph nodes but not more than 6 cms.

N2c-There is metastasis in bilateral or contralateral lymph nodes more than 6 cms.

N3c-There is metastasis in a lymph node more than 6 cms in the greatest dimension.

c) M-Distant metastasis:

MX-The distant metastasis cannot be assessed.

MO-No distant metastasis.

M1-There is distant metastasis.

Stage Grouping:

Stage 0: Tis N0 M0

Stage 1: T1 N0 M0

Stage II: T2 N0 M0

Stage III: T1, T2 N1 M0

T3 N0, N1 M0

Stage IVA: T1, T2, T3 N2 M0

T4a N0, N1, N2 M0

Stage4B: Any T N3 M0

T4b Any N M0

Stage3C: AnyT Any N M1

2) AJC (American Joint Committee) Staging:

It divides all cancers into stage 0 to 4 and takes into account all three previous TNM systems.

Stage 0: T0 N0 M0.

Stage 1: T1 N0 M0.

Stage 2: T2 N0 M0.

Stage 3:T3 N0 M0, T1N1M0, T2N1M0 and T3N1M0

Stage4 A: T4 N0 M0, T4 N1 M0, any T3 N1 M0

Stage 4 B: Any T N3 M0

Stage4C: Any T, Any N, M1.

Suggested reading:

1. Anil Govindrao Ghom, Textbook of oral Medicine, Neoplasm, 3rd ed., pg 12-13.
2. Sobin LH, Wittekind Ch. TNM classification of malignant tumors. 6th ed. New York: Wiley & Sons; 2002.

Q 3) Tumour markers

TNMGRU FEBRUARY 2005 (5 Marks)

Tumor Markers are biochemical substances that are synthesised or released by the tumourous cells either because of the cause or effect of malignancy. They may be normal endogenous products that are produced at a higher rate in cancer cells or can be the products of genes which are switched on newly and which remain dormant in the normal cells. When the tumour markers are produced by the tumour especially in significant quantities, suggests the presence of cancer.

They can be broadly classified as:

1. Oncofetal antigens, pancreatic oncofetal antigen.carcinoembryonic antigen, fetal sulfoglycoprotein.
2. Tumour associated antigens eg.CA125, CA19-9, CA15-3, CA72-4, CA50.
3. Hormones eg. calcitonin, beta human chorionic gonadotropin, placental lactogen etc.
4. Hormone receptors like estrogen and progesterone receptors.
5. Enzymes and isozymes like prostatic acid phosphtase, placental alkaline phosphatase, lysozyme, alpha amylase etc.
6. Serum and tissue proteins like, beta-2 microglobulin, protein s -100, fibrinogen degradation products.
7. Other biomolecules like polyamines.

The qualitative and quantative evaluation of these markers is possible due to modern techniques of sensitive immune assays, ELISA and RIA.

Ideal tumour markers should possess the following qualities:

(i) Must be highly sensitive with low false negative results.
(ii) Should be highly specific with low false positive results.
(iii) Should have high positive and negative values of prediction.
(iv) They should have 100% accuracy in bringing out the difference between healthy individuals and cancer patients.
(v) It should be able to differentiate between neoplastic and non-neoplastic disease and should be capable of showing positive co-relation with the tumour volume and extent.
(vi) It should have good prognostic value and be able to predict early recurrence.

(vii) Should be sensitive enough to be detectable at early stage of cancer.

(viii) Its levels should precede the neoplastic process and should be useful for early cancer screening.

(ix) It should be either a universal marker for all types of malignancies or should be specific to one type of malignancy.

(x) Assays should be possible and it should be able to indicate the changes occurring in cancer patients who are receiving treatment.

Tumour markers in oral cancer:

The classification of tumour markers for oral cancer:

(i) **Tumour growth markers:** Epithelial growth factor, Cyclins (cyclin A, B1, D1, E)They are essential in the control of cell cycle. Nuclear cell proliferation antigens which are nuclear proteins associated with DNA-polymerase Ki-67/MIB, AgNORs (, silver binding nucleolar organiser regions) proteins, Skp2, Bcl2/BAG1, HSP27 and 70 heat shock proteins, which happen to be associated with the mutations of p53 gene.

(ii) **Markers of anti-tumour response and tumour suppression:** The retinoblastoma protein, the dysregulation of which gives rise to abberations in various proteins of cells such as CD1 and CDK4, cyclin dependant kinase inhibitors, p53 genes, Bax, Fas/FasL, Dendritic cells (DC), Zeta chains.

(iii) **Angiogenesis Markers:** Vascular endothelial growth factor/ receptor (VEGF/VEGF-R), Nitric oxide synthase type II(NOS2) Platelet derived endothelial cell growth factor(PD-ECGF), FGFs (fibroblast growth factor).

(iv) **Markers of metastatic potential and tumour invasion:** Matrix-metallo proteases(Mmps), Cathepsins, Cadherins and catenins, Desmoplakin/placoglobin.

(v) **Cell Surface Markers:** Cytokeratins are epithelial cell proteins and there are 19 cytokeratins which are divided into two sub-families. The expression of CK 19 in the suprabasal cell layer of the oral mucosa can be used as a diagnostic marker of oral pre-cancerous lesions.

(vi) **Markers of Anomalous Keratinisation:** Filagrins, Involucrin, Desmosomal proteins, Intercellular substance antigen, Nuclear analysis.

(vii) **Arachidonic Acid Products.**

(viii) **Enzymes:** Glutathione S-transferase (GSTS) is an isoenzyme which acts in the second phase of cell metabolism. It can be used as a tumour marker of premalignant oral epithelial lesions.

Suggested reading:

1. Chimenos-Küstner E, Font-Costa I, López-López J, Oral cancer risk and molecular markers, Med Oral Patol Oral Cir Bucal 2004;9:377-84.
2. T. Malati Review Article Tumour Markers: An Overview Indian Journal of Clinical Biochemistry, 2007 / 22 (2) 17-31

Chapter 9

Malignant Tumours of the Orofacial Region

Q 1) Verrucous carcinoma:

RGUHS OCTOBER 2002 (5 Marks)

It is a slow growing, low grade malignancy of epithelial origin. Also called as snuff dipper's cancer or Ackerman's tumour. It was reported by Ackerman in 1948.

This tumour has been designated by several names like Ackerman's tumour, Buschke lowenstein tumour, epithelioma cuniculatum etc.

It is an uncommon variant of squamous cell carcinoma . Its a form of well differentiated squamous cell carcinoma and has specific clinical and histologic features.

It may occur in various head and neck regions and also in the genitalia.

Oral cavity is a very common site for occurrence of this tumour.

Etiology:

- Tobacco is the most important etiological factor. It occurs in individuals who have the habit of keeping the tobacco quid in the oral cavity, either in the buccal or labial vestibule.
- Betelnut chewing could be a major risk factor in causing verrucous carcinoma.
- Smoking, alcohol consumption and betel nut chewing may also cause this condition.
- Cigarette smoking seems to be the most important causative agent from among those mentioned above according to some studies:
- Alcohol consumption alone or in combination with tobacco increases the risk of this lesion.
- Human Papilloma Virus has been quoted as one of the reasons.
- Oral lichenoid reactions, leukoplakia, and poor oral hygiene can predispose to this lesion.

Clinical Features:

- Generally seen in older age group, most commonly between 60-70 years of age. Males are more commonly affected than females.
- The tumour is slow growing and is locally invasive but unlikely to metastasize.

- It occurs as a thick white plaque, which is painless and resembles a cauliflower.
- In the oral mucosa the common sites are buccal mucosa, alveolar crest of mandible, gingiva and tongue.
- Other regions that can be involved are the larynx, external auditory meatus, lacrimal ducts, skin, scrotum, penis, vulva, vagina, uterine cervix, scrotum and odontogenic cystic linings.
- Pain and difficulty in chewing are common complaints.
- They appear papillary, with pebble like surface and could be often covered with a film of leukoplakia. They may have rugae like folds & deep clefts, and some times may appear as warty fungating mass.
- They have large sessile base and elevate to varying degrees above the base. The margins of these lesions are well defined.
- The colour could be whitish or pinkish.
- Regional lymph nodes may be involved, which may be enlarged and tender, but usually are inflammatory in nature.
- Lesions on the mandibular mucosa grows into the overlying tissue and it gets fixed to the underlying periosteum of bone, gradually invading and destroying the bone.
- The lesions are slow growing, exophytic, and only superficially invasive and have low malignant potential.
- Prognosis is very good because of absence or late appearance of metastasis.

Histopathological features:

Verrucous carcinoma has a typically heavily keratinised, or parakeratinised, irregular surface with clefts, and parakeratin extending deeply into clefts. The prickle cell layer displays bulbous reteridges, but for a considerable time the tumour has a well defined lower border and basal lamina. There is usually a subepithelial inflammatory infiltrate and atypia is minimal.

Differential Diagnosis:

- Verrucous hyperplasia:It is a proliferative epithelial lesion with the epithelial hyperplastic folds extending above the surface of the mucosa, but in verrucous carcinoma the folds invade down into the connective tissue.
- Chronic hyperplastic candidiasis: Epithelial hyperplasia is not so extensive.
- Well-differentiated squamous cell carcinoma: The lesions are more extensive and lymph node metastases is common.

Management:

- Treatment by surgical excision which should be sufficiently radical to remove the entire lesion, gives good results and the prognosis is very good as there is almost absence of metastasis or very late metastasis if left untreated.
- Elective neck dissection was not necessary even in patients in the advanced stages:
- Combination of therapy can be used when the tumour extends to

the retro-molar area.

- When surgery is contraindicated, other treatment modalities such as cytostatic drugs may be preferred. Various doses of these drugs have shown to reduce the tumour size and alpha interferon has been found to support the therapy by delaying the growth of the tumour but doesnot replace surgery.
- Radiotherapy combined with chemotherapy is the next most preferred treatment.

Suggested reading:

1. Alper Alkan, Emel Bulut, Omer Gunhan, and Bora Ozden, Oral Verrucous Carcinoma: A Study of 12 Cases, Eur J Dent. 2010 Apr; 4(2): 202–207.
2. Anil Govindrao Ghom, Text Book Of Oral Medicine, 3rd edition, 323-324.
3. Yoshimura Y, Mishima K, Obara S, Nariai Y, Yoshimura H, Mikami T. Treatment modalities for oral verrucous carcinomas and their outcomes: contribution of radiotherapy and chemotherapy. Int J Clin Oncol. 2001 Aug;6(4):192-200.

Q 2) Hodgkin's disease:

RGUHS OCTOBER 2002 (2 Marks)

Hodgkin's disease or Hodgkin's lymphoma is the malignancy involving lymphocytes. It is the neoplastic proliferation of lymphopoietic portion of reticuloendothelial system. The exact cause is unknown and the role of Epstein barr virus is also indeterminate. It occurs when B-cell develops a mutation in its DNA.

The occurrence of the disease shows two peaks.

- First is in the young adulthood that is 15-35 years of age.
- The second peak in individuals of 55 years and above.

This disease was named after Thomas Hodgkin, who was the first to describe abnormalities in the lymph system in 1832.

Clinical features, signs and symptoms:

(i) **Age and sex:** It is characterised by the bimodal age incidence showing the peak one in young adults and the second peak in the 5th decade of life and affects males and females equally.

(ii) **Onset:** The onset is insidious, usually painless with the enlargement of one group of superficial nodes. The first to be affected are the cervical group of nodes but it could also start in the axillary, mediastinal, abdominal, pelvic and the inguinal lymph nodes. The cervical and supraclavicular group of nodes are very frequently involved, about in 80-90% of cases on an average. The lymph nodes of the chest are also affected which can be observed on chest radiographs.

(iii) Cough, dyspnoea, and anorexia.

(iv) Itchy skin

(v) Night sweats

(vi) Unexplained weight loss

(vii) Low grade fever.

(viii) In 30% of cases of this disease there is enlargement of spleen. The enlargement is rarely massive and the size may fluctuate during the course of treatment.

(ix) In about 5% of cases there is liver enlargement.

(x) There can be both liver and spleen enlargement also.

(xi) Pain as a result of alcohol consumption: Classically in such cases the involved nodes are painful. It is quite specific and can be considered a pathognomonic sign of Hodgkin's Lymphoma. The pain starts typically soon after alcohol consumption and occurs in the vicinity where there is an involved lymph node. The pain can be described as sharp and stabbing or dull and aching.

(xii) Non-specific back pain especially of the lower back has been reported.

(xiii) Low platelet count leads to red-coloured patches on the skin, and easy bleeding and petechiae are also observed.

(xiv) Patients may present with a cyclical pattern of high grade fever which is also known as the Pel-Ebstein fever.

(xv) In some cases nephrotic syndrome can occur.

Oral manifestations:

- Primary lesions involving the jaws is not common.
- Due to reduced host-immune response secondary effects in the form of infection in the oral cavity can be seen.
- Appearance: It may occur as an ulcer or a swelling or as an intrabony lesion presenting as a hard swelling.

Laboratory diagnosis: Microscopically the lymph node biopsy shows complete or partial effacement of architecture due to scattered large malignant cells called Reed-Sternberg cells.

Differential diagnosis:

The presence of Reed-Sternberg cells helps in differentiating Hodgkin's lymphoma from non-hodgkins lymphoma.

Treatment:

- Radiotherapy-irradiation treatment with 3500-4000 rads/week over the involved region plus all adjacent sites is given in stage I and II.
- **Chemotherapy:** Usually given in stage III and IV. Given in combination. One of the combinations is MOPP, ie mecchlorethamine, oncovin, procarbazine and prednisone.
- **Combination:** A combination of radiotherapy and chemotherapy may increase the overall response and long term survival rates.
- **Splenectomy:** It is advocated in many patients, except stage IV disease.

Suggested reading:

1. Anil Govindrao Ghom, TextBook Of Oral Medicine, Third Edition, 335-337.
2. Armitage JO (August 2010). "Early-stage Hodgkin's Lymphoma". N. Engl. J. Med. 363 (7): 653–62.
3. Hellman S (2007). "Brief Consideration of Thomas Hodgkin and His Times". In Hoppe RT, Mauch PT, Armitage JO, Diehl V, Weiss LM. Hodgkin Lymphoma (2nd ed.). Philadelphia: Wolters Kluwer Health/Lippincott Williams & Wilkins. pp. 3–6.

Q 3) Burkitt's lymphoma

(5 Marks)

Burkitt's Lymphoma, also called as African Jaw Lymphoma, was first described in last century by Denis Parsons Burkitt, a surgeon working in Africa.

It is a high grade B-cell neoplasm.

It is one of the fastest growing malignancies in humans, with a very high growth fraction.

A defining feature is the presence of translocation of c-myc gene and IgH gene [t(8;14)] in 80% cases or c-myc gene and kappa or lambda light chain [t(2;8) or t(8;22)] in remaining 20% cases.

WHO classified the disease into three clinical variations -

1. Endemic (African)
2. Sporadic (American)
3. Immunodeficiency – associated

Clinical Manifestations:

It occurs mostly in children and young adults.

Male: female predilection is approximately 2:1.

1) **Endemic:** It refers to cases occurring in African children, usually 4-7 years old.
   Nearly all are EBV associated.
   It involves primarily the jaws and other facial bones.
   It may also involve the gastro-intestinal tract, kidneys, breast, ovaries and other extra nodal sites.
2) **Sporadic:** It occurs worldwide.
   15 – 30% cases are EBV associated.
   In the abdomen the ileocecal region is most commonly involved.
   There may be malignant pleural effusion or ascites and involvement of lymph nodes, jaws, ovaries, kidneys, breasts, omentum, Waldeyer's ring and other sites.
3) **Immunodeficiency – associated:** It is often EBV associated.
   It mainly occurs in patients infected with HIV.
   It is also seen in organ transplant recipients and individuals with congenital immunodeficiency.
   Compared to other HIV infected patients with diffuse large B-cell type Non Hodgkin's Lymphoma, patients with Burkitt's Lymphoma are younger, less often cases are prior diagnosis of acquired immunodeficiency syndrome (AIDS) and have high CD4 counts >200 cells /µl.

Oral Manifestations:

Rapidly growing intraoral swelling of mandible and maxilla may be evident clinically.

Anterior open bite may be seen.

Pain is also usually associated.

Mobility of teeth may be present even if swelling is clinically not detectable.

Radiographic Features:

As seen on panoramic imaging-

- Resorption of alveolar bone.
- Loss of lamina dura.
- Enlargement of tooth follicles.
- Destruction of cortex around tooth crypts.
- Displacement of teeth and tooth buds by tumor resulting in "floating tooth appearance".

Histologic Features:

Monoclonal proliferation of uniform, small, non cleaved B lymphocytes with abundant cytoplasm is seen.

High mitotic rate can be seen.

Numerous scattered macrophages with abundant clear cytoplasm gives a characteristic "starry sky appearance".

Treatment:

Chemotherapy is the main stay of treatment which includes agents like cyclophosphamide, vincristine, methotrexate and corticosteroids.

Burkitt's Lymphoma is very sensitive to short duration and high intensity chemotherapy with survival rate as great as 50 – 70 %.

It may sometimes be combined with prophylaxis of central nervous system (intrathecal chemotherapy) in widespread diseases.

Surgical debulking and palliative low dose radiation therapy to local tumors are also considered.

Suggested reading:

1. Burket's Textbook of Oral Medicine, 11th edition, pg no. 407
2. Ferry JA. Burkitt's lymphoma a: clinicopathologic features and differential diagnosis. The Oncologist. 2006 Apr 1;11(4):375-83.
3. Shafer's Textbook of Oral pathology, 5th edition, pg no. 254-256

CHAPTER 10

Ulcerative and Vesiculobullous Lesions

Introduction:

Ulcerations are common phenomenon affecting the oral cavity and can pose a diagnostic challenge to the dental clinician. All types of ulcerations have similar appearance and distinguishing the cause can sometimes be difficult. As they can be infected easily by foods and the oral mucosa can be easily traumatised. They have non-specific appearance.

Vesicles are fluid filled blisters that are less than 1 cms in diameter. Bullae are fluid filled blisters and are more than 1 cms in diameter. Knowledge about ulcerative, vesicular and bullous lesions is important for the dentist as they are manifested frequently in the oral mucosa.

Q 1) Erythema multiforme:

RGUHS APRIL 2006 (4 Marks)

It is a acute self limiting disorder associated sometimes with recurring skin condition, thought to be a type-IV hypersensitivity reaction associated with certain medications, infections and various other triggers.

It is called multiforme because it manifests variety of skin lesions.

There are 4 types:

1. **Erythema multiforme minor:** Shows typical target lesions or raised, edematous papules distributed along the extremities.
2. **Erythema multiforme major:** Again showing the typical target lesions or raised edematous papules distributed on the extremities.
3. **Steven's Johnson's syndrome**: In case the vesicles and bullae affect the skin, eyes, mouth and the genitalia.
4. **Toxic epidermal necrolysis :** It is severe form and is seen as denudation of large areas of skin making it prone to infection and ultimately multisystem organ failure.

Precipitating factors:

- Herpes simplex virus (HSV) mostly HSV-1, histoplasmosis and Epstein Barr Virus.

- Medications such as barbiturates, sulfonamides, oral contraceptives.
- Other infections, such as mycoplasma.

Clinical Features:

(i) Seen most frequently in children and young adults and is rarely seen after the age of 50 years. It has an acute onset and it could even be explosive onset.

(ii) In severe cases generalised symptoms such as fever and malaise can occur.

(iii) Most common cutaneous areas of involvement are the hands, feet and extensor surfaces of elbows and knees and in severe cases the trunk.

(iv) Tyical skin lesions are target, iris or bulls eye lesions where in there are macules, papules and vesicles.

(v) There are petechiae in centre and bulla or pale areas surrounded by erythema (bull's eye).

Oral manifestations:

- The oral lesions begin as bullae on an erythematous base, however intact bullae are rarely seen in the mouth as they very quickly break down to form ulcers.
- In oral cavity, buccal mucosa and lips are commonly involved.
- There is difficulty in eating and swallowing and there is saliva drooling which could be blood stained.

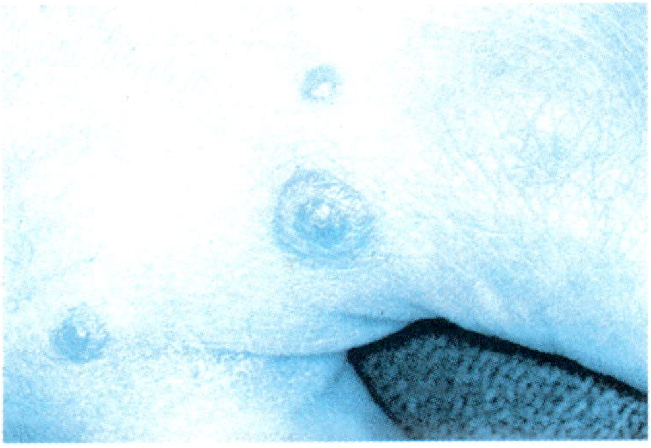

Fig. Figure showing Target or bulls eye lesion.

- Within a day or two the lesions on the lip begin to show crusting.
- Blood tinged crusty lesions of the lip are common.
- Though in majority of cases the healing starts within two weeks, in severe cases, extensive disease may continue for weeks.

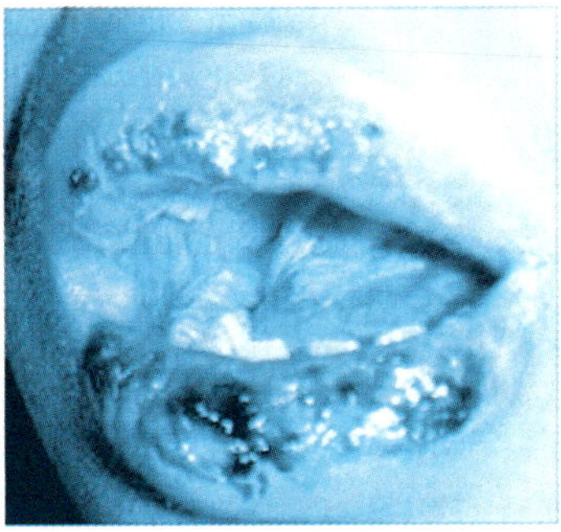

Fig. Bloody crusty appearance on lips

Treatment:

- Mild cases can be treated with supportive measures which includes topical anesthetics, mouth washes, and a soft and liquid diet.
- In severe cases antibiotics are used to prevent any secondary infections.
- Symptomatic : analgesics, antipyretics, antihistamines.
- Moderate to severe oral erythema multiforme can be treated with short course of systemic steroids.
- Application of topical steroid gels and ointment such as triamcinolone, flucinonide, clobetasol can be applied 3-4 times/ day with finger or cotton tip applicator.
- When the lesions are very serious so as to hamper the eating, routine functioning, and concentration, aggressive treatment with 40-60 mgs of prednisolone daily can be considered.
- Prednisone should be taken each morning with meals until the symptoms resolve.
- Morning doses are recommended because it mimics the body's diurnal release of endogenous cortisol and reduces the side effects. Tapering of dose is not required if the treatment is for less than two weeks.

Suggested reading:

1. Bastuji-Garin S, Stern RS, Shear NH, Naldi L, Roujeau JC. Clinical classification of cases of toxic epidermal necrolysis, Stevens-Johnson syndrome, and erythema multiforme. Arch Dermatol. 1993 Jan. 129(1):92-6
2. Burket's, Textbook of Oral Medicine, Edition 11th chapter 3; page. No.53-55.

Q 2) Angioneurotic edema:

RGUHS - APRIL 2000 (5 Marks)

Also called as 'Quincke's edema', 'Angioedema' and 'Giant urticaria', is a form of edema which involves subcutaneous submucosal connective tissue.

It is similar to urticaria and usually involves the upper dermis.

In many patients both urticaria and angioedema may be present.

Etiopathogenesis includes food allergy, physical stimuli, angiotensin converting enzyme inhibitors-captopril, enapril, lisinopril.

Swelling develops due to vasodilation due to release of histamine-like substances with subsequent transudation of plasma.

It is classified as:

(i) **Allergic angioedema:** This is the most common type and it usually affects those who have tendency to some kind of food allergy. and also by insect bites, contact with latex, certain medications like penicillin and aspirin. In severe cases there can be swelling of the throat, and it can become very hard for the patient to breathe. There can also be a sudden drop in blood pressure and a severe reaction like this is also known as anaphylaxis.

(ii) **Drug-induced angioedema:** Certain drugs can cause swelling of the deeper layers of skin, eg. angiotensin-converting enzyme inhibitors that are used for the treatment of hypertension. Symptoms may continue for a few months even after the patient ceases to take the medication. In some cases it might occur in patients taking COX-II inhibitors, non-steroidal anti-inflammatory drugs etc. Medication as a cause of angioedema is however not very common.

Idiopathic angioedema - idiopathic means the cause is uncertain. According to experts fear, anxiety, stress, infections, wearing tight clothes, and alcohol can precipitate this condition. Other causes can be dysfunction of thyroid, iron and vitamin B-12 deficiency.

(iii) **Hereditary angioedema:** Inheritance of faulty genes. In such cases urticaria is not common. This is the rarest where type C1-esterase inhibitor protein plays an important role in regulating the immune system and low levels of this protein can cause this disease. In this type the angioedema develops gradually. The symptoms usually start after puberty. It can also be triggered by pregnancy, infection, trauma, contraceptive pills. Patients can usually be treated effectively with medication.

Clinical features:

Clinically it is manifested as smooth diffuse edematous swelling, involving the face, around the lips, chin and eyes, the tongue and sometimes the hand and feet. Condition usually lasts for 24 to 36 hours, although some cases may persist for several days. It is generally only itchy if the individual develops urticaria. In some cases the swollen areas may feel hot, and even painful. If the lining of the throat and airways are affected there may be breathing problems.

Vision may also be affected in some cases.

Those with hereditary angioedema may have abdominal pain, nausea, diarrohea and vomiting. There may be difficulties while passing urine. As there is risk of suffocation rapidly progressing angioedema is treated as a medical emergency. When this condition occurs as a result of an allergic reaction the patient is usually injected with adrenaline. Some patients are given antihistaminics and steroid tablets, Diphenhydramine hydrochloride, 50-75mgs.

Suggested reading:

1. Anil Govindrao Ghom Textbook Of Oral Medicine, 5th Edition, chapter, 366.
2. National Health Service (NHS), UK, Medical News Today internal archives.

Q 3) Patch Testing:

MUHS MAY 2007 2 Marks

In the late 19th century patch tests were introduced as diagnostic tools Since then lot of improvisations have been done and hence today they are much more reliable and helpful. This test helps to identify whether a substance that comes in contact with the skin has the ability to produce inflammation of the skin(contact dermatitis)

Patch tests can detect sensitivity to a wide range of organic and inorganic drugs, inhalants, food allergens, natural allergens and solid allergens. Patch tests can detect full range of immunologic reactions, like Grill and Coombs type I-IV, they may be very helpful when other allergy tests are negative.

Two types of contact dermatitis exist: Irritant and allergic contact dermatitis.

1. The irritant type occurs when there is direct contact of the substance with the skin and the immune system is not involved.
2. An allergic reaction is when it is specific to an individual and to a specific substance or a group of related substances called the allergen.

Allergy is the hypersensitivity to a particular substance and it always involves the immune system.

The two can be differentiated by patch testing.

Prior to starting the application process the patients should be told about:

1. The objectives of the test.
2. Should be informed to not wet their back.
3. Not to do activities that will lead to excessive sweating.
4. Possibility of symptoms such as itching locally.
5. No exposure to UV radiations 15 days prior to the testing because it can have an immunosuppressive effect.

Before testing the skin needs to be normal and hence in case of eczema of the back, it will need to be controlled. However use of steroid creams should be avoided for at least 3-4 weeks before the test and exposure to sun should be minimal. High dosages of steroids like prednisolone more than 10mgs may interfere with the results.

The doctor can then decide the type of allergens the patient is sensitive to and identify those that can aggravate the dermatitis and will be able to advise on how to avoid those allergens.

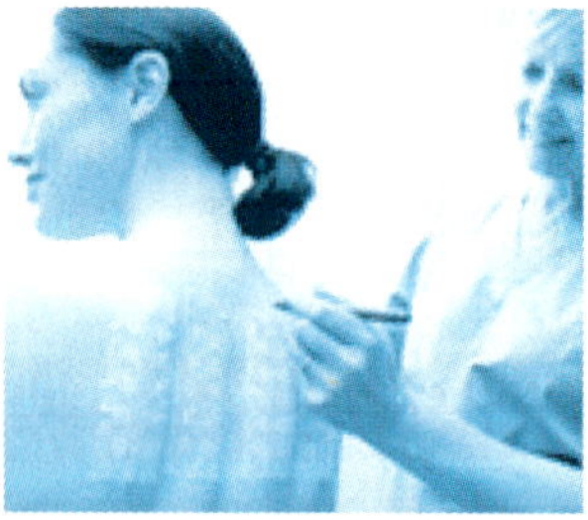

Fig. Patch testing

Method:

(a) A disc about 1cms in diameter is smeared with the chemical and then stuck to the patients back in strips of ten and is left in place for 48 hours.

(b) Allergy to 100 different substances can be tested for in each patient.

(c) Patient may also be asked to test himself with small sample of the substance he/she thinks is causing the allregic reaction eg. cosmetics.

(d) After another 48 hours the patient's skin is examined for any untoward response.

(e) Thus the doctor can then decide which particular allergen the patient is sensitive to and causing the dematitis and will be able to avoid the usage of that substance.

Suggested reading:

1. Gordon BR. Patch testing for allergies. Curr Opin Otolaryngol Head Neck Surg. 2010 Jun; 18(3):191-4.
2. Lazzarini R, Duarte I, Ferreira AL. Patch tests. An Bras Dermatol. 2013 Nov-Dec; 88(6):879-88.

Q 4) Behcets Syndrome

TNMGRU SEPTEMBER 2002 (5 Marks)

This syndrome is a classic triad of symptoms including recurring oral ulcers, genital ulcers, ocular inflammation-conjunctivitis, uveitis and keratitis.

As a systemic disease, it can also involve multiple organs like the pulmonary, gastrointestinal tract, musculoskeletal, cardiovascular and the neurological systems. The fatality in this syndrome is due to rupturing of vascular aneurysms and severe neurological complications.

It is more prevalent in the areas near the old silk trading routes of the middle east and in central Asia. It is hence referred to as the silk road disease.

To establish the diagnosis of this disease, the patient has to have oral (aphthous)ulcers, which can be any number, shape or size and occurring at least thrice in a year along with two out of the four significant symptoms:

(i) Genital ulcers (including anal ulcers and spots in the genital region and epididymitis in men).

(ii) Skin lesions which comprise of papules, pustules, erythema nodosum, and acne in post-adolescents who are not on steroids.

(iii) Inflammation of the eyes, including, iritis, retinal vasculitis, uveitis.

(iv) pathergy reaction that is a papule which measures more than 2mms in diameter, occurring 24-48 hours after a needle prick. The pathergy test is diagnostic of this syndrome with a specificity of 95-100%.

Etiology:

Immune complex formation leading to vasculitis of small & medium sized blood vessels, and inflammation of epithelium that is caused by immunocompetent T lymphocytes and plasma cells.

Clinical features:

- In this syndrome the most common site of involvement is the oral cavity.

- In above 90% of cases recurring oral ulcers appear.
- These lesions cannot be distinguished from recurrent aphthous stomatitis.
- In some patients there are mild recurring oral ulcers while in some cases there may be deep and large scarring lesions characteristic of major aphthous ulcers .They can affect the oral and pharyngeal mucosa anywhere.
- The second most common area of involvement are the genitals and the lesions appear as ulcers on the scrotum and penis in males and ulcers on the labia in females.
- The eye lesions include, conjunctivitis, keratitis, optic atrophy, uveitis edema and vascular occlusion.
- In about 50% of cases there is generalised involvement.
- Lesions on the skin are common and occur as large pustular lesions.
- In this syndrome the lesions may be precipitated by trauma and it is common for the patients to have hyper-reactivity to intracutaneous injections.
- Arthritis is a common phenomenon in about 50% of cases and affects commonly the knees and ankles.
- Affected joints may be red and swollen, but small joints of the hands are spared and there is no fear of permanent disability.
- Involvement of the central nervous system could be severely problematic aspect of the disease.
- It can involve the cranial nerves, brainstem syndrome, or neurologic degeneration resembling multiple sclerosis can occur.
- Other signs include, intestinal ulceration, thrombophlebitis, venous thrombosis, and renal and pulmonary disease.
- Arterial occlusions and aneurysms involving large vessels can be life threatening.
- In children this syndrome occurs between 9-10 years of age and the features are similar to those in adults, and oral ulcers are the commonest feature in over 95% of cases and uveitis is the least common.
- MAGIC syndrome which is a variant of the Behcet's syndrome is characterised by oral and genital ulcers with inflammation of the cartilage.

Investigations:

Depending upon the symptoms that are present, tests such as biopsy, MRI scan, lumbar puncture, and bowel tests are considered.

Treatment:

- Treatment depends on the severity and location of the lesions.
- Cortisone gels, kenalog in orabase, and creams can provide relief in oral and genital ulcers.
- Recurrent ulcers can be minimised by the use of colchicine.

- Pentoxyphylline has been tried for treatment of oral and genital ulcers.
- Patients in whom the eye sight is threatened who have central nervous system affectation may require more aggressive therapy with higher potential drugs having serious side efffects.
- Combination of prednisone and azathioprine has been shown to have a good scope of reducing ocular, oral and genital lesions.
- NSAIDs such as as ibuprofen and others or oral steroids can reduce the joint inflammation.
- Inflammatory involvement of the joints, skin, eyes and brain can be treated with colchicine and oral and injectable cortisone.
- In some cases sulfasalazine has been effective for treatment of arthritis and the bowel disease can be treated with oral steroids and sulfasalazine.
- In cases of severe Behcet's syndrome immunosuppressives such as chlorambucil, azathioprine, cyclophosphamide are used. In severe and resistant cases, cyclosporine is used for treatment.
- Systemic steroids help in rapidly controlling the disease and are helpful till the immunosuppresives begin to work.
- In emergency cases, plasmapheresis has been used successfully.
- Sometimes the oral lesions may not be controlled by systemic therapy and may require topical or intralesional high potency steroids like fluocinonide, betamethasone, clobetasol. When these drugs are placed directly over the lesion it reduces the healing time and size of the ulcers.
- Lesions that are large can be treated effectively by placing a gauze sponge containing topical steroids on the ulcers for 15-30 minutes so as to allow closer and prolonged contact with the medication.

Suggested reading:

1. Allen CM, Bouquot JE. (2008). Oral & maxillofacial pathology (3rd ed.). Philadelphia: W.B. Saunders. p. 336.
2. Bolster MB (2009). MKSAP 15 Medical Knowledge Self-assessment Program: Rheumatology. Philadelphia, Pa: American College of Physicians.
3. Criteria for diagnosis of Behçet's disease". Lancet **335** (8697): 1078–80.

Q 5) Describe management of Acute Necrotising Ulcerative Gingivitis:

MUHS WINTER 2013 (3 Marks)

1) Management of ANUG:

- Managing the underlying factors.
- Superficial cleaning in acute stage or use of oxygenating agents(H_2O_2 1.5-2% in water) or antibiotics(metronidazole & penicillin) coupled with local anesthesia.
- Gentle removal of the necrotic material with swab.
- 3% Hydrogen peroxide diluted with equal amounts of water and

used as mouth rinse every 2 hours on the first day and 3-4 times / day for next 4 days.

- In cases of extensive gingival involvement, lymphadenopathy or other systemic signs, and in cases where other mucosal surfaces than the gingiva are involved, antibiotics should be prescribed.
- Penicillin V (oral) 400000 units /day x 5 days or
- Amoxycillin 250-500mg TDS x 5 days.
- Metronidazole 400mg TDS x5 days.
- Well balanced diet and regular meals.
- Oral prophylaxis to be done after the acute symptoms subside.

2) Removal of pseudomembrane:

The involved areas are isolated with cotton and dried.

To remove the pseudomembrane, a topical anesthetic is applied and after 2-3 minutes its gently swabbed with a cotton pellet.

3) Maintenance of oral hygiene:

The patient is asked to rinse the mouth within every 2 hrs with a glassful of an equal mixture of warm water and 3% hydrogen peroxide. Twice daily rinse with 0.12% chlorhexidine are also effective.

4) Gingival curettage:

Oral prophylaxis is performed, if sensitivity permits. After the disease process is diminished a thorough gingival curettage and root planing is done.

5) Supportive care:

Supportive treatment consists of copious fluid consumption and administration of nutritional supplements, well balanced diet and regular meals.

Suggested reading:

1. Burket's Oral Medicine Diagnosis & Treatment Tenth Edition, page 61-63.

Q 6) How will you treat a case of Herpes Zoster?

MUHS MAY 2009 (2 Marks)

Three major objectives are important in the treatment of Herpes Zoster: 1) Treatment of acute viral infection. 2) alleviating the acute pain and 3) prevention of post-herpetic neuralgia.

To achieve these goals, antiviral agents, oral steroids, and adjunctive pain-management modalities are used to suit individual needs.

Antiviral agents:

They have been effective in reducing the duration of the rashes in herpes zoster along with the severity of pain associated with it.

(i) Acyclovir (Zovirax)-800mg orally x 5 times/day for 7 days.
(ii) Famciclovir (Famvir)-500mg orally TDSx 7days.
(iii) Valacyclovir (Valtrex)-1000mg orally TDSx 7 days.

Corticosteroids:

In treatment of herpes zoster corticosteroids that are orally administered are commonly used.A combination of prednisone and acyclovir has been shown to reduce the pain associated with this condition.

(i) Prednisone-30mgs orally BD from day 1-7.
(ii) After that 15mgs BD on day 8-14.
(iii) After that 7.5 mgs BD from day 15-21.

Analgesics:

In cases of mild to moderate pain, patients may respond to over the counter analgesics.In cases of very severe pain addition of narcotic analgesics may be required.

Calamine lotions may be used to soothe the open lesions to reduce pain and pruritus.

After the lesions start crusting capsaicin cream may be applied.

Topical application of lidocaine and nerve blocks have been found to be effective in reducing pain.

Ocular involvement:

Ocular lesions are also treated with orally administered antiviral agents and steroids.

Preventive treatment:

Prednisone in a daily dose of 40-60 mg for one to two weeks is given to prevent post-herpetic neuralgia.

Suggested reading:

1. Donahue JG, Choo PW, Manson JE, Platt R. The incidence of herpes zoster. Arch Intern Med. 1995;155:1605–9.

Q 7) Tzanck cells

TNMGRU APRIL 2001 (5 Marks)

Tzanck cells are a group of large hyperchromatic epithelial cells which can be seen lying free within the vesicular space in the spinous layer of the epithelium as a result of acantholysis. These multinucleated giant cells are seen in:

Herpes Zoster.
Varicella Zoster.
Herpes Simplex virus infections.
Pemphigus vulgaris.
Cytomegalo virus infections.

The Tzanck cells are so called as they were discovered by French dermatologist Arnault Tzanck.

These cells are keratinocytes that are large and round having hyperchromatic nuclei, with peripheral condensation of chromatin, having hazy or prominent nucleoli and abundance of basophilic cytoplasm.

On the periphery of the cell membrane the basophilic staining is deeper in colour because there is a tendency of the cytoplasm to show condensation at the periphery and this leads to formation of a perinuclear halo.

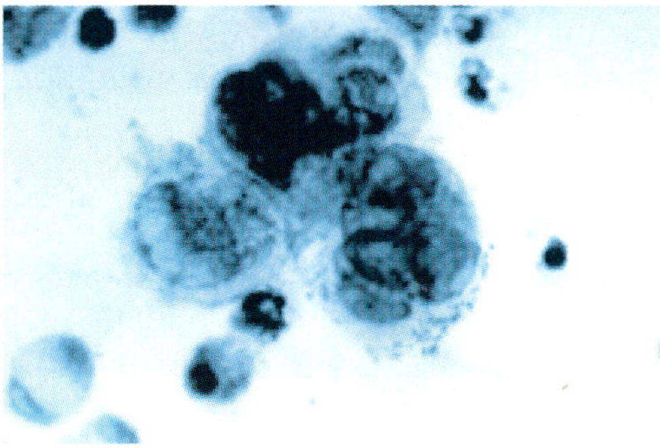

Fig. Multinucleated giant cells called Tzanck cells

Staining of tzanck smear:

The tissue is scraped from the base of a vesicle, and placed on a slide.

In order to prevent artifacts due to drying the smear should be fixed immediately.

Various methods can be used to stain the Tzanck cells like the Giemsa stain.They can also be stained very fast within a minute by stains like Hemacolory or Diff-Quiky. The other staining methods include the hematoxylin and eosin, papanicolaou, wright, methylene and toulidine blue.

(i) **Herpes zoster:** Tzanck test can be positive in cases of herpes zoster.The vesicles and their distribution unilaterally along the course of the nerve however helps in clinical diagnosis.

(ii) **Varicela zoster and Herpes simplex:** If the smear is obtained in the vesicular stage, the Tzanck test can be very reliable and useful in the diagnosis of varicella zoster and herpes simplex infections. When done by experts the sensitivity of this test is about 80% and specificity about 90%. The test however cannot differentiate between the varicella zoster and herpes simplex infections.This test is an important and age old technique to diagnose, vesicular, pustular and bullous diseases, especially herpes, however cytology will never be able to replace histopathology and cultures.

(iii) **Pemhigus vulgaris:** In the early stages of oral pemphigus where the biopsy is uncomfortable for the patient and of little help in diagnosis, Tzanck test is very useful for the diagnosis of this condition.It is characterised by intraepithelial bulla or vesicle and there is a suprabasilar split.The intercellular bridges between the cells are lost and thus there is loss of cohesiveness and results in acantholysis.Clumps of epithelial cells can be seen lying freely in the vesicular space. These multiple acantholytic cells are termed the Tzanck cells which is diagnostic of pemhigus vulgaris.

The cytologic features are similar in case of pemphigus vegetans, however there are more inflammatory cells present especially eosinophils.In pemphigus foliaceous and pemphigus erythematosus there is hyalinisation of cytoplasm which corresponds to the dyskeratosis seen in tissue sections.

(iv) **Hailey Hailey disease:** The Tzanck smear reveals multiple acantholytic cells.

(v) **Cytomegalovirus infection:** Involvement of skin in this condition is rare and a simple Tzanck preparation from the base of the blister will show multinucleated giant cells suggestive of viral infection.

Suggested reading:

1. Oranje AP, Folkers E. The Tzanck smear: old, but still of inestimable value. Pediatr Dermatol. 1988 May;5(2):127-9.

Q 8) Write the differential diagnosis of primary HSV and herpangina:

MUHS DECEMBER 2005 (2 Marks)

1) Primary HSV:

- Primary herpetic gingivostomatitis is a relatively common viral infection of the oral mucosa and is caused by HSV1 virus.
- Age: Children and young adults are commonly affected.
- Clinical Features:

This condition has an abrupt onset and has typical clinical characteristics like high fever, malaise, headache, anorexia, irritability, bilateral regional lymphadenopathy and sore lesions in the mouth.

There is redness of the affected mucosa and edema, with numerous vesicles that coalesce and rupture rapidly, leaving painful small, shallow round ulcers covered by yellow fibrin.

In the first 3-5 days newer lesions continue to develop and the ulcers heal in 10-14 days.

The typical feature of this lesion is the involvement of keratinized mucosa especially the attached gingva.

Another pathognomonic feature is generalized marginal gingivitis which helps in differentiating this condition from herpangina.

2) Herpangina:

This condition is caused by Coxackie A4 and is generally endemic condition that affects children between june-october.

Incubation period of 8-10 days.

There is fever, chills and anorexia.

Sore throat, dyspagia and sore mouth occurs.

In contrast to primary herpetic gingivostomatitis, where the vesicles and ulcers occur on attached gingival and anterior part of the oral cavity, the vesicles in herpangina occur most commonly on the posterior palate, soft palate, uvula, tonsillar pillars and posterior pharyngeal wall.

It is a self limiting disease and the ulcers heal between 7-10 days.

Suggested reading:

1. Burket's, Oral Medicine Diagnosis and Treatment, Eleventh edition, page 41.
2. Scully C. Orofacial herpes simplex virus infections. Current concepts in the epidemiology, pathogenesis and treatment.Oral Surg 1989;68:701–10.

Q 9) Discuss differential diagnosis of multiple ulcers in the oral cavity:

MUHS NOVEMBER 2011 (2 Marks)

I) Acute Multiple Ulcers:

1. **Primary herpetic gingivostomatitis:** Characterised by vesicular-ulcerative lesions on attached gingiva and typical is generalised marginal gingivitis.
2. **Coxsackievirus Infections:**
   (i) **Herpangina:** Lesions typically on the soft and hard palate and pharyngeal areas.
   (ii) **Hand-Foot and Mouth disease:** Ulcerative, vesicular lesions involving hands, feet and mouth.
3. **Varicella-Zoster Virus Infection:**
   (i) **Chicken pox:** Most commonly in children and young adults. Typical ulcerative-vesiculo-papular rashes, which are self healing.
   (ii) **Herpes zoster:** Ulcerative vesicular lesions along the course of involved nerve and are unilateral.
4. **Erythema Multiforme:** Have typical target or bulls eye lesions.
5. **Contact Allergic Stomatitis:** History of allergy will be present.
6. **Oral Ulcers Secondary to Cancer Chemotherapy:** Chronic ulcers with history of chemotherapy will be present.
7. **Acute necrotising ulcerative gingivostomatitis:** The lesions are typically punched out with grayish pseudomembrane on interdental papilla.

II) Recurrent Oral Ulcers:

1. **Recurrent aphthous stomatitis:** Recurrent oral ulcers with familial history.Ulcerations with an inflammatory halo which occur in crops and heal in about 14 days.
2. **Behçet's Syndrome:** Aphthous like ulcers but apart from mouth, skin, genital, eye lesions and multisystem involvement.Pathergy test is positive.
3. **Recurrent intraoral herpes:** History of previous infection will help in diagnosis.
4. **Recurrent herpes labialis;** Typical ulcerative lesions involving the lips, commonly seen in women.

III) Chronic Multiple Ulcers:

1. **Pemphigus :** Cyclical crops of bullous lesions breaking down into ulcers especially in the mouth, with involvement of trunk and limbs. Nikolsky's sign is positive.

2. **Bullous Pemphigoid :** Sub epithelial bullae are present.
3. **Mucous Membrane Pemphgoid (cicatricial pemphigoid**): Ulcerative, vesiculo-bullous lesions which heal by scarring.
4. **Erosive & Bullous Lichen Planus:** Ulcerative, bullous, erosive lesions along with presence of typical Wickham's striae.
5. Linear IgA Diseases:
6. **Epidermolysis bullosa aquisita:**

Suggested reading:

1. Burket's, Oral Medicine Diagnosis and Treatment 10th edi. 51-76.

Q 10) Pemphigus vulgaris

BFU MAY 2007 (5 Marks)

Pemphigus is serious and potentially fatal disease that causes bullae formation and erosions of the skin and mucous membranes.

Pemphigus vulgaris is the most common form of Pemphigus accounting to almost 80% of the cases.

Pemphigus Vulgaris is an autoimmune disorder of the mucocutaneous tissues that runs a chronic course and initially manifests as intra-oral lesions, which ultimately spreads to other mucous membranes and skin.

It is an autoimmune disorder where in the autoantibodies that are produced are directed against the intercellular bridges in the epithelium.

Etiology:

Most of the cases are idiopathic and the exact etiology is still unknown, however these lesions can be triggered by:

- Drugs: Catopril, penicillamine, rifampicin, phenobarbitone, and phenyl butazone.
- Radiation and surgery.
- Dietary habits and particularly the use of garlic.
- Emotional stress.
- Human herpes virus 8.
- High pesticide exposure.
- In females, pregnancy.
- Can occur in association with certain disorders like rheumatoid arthritis, myasthaenia gravis, lupus erythematosus, pernicious anemia.

Pathogenesis:

- Epithelial cells are attached to each other by desmosomes.
- Desmogleins that form the desmosomal component are desmoglein 1, desmoglein 2 and desmoglein 3.
- In Pemphigus vulgaris antibodies are directed against both desmoglein 1 and desmoglein 3 present in desmosomes resulting in the loss of desmosomes and therefore the loss of cohesion between keratinocytes in the epidermis, and it is classified as a type II hypersensitivity reaction.

Clinical features:

- The classical lesion of pemphigus is a thin-walled bulla which forms on the otherwise normal skin or mucosa.
- About 80-90% of cases of pemphigus vulgaris develop oral lesions and quite often oral lesions may appear first.
- Mean age of occurrence is 40-60 years and males and females could be equally affected.
- There may be single or multiple bullae which in the oral cavity may breakdown easily to form ulcers.
- The bullae are flaccid and thin walled and vary from few millimetres to several centimetres in size.
- Lesions bleed easily and may be very painful and cause difficulty in eating.
- Margins are ragged and they grow by peripheral extension.
- Intraorally the lesion can involve the palate, buccal mucosa, lips, and ventral surface of the tongue.Desquamative gingival lesions and bloody crusty lesions on lips are common.
- Apart from oral lesions there may be involvement of nasal, ocular, laryngeal and pharyngeal, upper respiratory and ano-genital lesions.
- Nikolsky's sign is positive, though not specific to pemphigus vulgaris.
- When the surface of the blister is pressurised vertically, the blister extends laterally, known as Nikolsky's sign II or Asboe-Hansen sign.

Histopathology:

The features include, acantholysis due to loss of intercellular adhesion, intercellular edema, suprabasilar split, formation of intra-epithelial bulla, presence of Tzanck cells which are free floating rounded acantholytic epithelial cells found within the vesicle or bulla.

Diagnosis:

- Clinically the presence of active blistering and positive Nilosky's sign can help in diagnosis.
- Tzanck smear will show acantholytic cells that float freely and are round or ovoid, having enlarged hyperchromatic nuclei.
- Direct and indirect fluorescence will show circulating anti-bodies, IgG type which is bound to the intercellular cement region of the oral mucosa.
- ELISA test can reveal DSG1 and DSG3 in samples of serum.

Treatment:

- The mainstay of treatment remains high doses of systemic corticosteroids, usually given in dosages of 1 to 2 mg/kg/d.
- Prednisone is used initially to bring the disease under control and once this is achieved it is given as low maintenance dose.
- Pulse therapy which is supra pharmacological dosages of prednisolone and cyclophosphamide may show good results.

- When only oral lesions are present lower doses of prednisone for shorter periods of time are used.
- Other therapies include, parentral gold therapy, dapsone, tetracycline and plasmapheresis.
- A new immunosuppressive mycophenolate has shown good results.
- 8 methoxypsoralen administration which is followed by exposure of the peripheral blood to UV radiation has also been used.

Suggested reading:

1. Anil Govindrao Ghom, Text Book Of Oral Medicine, 3rd edition, 371-374.
2. Burket's Oral Medicine Diagnosis And Treatment, 10th edition, 68-70.

Q 11) Clinical Features and Treatment of Herpes Zoster

BFU NOVEMBER 2009 (7½ Marks)

Herpes zoster also called as shingles is an acute viral infection which is extremely painful, and incapacitating characterised by inflammation of the dorsal root ganglion, that is associated with eruptions of vesicles involving the skin and mucous membranes of the region supplied by the nerve that is affected.

Clinical features:

- Affects adults and has no sex predilection.
- There is usually a prodromal phase where there is sharp shooting pain, burning, paresthesia, and tenderness occurring along the course of the affected nerve.
- The vesicles are unilateral on an erythematous base which occur in clusters mainly along the course of the affected nerve which is called zoster form pattern.
- Lesions appear unilaterally in linear or cluster pattern.The vesicles turn into scabs within about a week and healing occurs in 2-4 weeks.There can be scarring and hypopigmentation.
- Nerve commonly involved are C3, T5, L1, L2 and the first division of the trigeminal nerve. This can lead to lesions of the scalp, corneal scarring and blindness.
- Cutaneous zoster infection of the side of the nose is called as Hutchinson's sign.
- In immunocompromised patients zoster infection can occur bilaterally, and may be atypical due to involvement of multiple dermatome.
- In such patients varicella zoster virus infection may involve dorsal root ganglion as well as anterior horn cells resulting in paralysis.
- Retinitis, pneumonitis and encephalitis may occur as complications.

Oral manifestations:

- Herpes zoster involving 2nd and 3rd divisions of trigeminal nerve can cause oral manifestations.

- Involvement of 2nd division leads to lesions on the mid-face and upper lip, and of the third division leads to lesions of lower face, lip, mandibular gingiva and tongue.
- It could involve the buccal mucosa, tongue, pharynx and the larynx.
- There is burning sensation, pain and tenderness usually on the palate, unilaterally.
- Vesicles then develop which may rupture to leave behind ulcers or erosions, 1-5 mm.
- Healing occurs within 10-14 days.
- In some cases osteonecrosis of jaw bone may occur especially in immunocompromised patients.

Treatment:

There are three main objectives in the treatment of herpes zoster:

1. Treatment of the acute viral lesions.
2. Alleviation of the severe pain associated with the lesions.
3. Preventing precipitation of postherpetic neuralgia.
   - (i) Drugs like the anti-viral agents are known to reduce the duration of the rashes associated with herpes zoster, and severity of pain associated with it.However the benefits are seen in patients treated with these drugs within 72 hours of developing the rashes.
     - Acyclovir is given in doses of 800mg orally/5 time/day for 7-10 days.
     - Famcyclovir is given as 500mg orally, TDS for 7 days.
     - Valacyclovir is given in dose of 1000mg orally /three time/day for 7 days.
   - (ii) Corticosteroids may be used in treatment of herpes zoster with variable results.Prednisone combined with acyclovir has shown to reduce pain.
     - Prednisone is given as:
       30mg orally BD from day1-7.
       15mg BD on days 8-14
       7.5MG BD on days 15-21.
   - (iii) Analgesics have been used in herpes zoster to reduce pain.Patients with excruciating pain may require narcotic analgesics.
   - (iv) Local application of calamine lotion, capsaicin cream and lidocaine application have reported to reduce pain.

Prophylactic and preventive treatment:

A safe and effective preventive treatment can reduce the morbidity and mortality of herpes zoster if it is made available early.Herpes zoster usually occurs only once because the first reactivation of varicella-zoster usually provides future immunologic protection.Currently studies are being conducted on the development of vaccine against these viruses to evaluate its efficacy in preventing and modifying herpes zoster in the elderly.

Treatment of post-herpetic neuralgia:

Post herpetic neuralgia is generally a self-limiting condition but it can last indefinitely.The treatment is usually administered for controlling the severe pain associated with it.Multiple interventions like topical medications, analgesics, tricyclic antidepressants, anticonvulsants and a number of non-medical modalities are used .In some cases narcotic analgesics may be required.

Suggested reading:

1. Anil Govindrao Ghom, Text Book of Oral Medicine, 3rd edition, 719-722.
2. Donahue JG, Choo PW, Manson JE, Platt R. The incidence of herpes zoster. Arch Intern Med. 1995;155.

Q 12) Clinical differentiating points between primary herpetic gingivostomatitis and recurrent aphthous stomatitis:

MUHS NOVEMBER 2009 (2 Marks)

Primary herpetic gingivostomatitis	Recurrent aphthous stomatitis
Lesions are vesicular.	Lesions are ulcerative.
Most commonly affects the attached gingiva.	Can affect buccal mucosa, tongue, floor of the mouth or any other part of the oral mucosa.
There is prodrome of fever, malaise, before vesicular eruption.	Such a prodrome is not present.
Generally few millimetres in diameter.	May range from few millimetres to several centimetres in diameter.
These are acute ulcers.	These are recurrent ulcers.
There is typically generalised marginal gingivitis.	Generalised marginal gingivitis is absent.

Q 13) Pathergy test:

MUHS MAY 2013 (3 Marks)

Pathergy is a condition of the skin where even a minor trauma such as bruise or bump leads to development of skin lesions or ulcers which could be resistant to healing.

This reaction is unique feature of Behcet's syndrome and, according to the International Study Group (ISG) is the most important criteria for diagnosis. Various positive pathergy reactions rates in Behcet's Disease (BD) have been reported world wide.

A positive pathergy reaction can help to confirm the diagnosis of BD, but a negative reaction cannot necessarily exclude the presence of BD, because its important for the disease process to be active when the skin prick test is done to produce a reaction of pathergy.

The exact mechanism of the pathergy phenomenon is not known, but it seems that the skin injury caused due to needle prick, causes a cutaneous inflammatory response which is very prominent and extensive than that seen on normal skin, and it suggests the release of increased and aberrant cytokines from keratinocytes or other cells of the epidermis or dermis causing a perivascular infiltration that is observed in skin biopsy.

Types of pathergy tests:

I) Oral pathergy test:

1. **Site:** lower lip.
2. **Procedure:** The mucous membrane of the lower lip is pricked upto the submucosa using a 20 gauge blunt disposable needle.
3. **Assessment:** Readings are taken after 48 hours and if an ulcer or pustule develops, the test is considered positive.

II) Skin pathergy test:

1. **Site:** The test site is usually a hairless area on the flexor surface of the forearm.
2. **Routes for testing:** Subcutaneous, intradermal and intravenous.
3. Can be performed using 1-16 needle pricks.
4. Two needle pricks are sufficient for skin pathergy test.
5. Investigators generally use a sterile 20 gauge needle prick or an intradermal normal saline injection, monosodium urate (MSU) crystals or streptococcal antigens to perform the test. The procedure is carried out on the hairless part of the forearm and the needle is generally inserted vertically or diagonally which is at an angle of 45 degrees and depth of 3-5 mms.The needle has to reach the dermis to evoke a proper response.
6. After 48 hours of the needle prick, readings are taken. A 1-2 mms papule surrounded by an erythematous halo and which can be felt on palpation is formed on the skin. It may remain as a papule or convert into a pustule of 1-5 mms. The pustule becomes prominent in 24 hours and attains maximum size within 48 hours and takes around 45 days to disappear. A negative result is concluded when there is only erythema without any induration.

Suggested reading:

1. Fiona F Sequeira, Deepak Daryani, The oral and skin pathergy test, Indian Journal of Dermatology, Venereology, and Leprology, Vol. 77, No. 4, July-August, 2011, pp. 526-530.

Q 14) How do you clinically distinguish primary herpes simplex infection from herpangina:

MUHS, NOV 2006, (2 Marks)

Herpangina	Herpes simplex virus(HSV)
Coxsackie virus A4 has been shown to cause a majority of cases of herpangina, but types A1 to A10 as well as types A16 to A22 have also been implicated	Intraoral herpetic stomatitis is caused by HSV1 virus.
Vesicular lesions of Oropharyngeal area and soft palate involvement is prominent in herpangina.	Vesicular lesions of HSV occur in anterior part of the oral cavity especially the attached gingiva.
Mostly affects young children aged 3-10 years.	It affects both young children as well as young adults.
Herpangina occurs in epidemic usually in summer.	HSV does not occur in epidemic.
Clinical manifestations of herpangina are generally milder than HSV.	Lesions of HSV are larger and severe than lesions of herpangina.
Herpangina does not cause generalized acute marginal gingivitis.	Generalized acute marginal gingivitis is the typical characteristic feature of HSV.
Sore throat and pain on swallowing are present.	Sore throat and pain on swallowing is absent.
Lesions heal on their own and crusting is not seen.	As the lesions heal crusting can be seen.

Suggested reading:

1. Anil G. Ghom, Text Book Of Oral Medicine, 3 rdedi, chapter 28, pg no. 713-724.

Q 15) Steven Johnson's Syndrome:

RGUHS APRIL 2000 (5 Marks)

It was described in 1922 as an extraordinary generalized epidermal eruption which is accompanied by fever, inflammation of the buccal mucosa and purulent conjunctivitis. It comes under the category of erythema multiforme.

It is classified as steven's johnson's syndrome (SJS) when the generalized vesicles and bullae involve the skin, mouth, eyes and genitals.

Etiology:

It is classified as:

- **Iatrogenic:** Drug related and is caused by antibiotics, anticonvulsant, and variety of anti-inflammatory drugs like aspirin and phenylbutazone. Various drugs implicated are allopurinol, vancomycin, diclofenac, valdecoxib, penicillins, barbiturates, valproate, oxcarbazepine, azithromycin, sulfonamides, phenytoin lamotragine, ibuprofen, ethosuximide, carbamazepine, bupropion, and nystatin etc.

- **Idiopathic:** Occurs in 18-22% of cases.
- **Infectious:** Most commonly mycoplasma pneumonia and herpes simplex virus. Other infections include otitis media, upper respiratory infections, pharyngitis, Epstein-Barr virus, cytomegaloviruses, mycoplasma pneumoniae. Viruses reported to cause SJS are herpes simplex viruses, AIDS, coxackie, I nfluenza, influenza, hepatitis and mumps.

In children the viruses implicated in causing SJS are Epstein-Barr virus and entero viruses.

Bacterial infections supposed to cause SJS are group A beta-hemolytic streptococci, brucellosis, diphtheria, rickettsial infections, mycoplasma pnemoniae, tularemia and typhoid,

Fungal infections implicated in SJS are coccidiomycosis, histoplasmosis, dermatophytosis.

Trichomoniasis and malaria, protozoal infections have also been reported to cause SJS.

Pathophysiology:

The major pathologic change is a major lymphohistiocytic inflammatory infiltrate around blood vessels and degenerative changes in the endothelial cells of capillaries.

Clinical features:

More common in females. There is prodrome of flu like symptoms of 1-3 days after which there is eruption of skin and mucosal lesions.In the begining there is a nonspecific upper repiratory infection which may be accompanied with fever, malaise, sore throat, chills, headache, diarrhoea and vomiting.

- There is sloughing of mucosa in large sheets, and the patient may be dehydrated, with loss of electrolyte balance, hemodynamic shock, pulmonary edema and also possibility of coma.
- Though the skin lesions may erupt anywhere, the common sites are palms, soles, dorsum of hands, extensor surfaces. Most often the rashes are seen on the trunk.
- The rashes generally begin as macules and then convert into papules vesicles and bullae, urticarial plaques, or erythema.
- The central portion of the lesion could be vesicular, purpuric or necrotic.
- The typical lesion has a target or bull's eye appearance which is pathognomonic of this condition.
- Lesions develop into bullae and rupture and the skin may become prone to infections.
- Mucosal surfaces of mouth, genitals and eyes is severely involved. Tracheal and bronchial mucosa involvement can lead to bronchial tract inflammation and obstruction.
- Inflammation of eyes may lead to conjunctivitis, uveitis, scarring and blindness in some cases.

- Genital lesions can be balanitis, urethritis or vulvovaginitis.
- Atypical flat target lesions appear on skin and Nikolsky's sign is positive.
- Recovery takes long time and healing may occur with scarring.

Oral manifestation:

The oral lesions are widespread, erythematous, blisters, erosions and ulcerations. Hypersalivation is common. Typical bloody crusty lesions can be seen.

Treatment:

- Prompt identification and withdrawal of drug.
- This condition should be treated in the hospital and preferably in intensive care.
- Symptomatic treatment is provided with nutritional care and fluid therapy including electrolytes.
- Other measures include topical anesthetics, antiseptics, intravenous analgesics and maintaining a warm environment.
- High doses of corticosteroids are recommended and cyclosporine, and cyclophosphamide, are alternative drugs.
- Intravenous immunoglobulin administration and plasmapheresis are administered.
- For lesions in the eyes, an ophthalmologist should be consulted because SJS frequently leads to formation of scar tissue inside the eyelids, that leads to corneal vascularisation, impaired vision and a lot of other ocular problems.
- Surgical care and rehabilitation are sometimes required.

Suggested reading:

1. Bastuji-Garin S, Rzany B, Stern RS, et al; Clinical classification of cases of toxic epidermal necrolysis, Stevens-Johnson syndrome, and erythema multiforme. Arch Dermatol. 1993 Jan; 129 (1):92-6.
2. Van J. Stitt, Jr. Stevens-Johnson Syndrome: A Review of the Literature, J Natl Med Assoc. 1988 Jan; 80(1): 104, 106-108.

Q 16) Based on Clinical Features Alone, Differentiate Between Allergic Stomatitis and Erythema Multiforme:

MUHS NOVEMBER 2013 3 Marks

Sr. No	Erythema Multiforme	Allergic Stomatitis
1.	Age and sex: children and young adults, rare after 50 years. It affects males more than females.	Age and sex: it occurs at any age and gender.
2.	Preceeded by prodromal symptoms like fever, malaise.	No prodromal symptoms.
3.	Site: Apart from oral mucosal lesion, may involve genitals and conjunctiva. Skin lesions also present.	Site: Only oral cavity is involved.

4.	Appearance: it is characterized by macules, papules, vesicles, bullae and urticarial plaques 0.5 to 2 cm in diameter.	Appearance: in early stages of reaction, vesicle or even bullae may be found on the mucosa. Occasionally purpuric spots appear.
5.	Lip lesions are more extensive with presence of hemorrhagic crusting.	No hemorrhagic crusting on lips. Sometimes angioedema may involve lips.
6.	The pathognomonic lesion is the target or iris lesion, which consists of a central bulla or pale clearing area surrounded by edema and bands of erythema. The skin may feel itchy and burnt.	No target or iris lesion.
7.	Symptoms: mild discomfort to severe pain, patient cannot eat or swallow and blood tinged saliva .	Symptoms: Mild to moderate pain. Blood tinged saliva and drooling absent.
8.	The more severe vesiculobullous forms of the disease are Stevens-Johnson syndrome and Toxic Epidermal Necrolysis (TENS).	No such severe forms associated with allergic stomatitis.

Suggested reading:

1. Anil Govindrao Ghom, textbook of oral medicine, 3rd edition, 363-369.
2. Burket's, Oral Medicine, Diagnosis and Treatment, 10th edition, 57-61.

Q 17) Allergic stomatitis:

TNMGRU SEPTEMBER 2002 (5 Marks)

- Allergic stomatitis is a rare acute or chronic allergic reaction.
- External substances coming in contact with oral mucosa leading to inflammation is called contact stomatitis.
- Though the oral mucosa is exposed to a variety of antigenic stimuli it is less prone to contact allergic reactions than the skin.
- The potential allergens are solubilised, diluted and digested by the saliva thereby helping to wash them out and hence limits the duration and number of molecules coming in contact with the oral mucosa.
- The keratinisation being limited makes the binding of haptens more difficult and limits the number of antigen presenting cells.

Pathophysiology:

- In diagnosing allergic stomatitis, previous exposure with allergens is essential.
- Contact of the allergen with the mucosa causes the sensitisation.
- Soon after the initial exposure the Memory T cells are activated.

- When there is re-exposure to the same allergen, a typeIV hypersensitivity reaction occurs.
- The reaction can occur after 48 hours and the severity of reaction decides the clinical manifestation.

Etiology:

- Variety of substances which can act either as irritants or allergens can precipitate this condition.
- The substances include, dental materials, flavouring agents in food, preservatives, dentifrices, mouth washes, chewing gums etc.
- Clinical features:
  - In the acute form, the affected mucosa presents with diffuse erythema and edema, and occasionally small vesicles and erosions.In some cases there could be, erythema, edema, itching or stinging sensation.
  - In case of acute lesions there could be redness or burning sensation.
  - The lesions in contact allergy occur directly at the site of exposure of the causative agent.
  - Soon after the antigenic exposure, acute lesions develop and the diagnosis is easy because the cause and effect relationship can easily be established.
  - In case of chronic lesions, there may be areas of erythema, edema, desquamation and ulceration. The allergic contact stomatitis can present areas of erosions with rough surface, irregular borders, and are often surrounded by an erythematous halo.

Management:

- The first step in managing allergic stomatitis is avoiding contact with the identified or suspected irritant or allergen.
- It is advisable for the patients to avoid food with preservatives and coloring.
- Patient are instructed to avoid smoking. Toothpaste and mouth-washes with strong flavouring agents are best avoided.
- Pharmacologic agents used in the treatment are topical anesthetics, antihistamines, topical steroids.
- 10 mgs tablet of cetrizine hydrochloride HS, mixture of antacid liquid and diphenhydramine hydrochloride syrup in equal amounts to be swished and swallowed 3-4/day allows both local and systemic action to alleviate the symptoms.
- Topical triamcinolone acetonide or flucinonide 0.05% gel can be used.

Suggested reading:

1. P Lokesh, T Rooban, Joshua Elizabeth, K Umadevi, K Ranganathan Allergic Contact Stomatitis: A Case Report and Review of Literature. Indian Journal of Clinical Practice, Vol. 22, No. 9, February 2012.
2. Ravikiran ongle, textbook of oral medicine, oral diagnosis and oral radiology, second edition, chapter 8, page no. 208-209.

CHAPTER 11

Orofacial Pain

Introduction:

Pain is an unpleasant sensation and the fear of pain is a strong reason that patients seek dental care.The head and the face are very prone to chronic, persistent pain and the dentist becomes responsible to diagnose and treat the case to relieve the patient from this malady.Hence the accurate knowledge of this subject is very important.

The most frequent cause of oro-facial pain is the dental disease and in such case it is easier to diagnose and treat the pain.However when an obvious dental cause is absent is when the dentist is challenged to diagnose and treat the case.

Accurate case history, clinical examination and thorough knowledge can help the dental clinician to diagnose and treat this condition.

Q 1) Management of Tic Doloreaux:

RGUHS APRIL 2006 (4 Marks)

Tic doloreaux is a condition affecting one side of the face with severe stabbing, unbearable pain and which arises in one or more branches of the trigeminal nerve.

Known to be one of the most painful conditions to affect man kind.

So called because of painful jerking movement of the patient during pain episode.The pain lasts only for a few seconds to a few minutes.

The pain is so severe that the patient winces involuntarily and hence the name Tic. However between attacks there is no pain or numbness and no dysfunction of the facial muscles.

Management:

A) Medical Management:

(i) **Carbamazepine:** The anticonvulsant is the first line treatment; Dosage 100-1200mg/day
Start with200mg b.d. then 100mg every 2 days to a maximum of 1200 mg till pain disappears or side effects appear.

(ii) **Oxcarbazapine:** can be given in 2400-3000 mg /day.

(iii) **Baclofen:** Can be combined with carbamazepine to enhance the effects in dosages of 10-80 mg /day.

(iv) **Phenytoin:** 2nd drug of choice.
Dosage: 200-600mg/day
Blood Level: 10-20micro gm/Ml
Less effective than carbamazepine.

(v) **Gabapentin:**
It is a newer anti epileptic drug.
Dosage: 100-5000mg/day
Start with 300mg O.D.then increase to300-600mg TDS.

(vi) **Valproic Acid:**
Broad spectrum anticonvulsant.
Dosage: 125-2500mg/day

(vii) **Lamotragine:**
Causes prolongation of Na+ channel inactivation.
Dosage: 50-500mg/day

(viii) **Clonazepam:** 0.5-8mg/day

(ix) Capsaicin, lidocaine cream, misoprostol 600mcg/day, TENS and laser.

(x) Duloxetine is used in some cases of neuropathic pain, and it being an antidepressant, can be very useful when severe pain and depression both exist.

(xi) Effectiveness of morphine and oxycodone on neuropathic pain has been well established and especially so when combined with Gabapentin, TENS and Laser.

B) Surgical Management:

When the medical treatment proves futile surgery is recommended. Surgery can relieve the pain but there are chances of numbness after treatment.

(a) Best and longest pain relief is obtained by microvascular decompression.

(b) Treatment using percutaneous radiofrequency rhizotomy could also prove to be effective like the gamma knife radiosurgery, but the effectiveness decreases over time.

(c) Baloon compression which is a percutaneous surgical procedure has been reported to be effective.

(d) Glycerol injections that involves injection of an alcohol like substance which is corrosive for the nerve fibres and mildly injure the nerve so that the pain signals get hindered.

(e) Another form of surgery is to use an electrode to heat the selected divisions of the nerve, called radiofrequency rhizotomy, if performed accurately can target the exact regions of pain triggers and make them disable causing minimum numbness.

Suggested reading:

1. Lunn, MPT; Hughes, R.A.C; Wiffen, P.J (7 October 2009). "Duloxetine for treating painful neuropathy or chronic pain". In Lunn, MPT. Duloxetine for treating painful

neuropathy or chronic pain. The Cochrane Database of Systematic Reviews.
2. Sindou, M; Keravel, Y (April 2009). "Algorithms for neurosurgical treatment of trigeminal neuralgia." Neuro-Chirurgie 55 (2): 223–5.
3. Zakrzewska, JM; Akram, H (Sep 7, 2011). "Neurosurgical interventions for the treatment of classical trigeminal neuralgia". Cochrane database of systematic reviews.

Q 2) Ramsay Hunt syndrome:

RGUHS APRIL2003 (4 Marks)

Definition:

It is a syndrome with peripheral nerve palsy which is associated with an erythematous vesicular rash involving the ear or the mouth.This triad was discovered first by James Ramsay Hunt, happened to recognise other frequently occurring symptoms and signs such as loss of hearing, tinnitus, nausea, vomiting, nystagmus and vertigo. Features involving the 8th nerve also occur because of the close proximity of the geniculate ganglion to the vestibulo-cochlear nerve in the bony facial canal.

It is thus a triad of:

1. Acute peripheral facial neuropathy.
2. Vesicular rash that is erythematous involving the skin of the canal of the ear, auricle.
3. And/or vesicular rash of mucous membrane of the oropharynx.

It is now said that Ramsay Hunt Syndrome is caused by the varicella-zoster virus.

About 15% patients develop vesicles after the development of facial weakness hence it can be difficult to differentiate from bell's palsy.

Clinical Features:

(i) Patients suffer from paroxysmal pain in the depth of the ear.
(ii) The pain usually radiates to the pinna of the ear and could be associated with constant, diffuse, and dull pain.The pain onset occurs several hours or even days prior to the rash.

The classic features of Ramsay Hunt Syndrome are:

(a) In about 80% of cases vesicular eruptions of the ear or oral cavity.
(b) The rashes may occur prior to the onset of facial palsy/paresis.
(c) Presence of lower motor neuron facial paralysis of the affected side involving cranial nerve VII.
(d) Vertigo and hearing loss on the affected side.
(e) Tinnitus.
(f) Otalgia.
(g) Headaches.
(h) Difficulty in speech.
(i) Staggering gait.
(j) Fever and Cervical adenopathy.

Ramasay-Hunt Syndrome

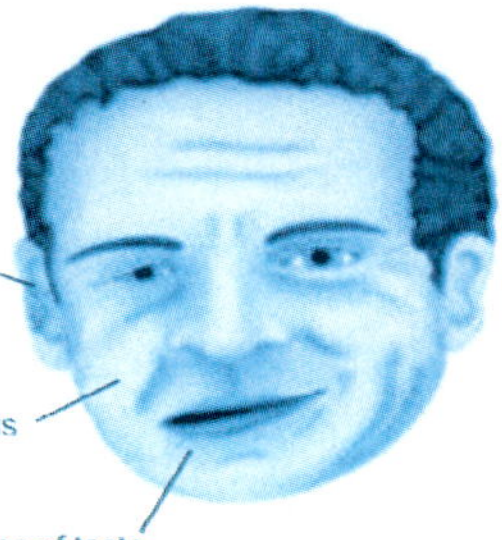

Fig. Typical features of Ramsay Hunt Syndrome

After the onset of symptoms the facial weakness usually reaches the maximum severity by 1st week.

The other cranial neuropathies involving cranial nerves V, VI, VIII, IX, X, may be present.

Complications:

In as many as 50% of the cases hearing loss on the affected side has been reported.

Secondary infections of the vesicles affecting the skin of the ear canals, auricle or both could be precipitated leading to cellulitis.

Good recovery that could be hindered by poor prognostic factors include:

(i) Age older than 50 years
(ii) Complete facial paralysis
(iii) Lack of cranial nerve VII excitability.

Treatment:

- To reduce the pain and neurologic symptoms and inflammation of the cranial nerves Corticosteroids are used.
- Prednisone dosepaks (packaged tablets with reducing dose) are usually the treatment of choice.
- Acyclovir can be used to treat infection caused by herpes viruses such as varicella zoster virus.
- When used within 48 hours of the onset of symptoms there is chance of less pain and faster recovery.
- May prevent recurrence of syndrome.
- Combined therapy using corticosteroids and intravenous acyclovir are also sometimes prescribed.
- However the benefit over corticosteroid alone is still not clear.
- It was concluded from other study that controlled release of oxycodone was safe and was well accepted by the patient who experienced severe and acute pain due to herpes zoster.
- In case the vestibular symptoms are severe vestibular suppressants can be helpful.

- Care must be taken to prevent corneal irritation and injury as in the case with Bell's Palsy.
- Local anesthetic or cocaine application to the trigger point if present in the external auditory canal can provide temporary relief from ear pain.
- The neuralgic pain associated with this syndrome can be dealt with giving carbamazepine and especially so in cases of idiopathic geniculate neuralgia.
- A specialist in infectious diseases should be consulted.
- If on imaging a structural lesion is discovered then a neurosurgeon or otolaryngologist should be consulted.
- An ophthalmologist should be consulted to take care of the eyes especially cornea related problems.
- Antihistamines are used to treat vertigo.
- In patients with this syndrome after starting the medical therapy follow-up should be done at 2-3-6 weeks and 3 months.
- Though the prognosis of resolution of symptoms is good, less than 50% of patients achieve complete recovery of facial functions.

Suggested reading:

1. Dworkin RH, Barbano RL, Tyring SK, et al. A randomized, placebo-controlled trial of oxycodone and of gabapentin for acute pain in herpes zoster. Pain. 2009 Apr. 142(3):209-17.
2. Sweeney CJ, Gilden DH, Ramsay Hunt syndrome. J Neurol Neurosurg Psychiatry. 2001 Aug; 71(2):149-54.
3. Uscategui T, Doree C, Chamberlain IJ, Burton MJ. Antiviral therapy for Ramsay Hunt syndrome (herpes zoster oticus with facial palsy) in adults. Cochrane Database Syst Rev. 2008 Oct 8.

Q 3) Eagle's syndrome:

RGUHS OCTOBER 1998 (5 Marks)

Also called as DISH syndrome/Elongated styloid process/stylohyoid syndrome/Carotid artery syndrome.

It was first described by Watt Eagle in 1937 and was divided into two subtypes:

(i) **"Classic syndrome":** because of fibrous tissue which causes distortion of the cranial nerve endings in the tonsillar bed after tonsillectomy.

(ii) **"stylo-carotid artery syndrome":** sympathetic chain compression in the carotid sheath.

Thus it is a condition which is characterised by presence of recurrent pain in the face and oropharyngeal region because of elongation of the styloid process or calcification of the stylohyoid ligament.

This condition is rare and mostly the patients are asymptomatic but when the ossified structures cause pressure on the structures of the head and neck region there can be a variety of symptoms manifesting.

At the base of the temporal bone, immediately posterior to the apex of mastoid is the styloid process which is a slender outgrowth and is placed caudally, medially and anteriorly towards the maxillo-vertebro-pharyngeal recess.

Clinical features:

Though the condition is usually unilateral rarely it could be bilateral.

It is common in patients between 30-50 years of age but can be seen in teenagers as well as in persons above 75 years of age.

It affects females more than males with a ratio of 1:2.

- Pharyngeal discomfort or pain.
- A sensation of foreign body in the throat.
- Pain on chewing.
- Painful neck movements.
- Elicits severe pain when the stylohyoid process is palpated in the pharyngeal wall.
- Pain along carotid artery distribution.
- Alteration in voice.
- Pain during tongue movements.
- Increased salivary secretions.
- Pain in the ear, and headache.
- Sore throat.
- Glossodynia.
- Dysphagia.

Establishment of diagnosis is by the typical clinical symptoms, physical examination and radiological findings.

Radiographic features:

Antero-posterior and lateral radiographs of the skull can reveal elongation of the styloid process, however in case of superimpositions of other structures the diagnosis can become difficult.

The advent of 3 dimensional CT has made the diagnosis easier and accurate.

Management:

1. Reassurance to the patient, and analgesics.
2. Local corticosteroid injection.
3. Topical anesthesia: Infiltration of local anesthesia around the styloid process, tonsillar area or tender areas.
4. Oral medication with antidepressants and anticonvulsants .
5. Physical therapy to relax the muscles constricted by styloid stimulation can reduce the pain.
6. Surgical treatment that is segmentation of elongated styloid process can be done using transpharyngeal or extraoral approach.

The extraoral approach seems to be better because it is less likely to cause deep space infections of the neck.

Suggested reading:

1. Deepika Raina, Rajesh Gothi, and Sriram Rajan. Indian J Radiol Imaging. 2009 May; 19(2): 107–108. Eagle syndrome.

2. Piagkou M, Anagnostopoulou S, Kouladouros K, Piagkos G, . Eagle's syndrome: a review of the literature, Clin Anat. 2009 Jul;22(5):545-58.

Q 4) Burning mouth syndrome:

TNMGRU FEBRUARY 2014 (5 Marks)
RGUHS APRIL 1999 (5 Marks)

Definition:

It is a idiopathic chronic, oral mucosal pain which is not associated with any clinical lesions or systemic diseases.

It is a dysesthesia or distortion of sense, described by patients presenting as a burning sensation involving the oral mucosa but in the absence of any mucosal alterations.

It is proposed that burning mouth syndrome (BMS) may be regarded as an oral dysesthesia or painful neuropathy based on neuropathological analysis.

Some describe it as condition which occurs in the absence of any particular or no apparent cause.

It is classified as three types:

- Type I: Symptoms not present on waking but increases through out the day.
- Type II: Symptoms on waking and present through out the day.
- Type III: No regular pattern of symptoms.

Classification according to etiology;

- Primary: Essential, idiopathic.
- Secondary: Underlying clinical abnormality.

Etiology:

Local factors:

- **Contact allergy:** Substances in denture material can be allergic to the patient, eg. Monomer, methyl methacrylate, epoxy resin, and glycol.
- **Chronic mechanical trauma:** Could occur from denture or clasps of restoration.
- **Habits:** Oral habits like clenching, grinding and chronic tongue thrusting habit.
- **Infections:** Infections with candida albicans and fusospirochetal organisms.
- **Xerostomia:** Due to irradiation, immunological deficiency, and other systemic causes.
- **Other factors:** Factors like TMJ dysfunction, geographic tongue, oral submucous fibrosis, esopageal reflux, angioedema, trauma to lingual nerve, and acoustic nerve neuroma.

Systemic factors:

- **Nutritional deficiency:** Pernicious anemia, deficiency of vitamin B-complex, folic acid, iron deficiency anemia, could cause burning mouth syndrome.

- **Psychological disturbances:** Depression, anxiety and stress.
- **Diabetes mellitus:** Could be an important cause of burning mouth syndrome.
- **Gastrointestinal problems:** Conditions like chronic gastritis and chronic gastric hypoacidity may cause this condition.
- **Endocrinal disturbances:** Hypothyroidism and estrogen deficiency could be causative factors.
- **Other causes:** Menopause, AIDS, Parkinson's disease, mercurialism, could be contributing factors.

Clinical Features:

(i) It occurs in patients over 50 years, and about 5.1% of the general population is affected. Females are affected more than males.

(ii) Tongue is most frequently affected followed by, denture bearing areas, buccal mucosa, floor of the mouth and throat.

(iii) Pain is present in the morning and it can persist or aggravate during the day, with maximum intensity in the evening.Some of the patients may have continuous burning and pain sensations during the day which can be mild, moderate or severe .Some patients may have waxing and waning patterns of pain occurring over several days or weeks.

(iv) Headache, insomnia, lethargy, mood changes (irritability, depression, and decreased desire to socialise) and decreased libido, could occur in patients with burning mouth syndrome.

(v) Factors like tension, fatigue or eating hot food can cause aggravation. Sleeping, eating and other distractions help to reduce the symptoms.

Diagnosis:

Diagnosis of this condition is done by presence of typical clinical features of burning and pain in the mouth which is lesser intensity in the morning and increasing during the day.

The typical waxing and waning patterns of pain and burning and the absence of any other particular systemic condition, helps in diagnosis.

Management:

(i) **Removal of cause:** Removing the cause that could cause burning like denture adaptation, allergy control, habit control and psychological counselling.

(ii) **Nutritional supplements:** Supplements like ferrous sulphate 300 mgs TDS, IM cyanocobalamine 250mgs/day, pyridoxine HCL 5-30 mgs /day, folic acid can bring relief.

(iii) Mood altering drugs like chlordiazepoxide has helped show improvement in some patients.

(iv) **Other drugs:** Amitryptilline, clonazepam, Alpha lipoic acid, Hydrocortisone locally, nystatin oral suspension, ketoconazole and diphenhydramine hcl as mouth rinse can be helpful.

Suggested reading:

1. Anil Govindrao Ghom, Text Book Of Oral Medicine, 3rd edition, page 403-404.
2. Patton LL, Siegel MA, Benoliel R, De Laat A. Management of burning mouth syndrome: systematic review and management recommendations.

Q 5) Atypical facial pain

RGUHS APRIL 1999 (5 Marks)

Pain is an unpleasant sensory and emotional experience created by a noxious stimulus and transmitted along a specialised neural network to the central nervous system where it is interpreted as such.

Atypical facial pain:It is a term used to describe an ill-defined group of cranio-facial pains which donot simulate any major neuralgia or pain that is secondary to disease of extracranial or intracranial structures.

It is also known as phantom tooth pain or atypical odontalgia.

In 1924 Frazier and Russel and then Glaser described the term atypical neuralgia so as to describe a heterogenous group of patients who suffer from facial pain but which is not typical of true neuralgia. Atypical facial pain, or atypical facial neuralgia as it used to be called, is characterized by an aching, burning, nagging pain which patients feel in the deep structures of the face or scalp and find difficult to describe. The pain is poorly localized and does not conform to the anatomical boundaries of sensory nerve supply. The areas affected may be one or more of those supplied by the fifth or ninth cranial nerves, or the second and third cervical nerves. In certain cases the pain is bilateral. Usually it is constant, but though exacerbations lasting for hours or days may occur the patient is never free from pain.

Etiopathology:

Generally occurs in patients who are chronic depressives, suffer from hysteria or schizophrenia.

Clinical Features:

- Commonly seen in sixth decade, and more common in females.
- The pain is deep, poorly localised and vague.
- Pain is boring, pressing or pulling type. The distribution of pain is not specific to a anatomical area.
- Pain is referred to temple, neck and occipital area.
- Patients often complain of pain onset after dental procedures.
- recurs in days or weeks.
- Some patients give a history of sinus procedures, some receiving multiple medication trials, which include antibiotics, steroids, decongestants, or anticonvulsant drugs.
- Pain is usually unilateral, may cross the midline in some cases, and may involve the maxillary and mandibular areas.
- Trigger zones are absent and lancinating pain is not a feature.

Management:

- Once the diagnosis has been made and other pathologies have been eliminated it is important to take the symptoms seriously and not to be dismissed as imaginary.

- Patients should be reassured.
- Consultations with other specialists like neurologists, psychiatrists and otolaryngologists is helpful when indicated.
- Amytryptillin, a tricyclic antidepressant, nor-triptyline, and doxepin when given in low or moderate dosages are quite effective in reduction or elimination of pain.
- Topical application of NSAIDs which go directly onto the skin at the affected site using rub on creams, gels, patches, and plasters. At the same time, side effects tend to be localized to the site of application, such as itching and rashes.
- Capsaicin used as topical creams in doses of 0.025%, 0.075%, 1%, 5% concentration applied 4 times/day for several weeks has been found to be effective.
- Gabapentin and clonazepam are other drugs prescribed.There can be benefit from topical desensitisation with capsaicin, topical anesthetics, or topical doxepin.
- Idiopathic facial pain is managed by a variety of other methods including psychological treatments and physical treatments such as acupuncture and TENS nerve stimulation.
- Surgical procedures are rarely effective and can aggravate the condition and may lead to a painful facial numbness called anesthesia dolorosa.
- Management of the patient is better achieved through a multidisciplinary approach intended to improve patient's quality of life as well as relieving the pain.

Prognosis and complication:

- In some patients, modern drug treatment can completely eliminate the pain. However the treatments, whether medical, psychological or physical, more commonly only reduce the intensity of symptoms and the consequent pain-related disability.
- In many patients the pain in some form will remain life long.
- The pain syndromes themselves rarely lead to any life-threatening complications although in severe cases severe depression must be assessed.
- Complications can follow multiple invasive treatments in an effort to abolish the pain, particularly destructive surgical procedures on nerves, which should be avoided.

Suggested reading:

1. Bells.Welden E, Orofacial pains classification, Diagnosis, Management third edition. Page 100-101.
2. Merskey H, Bogduk N, eds. Classification of chronic pain, Task Force on Taxonomy, International Association for the Study of Pain. 2nd ed. Seattle: IASP Press: 1994. p. 210–213.
3. Navneet Kaur Bhatia, M.S. Bhatia, Harpreet Grewal, Namita Katra, Case Report: Atypical Facial Pain and Depression, Delhi Psychiatry Journal Vol. 15 No.1 APRIL 2012.

Q 6) Post Herpetic Neuralgia:

BFU NOVEMBER 2007 (5 Marks)

In some cases of acute herpes zoster the patients experience severe pain beyond 4- week duration and about 10% develop unpleasant complication like postherpetic neuralgia, often defined as pain persisting for more than a period of 4 months after the beginning of the rash.

It is a complication of herpes zoster.

Elderly patients are at increased risk of post herpetic neuralgia.

Etiology:

- Injury to the peripheral nerve by zoster virus causing demyelination.
- Atrophy of the dorsal horn cells in the spinal cord.
- Low grade persistent infection of trigeminal ganglion.

Clinical features:

- Affects the older age group and more common in women than men.
- All the symptoms of herpes zoster infection are present like rash and severe pain.If the pain persists for more than six months it is called as post herpetic neuralgia.
- Main symptom is the pain along the course of the nerve.
- There can be sensitivity of the skin and itchiness as well.
- The pain and itching can be so severe that it may affect sleep.
- There may be paresthesia, hyperesthesia and allodynia.In some cases there may be sensory deficit.

Management:

- In patients older than 60 years of age the varicella zoster vaccine, may help prevent post herpetic neuralgia.
- Early in the course of episode of herpes zoster treatment with antiviral drugs can help prevent this condition.
- Topical agents like lidocaine patch, controlled release oxycodone, capsaicin can be used singly or in combination.
- Use of tricyclic antidepressants like amytryptilline, nortriptylline can be used to minimize the painful sequelae of this infection.
- In case of unacceptable feeling of sedation due to nortryptiline, Desipramine can be given.
- Patients who cannot be given tricyclic antidepressants can be treated with gabapentin and pregabapentin to minimize the pain.
- In some cases surgery at the level of peripheral nerve or dorsal root is indicated.
- Injectable steroids in patients above 60 years can provide relief from pain of post herpetic neuralgia.

Suggested reading:

1. Anil Govindrao Ghom, Textbook of Oral Medicine, third edition, 722.
2. Kanazi GE, Johnson RW, Dworkin RH Treatment of postherpetic neuralgia: an update. Drugs. 2000 May; 59(5):1113-26.

3. Argoff CE, Review of current guidelines on the care of postherpetic neuralgia. Postgrad Med. 2011 Sep; 123(5):134-42.

Q 7) Trigeminal Neuralgia:

TNMGRU FEBRUARY 2015 (5 Marks)

Definition: Trigeminal neuralgia is described as a unilateral painful affliction of the face, that is characterised by brief, electric shock like pain and which is limited to the distribution of one or more divisions of the trigeminal nerve.

Also called as Tic Doloreaux and Fothergill's disease.

Classification:

A) Paroxysmal:

(i) **Idiopathic:** (primary)

Here the exact cause is not known.

(ii) Symptomatic: (secondary)

This occurs due to specific cause like tumors, vascular abnormalities, demyelinating conditions.

B) Non-Paroxysmal:

(i) Post traumatic.

(ii) Post herpetic neuralgia.

(iii) Tumors of parotid gland, nasopharynx, and cerebellopontine angle tumors.

Etiology:

1. **Vascular compression theory, (**Peripheral mechanism)

   Pressure from blood vessels leading to demyelination of the nerve is considered as an etiologic factor.

2. **Central mechanism theory:**

   - The most widely accepted theory is that a majority of cases of TN are caused by an atherosclerotic blood vessel, especially the superior cerebellar artery, pressing on and grooving the root of the trigeminal nerve.This pressure results in focal demyelinization and hyperexcitability of nerve fibers, which will then fire in response to light touch, resulting in brief episodes of intense pain.
   - It postulates changes that result from peripheral focal demyelination & loss of segmental inhibition of afferent activity.
   - This allows paroxysmal stimulation & firing of low threshold mechanoreceptor interneurons in the nucleus oralis of the central trigeminal brainstem complex.
   - Once the attacks have been triggered from the periphery, they are self sustaining.

3. Multiple sclerosis {which causes a breakdown in the myelin sheath of the nerve}

4. Direct injury to the nerve.

5. Just the aging process.
6. Autoimmunity and hyper sensitivity are cited as causes of demyelination and hence neuralgia.
7. Ischemia affecting various portions of the trigeminal pathway could be responsible.
8. Aneurysms of the intrapetrous part of the internal carotid artery causing pulsatile irritation to the trigeminal ganglion.
9. Tumors of the maxillary antrum, cerebellopontine angle, nasopharynx, and of peripheral nerve root can lead to this condition.

Clinical features:

(i) Occurs most commonly in middle and old age, rarely below 35 years.
(ii) Pain located along the divisions of trigeminal nerve branches.Most commonly the maxillary division.
(iii) Almost always unilateral.
(iv) The pain is sharp, shooting, lancinating, electric shock like in nature and remains for a few seconds at a time.Complete remission between intervals.
(v) Presence of trigger zones is typical.They include supraorbital foramina, infraorbital foramina, inner canthus of eye, lateral to the ala, mental foramen, intraoral.
(vi) **Triggering Factors:** Talking Chewing, washing face, shaving, brushing the teeth, wind blowing on face, spontaneously.
(vii) Relieving factor is sleep.

Differential Diagnosis:

Migraine, sinusitis, tumors of nasopharynx, multiple sclerosis, tooth ache, postherpetic neuralgia , glossopharyngeal neuralgia.

Management:

(i) **Medical:**
- Carbamazepine-100-1200 mgs /day.
- Oxcarbazepine-2400-3000mg/day.
- Phenytoin -200-600mg/day.
- Baclofen-10-80 mg/day.
- Gabapentin-300mg OD.
- Other drugs include, valproic acid, lamotragine, clonazepam, pimozide, local application of capsaicin, lidocaine cream, laser treatment, TENS, tricyclic antidepressants, NSAIDs, opioids.

(ii) **Surgical:**
- Injection of nerve with anesthetic solution.
- Injection of nerve with alcohol.
- Peripheral neurectomy.
- Electrocoagulation of gasserion ganglion.
- Percutaneous radiofrequency trigeminal neurolysis.

- Trigeminal tractotomy and rhizotomy.
- Gamma knife radiosurgery.

Suggested reading:

1. Burket's, Oral Medicine Diagnosis and Treatment 10th edi.328-329.

Q 8) Give differential Diagnosis between pain characteristics of trigeminal neuralgia and acute pulpitis.

MUHS OCTOBER 2004 (2 Marks)

Sr. No.	Pain characteristics of Trigeminal Neuralgia	Pain characteristics of Acute Pulpitis
1.	Trigeminal neuralgia is a neuropathic pain syndrome characterised by "a sudden and usually unilateral severe brief stabbing recurrent pain in the distribution of one or more branches of the fifth cranial nerve.	Acute pulpitis is due to odontogenic origin and generally runs a precipitous, short, painful and sometimes violently painful course.
2.	Duration of pain: paroxysmal attacks of pain lasting from fraction of second to 2 minutes affecting one or more divisions of trigeminal nerve.	Duration of pain: No paroxysmal attacks. In acute reversible pulpitis pain is short duration that disappears when the stimulus is removed. In acute irreversible pulpitis pain lasts for few minutes to hours but lingering after removal of thermal stimulus. It can last for the day.
3.	Site: Most commonly on right side, and lower portion of face. It is unilateral and along the nerve involved nerve course.	Site: In acute pulpitis, pain is localised to the offending tooth. In acute irreversible pulpitis pain is diffuse.
4.	Nature of pain: Intense, sharp, superficial, or knife like, stabbing, lightening, electric shock or lancinating pain precipitated from trigger areas or by trigger factors.	Nature of pain: continuous and throbbing in nature.
5.	Trigger zones: are common on vermillion border of lip, ala of nose, cheeks, around the eyes.	There are no trigger points.
6.	Aggravating factor: cold, brushing, washing face, shaving, touching the trigger points	Aggravating factor: In acute reversible and irreversible pulpitis pain is on bending down, lying down, hot and cold stimulus.
7.	Relieving factor: Carbamazepine (tegretal) and Topical anesthetics, alcohol injection in ganglion.	Relieving factor: Root canal treatment and Antibiotics.
8.	No pain during sleep.	In acute irreversible pulpitis there is pain during sleep. In acute reversible pulpitis there is no pain during sleep.

Suggested reading:

1. Louis I grossman, ed: Endodontic Practice: Endodontic Emergencies, 11th ed. Varghese Publishing House, 1988 , 83-87.
2. Okeson J, ed: Orofacial Pain: Guidelines for Classification, Assessment, and Management, 3rd ed. Chicago: Quintessence Publishing, 1996.

Q 9) Gate control theory of pain:

TMNGRU AUGUST 2011 6 Marks

In 1965 Melzack and Wall proposed a theory to help explain and serve as a model to visualize pain modulation which they termed as gate control theory.

Noxious stimulation of the skin evokes the nerve impulses that are conducted to three spinal cord systems:

1. Cells of the substantia gelatinosa situated in the dorsal horn.
2. Dorsal column fibers that project towards brain.
3. First transmission cells in the dorsal horn.

This theory proposes that the substantia gelatinosa functions as a gate control system which modulates the afferent patterns prior to influencing the transmission cells.

The afferent patterns in the dorsal column system act as a control trigger, which activates the selective brain processes which influence the modulating properties of the gate control system.The transmission cells activate neural mechanisms that comprise of the action system responsible for the perception and response. Each of these systems receives nerve impulses initiated by noxious stimulation of skin.

Gate control system:

- When skin is noxiously stimulated, the impulses thus generated are transmitted centrally by both large A –delta and small C fibers.
- The large fibres have a much higher conduction rate than the small fibres.
- The nerve impulses via larger fibers arrive at the substantia gelatinosa well ahead of those transmitted by small fibres.
- Volleys of nerve impulses in large fibres are extremely effective in activating the transmission cells initially but these impulses also activate a negative feed-back mechanism, which reduces their effect on the transmission cells.
- These cells must be stimulated before the sensation is either perceived or acted upon.
- Volleys or nerve impulses in small fibres activate a positive feedback mechanism that exaggerates the effect of arriving impulses on the transmission cells.
- The effect of large fiber activity is to "close the gate".
- The effect of small fibre activity is to "open the gate" for passage of impulses to the transmission cells, the gate being the initial

synapses between peripheral neurons and secondary medullary neurons.

Three features of afferent sensory input are significant:

1. Ongoing activity that precedes the stimulus.
2. Stimulus evoked activity itself.
3. Relative balance of activity of the large fibers related to that of the small fibers.

The processes involved in the gate control mechanism of pain involves:

(i) **Presetting the gate:** There is continous, unceasing, ongoing bombardment by afferent nerve impulses, most of which are below conscious levels.This activity precedes the noxious stimulus and presets the gate before such noxious stimulation occurs.

(ii) **Resetting the gate:** The synaptic gate that permits the nerve impulses of the primary afferent neurons to fire the secondary transmission cells is affected or reset by the noxious stimulus itself, depending on the total number of active fibres involved, frequency of the nerve impulses, and balance of activity in large and small fibers.

(iii) **Critical firing level:** Another feature of this system concerns the critical level to which the out put of the transmission cells must rise before the action system is fired and the pain perception and reaction occur.Until this firing takes place there is neither perception of pain nor any reaction to it.

(iv) **Central control trigger:** Another feature of this theory has to do with the effect of the higher centers on both presetting and resetting the synaptic gate.The neurologic control of the gate-setting is by way of descending efferent fibres, which are activated by the brain.

(v) **Action system:** Another major element in this theory is concerned with reaction to painful nerve impulses transmitted to the higher centers by the firing of transmission cells, the second order neurons. Depending on the setting of the synaptic gate and the critical firing level, the action system is triggered, causing a sequence of responses that includes both conscious perception and physical reaction.

Suggested reading:

1. Welden E Bell, Orofacial Pains, 3rd edition, 45-51.

Q 10) How will you differentiate between dental pain and neuralgic pain

MUHS, MAY 2012 (3 Marks)

Odontogenic pain	Neuralgic pain
Pain is dull ache or occasionally sharp and severe.	Pain is usually sharp, shooting or lancinating..

Response to stimuli, such as hot, cold or percussion, is predictable and proportionate.	Response to hot, cold or percussion does not reliably relate to the pain and may be disproportionate.
Pain is usually inconsistent and tends to get better or worse over time depending on the stimulus and may be continuous.	In tic dolouреaux pain is paroxysmal sharp shooting lancinating lasting for few second to about less than two minutes. Pain is non-paroxysmal and more persistent in symptomatic neuralgia.
Pain may occur during sleep and may disturb it.	Sleep is a relieving factor.
There is often an identifiable source i.e., caries, deep restoration, periodontal disease, fractures, impacted teeth.	There is no obvious source of local pathology. Advanced investigations may reveal tumors of head and neck region or vascular compressions.
Local anesthesia of the suspect tooth eliminates the pain.	Local anesthesia of the affected branch of the nerve will eliminate pain.
Trigger zones absent.	Presence of Trigger zones is the most important characteristic feature of true neuralgia.
Pain can be controlled by anti-inflammatory or antibiotic drugs.	Anti-spasmodic and tricyclic anti-depressants will reduce the pain.
Treatment of the affected tooth will provide relief.	Nerve resection, decompression, rhizotomy or tractotomy will give relief.
Pain can be severe but doesnot invoke suicidal tendencies.	Pain can be so severe that patients may feel suicidal.

Suggested reading:

1. Anil G. Ghom, Text Book Of Oral Medicine, 3 rd edition, chapter 15, pg no. 390
2. Michael J. Matwychuk, Diagnostic Challenges of Neuropathic Tooth Pain; J Can Dent Assoc 2004; 70(8):542–6.

Q 11) Periodic migranous neuralgia:

RGUHS OCTOBER 2000 (5 Marks)

Synonyms: Sphenopalatine ganglion neuralgia, cluster headache, histamine headache, alarm clock headache etc.

Sphenopalatine neuralgia or periodic migranous neuralgia is characterised by paroxysms that are unilateral and are of intense pain in the region of the eyes, ear and mastoid, maxilla, base of the nose and below the zygoma. This condition is uncommon and different clinically, etiologically and genetically from migraine .The term "cluster" is used because individuals experience multiple headaches per day for 4 to 6 weeks and then may be without pain for months or even years. In some patients the pain appears at exactly the same time of the day and thus it is also referred as "alarm clock" headache.

Etiology:

- Vascular cause: The disease is caused by abnormal hypothalamic function, head trauma, and abnormal release from mast cells.
- Triggering factors: headache can be initiated by alcohol, cocaine and nitro-glycerine.

Clinical features:

1. Common in 3rd to 4th decade of life with strong male predilection. The pain is deep, intense may last for 15 min to 3 hrs, unilateral involves the periorbital area radiating to ipsilateral temple and maxilla, including teeth. Pain is present in the distribution of ophthalmic nerve.
2. Pain is paroxysmal, burning and lancinating without the trigger zone.
3. Symptoms such as lacrimation from the eye congestion of nose, rhinorrhea, swelling of the face and forehead, miosis, and eyelid oedema may be seen.
4. Paresthetic sensation of skin over the lower half of the face has also been reported in some cases.

Alarm clock headache without trigger zone will diagnose this condition.

Differential diagnosis:

- Paroxysmal hemicrania.
- Short lasting unilateral neuralgiform headache attacks along with conjunctival infection and tearing (SUNCT).

Management:

1. **Drug therapy:** Ergotamine-(2mg- sublingual tablets), prednisolone, lithium carbonate, indomethacin, methylsergide maleate, verpamil, sumatriptan-(50-100mg tablets) will give relief from symptoms.
2. **Oxygen inhalation:** inhalation of O_2 at 9l/min may shorten the attack symptoms.
3. Intranasal spray of 4% lidocaine is effective.
4. Surgical interventions such as trigeminal sensory rhizotomy, superficial petrosal neurectomy, gamma knife radiosurgery and decompression of the nervus intermedius.

Suggested reading:

1. Anil Govindrao Ghom.'textbook of oral medicine'; ch 15;pg 395
2. Matharu MS, Goadsby PJ; cluster headache: focus on emerging therapies; expert rev neurother. 2004 sep; 4(5):895-907.

CHAPTER 12

Oral Pigmented Lesions

Introduction:

Pigments are coloured substances, some of which are normally present in cells (eg.melanin) and some are abnormal and collect in cells under special circumstances.Pigments can be endogenous or exogenous. Exogenous pigmentation is usually due to deposition of foreign bodies in the oral mucosa.Endogenous pigments are due to melanin, haemoglobin, hemosiderin and carotene.

Pigmentation of the oral mucosal tissues is quite a frequent finding. Pigmentations can be physiologic (eg.racial pigmentation) or pathologic (like Addison's disease and malignant neoplasms like Kaposis sarcoma and melanoma.) Oral pigmentations may represent a systemic disease and hence its knowledge and understanding and ability to diagnose such conditions is must for a dental clinician.

Q 1) Endogenous Pigmentation:

RGUHS APRIL 2006 (4 Marks)

Pigmented lesions of the oral cavity and peri-oral tissue can be diagnostic challenge for the dental clinicians.

The oral pigmentations can be either physiological or pathological and it can exogenous or endogenous.As a part of differential diagnosis, the colour, location, distribution and duration as well as use of drugs, the family history and change in pattern is important.

Melanin, carotene, hemoglobin and hemosiderin are endogenous pigments.

These conditions are commonly found in the oral cavity and can be due to physiologic alterations eg racial pigmentation, systemic illnesses eg.Addison's disease and certain malignant neoplasms like melanoma and Kaposi's sarcoma.

Knowledge about them is thus essential.

(a) **Melanin Pigmentation associated disorders:** Brown, blue, gray or black areas could be due to increased melanin deposition depending upon the amount and location of melanin in the tissues.

Pigmented lesions due to melanin could be focal, multifocal, or diffuse and includes entities like racial pigmentation, blue nevus, melanotic macule, melanocytic macule, smoker's melanosis, oral melanoacanthoma, foreign body induced pigmentations or drugs. Peutz-Jegher's syndrome, Addison's disease and melanoma.

Causes:

(i) **Physiologic pigmentation:** More commonly affected are Individuals with dark skin.Light brown to black could be the colour range of physiologic pigmentation.
Physiological pigmentation can occur any where in the oral cavity but the attached gingiva is most commonly involved and may also occur on the tips of fungiform papillae on the dorsum of the tongue and can be easily diagnosed clinically.

(ii) Other causes can be idiopathic, developmental, neoplastic, reactive drugs, hormones and genetics, autoimmune and infectious conditions.

Manifestations:

Can range from ephelis, melanotic macule, melanocytic nevus, malignant melanoma, actinic lentigo, lichen planus pigmentosus, laugier-hunziker pigmentation, smoker's melanosis, oral submucous fibrosis, café au lait spots in Peutz-jegher's syndrome, adrenal insufficiency and HIV/ AIDS.

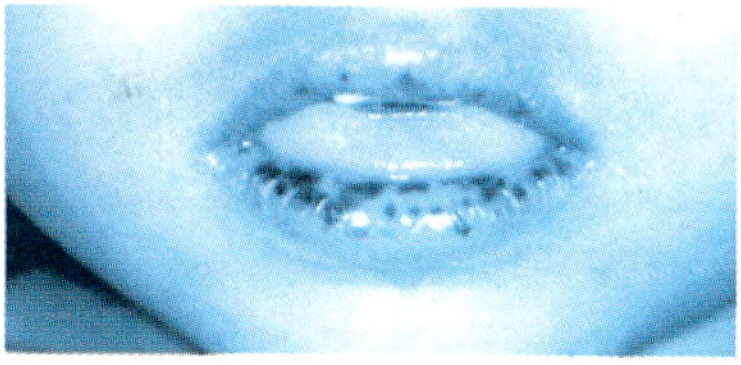

Fig. Brownish black pigmented lesions in the perioral area.

b) Hemoglobin/ hemosiderin associated disorders:

Causes:

Idiopathic, trauma, genetic, inflammatory and autoimmune.

Manifestations:

Hematoma, ecchymosis, purpura, petechiae, vasculitis, hemochromatosis.

c) Bilirubin associated disorders:

Causes:

Alcohol, trauma, infection, neoplasia, genetic and autoimmune.

Manifestation:

Jaundice:

Causes yellowish discolouration of skin and mucous membrane due to bile pigments when the serum bilirubin levels exceed 2-5mg/dl.

Oral cavity may show yellow discoloration in severe cases.Intraorally the discoloration is more pronounced on the buccal mucosa and palate.

d) Carotene Pigments associated disorders:

Causes:

Excess use of food containing carotenides might lead to carotenemia or excess deposition of carotene pigments.In oral cavity it can be seen as yellowish, orangeish discoloration especially of the soft palate.

e) Vascular associated disorders:

Causes:

Developmental, hamartomatous, neoplastic, autoimmune.

Manifestations:

Hemangioma, varix, lymhangioma, angiosarcoma, kaposi's sarcoma, hereditary hemorrhagic telanjiectesia, CREST syndrome.

f) Iron pigmentation(Hemochromatosis):

Causes:

Idiopathic, dietary excess, or the result of iron overload due to repeated blood transfusions. Pigmentations of oral mucosa occurs in 15-20% of cases.

Suggested reading:

1. Adel Kauzman, Marisa Pavone, Blanas Nick, Grace Bradley: Pigmented Lesions of the Oral Cavity: Review, Differential Diagnosis, and Case Presentations.
2. Anil Govindrao Ghom, Textbook of Oral Medicine, Third Edition, 457-476.

Q 2) Café' au lait spots

RGUHS OCTOBER 2005 4Marks

Solitary, idiopathic cafe au lait spots are occasionally seen in the general population, however multiple cafe au lait spots are indicative of an underlying genetic disorder.

They are so called because they resemble the colour of coffee mixed with milk.

They are also known as Giraffe Spots and are caused by a collection of pigment producing melanocytes in the skin epidermis.

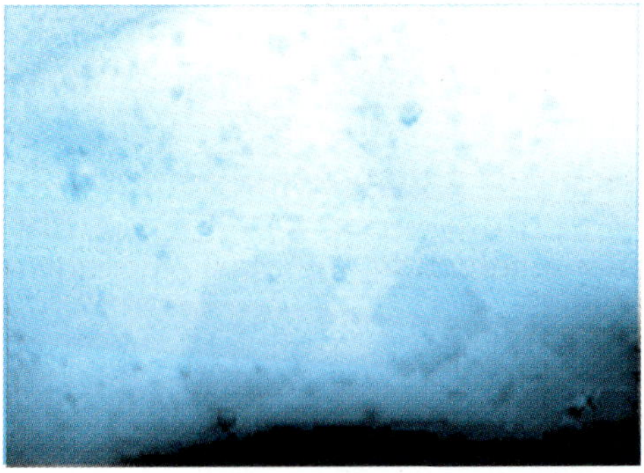

Fig. Cafe Au Lait spots on skin

They are generally permanent and could grow or increase in number over a period of time. They are quite often harmless but could also be associated with syndromes like neurofibromatosis type 1.McCune-albright and Noonan's syndrome.

(a) Neurofibromatosis is an autosomal dominant disease that is caused by the mutation or deletion of NF1 gene which is located on chromosome 17.
It is associated with multiple neurofibromas, inguinal and axillary freckles and pigmented lesions of the iris.
If there are 6 or more cafe-au-lait spots which are greater than 5 mms before puberty or greater than 15 mms after puberty, it can be diagnostic of neurofibromatosis type1 but other features should also be present to confirm the diagnosis.

(b) McCune-Albright syndrome is characterised by polyostotic fibrous dysplasia, various endocrinopathies and soft tissue myxomas.
The cafe-au-lait spots in MCcune-Albright syndrome has pigmented macules with irregular borders, as compared to the smooth borders of macules of Neurofibromatosis Type 1.

(c) Pigmented muco-cutaneous macules and multiple melaontic nevi are seen in Noonan's syndrome and the Allelic Leopard syndrome. Leopard phenotype is usually associated with several small freckles like macules often involving the facia.
The pathogenesis is not clear but a recent study suggests that colocalization of neurofibromin (the neurofibromatosis type 1 gene) and amyloid precursor protein in melanosomes may be important for the development of the pigmented lesions in Neurofibromatosis Type 1.

Diagnosis is done by measuring spot size and number of spots to confirm the associated disorders such as Neurofibromatosis type I which usually shows, more than 6 spots more than 3 cm in diameter

Diagnosis requires the presence of 2 or more major criteria, 6 or more cafe-au-lait spots, inguinal or axillary freckling, 2 or more cutaneous neurofibromas, 1 plexiform neurofibroma, characteristic bony lesions, (pseudarthrosis, sphenoid wing hypoplasia), an optic glioma, 2 or more iris, Lisch nodules, or a first degree relative neurofibromatosis -1.

These spots are usually present at birth, and are permanent and could grow or increase in size over a period of time and are benign and donot cause any problems or illness.

These spots can be removed with lasers. Unfortunately they may not be completely removed and may recur after treatment. Many a times just one spot is treated so as to predict the outcome of treatment.

Suggested reading:

1. Burket's Oral Medicine, Diagnosis And Treatment 12th Edition, 120.

Q 3) Albrights Syndrome:

TNMGRU FEBRUARY 2006 (5 Marks)

Albright's syndrome is a genetic disorder affecting bones, skin pigmentation, hormonal imbalances, and premature sexual development.It is also known as McCune-Albright syndrome.

It is the result of a genetic change (mutation) in the GNAS1 gene that occurs randomly, for no apparent reason, that is it occurs sporadically. In individuals with the disorder, this sporadic genetic mutation is present in only some of the body's cells.

Thus, this syndrome happens when Polyostotic fibrous dysplasia occurs in association with cafe-au-lait spots and multiple endocrinopathies like sexual precociousness, hyperthyroidism and pituitary adenoma.

It could be associated with other endocrine syndromes like Cushing's syndrome, hyperthyroidism and acromegaly.

The syndrome shows a variable range of severity.In children, in some cases diagnosis can be done in early infancy with frank bone disease, and increased secretion from several endocrine glands.In some children there may be no outward evidence of bone disease or endocrine involvement and may appear healthy.They may achieve puberty at almost normal age and have no unusual skin pigmentations.

Signs and symptoms:

The clinical presentation of Albrights syndrome varies depending upon which component of the syndrome is predominant.Major manifestations include:

(i) **Precocious puberty:** Which includes early breast development, genital maturation, speedy increase in height and abnormally large testes in males.

(ii) **Cafe-au-lait- pigmentation:** The colour of the spots range from light to dark brown and can show segmental distribution, and affects quite often only one side of the body and may not cross the midline and should be differentiated from those of neurofibromatosis .

(iii) **Polyostotic fibrous dysplasia:** Multiple pathologic fractures which may be prominently present in the early stages.

In quite a few cases involvement of bone may be present involving only one side. Prominently there might be manifestations like abnormal gait, bony deformities, bone pain and joint stiffness and pain.

Symptoms may start in childhood, but in some cases the disease is clinically silent and can be discovered on routine radiographic examination for other reasons.

The bony lesions do not show spontaneous improvement .The existing bony lesions can slowly get worsened or could remain static, and chances of new lesions may be there.During pregnancy the bony lesions worsen. This effect could be due to the trophic effects of estrogen on the fibrous dysplastic bone which may possess estrogen receptors.

(i) presence of hyperthyroidism is rare with out several other findings of Albright's syndrome being present.

The findings could include, arrythmias, tachycardia, hypertension, sleeplessness, tremors, weight loss hyperthermia, and in infants there could be failure to thrive.

(ii) Infantile Cushing's syndrome can be seen initially without any signs of Albright's syndrome.

(iii) Other manifestations could be:

Growth hormone excess, gigantism, acromegaly, pituitary tumours, ovarian cysts, thyroid tumours, hypophosphatemia, hypogonadotropic hypogonadism especially in the setting of hyperprolactemia.

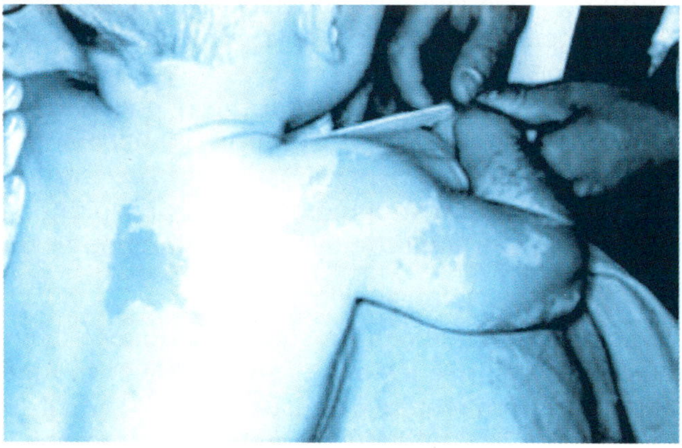

Fig. Cafe au lait spots in an infant with Albrights syndrome

Oral manifestations:

Dental findings include malocclusion, delayed eruption, tooth displacement and tooth anomalies like tooth rotation, oligodontia and taurodontism.

In cases when the jaws are first involved, patients may complain of unilateral swelling of face or enlarging of the alveolar process.

Pain and pathologic fractures can be seen rarely.If the extensive lesions involving the craniofacial region, impinge on the nerve foramina, certain neurologic symptoms like loss of sense of smell, deafness or blindness may occur.

Expansile lesions of jaw bones are seen and radiographically show osteolytic and mixed radioopaque, radiolucent lesions.

Management:

Though no specific treatment exists for this condition, certain drugs that block the estrogen production like testolactone have been tried with some amount of success. In Cushing's syndrome, surgery is done to remove the adrenal glands.Gigantism and pituitary adenoma may be treated with hormone inhibitors or surgery.There are no specific medications to treat the bony lesions.The role of anti-resorptive agents like alendronate and bisphosphonates have been tried which have a palliative effect due to their pain controlling feature, in this disease.

Calcium, vitamin D and phosphorus supplements may be useful in some patients.

Surgery is helpful to prevent and treat fracture and deformities.

Trans-sphenoidal surgery remains difficult due to severe thickening of the base of the skull.

Irradiation should be avoided unless important, as it may lead to sarcomatous degeneration.

Gonado-tropin releasing hormones donot have any effect on the precocious puberty associated with this syndrome and the short acting aromatase inhibitors have limited effects.The results with the use of bromocriptine, abergoline, octreotide or their combination have shown inconsistent results.

Hormone replacement therapy can treat the Hypogonadism.

Aggressive treatment with oral phosphorous replacement is useful for treating hypophosphatemia with hyperphosphaturia.

Sufficient doses of calcium supplementation, phosphate repletion and calcitriol administration can treat the hypophosphatemic rickets.

Treatment of oral manifestations:

Smaller lesions in mandible can be surgically removed completely, but the more extensive and diffuse lesions of the maxilla can make treatment with surgery difficult and may require extensive surgery.Though in some cases the disease tends to stabilise and stops enlarging with skeletal maturity, in some cases the lesions continue to grow though slowly especially in adults. Cosmetic deformity with associated psychologic problems or functional deformity may warrant surgical intervention in young patients.In such cases surgical contouring by bone reduction is done without attempts to remove the entire lesion.The cosmetic outcome is good but the regrowth of the lesion occurs over time.

Suggested reading:

1. Chapurlat RD, Orcel, PBest Pract Res Clin Rheumatol. 2008 Mar;22(1):55-69. Fibrous dysplasia of bone and McCune-Albright syndrome.
2. Christoforidis A, Maniadaki I, Stanhope R. McCune-Albright syndrome: growth hormone and prolactin hypersecretion. J Pediatr Endocrinol Metab. 2006 May. 19 Suppl 2:623-5.

Q 4) Argyria:

TNMGRU AUGUST 2005 (5 Marks)

Synonyms : Argyrosis.

This condition results due to prolonged contact with or injestion of silver salts.It is characterised by gray to grayish-black staining of the skin and mucous membrane due to deposition of silver.The deposition of silver can occur due to industrial exposure or injestion of medications containing silver salts.

Argyria may cause toxic effects on liver, kidney, spleen, intestinal tract and respiratory system.

Etiology:

- It is commonly caused due to impregnation of the skin or mucosa by small silver particles in the workers who are in silver mining and refining, silverware and metal alloy manufacturing, putting metallic films on glass and china, dealing with electroplating solutions and photographic processing.

- Dietary supplements of colloidal silver are used widely for cancer, AIDS, diabetes and herpetic infections.
- Some cases occur due to prolonged use of silver salts for nasal or urethral mucous membrane irrigation, in eye drops, wound dressing and extensive use of oral smoking remedy that contains silver acetate.
- Some cases of argyria are seen in dental and surgical procedures eg.amalgam tattoo, silver sutures used in abdominal surgery etc. blue macules can appear at sites of acupuncture needles and at sites of silver earrings.
- It occurs from local & systemic absorption of silver compounds. Silver present in certain nasal drops or sprays, used in the treatment of aphthous ulcer, silver arsphenamine injection used in the treatment of syphilis.
- Chewing pieces of photographic films over extended period can also result in argyria.
- Industrial exposure.

Clinical Features:

- In the early stages, gray-brown staining of the gingiva develops and later progresses to involve the skin diffusely.The skin pigmentation appears slate-gray, metallic or blue-gray in colour and generally is apparent clinically after a few months.The clinical appearance of this condition usually takes many years and depends on the degree of exposure.
- The skin exposed to sun especially the forehead, nose and hands shows the hyperpigmentation to the greatest extent.
- In some cases the large areas of skin may acquire a slate-blue colour.
- Hyperpigmentation may be seen in the sclerae, nail beds and mucous membranes.
- During abdominal surgery or post mortem examination, the viscera may show a blue discolouration, including the spleen, liver and gut.

Oral manifestations:

- diffuse pigmentation of the gingiva & mucosal tissue.
- stale blue line along the gingival margin.
- diffuse bluish back discolouration of the oral mucosa seen.

Treatment:

5% hydroquinone treatment may reduce the number of silver granules within the upper dermis and surrounding the sweat glands and reduce the number of melanocytes.

Chelation therapy to remove silver granules have proven unsuccessful.

Sun screens and certain other opaque cosmetics may help in preventing further darkening of the pigment and help in masking the discolouration.

Selenium and sulfur form complexes with silver and have favourable modifying effects on the metabolism and toxicity .Silver selenide is highly insoluble in vivo and thus reduces the availability of mono-valent silver to interfere with normal enzymatic activities in the tissues.The silver-sulfur complexes that are formed in vivo are not as stable as silver-selenium complexes.

Suggested reading:

1. Brad W. Neville, Douglas D. Damm, Angela C. Chi, Carl M. Allen, Oral and Maxillofacial Pathology, 288.
2. Gaslin MT, Rubin C, Pribitkin EA. Silver nasal sprays: misleading Internet marketing. Ear Nose Throat J. 2008 Apr. 87(4):217-20.
3. Menaguale G, Fazio R, Fazio M. Argyria: a case following the prolonged use of a rhinologic drug. Esper Dermatol (Roma). 2003. 4:299-303

Q 5) Melanoma:

TNMGRU AUGUST 2016 (5 Marks)

Also known as melanocarcinoma.

It is a malignant neoplasm of melanocytic origin.

It is the third most common cancer of the skin and rarely involves the oral mucosa about 0.2%-8% of all melanomas.

There is a dramatic increase in incidences of melanoma and it is continuing. In men the incidence is increasing rapidly than any other malignancy and in women rapidly than other malignancies except lung cancer. The median age at diagnosis is 59 years. Therefore, melanoma ranks second to adult leukemia in terms of loss of years of potential life, per death.

Risk factors:

A positive family history of melanoma, prior melanoma, multiple clinically atypical moles or dysplastic nevi.

Inherited genetic mutations.

Sun exposure may also contribute to the development of melanoma.

Individuals with an inability to tan and fair skin that sunburns easily have a greater risk of developing melanoma.

However, melanoma can occur in any ethnic group and also in areas of the body without substantial sun exposure.

Clinical features:

- More common in men and average age group is 40-70 years.
- Most frequent site in the oral cavity is the palate and maxillary gingiva.
- It develops slowly into a well defined, elevated pigmented patch.It is tan, brown or blackish in colour.

- Can appear as a nodular pigmented lesion on skin and mucous membrane or flat pigmented patch known as lentigo-maligna.

Oral manifestations:

- Occurs most commonly on the palate and the maxillary gingiva.
- In the oral cavity it begins as a brown to blackish macule with irregular borders. May become nodular and also grows laterally.
- Ulceration may or may not occur and they exist as dark brown or black lobulated exophytic masses.
- They are usually painless unless ulcerated and are relatively soft on palpation.

Radiological features:

When melanomas affect the jaws the radiographic features are almost similar to osteomyelitis.

It appears as areas of irregular bone destruction giving a moth eaten appearance.

Differential diagnosis:

- Melanotic macule: The irregular borders, colour variations, asymmetry and diameter greater than 0.5 cms helps in differentiating.
- Ecchymotic patch: It disappears in a few days.
- Melanoplakia: It occurs in infancy and appears as a firm patch without change.
- Intramucosal blue nevus: It can be differentiated as a melanotic macule is differentiated.
- Pigmented fibroma: Biopsy will help in diagnosis.

Management:

- Surgical excision along with regional lymph nodes dissection in case of their involvement.
- Patients unable to undergo surgery are treated with radiotherapy.
- Preoperative radiotherapy is given to reduce the size of the tumour for better management before surgical excision. The commonly used chemotherapeutic agents are, dimethyltiazeno, imidazole carboxamide, solely or in combination with vincristine or dactynomycin. Other immunotherapeutic drugs used are Interferon and cimetidine.
- Intra lesional injections of interferon and polyvalent melanoma antigen vaccine.

Suggested reading:

1. Anil Govinrao Ghom, Textbook Of Oral Medicine, 3rd edition, 464-465.
2. Coit DG, Andtbacka R, Anker CJ, Bichakjian CK, Carson WE 3rd, Daud A, Dilawari RA, Dimaio D, Guild V, Halpern AC, Hodi FS Jr, Kelley MC, Khushalani NI, Kudchadkar RR, Lange JR, Lind A, Martini MC, Olszanski AJ, Pruitt SK, Ross MI, Swetter SM, Tanabe KK, Thompson JA, Trisal V, Urist MM; Melanoma, J Natl Compr Canc Netw. 2012 Mar; 10(3):366-400.

CHAPTER 13

Diseases of Tongue

Introduction:

Tongue is an important organ of the oral cavity.It has several functions like speech, deglutition, mastication, taste, digestion, jaw development, maintenance of oral hygiene, defense mechanism , sucking, thermal regulation etc.The tongue may be affected in oral disease or even in systemic disorders and it is referred to as mirror of oral and general health. It is composed of body which is movable and base which is attached.It is important to understand and recognise diseases affecting the tongue.

Q 1) Benign migratory glossitis:

SEPTEMBER 2002 TNMGRU (5 Marks)

This condition is referred by terms like geographic tongue, erythema migrans, and benign migratory glossitis etc.and is a benign condition that affects the dorsum of the tongue primarily.

So called because the circinate lesions keep shifting locations on the tongue by healing of old lesion and formation of new one at another place.

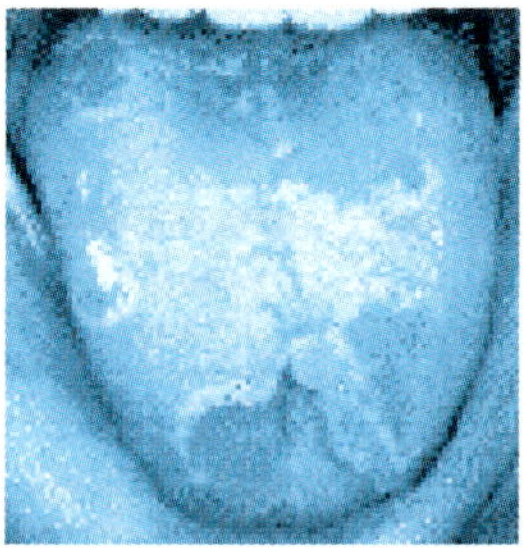

Fig. Circinate lesions with white borders

Etiology:

- Although it is an inflammatory condition it is seen in clusters in families and hence Genetic predisposition is considered.
- Its association with HLA-DRW6 and HLA-Cw6 has been reported.
- It is quite often seen with high frequency in patients with psoriasis, fissured tongue and chronic granulomatous diseases.

- Stress
- Hormonal changes.
- Vitamin deficiency.
- Excessive consumption of processed, spicy and acidic foods.
- Allergies and asthma.

Clinical Features:

- The general population up to 3% is seen to be affected.
- Areas of atrophy surrounded by grayish or whitish margins give a map like appearance and hence called geographic tongue.
- The terms such as geographic stomatitis, stomatitis erythema migrans, ectopic geographic tongue etc are used when other mucosal surfaces in addition to the tongue surface like the ventral surface of tongue, buccal mucosa, soft palate, floor of the mouth, lips are involved.
- The lesions in this condition may start as a white patch, prior to the occurrence of depapillation. Though a single lesion can be present, it is usual to have multiple lesions on the tongue and they coalesce in some time to give a map like appearance.
- Though the lesions are usually asymptomatic, in some cases there can be increased sensitivity to hot and spicy food.
- Though it doesnot cause pain it does cause a feeling of tingling and numbness.
- Geographic tongue affects both males and females and occurs more commonly in adults than children.
- Females are more prone, almost three times as commonly than males.
- The typical appearance of this lesion is an area of erythema, with atrophy of filliform papillae, surrounded by a white serpiginous, hyperkeratotic border.
- There could be spontaneous resolution of one lesion followed by occurrence of another lesion in another location on the tongue.
- The activity of the lesions could increase or decrease with time and the patients may have lesion free intervals.
- It occurs more commonly in patients with psoriasis, fissured tongue and chronic granulomatous diseases.
- The lesions may appear annular, circinate or serpiginous, having depressed atrophic centers, are devoid of filliform papillae and have raised white borders.
- Histopathology:
- Hyperkeratosis.
- Acanthosis.
- T lymphocyte inflammatory infiltration in the sub epithelium.
- Neutrophilic granulocyte migration in the epithelial layer, creating superficial microabscesses, which are similar to Munro's microabscesses that are described in pustular psoriasis.

Differential diagnosis:

- Cancers of the Oral Mucosa: Typical induration and biopsy will help in diagnosis.
- Chemical Burns: History of keeping tablet or ingestion of some chemicals can be elicited.
- Contact Stomatitis: Absence of map like lesions and history of contact with allergens can help differentiate.
- Fissured Tongue: The typical fissures will help in diagnosis.
- Lichen Planus: Presence of white lacy pattern and wickham's striae will help in diagnosis.
- Mucosal Candidiasis: These lesions can be easily scraped off and smears will show candidal hyphae.
- Plaque Psoriasis: Skin lesions will also be present which is not the case in geographic tongue.

Treatment:

Though most of the lesions are asymptomatic, in cases of burning and pain over the counter analgesic and anti-inflammatory drugs can be used.

Topical steroids and tacrolimus, have shown beneficial results.

As it is seen to occur following stress anxiolytics can also be given.

Topical anesthetics to relieve pain and zinc supplements are given.

Treatment with cyclosporin and topical antihistaminics have been successful giving good results according to some studies.

Mouth rinses with anesthetics.

It is best to avoid tobacco, spicy foods, acidic foods and nuts.

Suggested reading:

1. Kleinman DV, Swango PA, Pindborg JJ. Epidemiology of oral mucosal lesions in United States schoolchildren: 1986-87. Community Dent Oral Epidemiol. 1994 Aug. 22(4):243-53.
2. Shulman JD. Prevalence of oral mucosal lesions in children and youths in the USA. Int J Paediatr Dent. 2005 Mar. 15(2):89-97.
3. Sigal MJ, Mock D. Symptomatic benign migratory glossitis: report of two cases and literature review.Pediatr Dent. 1992 Nov-Dec. 14(6):392-6.
4. Zargari O. The prevalence and significance of fissured tongue and geographical tongue in psoriatic patients. Clin Exp Dermatol. 2006 Mar. 31(2):192-5.

Q 2) Melkersson-Rosenthal syndrome:

RGUHS APRIL 1998 (5 Marks)

This syndrome is a neurological disorder that is rare and of unknown etiology which is characterised by triad of:

- Swelling of the face and lip, especially the upper lip and is recurrent.
- Recurrent facial paralysis.
- Fissured tongue.

There is firm edema of the face and fissured, reddish brown, swollen, non-pruritic lips.

The facial palsy is similar to Bell's palsy.

The fissured tongue is manifested in $1/3^{rd}$ to 50% of cases and is least common of the features, but when present, very helpful in diagnosis.All the three features are rarely present together, making diagnosis difficult.

Though the exact cause is unknown, genetic predisposition could play a role. It has been found to be prevalent in the ethnic groups in Bolivia.

Various theories put forth to explain the origin of this syndrome include allergic reaction, syphilis, lymphogranuloma inguinale, basal arachnoiditis, benign lymphogranulomatosis and bacterial infection of the oral cavity or oropharynx.

However, all these have failed to explain the peculiar manifestations of this syndrome and hence the exact aetiology still remains obscure.

Neurologic dysfunction and autonomic imbalance are suggested etiological factors.

Clinical features:

- This syndrome commonly affects females and is seen usually in the second decade of life.
- Onset can be in childhood or early adolescence. The edema is non-tender and non-pitting and the skin appears darker than normal.
- It commonly affects the lips and may be unilateral or bilateral.
- After recurrence of attacks the swelling may coexist and increase in size and could become permanent.The lip may become, hard, fissured and cracked resulting in a reddish brown discolouration.
- The lingua plicata is considered by some to be a congenital stigma and not the result of the oedema.
- The most dominant manifestation of MRS is facial edema, which is acute, painless and mostly confined to the lips. The upper lip seems to be affected more frequently, and the edema tends to be recurrent and lasts from hours to several weeks. It usually mimics angioedema, but is more persistent than it and it does not respond to the antihistaminics and can lead to fibrosis of the involved tissues.
- Facial paralysis associated with MRS may occur months to years before or after the onset of facial edema. Peripheral facial paralysis may be unilateral or bilateral, and it may be partial or complete.
- Lingua plicata has been accepted to be congenital in 30% to 80% of the reported patients. This anomaly is present in only 0.5% to 5% of the general population, and it is considered a developmental malformation.
- A monosymptomatic variant of Melkersson-Rosenthal syndrome (MRS) is the Cheilitis granulomatosa of Miescher.
- Histopathology shows non-caseating, sarcoidal granulomas which support the diagnosis.As these granulomas are not always present, their absence cannot exclude the diagnosis of this syndrome.Thus MRS is a disorder with elements of oro-facial granulomatosis.

Treatment:

Several modalities of treatment like thalidomide 100 mgs daily for 3-6 months and steroids both systemic and intralesional.

Long-term remission after three-intralesional administration of triamcinolone has been observed.

Recently, oral Clofazimine has been successfully used.

Symptomatic treatment could include NSAIDs and steroids to reduce the swelling, antibiotics and immunosuppressants.

Though surgery could be attempted to reduce the pressure on facial nerve and decrease the swelling, its effectiveness is uncertain.

Electrical stimulation and massage could be advised.

Laser beam acupuncture using the traditional chinese medicine could be helpful.

Suggested reading:

1. Bachi T. Hathiram, D. S. GrewaP, Rohan Waivekar, Ashwin Dwivedi, Lovneesh Kumar s, Alok Mohorikar:The melkersson - rosenthal syndrome as a rare cause of facial nerve palsy - a case report, Indian Journal of Otolaryngology and Head and Neck Surgery Vol. 52 No. 4, 375-376, October - December 2000.
2. Andreea Liana Răchişan, A. Hruşcă, D. Gheban, Simona Căinap, T. L. Pop, A. Băican, L. Fodor, N. Miu, Mariana Andreica :Granulomatous cheilitis of Miescher: the diagnostic proof for a Melkersson–Rosenthal syndrome- case report, Rom J Morphol Embryol 2012, 53(3 Suppl):851–853.
3. James, William D.; Berger, Timothy G.; et al Melkersson-Rosenthal syndrome and orofacial granulomatosis: Andrews' Diseases of the Skin: Clinical Dermatology. Saunders Elsevier.
4. Rogers RS 3rd, Melkersson-Rosenthal syndrome and orofacial granulomatosis. Dermatol Clin. 1996 Apr; 14(2):371-9.

Q 3) Differential diagnosis of depapillation of tongue:

TNMGRU FEBRUARY 2012 (5 Marks)

I) Local causes of depapillation:

(i) **Traumatic injuries:** The tongue could be repeatedly traumatised either mechanically or chemically.Mechanical injuries include sharp teeth, rough margins of restorations, and broken restorations can cause ulcers and depapillation.
Chemicals such as phenol and eugenol can come in contact with tongue and cause localised area of depapillation.
Prolonged intubation, cotton roll ulcers, and trauma during epileptic seizures can cause depapillation.
Proper history and clinical examination will help in diagnosis.

(ii) **Traumatic granuloma(ulcerated granuloma eosinophilicum diutinum)**: It can occur at any age and is located on dorsum, margin or inferior surface of tongue, and is characterised by well demarcated proliferative ulceration covered by thick masses of fibrin and debris.Can be confused with squamous cell carcinoma, but it is not indurated and spontaneous remissions can occur.

(iii) **Selfinflicted bites:** Can cause ulceration and depapillation especially in mentally handicapped patients.

(iv) **Allergic stomatitis:** Hypersensitivity reactions to antibiotics, chemotherapy, anticholinergics and other allergy causing materials like monomer of denture, mouth washes, chewing gum, lipstick etc can cause edema and depapillation.The edema associated with atrophy of tongue and previous history of allergy to the above agents can help in diagnosis.

(v) Facial hemiatrophy is associated with atrophy of half part of the tongue.

(vi) **Cranial arteritis:** Seen in elderly patients, can lead to painful ulceration and gangrene of the tongue due to arteritis.The associated symptoms of fever, sweating, malaise, anorexia and weight loss and old age of patients can help in diagnosis.

(vii) **Chronic candidiasis:** Chronic atrophic candidiasis can cause depapillation of tongue.Scraping and cytological examination can help diagnose candidiasis.

(viii) **Benign migratory glossitis:** Benign migratory glossitis (BMG) is an intraoral benign condition of dorsal tongue, and is usually asymptomatic. Clinically it appears as red patches, which peripherally are often surrounded by well defined, raised, yellowish white lines on the dorsum of the tongue. The red patches are the depapillated filiform papillae.The frequent change in locations of the lesions by healing in one area and beginning in the other helps in diagnosis.

(ix) **Median Rhomboid Glossitis:** It is a condition characterised by an area of redness and atrophy of lingual papilla, which is seen on the dorsum of the tongue in the midline immediately in front of the circumvallate papillae.It is thought to be caused by a chronic fungal infection.It is thought to be a type of oral candidiasis.The rhomboid shape and location helps in diagnosis.

II) Systemic causes:

(i) **Iron deficiency anemia**: Atrophic changes on the dorsum of the tongue can occur and in severe cases can cause bald, smooth, painful fiery red tongue.

(ii) **Plummer Vinson syndrome:** Can cause, red or pale, painful, fissured tongue, and atrophic glossitis.Presence of other symptoms like dysphagia and spoon shaped nails can help in diagnosis.

(iii) **Pernicious anemia:** There can be complete atrophy of tongue and it may become flabby.There is generalised weakness, burning of mouth, and along with changes in blood tests can be diagnosed .

(iv) **Niacin deficiency:** Results in pellagra.There is fiery red tongue which is atrophic.Later on the tongue can become swollen and indentations of teeth along the lateral border of the tongue can be seen.

(v) **Folic acid deficiency:** There can be severe atrophy with loss of filliform and fungiform papillae.The tongue can swell and small cracks may appear on the dorsum of the tongue.

(vi) **Scleroderma:** There is scarred, shrunken and atrophic appearance of tongue, due to fibrosis of submucosal tissue due to obliteration of small blood vessels.The tongue loses mobility and becomes stiff which is typical of scleroderma.

(vii) **Lupus erythematosus:** Irregular areas of atrophy and ulceration caused by arteritis are typical of this condition.

(viii) **Polymyositis:** It is a syndrome consisting of polymyositis and associated with skin lesions.In early stages tongue is very much swollen and later becomes harder and atrophic.

(ix) **Diabetes:** Due to vascular changes associated with diabetes, it results in atrophic glossitis.Central papillary atrophy of the dorsum just anterior to the row of circumvallate papillae is typical of atrophic tongue associated with diabetes.

(x) **Syphillis:** Depapillation is seen in the secondary and tertiary stage of syphilis.Gumma may also form. The typical clinical features and signs can help in diagnosing syphilitic tongue atrophy.

(xi) **Herpes zoster:** Unilateral vesicles along the ventral surface of the tongue associated with atrophy can be seen.

(xii) **Tuberculosis:** There is ulceration with irregular outline and undermined margins and thus atrophy, which can be seen on the dorsum of the tongue in tuberculosis.

Suggested reading:

1. Anil Govindrao Ghom, Text Book Of Oral Medicine, Third Edition, 514-515.
2. Daud Mirza, Navid Rashid Qureshi, Kashif Naqvi, Benign Migratory Glossitis An Unusual Enigmatic Lesion, Pakistan Oral & Dental Journal Vol 33, No. 3 (December 2013).
3. Rapini, Ronald P.; Bolognia, Jean L.; Jorizzo, Joseph L. (2007).Dermatology: 2-Volume Set. St. Louis: Mosby.

Q 4) Glossodynia:

TNMGRU AUGUST 2014 (5 Marks)

Glossodynia means pain in the tongue. Many a times it is considered as burning mouth syndrome and is described as such.However according to certain literature glossodynia is considered a separate entity especially when it is not associated with xerostomia or altered taste sensation as is seen in cases of burning mouth syndrome.

It is thus being discussed as a separate condition from burning mouth syndrome.

Etiology:

Local factors:

- Habits: Excessive use of tobacco, alcohol, uncontrolled movements of the tongue, or bruxism.
- Dental causes: Dentures, irritating clasps, or fixed bridges.
- Referred pain: Especially from infected teeth and tonsils.
- Tongue disorders: Geographic tongue, lichen planus involving tongue, and median rhomboid glossitis can cause glossodynia.

- Electrogalvanic currents: Presence of dissimilar metals in the oral cavity can result in painful tongue due to production of electrogalvanic currents.
- Atherosclerotic changes in the lingual arteries can cause glossodynia.
- Allergic reactions: Various agents like food, mouth washes, metals of restorations, denture base materials, and dentifrices can cause allergic reactions and glossodynia.

Systemic factors:

Diseases like multiple myeloma, amyloidosis, pellagra, vitamin B deficiency, diabetes can cause glossodynia.Gastrointestinal disturbances, prolonged antibiotic therapy, psychological problems, xerostomia can also cause glossodynia.

Neurological factors:

Trigeminal neuralgia, glossopharyngeal neuralgia, damage to lingual nerve due to surgery can cause glossodynia.

Idiopathic:

Where no particular cause can be identified .In such cases it could be due to depression or neurosis.

Clinical Features:

The symptoms vary and could be described as painful, burning or tingling sensation or numbness of tongue. It could be a singular symptom or one among a group of symptoms.

Clinically observable changes on the tongue may or may not occur.

Management:

- Removing the causative factor could be the best form of treatment.
- Muscle relaxants and sedatives could help reduce the symptoms.
- Treatment of underlying systemic causes can help resolve the symptoms.
- Topical use of 0.5% diphenhydramine hydrochloride alone or in combination of lidocaine cream can give relief.
- Treatment with olanzapine showed complete relief from pain in some studies.
- Use of Topiramate, an anticonvulsant drug has shown very good results for glossodynia.

Suggested reading:

1. Anil Govindrao Ghom, text book of oral medicine, 3rd edition, 516.
2. Gick CL Mirowski GW, Kennedy JS, Bymaster FP, Treatment of glossodynia with olanzapine, J Am Acad Dermatol. 2004 Sep; 51(3):463-5.

Q 5) Developmental anomalies of tongue:

MUHS MAY 2015 (3 Marks)

Developmental anomalies include:

Cleft, bifurcated, tetrafurcated and lobed tongue:

- Bifurcation of tip of the tongue is sometimes seen in apparently normal individuals.
- Clefting of anterior 2/3rd of the tongue is rare and usually associated with defined congenital syndromes.
- Lobulated tongue is usually associated with lingual hamartomas.

Ankyloglossia:

- There is absent or shortened lingual frenum.Causes difficulty in sucking and swallowing.May also lead to traumatic ulcerations and reduced self cleaning activity.

Macroglossia:

Large tongue is component of various syndrome.

True macroglossia is seen in:

(i) Cretinism.
(ii) Mongolism.
(iii) Amyloidosis.
(iv) Hemangioma.
(v) Lymphangioma of tongue with cystic hygroma is the most common of congenital macroglossia.

Can cause slurred speech and defective development of maxilla and mandible.

Aglossia (Hypoglossia):

Aglossia is a condition which is a congenital defect and can have partially developed or complete absence of tongue.It is often associated with craniofacial and limb defects. It is thought to belong to a family of oro-mandibular limb hypogenesis syndrome.Heat induced vascular dysruption near the fourth week of embryonic development is thought to be the cause.

Fissured tongue:

It is a developmental variation where in several deep fissures are seen on the dorsal surface of the tongue.It often goes unnoticed unless there is trauma or infection causing pain and burning sensation. It is an important feature of Melkersson-Rosenthal syndrome.

Bald or depapillated tongue:

Depapillation or absence of fungiform and vallate papillae could be caused due to congenital anomaly or may develop as a secondary feature.

Localised enlargement and papillomatosis:

In some congenital disorders, the surface of the tongue dorsum is either papilomatous or may exhibit other localised enlargements.When severe may be described as pebbly, cobblestoned or lumpy tongue.

Suggested reading:

1. Burket's Oral Medicine Diagnosis And Treatment, 9th edition, 256-257.

CHAPTER 14

Gingival and Periodontal Diseases

Introduction:

Gingival and periodontal diseases are the most common maladies witnessed by a dental clinician.They have been found to be a major cause of tooth loss after dental caries.

Periodontal disease appears to be a global public health problem affecting adults after the age of 35 to 40 years.The disease starts as gingivitis and if left untreated leads to a progressive periodontitis. More than 90% of variance in severity of periodontal diseases can be attributed to age and oral hygiene.

It is important for dental clinicians to have knowledge about the local and systemic causes of these conditions so that they can be treated effectively.

Q 1) Drugs causing gingival enlargement:

RGUHS APRIL 2003 (2 Marks)

Certain drugs are known to cause gingival enlargement. Drug Induced Gingival enlargement was reported first by Kimball in 1939, associated with chronic usage of the anti-epileptic drug Phenytoin.

The drugs that are implicated in Gingival enlargement are:

1. **Anticonvulsants:** Phenytoin, sodium valproate, phenobarbitone, vigabatrin. primidone, mehenytoin, ethotoin, ethosuximide, methosuximide.
2. **Immunosuppressants:** Cyclosporin, tacrolimus, sirolimus.
3. **Calcium channel blockers**: Nifedipine, Diltiazem, Felodipine, Nitrendopine, Verapamil, Amlodipine, Nicardipine.
4. **Miscellaneous:** Erythromycin, Cannabis, Pencillium, Eltroxin, dilitazem, sertraline.

1) Phenytoin induced gingival enlargement:

- This antiepileptic drug most commonly causes gingival enlargement.
- Gingival enlargement may begin as early as two weeks after the Dilantin therapy.

- The enlargement is usually generalized throughout the mouth being most severe in the maxillary and mandibular anterior regions. It occurs in areas in which teeth are present, not in edentulous spaces, and there is disappearance of the enlargement in areas of extracted teeth.
- The gingival enlargement begins as a bead like growth which is painless involving the inter-dental papilla and then gradually extends to the facial and lingual gingival margins.
- The surface of gingiva shows an increase in stippling and finally a cauliflower like, warty or pebbled surface.
- With the progress of the condition, the marginal and papillary enlargements fuse and could develop into massive tissue fold that may cover a considerable portion of the crown and also interfere with occlusion.
- The enlargement characteristically appears to project from beneath the gingival margin, from which it is separated by a linear groove. The enlargement is chronic and slowly increases in size. When surgically removed, it recurs.
- Spontaneous disappearance occurs within a few months after discontinuation of the drug.

2) Cyclosporin induced gingival enlargement:

It is an immunosuppressive agent administered intravenously or by mouth and dosages greater than 500mg/day has been reported to induce gingival enlargement.

- It is more vascularized than the Dilantin induced gingival overgrowth.
- Occurs in approx 30% of patients receiving the drug.
- More frequent in children.
- Clinically it is similar as seen in Dilantin induced gingival enlargement.
- The lesion is mulberry shaped, firm, pale pink in colour and resilient with minute lobules on the surface till it is not complicated by inflammation with little tendency to bleed.
- Mandibular incisors and canines have higher rate of gingival enlargement than other teeth.
- Papillary gingiva more affected than marginal gingiva.

3) Calcium channel blockers induced gingival enlargement (Nifedipine)

- Nifedepine, the most commonly used, induces GE in 20% of the cases.
- Clinically it is similar as seen in Dilantin induced gingival enlargement.

4) Erythromycin and certain hormone may also cause gingival enlargement similar to those caused by anticonvulsants antihypertensives and imunosuppressants.

5) The other drugs in the miscellaneous category may also cause gingival enlargement.

Suggested reading:

1. Anil Govindrao Ghom, Textbook of oral medicine, 3rd edition. Page no. 546-7.
2. Vipin Bharti, Chhaya Bansal, Drug-induced gingival overgrowth: The nemesis of gingiva unravelled, J Indian Soc Periodontol. 2013 Mar-Apr; 17(2): 182–187.

Q 2) Gingival hyperplasia:

RGUHS APRIL 2006 (2 Marks)

Gingival hyperplasia is defined as increase in number of gingival epithelial cells.

Classification:

A) Depending on the etiologic factors and pathologic changes:

I) Inflammatory Hyperplasia:

(a) chronic

(b) Acute

The formation and collection along with the retention of plaque is the main cause of inflammatory gingival enlargement.Poor oral hygiene, improper restorations causing irritation of the gingiva and orthodontic appliances are the risk factors.

Mouth breathers often suffer from gingivitis and enlargement due to irritation caused by surface dehydration.

Chronic inflammatory gingival enlargement is most common and in such cases the gingivae are soft and discoloured.The reason is edema of the tissues and infective cellular infiltration caused due to prolonged exposure to the bacterial plaque and these cases are treated by conventional scaling and root planing.

II) Drug induced hyperplasia: They can be basically caused due to three groups of drugs:

Anticonvulsant drugs:

Phenobarbital, phenytoin, lamotrigine, vigabatrin etc.

Calcium channel blockers:

- Antihypertensive medications that include nifedipine, amlodipine, and verapamil.
- Cyclosporin, which is an immunosuppresant.

III) Systemic disease associated hyperplasia:

a) Conditioned gingival enlargement:

1. Pregnancy.
2. Puberty.
3. Vitamin C deficiency.
4. Plasma cell gingivitis.
5. Pyogenic granuloma which is a non-specific conditioned enlargement.

b) Systemic diseases:

(i) Leukemia:

(ii) Granulomatous diseases: Sarcoidosis, orofacial granulomas, granulomatosis with polyangitis.

IV) **Neoplastic enlargement:**
   (a) Benign tumors: Fibromas, papillomas, giant cell granuloma.
   (b) Malignant tumors: such as a carcinoma or malignant melanoma.

V) **False enlargement:** In case of underlying bony or dental tissue lesion.

B) According to location and distribution:

Localized: gingival enlargement limited to one or more teeth.
Generalized: entire mouth gingiva is enlarged.
Marginal: limited to marginal gingiva.
Papillary: Which is confined to the interdental papilla.
Diffuse: Involving all parts of gingiva.
Discrete: Isolated sessile or pedunculated tumor like enlargement.

Q 3) Mobility of tooth:

RGUHS APRIL 2003 (2 Marks)

Tooth has the tendency for a slight degree of physiologic mobility which varies between different teeth at different times of the day.

Mobility beyond the physiologic range is called abnormal or pathologic mobility.

Thus tooth mobility can be defined as the movement of tooth in its socket resulting from applied force.

Normal physiologic mobility of tooth of about 0.25mm is considered normal.The reason is that the tooth is not fused to the bone but is connected to the socket through the periodontal ligament. The slight mobility, the tooth possesses is to accommodate the forces acting on teeth during chewing without causing any damage.Tooth mobility becomes abnormal when the attachment of the periodontal ligament to the tooth is reduced. or if the periodontal ligament is inflammed.

Classification by Preston D. Miller:

- Class 0: Normal movement when force is applied.
- Class 1: Less than 1mm(horizontal)
- Class 2: More than 1mm(horizontal) and inability to depress in vertical direction.
- Class 3 : More than 1mm(horizontal+vertical mobility)

Etiology:

1. The most common cause is periodontal disease.It is a painless, slowly progressing, bone loss around the tooth.It worsens by smoking and improves by maintaining oral hygiene above and below the gingival line.
2. Apical alveolar abscesses can cause bone resorption and loss of attachment. If the abscess is treatable then the loss of attachment can be restored, if not the condition could be permanent.
3. **Trauma from occlusion:** Results in mobility of teeth. It occurs initially as a result of resorption of cortical layer of bone which leads

to reduced fiber support and later leads to widened periodontal ligament space.

4. **Loss of tooth support:** mobility depends on severity and distribution of bone loss.
5. **Inflammation:** extension of inflammation from gingiva or periapical region into the periodontal ligament space may lead to mobility.
6. Periodontal surgery may temporarily increase tooth mobility.
7. Some systemic diseases, pregnancy, conditions like langerhan's cell histiocytosis can cause tooth mobility.
8. Destruction of surrounding alveolar bone due to osteomyelitis or tumours of the alveolus and other oral squamous cell carcinomas can lead to mobility of teeth.
9. Bruxism can cause aggravation of loss of attachment and tooth mobility especially if periodontal disease is present.Once the bruxism is controlled, the tooth mobility will reverse and become stable.
10. **Trauma to teeth:** Luxations, fractures of teeth can result in sudden mobility after a blow.
11. High biting force on one tooth can cause temporary mobility but once corrected the tooth can become stable. Another reason could be a filling or crown restoration which is a little high and prominent in the bite, if not corrected can lead to periodontal pain in that or the opposing tooth and mobility.

Radiographic features:

1. PDL space widening:- widening of PDL space and single root may develop an hourglass shape.In multirooted teeth widening of the periodontal ligament space at apices and in the region of furcation is seen.
2. Angular bone loss: bone loss which surrounds the tooth is also present.

Treatment:

- Control of inflammation and its causes.
- Occlusal adjustment and splinting to stabilize the tooth.
- Treatment of infections like osteomyelitis and periodontitis.
- Treatment of trauma from occlusion.
- Appliances to correct bruxism.
- After filling, if high points are present, they should be reduced.

Suggested reading:

1. Anil Govindrao Ghom, Textbook Of Oral Medicine, 3rd Edition, 561.
2. Odell EW (Editor) (2010). Clinical problem solving in dentistry (3rd ed.). Edinburgh: Churchill Livingstone.

Q 4) Scorbutic gingivitis:

TNMGRU APRIL 2000 (5 Marks)

Scurvy is a disease resulting from a deficiency of vitamin C, which is required for the synthesis of collagen in humans.

Scorbutic gingivitis is a condition caused by severe vitamin C deficiency leading to severe periodontal condition which is characterised by ulcerative gingivitis and rapid periodontal pocket development leading to tooth exfoliation.

There is often fetid odour and poor oral hygiene.

Although vitamin C deficiency is a rarity today, in case of lack of fresh fruits and vegetables in the dietary intake can lead to this condition.

Etiology:

(i) It is seen in elderly people who are alcoholics, smokers or drug addicts.
(ii) Seen in people staying in warm climatic areas.
(iii) This generally leads to lack of availability of fresh fruits and vegetables.
(iv) Along with these factors, it affects people who are socially and financially compromised and have poor dietary intake.

Oral manifestations:

- Interdental and marginal gingiva is swollen, bright red, shiny, smooth and bleeds easily.
- There is gingival bleeding on slightest provocation and can result in haemorrhages, purpura and bruising.
- Scurvy siderosis is a condition in which there is general discolouration which results from bleeding and breakdown of blood.
- Severe periodontal pocket formation and ulcerative gingivitis causing tooth exfoliation occurs.
- Poor oral hygiene with fetid breath is present.
- Severe pain can interfere with normal food intake as there is difficulty in chewing and eating spicy food.
- In severe case hemorrhage, periodontal ligament space widening followed by loss of bone can be seen.
- Anemia in scurvy is mild to moderate but can be severe.

Diagnosis:

This condition can be misdiagnosed as vasulitis, ulcerative gingivitis or blood dyscrasias.

However a thorough physical examination, proper past medical and dietary history in combination with blood examination and histopathologic tests can help in diagnosis.

Histopathology:

There is intra-epidermal vesicles and spongiosis involving the squamous epithelium.There are also koilocytic changes. In the deeper connective tissue there is increased vascularity and acute or chronic inflammatory exudation.Some areas can show subepithelial hemorrhages and fibrin thrombi in capillaries.

Management:

- Antibiotics: Metronidazole 400mg, amoxycillin 500mg and

ibuprofen 400mg is given for 5 days. Vitamin C supplements 250mg QID for 2 weeks is also included.

- The necrotic slough is slowly and gently swabbed with 3% hydrogen peroxide solution and thus removed.
- Irrigation with solution containing povidone and iodine is done.
- The superficial calculus and other deposits are gently removed with curettes without hurting the gingiva.
- Scaling and root planing of the subgingiva is done when the patient is recalled after 1 week.
- Counseling of the patient is done for proper oral hygiene maintenance and is explained the importance of including fruits and vegetables in the diet.

Suggested reading:

1. Sharanabasappa R. Japatti, Anuradha Bhatsange, Manjunath Reddy, Y.S. Chidambar, Satish Patil, and Priyanka Vhanmane Scurvy-scorbutic siderosis of gingiva: A diagnostic challenge - A rare case report Dent Res J (Isfahan). 2013 May-Jun; 10(3): 394–400.
2. Touyz LZ S Vitamin C, oral scurvy and periodontal disease. Afr Med J. 1984 May 26; 65(21):838-42.

CHAPTER 15

Granulomatous Diseases

Q 1) Heerfordt's syndrome:

RGUHS OCTOBER 2002 (5 Marks)

Definition:

This syndrome is a rare manifestation of sarcoidosis and is also referred as, uveoparotid fever, Heerfordt-Mylius, Heerfordt-Waldenstrom syndrome etc.The symptoms consist of uveitis, swelling of the parotids plus or minus other salivary/lacrimal glands, chronic fever and in some cases palsy, of the facial nerves.

Paralysis of the facial nerve may be a feature but is not necessary to confirm the diagnosis.

Sarcoidosis occurs throughout the world, affecting individuals of all ages, genders and race. This syndrome shows a predilection for adults below 40 years and there is a peak incidence in ages 20-29 years.

Etiology:

Though the exact cause is not known, it is thought to be a combination of an environmental agent and hereditary predisposition.Though inconclusive, the mycobacterium and propionibacteria species have been implicated as the environment agent in this syndrome.

The prevalence of sarcoidosis is about 10 persons in 100000 whites and 36 cases per 100000 in blacks in the united states.The Heerfordt's syndrome is present in about 4.1-5.6% of cases with sarcoidosis.

Clinical features:

In cases already diagnosed with sarcoidosis, presence of major symptoms like parotitis, fever, and facial nerve paralysis can confirm heerfordts syndrome:

Other features such as skin lesions and thoracic involvement which are features of sarcoidosis can co-exist with this syndrome. As it represents a form of neuro-sarcoidosis, there could be presence of other neurological involvement such as meningism or other cranial lesions causing ophthalmoplegia, pupillary reflex dysfunction or other abnormalities.

There is swelling of submandibular and sublingual glands, and the lacrimal glands may also be swollen.

The eye involvement includes uveitis, but conjunctivitis, keratitis and corneal herpes may also occur.

Although the uveitis may begin unilaterally it may eventually become bilateral.In many cases it may lead to visual impairment.

There may be chronic low grade fever and there could be complaints of lassitude, malaise and vague gastrointestinal disturbances, nausea and vomiting.

The common nerve paralysis is of the seventh nerve which may be unilateral or bilateral and may occur in 1/2-1/3 rd of cases.

The signs and symptoms of this syndrome usually disappears with time, though some swellings of the parotid glands and visual disturbances may persist.

The summary of signs and symptoms include:

- Uveitis.
- Enlargement of salivary glands(Parotid)
- Facial paralysis.
- Weakness.
- Cough.
- Increased urination
- Dry mouth
- Gastrointestinal disorders
- Mild fever
- Light sensitivity
- Blurred vision
- Floaters in vision
- Red eye

Less common symptoms:

- Headache.
- Loss of weight.
- Puffiness of eyelids.
- Altered taste sensation.

Diagnosis and management:

In patients with confirmed diagnosis of sarcoidosis, the presence of parotitis, fever and facial nerve palsy can be helpful in diagnosis of Heerfordt's syndrome.

The diagnosis is confirmed by histology of minor salivary gland biopsy which shows pathognomonic noncaseating granulomas.

Other diagnostic aids include fibreoptic bronchoscopy along with bronchoalveolar lavage, or the gallium-67 scan along with the blood test findings.

To exclude lymphoma in cases of parotitis, ultrasound guided biopsy is performed.

Treatment: In 50-60% of cases the sarcoidosis undergoes spontaneous remission and may not require specific management. However the course of the disease is variable and difficult to predict.

Medical management:

Uveitis which might lead to eyesight problems of severe proportions, is the most difficult problem in this syndrome.Consultation of an ophthalmologist and proper assesssment and monitoring is of utmost importance.

The most important way of managing the ocular sarcoidosis is the use of topical or systemic steroids.

Other immunomodulatory drugs can be used which can modify the disease and help in reducing the steroid intake.

In case the facial nerve palsy is causing trouble and not easily resolvable, systemic steroids can be used.

Surgical management:

Once the active disease is in control, surgical intervention can be done to treat complications like cataracts or vitreous opacification.

The risk of developing glaucoma increases in the presence of uveitis and hence some patients may require trabeculectomy or devices for drainage of glaucoma.

Suggested reading:

1. Anil Govindrao Ghom, Text book Of Oral Medicine, Third Edition, page 711-712.
2. Evanchan, Jason; Barreiro, Timothy J.; Gemmel, David (May 2010). "Uveitis, salivary gland swelling, and facial nerve palsy in a febrile woman".Journal of the American Academy of Physician Assistants **23** (5): 46–50.

Q 2) The Kveim test

TNMGRU AUGUST 2015 (5 Marks)

The skin test for sarcoidosis is known as Kveim test and was introduced by A.Kveim.

The first published report of the use of a particulate suspension prepared from human sarcoid tissue(lymph node) and used as an intracutaneous test, including an account of the histological features obtained by biopsy of the test site, was given by Kveim in the year 1941.

This test was later popularised and extensively studied by Dr.Louis Siltzbach. This is the only test, which in case is positive is diagnostic of sarcoidosis.

For the clinical research of etiology and pathogenesis of sarcoidosis this test is of great importance.

At the present time an unequivocal diagnosis of sarcoidosis is difficult since clinical, laboratory and pathologic studies cannot always be relied on, to differentiate sarcoidosis from tuberculosis, beryllium poisoning and other granulomatous diseases.

Hence the desire to obtain a specific test for sarcoidosis has prompted many studies of a diagnostic skin reaction usually referred to as the Kveim test.

This test is a skin test to detect sarcoidosis, in which a part of the spleen from a patient with sarcoidosis is injected into the skin of the patient who is suspected to have the disease.In case non-caseating granulomas are found about 4-6 weeks later, then this test is considered positive.

Also it can be done by using a fine suspension in saline made of material from a granulomatous lymph node taken from a patient with active disease which is injected intradermally in quantity of 0.15-0.20 ml.

A positive reaction which takes about 4-6 weeks to form, appears as a firm nodule 3-8mm in diameter.

Histological examination shows it to be composed of collections of epitheloid cells in small tubercles, usually associated with multinucleate giant cells and a few lymphocytes.

The test material is important for the reliability of the test and the batches of test material, though prepared in apparently identical way could vary widely in their activity.

Hence adequate standardisation of the test material used for the diagnostic purpose against material of known activity is important.

If the reagent is satisfactory positive reactions are obtained in about 80% of patients in whom the diagnosis has been histologically confirmed, and in 50%, in whom the diagnosis has been made on only clinical grounds.

False positive reactions have been reported in only 2% of persons tested.

The highest incidence of positive reactions is said to occur in acute cases, lower in subacute and chronically active cases and only about 33% in the inactive cases.

The Kveim test when positive is considered as evidence of sarcoidosis but the mechanism of the test is obscure.

There is at present almost no evidence that supports the view that a positive reaction is based on an immune response to a etiological agent that is unique though this test was probably the theoretical basis of the original test.

The Kveim test has been replaced by transbronchial biopsy for the diagnosis of sarcoidosis because of the problems involved in the preparation.

Summary

Since 50 years the Kveim-Siltzbach test is being used world wide.Its a safe and reliable, simple and specific test to confirm the diagnosis of sarcoidosis.It provides evidence of the activity of the disease.Sarcoidosis as a cause of erythema nodosum, hyperclaciurea, meningitis, uveitis and liver granulomas can be confirmed with the help of this test.When the patient is confronted with a choice between, the skin test and bronchoscopy, lung biopsy or aspiration biopsy of liver, its the patients choice generally to go with the skin test.The disadvantage is that it takes about a month to give results.

Suggested reading:

1. J. R. Mikhail and D. N. Mitchell The Kveim test in sarcoidosis postgrad Med J. 1970 Aug; 46(538): 484–485.
2. James DG, Williams WJ, Kveim-Siltzbach test revisited, Sarcoidosis 1991 Mar; 8(1):6-9.

Q 3) What is Hutchinson's triad?

MUHS OCTOBER 2003 (2 Marks)

In 1856 Sir Jonathan Hutchinson reported typical defects in congenital syphilis, of permanent incisors and in 1959 he described the diagnostic triad.

It includes:

(i) The characteristic defects (hypoplasia) of permanent incisors and first permanent molars.
(ii) Eighth nerve deafness.
(iii) Interstitial keratitis.

Complete triad occurs in less than 1% of cases of congenital syphilis.

The dental hypoplasia in this triad affects the permanent incisors, cuspids and first molars.

There is general constriction of the crown towards the incisal edge, which produces the screw driver and peg shaped incisors associated with this disease. There is also rounding off of the mesial and distal incisal line-angles.The tip of the cuspid is frequently involved.

The molar lesions are characterised by a positioning of the cusps towards the central portion of the crown giving the tooth a bud shaped or a shrunken occlusal form (mulberry molars).

The enamel covering the cusps may be intact, although marked defects are present in the grooves and the fissures of the tooth.

The characteristic notching of the incisal edge of the permanent incisors has been demonstrated by means of a radiographic examination before the eruption of this tooth.

Suggested reading:

1. Burket's Oral Medicine Diagnosis and Treatment, 9th edition, 648-649.

Q 4) Cheilitis Granulomatosa

TNMGRU APRIL 1999 (5 Marks)

Cheilitis granulomatosa (GC) which was first described in 1945 by Miescher, describes a persistent, painless swelling that involves one or both lips.When the granulomatous changes are confined to the lips only, it is termed as Miescher's cheilitis. It is regarded as a monosymptomatic manifestation of Melkersson Rosenthal syndrome.

It could be considered as part of Orofacial granulomatosis (OFG) which is a rare condition of unknown aetiology which is used to describe the swelling involving the lips, other areas of the mouth and face, and there is absence of any other recognised systemic condition.

Etiology:

1. Local causes:

- Chronic oral/dental infection.
- Embedded foreign material.
- Allergy to cosmetics, food etc. especially benzoates, cinnamon

aldehyde, butylated hydroxyanisole, menthol, mono sodium glutamate etc.
- Cobalt, mercury and gold that can act as contact antigen.

2. **Systemic causes :**
   - Chronic granulomatous disease.
   - Crohn's disease.
   - Sarcoidosis and Tuberculosis.
   - Genetic-Debate about link with HLA antigen
   - Immunological.

Clinical features:

- It is seen in children as well as adults .
- More commonly seen in females than males.
- Diffuse swelling on lips, especially the lower lip.
- First episode consists of severe edema of the lips which may subside within hours or days, completely.
- After several recurrent attacks, which may range from days to years, swelling may persist and progressively increase, eventually becoming permanent.
- Sometimes there may be mild constitutional symptoms like headache, visual disturbances and fever. Regional lymph nodes are enlarged in some cases.
- The swelling is usually soft and may show pitting on pressure.If it persists it can become firm and hard and rubbery in consistency.
- It is associated with Melkersson-Rosenthal syndrome.
- In about 30% of the cases with granulomatous chelitis, there is facial lower motor neuron paralysis. Though the facial palsy commonly develops later, it could precede the facial swelling by months or years. Though the facial palsy is intermittent in the beginning, it could later become permanent.It can be partial or complete and unilateral or bilateral. Other cranial nerves occasionally affected are the olfactory, glossopharyngeal, auditory, or hypoglossal.

Differential Diagnosis:

- Cheilitis glandularis- In this condition there is involvement of labial salivary gland.
- Angioedema- It is recurrent condition and subsides after giving antihistaminics.
- Sarcoidosis.
- Crohn's disease.
- Lymphangioma.
- Dental abscess or infection.
- Trauma.

Investigations:

Evaluation includes a complete blood count, ACE levels, C1 esterase level, tuberculosis skin tests and patch tests. Patch tests have identified sensitivities to various foodstuffs and additives, most commonly to benzoic acid.

Gastrointestinal endoscopy, gallium scan or PET (positron emission tomography) scanning can be performed. A panoramic scanning dental X-ray may be obtained to exclude chronic dental abscess.

Treatment:

- When the offending substances are excluded, it could help to resolve the facial swelling.
- Procedures like simple compression every day can produce some temporary relief. The lip edema could be reduced by compression devices.
- Advising a cinammon and benzoate free diet can be helpful.
- Corticosteroid injection-0.1% triamcinolone acetonide inj. given weekly for 7-10 weeks. Apply topical anesthetics gel over the lesion before giving steroids.
- Cheiloplasty-surgical stripping of lip.
- Intralesional triamcinolone and systemic tetracycline given along with reduction cheiloplasty can give very good results.
- Recurrent nerve palsy has been successfully treated with nerve decompression.

Suggested reading:

1. Kruse-Losler B, Presser D, Metze D, Joos U. Surgical treatment of persistent macrocheilia in patients with Melkersson-Rosenthal syndrome and cheilitis granulomatosa. Arch Dermatol. Sep 2005; 141(9):1085-91
2. MF Baqai, MT Baqai, T Kashif, Granulomatous cheilitis, J R Coll Physicians Edinb 2013; 43:312–4.
3. William Austin Critchlow and David Chang, Cheilitis Granulomatosa: A Review, Head Neck Pathol. 2014 Jun; 8(2): 209–213.

CHAPTER 16

Temporomandibular Joint Disorders

Introduction:

T.M.J is a gynglimodiarthroidial joint and is unique in that, it has a rotational as well as translator movements, and where both ends of the bone articulate, in the same plane, with that of other bone.It has a sliding type of movement between the bony surfaces and also a hinge movement.

It is important to know about the disorders of the T.M.J as the pain and other symptoms can be chronic and distressing for the patient.

Q 1) MPD Syndrome

TNMGRU APRIL 2004 (5 Marks)
RGUHS APRIL 1998 (5 Marks)
MUHS MAY 2010 (2 Marks)

A pathophysiologically altered condition, involving the muscles of mastication and the cervical group of muscles is called Myofacial Pain Dysfunction Syndrome. (MPDS)

The MPDS is typically characterised by, dull, aching, radiating pain which often results in muscle spasm and restricted movements of the jaws.

Etiology:

(i) Abnormal occlusion: Painful and damaging contacts lead to modifications in closure pathways and may result in muscle strain and spasm and abnormal pressure on temporo mandibular joint.

(ii) Occlusal abnormalities of teeth causing interference and incoordination and spasm of muscles of mastication.

(iii) Prosthetic problems like ill fitting partial dentures, increased vertical height in partial and complete dentures can lead to MPD syndrome.

(iv) Stress and emotional problems leading to clenching and grinding habits which result in muscle spasm, are thought to be major cause of MPD syndrome as suggested by Laskin in 1969 who then proposed the psychophysiological theory. According to this theory, psychophysiologically motivated oral parafunctional habits, is the frequent cause of muscle spasm, though it is thought that mechanical factors related to occlusion may cause this condition by causing over-extension or over-contraction of the muscles leading to fatigue.

Factors like improper dental restorations, loss of teeth leading to over contraction, dentures, either partial or complete, parafunctional oral habits like clenching and grinding, and dental irritation caused by malocculding restorations or overhanging margins of restoration all lead to this dysfunction syndrome.

(v) Temporomandibular joint problems like hypermobility due to laxity of ligaments and degenerative changes in the joint due to parafunctional habits, or overclosure of the joint due to bilateral loss of molars can ultimately lead to MPD syndrome.

According to Laskin the role played by stress along with occlusal abnormalities leading to strain and spasm of muscles of mastication, the term myofacial pain dysfunction syndrome is more appropriate term than temporomandibular joint dysfunction syndrome.

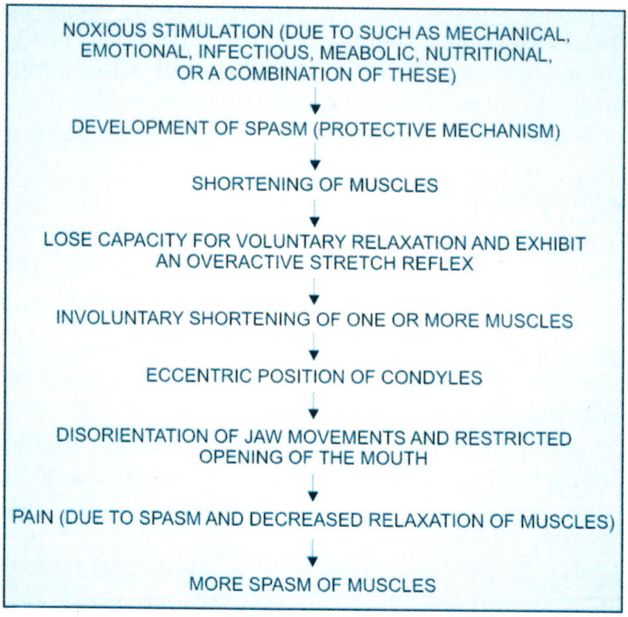

Fig. The Pathopysiology of MPDS

Clincal features:

(i) Seen in middle aged group with predilection towards women.

(ii) The symptomatic episodes of pain can occur several times a day and between intervals patient is symptom free.The episodes increase during increased emotional strain and stress.

There is pain in a zone of reference which usually causes patient to seek treatment.

(iii) Pain on stimulation can be caused by the trigger points on the muscles.

(iv) Taut muscle bands are present.

(v) Restricted jaw opening and associated symptoms.
(vi) No tenderness in the temporomandibular joint.
(vii) Ringing and pain in the ear and tooth ache are also manifestations of this condition.
(viii) Presence of bruxism, indentations on lateral border of tongue, ridging of buccal mucosa and excessive attrition of teeth are present.

Laskins diagnostic criterion:

(a) Unilateral dull aching pain in the ear or preauricular area or at the angle of mandible.
Pain is severe on arising in the morning.
(b) Muscle tenderness in the region of neck of the mandible and distal and superior to maxillary tuberosity.
(c) Clicking or popping noise in the TMJ.
(d) Limitation of jaw movement or deviation of mandible on opening.

Treatment:

(i) The treatment of MPDS should be directed towards a complete management and not only curing the symptoms.
(ii) The probable etilogy and the problems associated with this syndrome should be explained to the patient.Rather than discussing the psychophysiologic aspect, it should include information dealing with muscle fatigue, spasm and explanation about the condition.
(iii) Soft dietary intake and food cut in small pieces should be taken.
(iv) The patients should be made aware and asked to avoid parafunctional habits like, clenching and grinding, and other habits like nail biting, lip biting should be avoided.
(v) Muscle relaxation exercises which include tongue, mouth opening and voluntary resistance exercises.
(vi) Moist heat application for half an hour two time /day is advised.
(vii) The affected area should be massaged with gentle kneading motion, which helps in return of venous blood, lymph and catabolites and helps in reducing muscle pain and spasm.
(viii) Splint therapy especially if there is clenching and other forms of therapy are unsuccessful, like: Stabilisation splint, Relaxation splint, Resilient splint and Pivoting splint.
(ix) Physical therapies like ultrasound, high voltage electrogalvanic stimulation, cryotherapy, vapour coolant spray like ethyl chloride, applying over the involved muscle, ice pack application.
(x) Biofeedback which involves visual or auditory information about the contraction status of the muscle being monitored.
(xi) Tens therapy, acupuncture, diathermy, restorations, prosthodontic and orthodontic therapy are other modalities of treatment.
(xii) Pharmacotherapy includes analgesics like aspirin mostly, tranquilisers like benzothiazine derivatives, antidepressants like lithium carbonate, monoamineoxidase inhibitor, sedatives and hypnotics.

(xiii) Anesthetics like injection of local anesthesia in the trigger zones, intra articular anesthetic and hydrocortisone combination to be injected in the TMJ.

Suggested reading:

1. Anil Govindrao Ghom, Text book of Oral Medicine Third Edition page,
2. Ravi Patel, Himanshu Arora, Sarfaraz Memon, Usha Sharma, RamjeeLal Raigar Anant Raghav Sharma, Myofascial Pain - Dysfunction Syndrome: A Dilemma for the Clinicians : J Pre Clin Dent Res 2015; 2(5):38-43 January-March.

Q 2) Subluxation of TMJ

RGUHS APRIL 2003 (2 Marks)

The positioning of the condyle unilaterally or bilaterally anterior to the articular eminence, with the ability to repositioning to normal accomplishment of physiologic activity is called TMJ subluxation.

It is also called as hypermobility.

Its an incomplete dislocation with the ability to self-reduce and which generally occurs due to stretching of the capsule and ligament.

Partial dislocation of the TMJ occurs repeatedly.

Etiology

- Congenital weakness of the capsules or malformations of the condyles or both.
- Structural deficit or neuromuscular function:As a result of looseness of the articular disc and the capsular ligament, internal derangement of long standing, and spasm of the lateral pterygoid muscles which occur due to alteration in neuromuscular function.
- Arthritic changes in the condyle like, flattening and narrowing, reduction in the height of the articular eminence, changes in the morphology of the glenoid fossa, zygomatic arch, and squamo-tympanic fissure are the structural deficit that occurs.
- Effect of age and changes in the dentition also play a definite role.
- Keeping the mouth open for a long time on the dental chair, yawning widely, singing or sleeping on one arm.
- Long drawn procedures of oral surgery causing excessive stretching of ligament of TMJ.
- Chronic degenerative changes like osteoarthritis.
- Psychiatric problem.
- Use of phenothiazine derivatives, may also be responsible for subluxation due to the adverse effect of this drug.
- Certain syndromes like Ehlers-Danlos, oro-facial dystonia and the Marfan syndrome are also associated with it.

Clinical features:

- It may be unilateral or bilateral.
- Temporary locking and immobilization of jaw.
- o When the mouth is wide open the condyle may get locked and

while closing the mouth it may return to place accompanied with cracking noise.

- On palpation a click on opening and sliding movements of condyle is common.
- Patient may describe weakness of joint while yawning.
- Pain may be associated with wide opening of mouth.

Radiographic features:

- The radiograph will show excessive translation of the condyle from rest position to position when jaw is wide open.

Management:

1. **Injections of sclerosing agents:** 5% sodium psylliate or 5% oil based intracaine or mixture sodium psylliate aqueous solution 5% and 0.5% eucupine in oil.
   Sclerosing agents cause the fibrosis of the capsule, so that the capsule shrinks.
   It limits the excursion of the condyle without any bad effects on the motion and the cartilage part of the articulating surface.
   Repetition of injectables every 2-3 weeks may be required till fibrosis occurs.
2. Elastic rubber traction, traction with arch bars and ligature wire, intermaxillary fixation with elastic bands are helpful in achieving the reduction.
3. Another latest method is the use of Botulinum toxin in the treatment of recurrent TMJ dislocation.
4. **Surgery:** The joint is surgically opened and a vertical incision is given in the outer part of the capsule. The edges are overlapped and then suturing is done so as to make the capsule tight in the antero-posterior plane.Insertion of bone graft is done. Intermaxillary fixation for 7 days is done and after that the clicking and subluxation both are relieved.

Temporalis muscle tendon is shortened as part of treatment.

Suggested reading:

1. Naresh Kumar Sharma, Akhilesh Kumar Singh, Arun Pandey, Vishal Verma, andShreya Singh, Temporomandibular joint dislocation, Natl J Maxillofac Surg. 2015 Jan-Jun; 6(1): 16–20.

Q 3) Differential diagnosis of trismus:

MUHS MAY 2012 (2 Marks)

The word trismus is derived from the greek word Trismos, which means restricted mouth opening.

Differential diagnosis:

- Congenital disorders: Birth injury, hemifacial microsomia, craniocarpotarsal dysplasia, and other disorders can cause trismus. History will help in diagnosis.

- Traumatic: Removal of impacted third molars by surgery, fractures of mandible, fracture with dislocation of condylar head, and fractures of zygomatico-facial complex, haemarthrosis, trauma and inflammation of medial pterygoid, anterior dislocation of TMJ meniscus may cause trismus. Proper history and clinical examination will help in diagnosis.
- Neoplastic: Benign tumours like osteochondromas, osteomas, involving the condyle and coronoid process can cause trismus. Malignant tumours involving the jaws, muscles of mastication, and associated structures can cause trismus.Nasopharyngeal and oropharyngeal carcinomas may give rise to coronoid locking.
- **Infections:** Tetanus, abscesses involving the spaces surrounding the muscles of mastication, facial cellulitis, acute parotitis, Ludwig's angina, peritonsillar abscess, pharyngeal spread of infections can cause trismus.
- Chronic reactive conditions: TMJ ankylosis, degenerative disease of the joints, rheumatoid arthritis, post radiation fibrosis of muscles of mastication and MPD syndrome can lead to trismus.
- **Psychogenic:** Hysteria may commonly cause trismus.Psychiatric assessment will help in diagnosis.
- **Drug induced:** Neuroleptic and antiemetic medication may often cause trismus.Strychnine poisoning may cause trismus.
- **Other causes:** Submucous fibrosis, post-burns scar, post surgical scarring, scleroderma, tuberculous meningitis, epilepsy, myositis ossificans, tetany, rabies may lead to difficulty in opening the mouth.

Suggested reading:

1. H R Umarji, concise oral medicine, 1st edition, 249-251.

Q 4) Internal derangement of TMJ:

TNMGRU FEBRUARY 2007 (5 Marks)

- A change in the internal aspect of the TMJ where in there is a displacement of the disc from its normal functional relationship with the condyle and the articular portion of the temporal bone is called internal derangement of the TMJ.
- There is characteristic displacement of the intra-articular disc with clicking and popping sounds.
- It is usually displaced in anteromedial, medial and lateral direction and rarely in the posterior direction.
- The articular disc displacement always doesnot cause mechanical obstruction.
- The internal disc derangement can be painless or some times cause pain during function.

Etiology:

1. Parafunctional habits e.g. Bruxism, dental clenching, mandible

trauma, excessive mastication, abnormal dental occlusion, very steep articular eminence.

2. Osseous morphologic changes and alteration in the disc morphology –causes elongation of ligaments & disc displacement and inflammation from the neighboring regions (otitis, maxillary sinusitis, tonsillitis).
3. Lack of lubrication, disc modifications, degenerative articular disorder, hyperactivity of the lateral pterygoid muscle, ligament sprains, mandible hypoplasia, loss of posterior teeth, hypermobility and occasionally, whiplash injury, are also considered as possible risk factors.

Classification:

1. Anterior disc displacement with reduction.
2. Disc displacement anteriorly without reduction.
3. Posterior disc displacement
4. Disc displacement with intermittent locking
5. Disc displacement with perforation

1. Disk Displacement With Reduction:

- It represents the early stages of disc derangement disorders, associated with a clicking sound over the joint with or without pain and results from elongation of the capsular and discal ligaments along with thinning of the articular disc.
- Till the mouth is closed the disc remains in this position.However once the mouth is opened, the disc gets resituated on the head of the condyle.The movement of the disc onto and off the head of the condyle results in a clicking, snapping or popping sound.
- The clinical examination reveals normal range of motion with restriction occurring only in association with the pain.
- Deviations in the opening pathway are commonly seen.
- Reciprocal clicking i.e. an opening and a closing click is present.
- Deviation of the jaw towards the side of click till it occurs and then returns to the midline.

2. Disk Displacement without Reduction (Also Known As Closed Locking)

- TMJ disc displacement without reduction is a temporomandibular disorder that usually cause TMJ pain and limited mouth opening (painful locking), sometimes called a "closed lock" (Okeson, 2007).
- Its incidence among TMD patients is estimated at 2% to 8%.
- Disc Displacement without reduction, depending on the duration of locking is subdivided into 3 forms:
    1) Intermittent lock- lasts for seconds to minutes.
    2) Acute lock–persistent in the absence of treatment
    3) Chronic closed lock-resolution of acute lock.

3. Posterior Disc Displacement:

It is the condition in which the condyle slips in the anterior rim of the disc while opening with the disc being caught and brought backward in an abnormal position while closing. The disc is folded in the dorsal part of the joint space.

- Sudden inability to bring the upper and lower teeth together in maximum occlusion .i.e. disocclusion of approximately 1 mm on the affected side.
- Pain in the affected joint while trying to get the teeth firmly in occlusion.
- Forward displacement of mandible on affected side.
- Restricted lateral movements on the affected side.
- No restriction of mouth opening.
- Midline deviation to the affected side.

4. Disc displacement associated with intermittent locking.

Disc displacement with reduction is a similar condition as this but there is an additional feature of intermittent limited mandibular movements as at times the disc does not reduce.

5. Disc displacement with perforation:

- Perforations between the superior and inferior compartment occurs in the retrodiscal tissue.
- There is loss of joint space, that results in bone- to- bone contact between the osseous compartment.
- There is joint pain associated with clicking with intermittent locking, and closed lock.
- Crepitus and grinding noise is present.

Management:

Internal derangement of TMJ are treated with nonsurgical methods which includes, medical treatment, physiotherapy and occlusal splints in the initial stages.

A. Conservative (or non invasive)
B. Surgical (or invasive)

A. Conservative (or non invasive):

Patient with TMJ clicking and popping that is not associated with pain does not require any treatment. The painful clicking is treated with:

- Avoiding extreme jaw movements.
- Pharmacotherapy:
- Nonsteroidal anti-inflammatory and muscle relaxants drugs such as
  - Tab Ibuprofen in a dose of 800 mg, 3 times per day up to 6 weeks.
  - Muscle relaxants- Tab Cyclobenzaprine in dose of 10 mg, once a day, at bedtime for the initial 1–2 weeks.
- Splints:
- Flat plane stabilization splints.
- Anterior repositioning splints.

Exercise Therapy:

- Active movements includes lateral motion towards right and left side, protrusion and wide mouth opening for 10-min.
- Passive exercise – opening mouth by pushing simultaneously the thumb against the upper anterior teeth and forefinger against the lower anterior teeth.

Intra Articular Injections of:

- Corticosteroids, ozone gas injection, sclerosing agent (alcohol, 5%sodium psylliate), autologous blood injection into the TMJ, use of botulinum toxin Injections for dislocation in to the upper joint cavity guided by arthroscopy.

  Cognitive- Behavioral Therapy, Hot And Cold Therapy, Biofeedback, Ultrasound, Transcutaneous Electrical Neural Stimulation, Teeth Selective Grinding, Physical Auto-Regulation, Low level laser therapy.

B. Surgical:

- Arthroscopy-irrigation and lubrication of the TMJ.
- Reconstruction Arthroplasty (Disk Repositioning)
- Meniscectomy.
- Repair of Perforation of Disk.

Suggested reading:

1. Andrew L. Young, Internal Derangements Of The Temporomandibular Joint: A Review Of The Anatomy, Diagnosis, And Management ; Journal Of Indian Prosthodontic Society; Jan-Mar 2015 ; 15 :1.
2. Burket's, Oral Medicine Diagnosis and Treatment Edi; 12 Th, Ch:1; Pg: 301-303.
3. Freny R Karjodkar, Essentials Of Oral Maxillofacial Radiology-, Edition: Ist; Ch: 25; pg: 471-475.
4. Sharmila Devi Devaraj, Dr. Pradeep D, Internal Derangement Of Temporomandibular Joint - A Review Volume 13, Issue 3 Ver. II. (Mar. 2014), PP 66-73.
5. Stuart C White, Michael J Pharoah, Oral Radiology, Principles and Interpretation. Edi: 1st South Asia; Ch: 27; Pg: 505-506.

CHAPTER 17

Salivary Gland Disorders

Introduction:

Major salivary glands include the parotid, submandibular and sublingual glands.The minor salivary glands are distributed in the mucosa and submucosa of the oral cavity.The disorders of these glands come under the perview of the dental clinician and hence the knowledge about these glands and their disorders is of great importance in dentistry.

Q 1) Sjogren's Syndrome:

RGUHS APRIL 2001 (5 Marks)
TNMGRU APRIL 2003 (5 Marks)

Q) Write clinical diagnostic triad and investigation for sjogren's syndrome:

MUHS NOVEMBER 2009 (2 Marks)

Sjogren's syndrome is a chronic autoimmune disorder in which the white blood cells of the body destroy the exocrine glands, especially the lacrimal and salivary glands which produce, tears and saliva respectively. The attack on the salivary and lacrimal glands due to immune -mediated process, causes xerostomia or dry mouth and keratoconjunctivitis sicca or dry eyes, which occurs in association with the infiltration of the glands by lymphocytes and this inflammatory process ultimately damages or destroys the glands severely.

Sjogren's syndrome can be classified as primary or secondary.

Primary sjogren's syndrome: is a systemic disorder that includes both lacrimal and salivary gland dysfunctions without another autoimmune condition.

Secondary sjogren's syndrome: salivary and/or lacrimal gland dysfunction along with the presence of another connective tissue disorder.

Etiology:

1. **Genetic factors:** In families with Sjogren's syndrome high prevalence of auto-immune disorders have been observed and hence this syndrome is thought to have genetic predisposition.

2. **Hormonal causes:** Since Sjögren's syndrome is seen with high frequency in women, sex hormones, especially, estrogen is thought to affect humoral and cell-mediated immune responses and affect the susceptibility to this syndrome.
3. **Michrochimerism factors:** The presence of offspring lymphoid cells in maternal circulation is michrochimerism and it is thought to generate autoimmunity in females who have been pregnant earlier.
4. **Environmental factors:** Degraded self structures, viral proteins, engulfed molecules, could initiate autoimmunity by molecule mimicry and cause increased chances of Sjögren's syndrome development.

Clinical Features:

Symptoms of Sjogren's syndrome include, generalised dryness especially, xerostomia and keratoconjunctivitis sicca and is also termed the sicca syndrome.

- The sicca syndrome also consists of vaginal dryness and chronic bronchitis.Sjogren's syndrome may also involve dryness of the nose, skin, vagina and may also affect other organs of the body, which can include, kidneys, liver, lungs, blood vessels, biliary system, pancreas, peripheral nervous system and brain.
- Skin dryness in some Sjogren's syndrome cases could be a result of lymphocytic infiltration of the glands of the skin.
- Patients experience the full spectrum of oral complications that result from decreased salivary function.
- Virtually all patients complain of dry mouth and the need to sip liquids throughout the day.
- Oral dryness causes difficulty with chewing, swallowing, and speaking without additional fluids. Patients often have dry cracked lips and angular cheilitis.
- Intraorally, the mucosa is pale and dry, minimal salivary pooling is noted, and the saliva that is present tends to be thick and ropy.
- Mucocutaneous candidal infections are common in these patients.
- Decreased salivary flow results in increased dental caries and erosion of the enamel structure.
- Patients with this syndrome can experience chronic salivary gland enlargement. They are also susceptible to salivary gland infections.

Investigations and diagnoses:

(i) **Eye test:**

(a) Dryness of the surface of the eyes can be revealed by the slit-lamp examination.

(b) Shirmer's test: Schirmer's test uses paper strips inserted into the eye for several minutes to measure the production of tears.

(c) Rose Bengal dye test: In this test the physician instills a red vegetable dye on the surface of the eyes that stain cells that have lost mucin coating.

(ii) **Salivary flow test:** Flow rate of saliva test is done to check the status of salivary glands and the production of saliva.The patient is asked to spit into a cup and the saliva sample is collected and weight is taken to assess the result.

(iii) **Lip/ minor salivary gland biopsy:** The presence of a salivary gland biopsy specimen demonstrating characteristic histopathologic findings the presence of autoantibodies against the extractable nuclear antigens SS-A/RO or SS-B/La, in addition to objective evidence of lacrimal dysfunction.

(iv) **Sialography** shows characteristic changes and may be useful in the evaluation of SS.It may show a cherry blossom appearance of salivary gland and duct.Parotid gland involvement may show honey comb or salt and pepper appearance.

(v) **MRI or CT:** Can be helpful also, particularly in the assessment of enlarged glands and potential lymphadenopathies.

(vi) **Ultrasound scans**: These are commonly performed now to help diagnose Sjogren's syndrome.

(vii) **Blood tests**: Patient's with Sjogren's syndrome often have high levels of antibodies in their blood.

Treatment:

1. **Eye care:** Eye drops containing artificial tears is a liquid that can mimic tears and can be given for mild to moderate cases of dry eyes and treatment is often successful.
   In case of irritation of eyes, eye-drops containing corticosteroids could be recommended.
2. **Oral care:**
   (i) Caries can be prevented by maintaining good oral hygiene.
   (ii) Increasing fluid intake and regular sipping of water.
   (iii) Sugar-free chewing gum can be given to stimulate saliva flow.
   (iv) Lubrication of mouth can be done by sucking ice cubes that can also reduce dryness.
   (v) regularly using mouth rinses for soothing effects and protect it against infection.
   (vi) Use of Saliva substitutes can be given that are available in the form of sprays, lozenges, gel or gum.
   (vii) Avoidance of anticholinergic drugs if possible.
   (viii) Professional topical fluoride application.

Medical treatment:

- The symptoms of dry eyes and dry mouth can be treated with pilocarpine.
- The use of hydroxychloroquine has been observed to reduce the effect of attack of immune system on the lacrimal and salivary glands.

- o Systemic muscarinic agonists are being currently used in the USA for treatment of Sjogren's syndrome.
- o Cevimeline, a newer drug that stimulates muscarinic M3 receptors on the salivary and lacrimal glands and is being given three times/ day as oral tablet.

Suggested reading:

1. Borchers, A. T., Naguwa, S. M., Keen, C. L. & Gershwin, M. E. Immunopathogenesis of Sjögren's syndrome. Clin. Rev. Allergy Immunol. 25, 89-104 (2003)
2. Delaleu, N., Jonsson, R. & Koller, M. M. Sjögren's syndrome. Eur. J. Oral Sci. 113, 101-113 (2005)
3. K Bayetto, R.M Logan, Sogren's syndrome: A review of etiology, pathogenesis, diagnosis and management, Australian Dental Journal 2010; 55: (1 Suppl): 39–47.

Q 2) Sialosis

TNMGRU FEBRUARY 2010 (6 Marks)

Sialosis is a term which is non-specific and is used to describe a condition that is uncommon, benign, non-inflammatory, non-neoplastic enlargement involving the salivary gland, usually the parotid but some times involving the submandibular and rarely minor salivary glands.

This enlargement is bilateral, symmetrical and often painless.The enlargement is generally asymptomatic and usually idiopathic.In this condition, both the parotids may be diffusely enlarged and the symptoms may be moderate.The general age of the patients is between 30-69 years and both the sexes are affected equally, and the glands are soft and painless.

Etiology:

1. **Systemic disease:** This condition is associated with diseases especially cirrhosis, diabetes, ovarian and thyroid insufficiency, alcoholism, malnutrition, and anorexia nervosa.
   Whenever digestion of food or its absorption is affected for a prolonged period of time, can result in sialosis.Malnutrition in alcoholics can lead to sialosis.
   Recently bulimia and anorexia nervosa have increasingly become recognised causes.
2. **Neurogenic medication:** Antihypertensive drugs, psychotropic drugs and sympathomimetic drugs can cause sialosis.
3. It is now recognised that many of its causes may produce sialosis through the common feature of autonomic nerve dysfunction, causing an aberrant intercellular secretory cycle, and it is possible that there are functional alterations in salivary aquaporin water channels.

Clinical features:

(i) **Age and sex distribution:** It more commonly affects females, however there is no particular age predilection.

(ii) **Site:** The enlargement is usually bilateral and may present with recurrent painless enlargement of the glands .The parotid is most commonly affected.

(iii) **Appearance:** Swelling of the preauricular area of the parotid gland is the most common sign but the retromandibular part of the gland may also be involved.

Radiological features:

Sialography shows leafless tree like appearance which is caused by compression of finer ducts by hypertrophic acinar cells.

Diagnosis:

The diagnosis of sialosis requires exclusion of inflammatory causes of salivary swelling particularly Sjogren's syndrome, HIV infection, sarcoidosis, and lymphoepithelial disease, by the relevant investigations.

(a) **Clinical diagnosis:** Bilateral non-inflammatory and usually painless enlargement of the parotid gland gives a clue to diagnosis.

(b) **Radiological diagnosis:** Sialography will show leafless tree like appearance.

(c) MRI is one of the best methods for investigating conditions of the salivary gland and is valuable for excluding other diseases.

(d) Salivary sonography is also useful to exclude other diseases is noninvasive, and often more readily available than other methods of imaging.

(e) **Laboratory diagnosis:** There is significant elevation in salivary potassium and decrease in salivary sodium. This salivary chemistry is typical of sialosis.

(f) Fine needle aspiration or open biopsy examination may aid diagnosis, but are rarely needed.

Management:

Treating and controlling the underlying causes is the mainstay of treatment.

Partial parotidectomy in cases of bad esthetic appearance, may have to be performed.

Suggested reading:

1. C. Scully et al. British Journal of Oral and Maxillofacial Surgery 46 (2008) 468–472.
2. Som PM, Curtin HD. Head and Neck Imaging Vol 2, 3rd ed Chicago: Mosby; 2003. p.912.

Q 3) Sialolithiasis

TNMGRU FEBRUARY 2014 (5 Marks)

Sialolithiasis is the formation of calcific concretion involving the ductal system or parenchyma of the major or minor salivary glands.It is also known as salivary calculus or salivary gland stone.They are the most common calcifications seen in the soft tissues of oro-orbital region.

Composition:

- **Calculus:** It consists of inorganic material arranged in laminated form and covered with concentric shells of calcific material.
- **Crystalline structure:** It is chiefly made up of hydroxyapetite and consists of octacalcium phosphate.
- **Chemical composition:** It consists primarily of calcium phosphate and carbon with traces of magnesium, potassium, chloride and ammonium.
- **Etiopathogenesis:**
- **Neurohumoral mechanism:** A neurohumoral condition that leads to stagnation of saliva, and results in a nidus and matrix formation.
- **Metabolic mechanism:** When there is coexisting inflammation, a mechanism favors precipitation of salts in to the matrix.

Prevalence:

The submandibular gland is affected the most, about 85% followed by parotid, 10%, sublingual gland, 7% which is due to following factors:

Anatomic conditions:

- The wharton's duct which has an irregular course and is lengthy.
- The submandibular gland is situated in a dependant position.
- The size of the orifice is big and the position favours the caculi formation.
- But the size of the orifice is much smaller as compared to the ductal lumen.

Physiochemical factors:

- Saliva contains high mucin.
- Saliva is highly alkaline with high percentage of organic matter.
- There is higher concentration of calcium and phosphate salts.
- Low carbon dioxide content.
- Rich in phosphatase enzyme.

Varieties:

- Ductal sialoliths: The calculi are located in ducts.
- Glandular sialoliths: The calculi are present within the glands.

Clinical manifestations:

- Usually found in the middle aged patients and has slight predilection for men.
- The intraglandular stones cause less severe symptoms than the extraglandular or the ductal types.In some cases, there may be absence of any symptoms.
- Many patients complain of moderate pain due to the occlusion of ducts that obstruct the free flow of saliva and this stagnation results in pain.
- There is tendency for swelling which can be intermittent or transient during meals and reduces after meals.When the salivary demand

reduces the swelling subsides as the saliva sweeps past the partial obstruction.

- Systemic symptoms: If left untreated suppurative process may ensue and there can be fever and malaise.

Signs:

- There could be exudation of pus from the duct orifice.
- The soft tissue surrounding the duct generally shows a severe inflammatory reaction.There may be swelling, redness and tenderness.
- If the size is sufficiently big the stones can be palpated within the peripheral portion of the duct.
- In some cases the mucosa overlying the stone may ulcerate and the calculus may extend to the floor of the mouth.
- The size may vary from few millimeters to several centimeters and usually occurs as a solitary mass.
- Salivary stones in the minor salivary gland is rare but may occur near the commisure in the buccal mucosa or near the mandibular mucobuccal fold.

Radiographic features:

- The radiograph for submandibular gland stone is the mandibular occlusal view and for parotids its an IOPA in the buccal vestibule. The exposure is reduced to avoid burnout of sialoliths.
- Sialography is indicated when the stones are radiolucent and there is dilatation due to sialodochitis.The contrast medium on the film will be seen behind the stone.
- They are almost always radiopaque and even very small stones are visible in good radiographs.
- They are usually oval in shape and is cylindrical and has multiple layers of calcification.
- They have smooth borders and are of even radiodensity.
- As mentioned above the size varies from that of pin head to almost an inch in length and width may be about 5mms.
- CT scan will show dense radiopaque structure in contrast study.
- Ultrasonography: Can also reveal salivary calculus.

Diagnosis:

- Palpation is an important diagnostic tool and will reveal the affected gland to be larger and firmer than the opposite side normal gland. Digital palpation will allow the saliva to flow through the orifice which can be seen visually.The physical distortion of the affected duct may be apparent and the yellowish colour of the calculus may be apparent through the thinned mucosa.
- Probing with a metal probe will show the presence and location of the calculus.
- Radiographs will help in confirming the presence of calculus.
- Sialography will help reveal the calculus not seen on conventional intra and extra-oral radiographs.

Differential diagnosis:

- Patient comes with pain and swelling of salivary gland, there should be immediate consideration of inflammatory, infectious and non-neoplastic etiologies.
- Chronic sialadenitis occurs in quite a few patients with chronic sialadenitis.They may also be associated with acute sialadenitis. Mumps should be ruled out in acute infectious cases.
- Gas bubbles which can be introduced into the ducts while sialography could mimic sialoliths but can be easily removed and are more round than the calculi.
- In panoramic radiography the hyoid bone though opaque will appear bilaterally.
- In myositis ossificans there will be restriction of mandibular movements.
- In case of phleboliths the sialadenitis will be absent and are more round and may present central dark areas.
- Calcified submandibular lymph nodes should be differentiated from sialoliths, but if the calcified mass is accompanied by pain and swelling they are mostly sialoliths.

Treatment:

- Initial management is conservative, with penicillinase-resistent staphylococcal antibiotic coverage, moist heat, sialogogues, and gentle massage.
- Most cases will respond to this treatment, followed by simple sialolithotomy, when required.
- In case of small stones gentle massage of the gland will promote the stones to move forward towards the orifice. Moist heat application, increased fluid intake and sialogogues will help the passage of stones.
- Salivary calculus in the submandibular duct near the orifice can be removed by an incision made directly over it.
- In case of stone within the submandibular gland, excision of the gland is advised.
- In case of acute infection, antibiotics are advised.
- Salivary gland endoscopy is the newer technique for removal of sialoliths.
- Fragmentation of the stone within the gland by lithotripsy and extra-oral shock wave lithotripsy have been used with success.

Suggested reading:

1. Anil G. Ghom Textbook of Oral Medicine, Page no. 609 – 613.
2. Charles V Pollack, Harry W sEverance, Sialolithiasis: Case studies and Review, The Journal Of Emergency Medicine, volume 8, 561-565, 1990.
3. Felix Grases· Cristina Santiago, Bartolomé M. Simonet, Antonia Costa-Bauzá, Sialolithiasis: mechanism of calculi formation and etiologic factors, Clinica Chimica ActaVolume 334, Issues 1–2, August 2003, Pages 131–136.

Q 4) Necrotising sialometaplasia:

RGUHS APRIL 1999 (5 Marks)

Necrotizing sialometaplasia (NS) is an inflammatory, non-neoplastic condition, of the salivary glands.It was first reported by Abrams etal in 1973. It is self healing and clinical and histopathologic features mimics salivary gland malignancy. Usually involves the minor salivary glands.

It is very important to recognise and understand this condition to avoid misdiagnosis and wrong treatment.

Etiology and pathogenesis:

- **Local ischemia:** Could be due to physical, chemical, infective or local vasculitis.
- **Trauma:** Various causes such as pressure from dental prosthesis or recent oral surgical procedures, local anesthesia, could precipitate this condition.
- **Other factors:** In some cases upper respiratory tract infection, smoking and alcohol intake can cause this condition.Allergy, diabetes, infections, ionising radiation can cause this condition.

Clinical features:

- **Prevalence:** It is more common in males and in the 4th or 5th decades.
- **Location:** 75% of cases have been reported on posterior palatal area. Most cases are unilateral but may occur in midpalatal area. Minor salivary glands of retromolar region, tongue, labial mucosa, buccal mucosa, incisive canal have been reported to be involved.
- **Onset:** There may be early mild swelling which could be nonulcerated.
- **Symptoms:** Generally painless but could cause mild pain. Numbness in the palatal region can be present.Pain may be referred to ear or pharynx.
- **Signs:** Lesion begins as ulcer or ulcerated nodule, and may be unilateral or bilateral. The ulcer is well demarcated and may have inflammed margins and edges could be indurated. The lesion is covered with inflammatory exudates and necrotic debris.
- **Size:** The lesion can be deep, crater like, non-draining ulcer about 1-3 cm in size.

Diagnosis:

- **Clinical:** Lesion on the posterior palate that is ulcerative will help in diagnosis.
- **Histopathology:** Biopsy will show necrosis of the acini and salivary ductal squamous metaplasia.

Differential diagnosis:

- **Traumatic ulcers:** Can be related to source of trauma and will be of short duration.
- **Aphthous ulcers:** Especially the major ulcers and sutton's disease

may appear similar, but are painful and heal in about 14 days.

- **Squamous cell carcinoma:** Occurs in older age group, and is associated with habits, biopsy will help in diagnosis.
- **Syphilis:** There is painless edematous induration and painless lymph node swelling.The other clinical features and serology tests will help in diagnosis.
- **Non-hodgkin's lymphoma:** The lymph nodes are painless, swollen and rubbery in consistency and the biopsy will help in differentiating.

Treatment:

The disease is self-limiting and generally requires no treatment.The healing occurs in 6-12 weeks by secondary intention.

Debriding and saline rinses may help in healing process.

Suggested reading:

1. Schmidt-Westhausen A, Philipsen HP, Reichart PA. [Necrotizing sialometaplasia of the palate. Literature report of 3 new cases].Dtsch Z Mund Kiefer Gesichtschir.1991 Jan-Feb. 15(1):30-4.

Q 5) Diagnostic importance of saliva

TNMGRU FEBRUARY 2012 (5 Marks)

Saliva has been used in the past few decades as a new diagnostic fluid.Increasing number of dentists, clinical and forensic pathologists, pediatricians, endocrinologists, immunologists are realising that saliva is an easily available, non-invasive diagnostic medium which can be used in a wide range of diseases and clinical situations.

The diagnostic importance is as follows:

1 Genetic disorders:

A) Cystic fibrosis: (CF)

- Its a disorder of children and young adults which is genetically transmitted.
- In these patients, increased levels of electrolytes like sodium, chloride, and phosphorous, uric acid and urea, and total lipid and proteins was observed in the saliva of submandibular salivary glands in the CF patients.

B) Ectodermal Dysplasia:

- It was observed that there was reduction in flow of whole saliva and increased concentration of inorganic constituents and total protein.
- There was reduced activity and concentration of the alpha-amylase in the saliva.

2. Autoimmune disorders:

A) Sjogren's syndrome:

- There are elevated levels of rheumatoid factor, polyclonal hypergammaglobulinemia, antinuclear antibody, anti-SS-A and anti-SS-B antibody.

3. Malignancies:

- Early detection improves the prognosis and saliva has been used as a diagnostic medium in oral squamous cell carcinomas(OSCC) where in the salivary amylases such as proteins, mRNA, and DNA have been used for diagnosis.
- In saliva of patients diagnosed with OSCC, p53 antibodies can be detected.

4) Infectious diseases:

A) Viral infections:

- The advantage of diagnostic tests for viruses are the identification of a single target and the oral mucosal transudate which is obtained by swabbing the tongue and buccal mucosa contains a mixture of IgG, IgM, IgA and a rich source of antibodies.
- The diagnosis of HIV causing AIDS can be done by a confirmatory test using a reactive antibody assay which can be a Western blot test via blood or saliva and can also be detected by a polymerase chain reaction through blood.

B) Fungal infections:

- Saliva can be used to detect the oral fungi.In cases of oral candidiasis, the salivary fungal count can provide valuable information.
- In these cases alterations in the proteins of saliva like the immunoglobulins, histatins, mucins, Hsp70, proline rich proteins, and peroxidases have an important diagnostic value.

5) Detection of drugs:

- Saliva can be used for detection of various drugs like antiepileptics, amphetamines, dexodiazepines, cocaine, phencyclidine, opioids, anticancer and psychiatric drugs.
- Nicotine levels can be determined to monitor smoking habits.

6) The Monitoring of Hormone Levels:

- Cortisol, projesteron, insulin levels can be detected by saliva.
- However the leves of serum and salivary protein hormones cannot be well co-related.

7) The turn over of bone markers in saliva:

- The bone turn over can be measured with the use of saliva.The ELISA test can be used to detect the presence of osteocalcin and pyridinoline in whole saliva in women.

8) Dental Caries and Periodontal Disease:

- The levels of oral bacteria can be monitored by the use of saliva and there are increased numbers of Streptococcus mutans and lactobacilli with increased caries and root caries incidences.

- The levels of asparate aminotransferase and alkaline phosphatase is increased in periodontal diseases and these can be used as markers for monitoring the periodontal disease process.

9) Forensic odontology:

- Saliva can be found frequently on victims of violent crimes.It can be recovered from bite marks, glasses, stamps, envelops, cigarette butts, cigarettes, food products and other objects.
- Blood group antigens are secreted in to the saliva of several individuals and can be used for identification of suspected criminals or in cases of paternity law suits.
- DNA testing can be done from salivary samples as it is relatively stable in dry state. In cases of sexual abuse and harassment identification of DNA from salivary samples can help in identification by doing genetic profiling.

Suggested reading:

1. NarasimhanMalathi et al. Salivary Diagnostics: A Brief Review. ISRN Dentistry, 2014; Article ID 158786:1-8.
2. Vijayalaxmi B Madalli et al. Saliva – A diagnostic tool. Journal of dental and medical sciences.2013;11(6):96-99.

Q 6) Mucocele:

TNMGRU AUGUST 2011 6 Marks

Definitions:

(i) Accumulation of mucous secretion with dilation of a cavity.

(ii) Mucocele is a localized swelling caused by the pooling of saliva in the submucosa at the site of trauma or because of obstruction of the minor salivary gland ducts.

They can occur in the mouth, lacrimal sac, paranasal sinuses, gall bladder, appendix.

I) Intraoral mucoceles:

Can be of two types:

- Extravasation
- Retention:

Ranula is a large mucocele, bluish in colour, occurring on the floor of the mouth.

Etiology:

(i) Extravasation cyst is caused by traumatic injury to the excretory duct of the minor salivary glands.Injury or laceration of the duct results in pooling of the saliva in the adjoining submucosal tissue resulting in swelling.This is the commonest form.

(ii) The retention cyst is the result of obstruction of the minor salivary gland duct by calculus or contraction of scar around the injured ducts. Due to blockage of flow of saliva there is accumulation of the same and dilatation of the duct forming a mucocele.

Clinical features:

- Extravasation mucoceles occur most commonly on the lower lips, tongue, floor of the mouth, buccal mucosa and the retro-molar regions, which can be easily traumatized.
- Mucous retention cysts are more common in the floor of the mouth or palate.
- They follow an episode of trauma.
- They occur as smooth, painless, discrete swellings which can measure from few millimeters to centimeters in diameter.
- A typical blue hue is present with superficial lesions.
- When the lesions are deeper they appear more diffuse and may lack the blue colour.
- If it gets traumatized it drains and deflates.
- Recurrence is common.

Differential diagnosis:

Neoplasms of the salivary glands, soft tissue tumours, vascular malformations and vesiculo-bullous lesions.

Treatment:

Surgical excision is the treatment of choice.

Removal of associated salivary gland is necessary to prevent recurrence.

However surgical removal can lead to trauma of adjacent minor salivary glands and development of a new mucocele.

In some cases corticosteroids given intra lesionally have met with some success.

Ranula:

It is a large mucocele which occurs on the floor of the mouth and can be mucous retention or extravasation phenomenon.It is mostly associated with sublingual salivary gland duct.

The etiology is trauma or obstruction of the gland or ductal aneurysm.

Clinical feature:

Occurs on the floor of the mouth generally on one side of the lingual frenum but may be big enough to cross the midline.

It is slow growing, painless and movable.

It resembles the belly of a frog and hence the term Ranula.

Some times a deep lesion may be herniated through the mylohyoid muscle, which may extend along the fascial planes and is termed as plunging Ranula.

Treatment:

Surgical treatment is done. Marsupialisation is the method of choice.

Excision of the lesion along with removal of the gland may be needed.

Intralesional injections of corticosteroids have met with some success.

II) Mucocele of maxillary antrum:

Though less commonly involved than the other paranasal sinuses, mucoceles do occur in maxillary antrum.

As a result of blocked sinus ostium, an expanding, destructive lesion can occur.

Clinical Features:

Radiating pain can occur due to a mucocele in the maxillary sinus which can exert pressure on the superior alveolar nerves.

There can be loosening of the posterior teeth in the area where the lesion expands inferiorly.

In case of expansion of the medial wall of the sinus, there can occur deformity of the lateral nasal wall, causing nasal airway obstruction.

Expansion into the orbit can cause diplopia, (double vision) or proptosis(protrusion of the globe of the eye).

Radiographic features:

The lesion may cause the shape of maxillary antrum to change to a more round shape.The lesion appears uniformly opaque.May cause displacement of teeth and root resorption.

Treatment:

Surgical excision of the lesion using Caldwell-luc technique is treatment of choice.

Suggested reading:

1. Burket's Oral Medicine Diagnosis And Treatment, 10th Edition, 246-247.
2. Stuart.C White, Michael.j Pharaoh, Oral radiology, principles and interpretation, 5th edition, 584-585.

Q 7) Mumps

RGUHS APRIL 1998 (5 Marks)

It is also known as epidemic parotitis and is a contagious infection caused by paramyxovirus, involving the major salivary glands especially the parotids.

In about 50% Of cases there is evidence of central nervous system infection as the virus is highly neurotropic.

It may also affect testis, mammary glands, pancreas, heart and meninges.

Transmission is usually through airborne infection, mainly the infected saliva.

Painful inflammatory symptoms like parotitis and orchitis are characteristic of mumps.

Though mumps was first described by Hippocrates, the viral etiology was demonstrated in 1930 by Johnson and Goodpasture.

Clinical features:

- Mumps is spread through inhalation or oral contact with droplets or secretions of the respiratory tract.
- Occurs between age of 5-15 years and is more common in boys than the girls.

- There is about 2-3 weeks of incubation period.
- It is clear that mumps virus can systemically disseminate within the body and hence it is assumed that after the infection of the upper respiratory mucosa, the virus infects the regional lymph nodes and causes viremia in the acute phase.
- Progression of disease is as follows: i) Prodromal phase-headache, malaise, myalgia and fever. ii) early acute-meningitis and parotitis. iii) Established acute-encephalitis, deafness, pancreatitis, orchitis, viruria.
- Parotid gland is more commonly involved. Submandibular salivary gland may be involved.
- Parotids are generally bilaterally involved and some times one gland is involved followed by the other.
- There is prodrome of fever, chills, malaise, pain below the ear a week before the onset of swellings.
- This is followed by enlargement of salivary glands which are firm, rubbery or elastic in consistency and there is no purulent discharge from the duct of the involved salivary gland.
- The swellings are painful especially while mastication and eating sour foods.
- The skin over the involved glands is edematous.
- Enlargement of the parotid may cause ear lobule elevation.
- Involvement of sublingual glands may cause elevation of floor of the mouth.
- Parotid papilla may be reddened and swollen.
- Unilateral orchitis is the most common, occurence apart from the salivary gland involvement and occurs in about 10-20% of cases in postpubertal men.
- In post pubertal women in about 5-10% of cases Mastitis and oophoritis which manifests as pelvic pain occurs.
- In the acute phase of the disease the viruses often disseminate to the kidneys as suggested by presence of viruria.
- Meningitis occurs in approximately 5–10% of cases and encephalitis in less than 0.5%.cases.
- In 4% of cases deafness has been reported and leads to unilateral hearing loss in children.Though it can be transient can become permanent.
- The course of disease is self limiting and the lesion subsides in a week.

Complications: Orchitis, meningitis, pancreatitis, deafness, mastoiditis, epididymitis, cerebellar ataxia, autoimmune haemolytic anaemia, thyroiditis, thrombocytopenia, retinitis and corneal endothelitis.

Diagnosis: The typical parotid swellings along with the other clinical features helps in diagnosis.

Laboratory diagnosis will reveal increased salivary amylase levels, and isolation of paramyxovirus from saliva.

Management:

- When there are no major complications, the patients can be managed in the out patient basis but with constant guidance, support and care.The patients should be isolated for 5 days from the onset of the disease to prevent the risk of spreading the infection.
- The treatment of this condition is conservative with supportive medical care and no antiviral agent is prescribed as it is a self limiting disease.
- Symptomatic treatment with analgesics and antipyretics can provide relief.
- Adequate hydration by sufficient oral fluid intake is important to maintain hydration of the patient and they should avoid acidic food intake which may cause difficulty in swallowing and gastric irritation.
- Maintenance of nutrition and electrolyte balance.
- To treat the discomfort due to parotitis and headaches, ibuprofen or acitaminophen can be given.Warm or cold fomentation to the affected gland may soothe the symptoms.
- In patients with orchitis, stronger analgesics may be required. Bed rest, support to the scrotum and ice packs are recommended.
- In patients with complications IPD care will be required with intravenous fluids administration, management of pain and close observation.
- Higher level of IPD care may be required in patients with complications like encephalitis, nephritis, myocarditis, or pancreatitis.
- Bed rest is advised to prevent complications.
- In infants and young children the prime motive is to prevent mumps by achieving and maintaining high levels of immunization. To prevent and give good health care universal imunization should be routinely carried out in physician's office and public health care units.
- Prevention with vaccine is the best form of treatment .Doses given in the 12-15 months of life is repeated in the 4th-5th year.

Suggested reading:

1. Anil Govindrao Ghom, Textbook Of Oral Medicine, 3rd edition, 618-619.
2. Steven Rubin, Michael Eckhaus, Linda J Rennick, Connor GG Bamford, W Paul Duprex, Molecular biology, pathogenesis and pathology of mumps virus, The journal of pathology, Volume 235, Issue 2 January 2015 Pages 242–252.

Q 8) Write about the complete treatment plan for acute bacterial sialadenitis:

MUHS NOVEMBER 2012 (3 Marks)

Also called as 'acute suppurative parotitis'.

Ascending bacterial inflammation from oral cavity most frequently localises to the parotid gland. This condition occurs due to a septic focus in the mouth like chronic tonsillitis or dental abscess.

Treatment should commence after a culture from the appropriate duct on suspicion of the disease. A blood culture should be obtained and fluid and electrolyte balance should be assessed in surgical patients.

Treatment plan:

- In any patient with a high fever, with an inability to open the mouth, or with any signs of cranial nerve involvement (cranial nerves VII, IX, and XII may be affected by glandular swelling) hospitalisation and inpatient treatment becomes mandatory.
- These patients need careful observation for any signs of airway compromise, general supportive care, and empirical broad-spectrum antibiotics after appropriate cultures (blood and pus from ductal orifice if present) have been taken.
- For the first 48 hours intravenous antibiotics are given and then could be continued or treatment could be switched to oral medications in case of resolution of fever and clinical improvement.
- Beta-lactams or vancomycin are generally considered first-line options. Clindamycin or metronidazole are acceptable alternatives.
- Most often the treatment is done in OPD and there is administration of a single dose of parenteral antibiotics, which is followed by oral antibiotics for 7-10 days.Intravenous clindamycin 8 hourly or 300mgs PO 8 hourly is a very good choice against the causative organisms.
- Cephalosporins and fluoroquinolones have been studied and found to have favourable pharmacokinetics in saliva.
- If the patient has no fever without the cranial nerves being affected, then out patient antibiotic therapy is effective. However review after 24 hours is recommended.
- If the condition is worsening, inpatient treatment with intravenous antibiotics may be necessary.
- Older patients with this condition need special care as morbidity may be associated with this condition due to age factor. They may benefit from a short period of inpatient treatment even in the absence of fever, trismus or cranial nerve involvement.
- Other medical treatments include conservative therapies such as hydration, analgesia with NSAIDs, for salivary stimulation, use of sialogogues, and regular, gentle massage of the glands.
- In some patients topical application of ice cubes provides relief. Corticosteroids can be of benefit in reducing soft tissue swelling.
- In case of presence of abscess, surgical incision and drainage is important.
- For mature and fluctuant abscesses surgical intervention is required.
- Surgical approach is decided by the location of abscess. In case of involvement of submandibular gland an intra or extra-oral approach or a combination may be effective but in parotid involvement an extra-oral approach is necessary.

- Care should be taken to avoid injury to the facial nerve.
- Maintenance of oral hygiene is of utmost importance and if necessary debridement and irrigation should be done.
- Proper electrolyte balance should be maintained and if necessary intravenous fluids should be administered.
- When cases dont respond to antibiotics the atypical bacterial or viral causes should be considered.

Suggested reading:

1. Patrick J, Bradley, Microbiology and management of sialadenitis, Current infectious disease reports, 2002, 4: 217-224.
2. Raad II, Sabbagh MF, Caranasos GJ Acute bacterial sialadenitis: a study of 29 cases and review. Rev Infect Dis. 1990 Jul-Aug; 12(4):591-601.

Q 9) Ptyalism:

TNMGRU APRIL 1999 (5 Marks)

Increased salivary production is known as Sialorrhea or Ptyalism.

It can be due to increased production of saliva due to idiopathic or drug related reasons or due to mechanism failure for clearance of saliva from the oral cavity. In coordination between the oro-facial and the palato-lingual musculature could be one reason that leads to collection of saliva at anterior portion of the mouth. Finally the muscle incoordination hampers the initiation of the swallow reflex and hinders the passage of saliva from the mouth to the oro-pharynx.

Etiology:

- Conditions like Rabies, gastro-esophageal reflex disorder known as water brash, leads to accumulation of sour fluid or tasteless saliva in the mouth.
- Pregnancy, Pancreatitis, Liver disease, Mouth ulcers, Serotonin syndrome and oral infections.
- **Medications that lead to increased production of saliva:**
- Pilocarpine, ketamine, clozapine, potassium chlorate, rabeprazole, risperidone etc.
- Toxins causing sialorrhea are:
- Mercury, copper, arsenic, insecticides.
- **Reduced clearance:**
- Tonsillitis, peritonsillar and retropharyngeal abscess, epiglottitis and mumps.
- Dislocations or fractures or trauma to the jaws.
- Radiotherapy
- Neurological conditions like Parkinsonism, myasthenia gravis, rabies, bulbar paralysis, bilateral facial and hypoglossal nerve palsy, epilepsy, autism and mental retardation.
- In neurologic disorders the increased salivation is due to improper swallowing because of impaired neuromuscular function.
- In adults 70-80% of cases of Parkinon's disease is associated with sialorrhoea.

- In schizophrenics about 30-80% suffer from excessive salivation while taking clozapine.

Clinical Features:

There is excessive drooling of saliva and there could be difficulty in swallowing and speech.

Feeling of discomfort and social awkwardness can be a problem.

Excessive salivation may lead to scarring of the buccal mucosa, lip chapping or infections of the oral cavity.

It can lead to aspiration, skin breakdown and bad odour.

Management:

It is a difficult condition to treat.The treatment could be conservative or invasive.In conservative treatment, changes are made in diet or habits, palatal training devices are given, and botulinum toxin injections.

Modification of behavior has been tried with little success.

Invasive treatments include surgery or radiation.Though surgery is effective and more long lasting, it has its side effects.

Radiotherapy is reserved only for older patients who cannot tolerate surgery or medications.

- Oral therapy for sialorrhea consists anticholinergics like glycopyrrolate, benztropine, scopolamine and tropicamide.The use of Biperiden is known to have an adverse effect on cognition, and hence its use has been limited.
- The use of anticholinergics help by down regulation of acetylcholine resulting in decreased saliva secretion by way of parasympathetic nervous system.
- Glycopyrrolate use has been found to be safe and effective in dosages of 1mg TDS.
- Intra-oral tropicamide films are known to provide short term relief from sialorrhea.
- In cases of drooling anti-reflux medications have been suggested.
- Transdermal scopolamine has been used effectively in cases of cerebral palsy, Down's syndrome, mental retardation, epilepsy and autism.
- Botulimun toxin which is a potent neurotoxin helps in blocking the release of acetylcholine and other neurotransmitters from synaptic vesicles and its use in treatment of ptyalism is being studied.
- The surgical procedures for sialorrhea include, alteration of anatomy of salivary glands and some times excision, denervation and ligation or transposition of salivary ducts. These procedures are reserved for severe cases and are associated with side effects.

Suggested reading:

1. Amanda Amrita Lakraj, Narges Moghimi, and Bahman Jabbari, Sialorrhea: Anatomy, Pathophysiology and Treatment with Emphasis on the Role of Botulinum Toxins, Toxins (Basel). 2013 May; 5(5): 1010–1031.

CHAPTER 18

Disorders of Maxillary Sinus

Introduction:

Paranasal sinuses are air filled spaces around the nasal cavity.The sinuses are frontal, maxillary, sphenoidal, and ethmoidal.Due to close proximity of the teeth with maxillary sinus, they are important from dentistry point of view.

Q 1) Causes of oro-antral fistula and enlist the investigations:

MUHS NOVEMBER 2010 (2 Marks)

It is pathologic, undesired communication between the oral cavity and the maxillary sinus which can be caused by iatrogenic, dental infections, osteomyelitis, trauma or radiation therapy.

Dental factors including extraction:

- While extraction of maxillary teeth it is often possible to cause an opening in the maxillary sinus due to traumatic procedure.
- The root of a tooth could be forced into the sinus accidentally causing an oro-antral fistula.
- Maxillary implants that are associated with contamination or disease can lead to this condition.
- Breaking of the palatal root of maxillary tooth can lead to an opening between the oral cavity and antrum.
- A small sized conical maxillary molar can accidentally slip in to the antrum while extraction especially along the tuberosity fracture leading to this condition.
- A periapical alveolar abscess may destroy the antral floor leading to communication between it and oral cavity.
- A chronic periapical abscess can erode the lamina dura and the root apex and sinus membrane can come in direct contact.

Surgical procedures:

- After a Caldwell-luc procedure if the incision does not heal it can lead to a fistula.
- Instrumentation done carelessly during maxillary sinusitis surgery can perforate the antral mucosa.

- A big cystic lesion very close to the sinus, during its removal can cause fistula formation.
- Marsupialisation involving a defective alveolar antral wall can result in a fistula.

Severe facial trauma:

Sharp objects or missiles can lead to extensive facial trauma and can get inserted into the sinus through the oral cavity causing a fistula.Even the gunshot injuries affecting the sinus walls can create a fistula.

Malignancies:

- Malignant lesions or granulomas of the maxillary sinus can erode the oral cavity.
- Tumours of the maxilla can encroach upon the sinus causing a fistula.

Investigations:

- Intraoral periapical radiograph of the affected region can show break in continuity of the sinus lining.
- Waters projection taken twice: The second radiograph with head tilted can clearly show the displaced root/tooth.
- Silver probe introduction into the orifice and radiograph taken, can show the oro-antral fistula.
- Blunt probe introduced in to the socket can confirm the bone defect.
- Patient asked to blow air with pinched nose and mouth open can show air bubbles in the extraction socket confirming the diagnosis.
- Computerised tomographic scan can help confirm the diagnosis.
- Cone beam computerised tomography (CBCT) of the affected region can reveal oro-antral fistula.

Suggested reading:

1. Frederick Valerio Berardinelli, Marco Favale, andCarlo Maiorana, Andrea Enrico Borgonovo, Surgical Options In Oroantral Fistula Treatment, Open Dent J. 2012; 6: 94–98.
2. Neelima Malik, Text book of oral and maxillofacial surgery, 2nd edition.page 572-584.

CHAPTER 19

Infections of Oral Cavity

Introduction:

Infection is a clinicopathological entity involving invasion of the body by pathogenic organisms and reaction of the tissues to them and their toxins.Orofacial infections are commonly encountered by the dentists. Most originate in the superficial structures and are often easily diagnosed and treated.However infections originating in the deeper structures can be severe, rapidly progressive, and may take long time to heal and could be associated with morbidity.Accurate diagnosis is hence very important with early aggressive medical treatment and decisive surgical treatment.

Infections can be odontogenic or non-odontogenic.The odontogenic infections can become serious life threatening facial space infections.The key to successful management is sound surgical principles.

Q 1) Pericoronitis:

TNMGRU APRIL 1993 (4 Marks)

Pericoronitis means inflammation around the coronal part of tooth.It is usually associated with impacted or partially erupted teeth.

The growth of microorganisms that develop in the distal pseudopocket is the major cause.

These microbes are mainly anaerobic.

Clinical features:

- It is usually associated with mandibular third molar which is prone to being impacted and is so positioned that its pericoronal flap gets traumatised easily and thus is the most affected region.
- It also occurs in infants in whom the tissue above the erupting tooth gets affected. The infection is associated with the supradental tissue, involving the superior portion of the follicle and the overlying mucoperiosteum which may become inflammed. It ultimately develops into a soft fluctuant abscess.Incision and drainage may have to be carried out followed by warm saline gargles at regular intervals.
- The patient can have toxic systemic complications like fever and

malaise and pain that may radiate to the throat, ear and floor of the mouth.There may be leucocytosis.

- There is usually swelling in the affected area and pain and difficulty in opening the mouth.There is cellulitis and muscular trismus.
- Sometimes it can be severe and complete mouth opening may be affected and difficulty in swallowing.
- The operculum can get traumatised by opposing teeth during mastication and there can be edema which is visible in the submandibular area and peritonsillar region. The abscess can be extremely tender.
- Submandibular lymphadenopathy is present and are enlarged, and tender.
- Complications include peritonsillar abscess, cellulitis and Ludwig's angina.

Radiographic features:

- There can be mesial or distal bone loss appearing as a step like defect.
- In the mandibular third molar area there can be circumferential bone loss around the tooth.
- Follicular crypt may show sclerosing osteitis.
- Medially inclined impacted teeth can show semilunar shaped bone resorption mesial to the crown and distal resorption in distally tilted crowns.

Diagnosis:

Clinically inflammation of pericoronal tissue around the third molar with pain and difficulty in opening the mouth and swallowing will help in diagnosis.

Radiographiclly, semilunar shaped bone loss will help in diagnosis.

Management:

- Antibiotics like phenoxymethyl penicillin is given 250mgs four times a day.
- Metronidazole 200mgs TDS for 7 days can be given.
- Evacuation of pus and septic material from the affected area.
- Once the acute condition subsides, extraction of the impacted third molar can be carried out.
- If the third molar can be retained, operculectomy, that is excision of the inflammed tissue around the affected tooth can be done.
- The pericoronal flap is excised with periodontal knife.
- The occlusal flap and the distal portion of the tissue is excised.
- In case only the occlusal flap is excised a deep distal pocket remains which can invite recurrence of acute pericoronal infection.
- After the tissue is removed a periodontal pack is applied which is removed after 1 week.
- In some cases the maxillary third molar can be a contributing factor in pericoronitis of the mandibular third molar.In such cases,

if the mandibular molar is fully erupted and in place, the maxillary third molar may be extracted to prevent further infection and complications.

Suggested reading:

1. Anil Govindrao Ghom, Textbook Of Oral Medicine, 3rd Edition, 420-421.
2. Jean-Louis Sixou, Christophe Magaud, Anne Jolivet-Gougeon, Michel Cormier, and Martine Bonnaure-Mallet, Evaluation of the Mandibular Third Molar Pericoronitis Flora and Its Susceptibility to Different Antibiotics Prescribed in France, J Clin Microbiol. 2003 Dec; 41(12): 5794–5797.

Q 2) Garre's osteomyelitis:

RGUHS APRIL 2001 (5 Marks)

Carl Gaffe in 1893 described Garre's osteomyelitis as focal gross thickening of the periosteum with formation of peripheral reactive bone formation due to infection.It was initially reported only in long bones like the tibia but in 1948 Berger reported a case involving the mandible.

Children and young adults are most commonly affected by this typical chronic type of osteomyelitis.It is commonly associated with an odontogenic infection due to caries.

Is is also known as 'proliferative periostitis'.

This is non-suppurating sclerosing osteomyelitis characterized by formation of hard, bony swelling at periphery of jaw.

It is induced by a mild infection below the periosteum from cancellous portion of jaw that penetrates the cortex.

For lesion to develop following conditions should be satisfied:

1. Periosteum must possess a high potential for osteoblastic activity.
2. Mild infection should be present to serve as a stimulus.
3. A fine balance has to be maintained between resistance of host and number and virulence of organism.

Etiology:

Staphylococcus pyogenes especially the aureus and albus type are isolated but variety of streptococci and mixed organisms can also be responsible.

Typical evolution of this lesion can be because of the high osteogenic potential of the young patients which allows the osteoblastic process superior to the osteolytic one and the pattern is identical to the condensing osteitis which can be seen periapical to a carious tooth, only that the proliferation of bone is of periosteal origin rather than endosteal.

Clinical features:

(a) Males affected more than females and generally below below 30 years of age.

In the younger patients as mentioned earlier, the osteoblastic process predominates in the periosteum, leading to a condensation of bone rather than a osteolysis. It affects the mandible more commonly and results in a hard swelling of the jaws causing facial asymmetry and mild or no pain.

(b) Mandible is more often affected than the maxilla especially inferior border of mandible and 1st molar region.
(c) Presents as hard non tender swelling with medial and lateral expansion of jaw.
(d) Size vary from 1-2 cm to involvement of the entire length of affected side. Cortex may become 2-3 cm thick.
(e) If secondarily infected it causes considerable discomfort.
(f) Usually the overlying skin appears normal unless there is inflammation and pain.
(g) Other associated symptoms: lymphadenopathy, hyperpyrexia, leukocytosis. However these findings are milder than the other forms of osteomyelitis where there could be high fever, increased WBCs count, ESR or alkaline phosphatase levels.

Radiographic features:

(a) An intra oral periapical radiograph will show a carious tooth opposite the hard bony mass.
(b) Layers of bone forming a thin convex shell on the cortex with radiolucent space between the two is seen.
(c) Panoramic and occlusal views will reveal a localised bony growth on the outer surface of the cortex.This bony mass is subperiosteal and supracortical, smooth, fairly calcified, and is often described as a duplication of the mandibular cortical layer.
(d) Panoramic radiographs will show vertical and the occlusal radiographs will show a lateral apposition of bone, but a lateral oblique view can show the expansion of the lesion which can be inferior and lateral to the lower border of the mandible.
(e) As infection persists cortex becomes thick and becomes laminated showing alternate radiolucent and radiopaque layers giving an onion peel like appearance.
(f) Adjacent cancellous bone may remain normal.
(g) Following removal of irritation cortical bone may remodel to a normal appearance.

Histopathologic findings:

The typical feature is the formation of new bone, or osteoid tissue, bordered with osteoblasts and some areas of bone reorption.Lymphocytes predominate in marrow spaces.

Differential diagnosis:

1. Ewing's sarcoma
2. Caffey's disease (infantile cortical hyperostosis)
3. Osteosarcoma.
4. Peripheral osteomas, tori, exostoses should clinically distinguished.
5. Ossifying subperiosteal hematoma.

Treatment:

The usual treatment options can be careful observation, use of analgesics and NSAIDs and curettage of bone.

Removal of the offending teeth or source of infection along with antibiotic therapy will help in resolution of the condition.

The treatment for this condition could be resection of bone and transport with the use of a circular external fixator which could be a safe and effective method.

Suggested reading:

1. McWalter GM, Schaberg Garre's osteomyelitis of the mandible resolved by endodontic treatment.SJJ Am Dent Assoc. 1984 Feb; 108(2):193-5.
2. Nikomarov D, Zaidman M, Katzman A, Keren Y, Eidelman M., New treatment option for sclerosing osteomyelitis of Garré, J Pediatr Orthop B. 2013 Nov;22(6):577-82.
3. Stephane Schwartz, Huan Pham, Garre's osteomyelitis: a case report, The American Academy of Pedodontics/Vol. 3, No. 3, 283-285.

Q 3) Ludwig's Angina:

5 Marks (not specific to any university)

1. Ludwigs angina is a condition characterized by cellulitis of the submandibular, sublingual and submental spaces bilaterally.
2. This condition was first described by Wilhelm Friedreich Von Ludwig in 1836.
3. It is also known as marbus strangulatorius, angina maligna, Garotillo.

Etiology:

1. **Odontogenic infections:** It is the most common cause of Ludwigs angina. It mainly arises due to infection through second and third molar teeth.
2. **Traumatic injuries:** Compounded and comminuted mandibular fractures, lacerating and penetrating injuries to the orofacial region can develop into ludwigs angina.
3. **Sialadenitis:** Acute or chronic infection of submandibular and sublingual gland may involve submandibular, sublingual and submental spaces.
4. **Osteomyelitis:** Mandibular fractures may precipitate in osteomyelitis further resulting into ludwigs angina.
5. Secondary infection due to malignancies.
6. **Iatrogenic:** Due to use of contaminated needle during local anesthesia.
7. **Miscellaneous:** a) Purulent tonsillitis
   b) Foreign bodies such as fish bone etc.

Microbiology:

In early stages of the condition, mixed aerobic and anaerobic flora exists while in later stages the infection becomes more anaerobic. The most commonly involved organism is streptococci while the staphylococci, gram negative micro-organisms such as E-coli, pseudomonas, bacteriods, peptostreptococcus and fusospirocheates are also isolated.

Clinical Features:

1. General symptoms: General symptoms include fever accompanied

with chills, fatigue, weakness, excessive tiredness, mental confusion. Patient looks ill, toxic, dehydrated.
2. Respiratory distress due to airway obstruction may be present.
3. Swelling is diffused, firm/hard present bilaterally in submandibular, sublingual region with presence of severe tenderness associated with the swelling.
4. There is pain, stiffness and redness of neck.There is tenderness and enlargement of the neck region above the hyoid bone due to submandibular gland involvement and is called as bull's neck.
5. Involvement of sublingual space leads to posterior enlargement, protrusion and elevation of the tongue. Patient complains of excessive salivation and inability to eat and swallow.
6. Severe muscle spasm may lead to trismus and difficulty in mouth opening.
7. Floor of mouth, larynx and glottis becomes edematous.
8. Fatal death may occur in untreated cases with ludwigs angina.

Management:

Management of Ludwig's angina includes combination of following interventions:

1. **Surgical drainage of facial spaces:** Incisions are made in the submandibular and submental region 1 cm below the inferior border of mandible to drain the facial spaces.A through and through drain is placed to drain the edematous area.
2. **Maintenance of airway:** Due to respiratory distress tracheostomy is advised in patients with ludwigs angina.Nasoendotracheal intubation is the most reliable method for maintaining the patients airway.
3. Extraction of the offending tooth.
4. **Prolonged antibiotic therapy:** Penicillin is the drug of choice for patients with Ludwig's angina it should be given IV or IM 2 to 4 million units 4-6hrly or 500mg 6hrly orally.In case of allergy to penicillins, erythromycin 600mg 6-8hrly is advised. In case of penicillinase resistant staphylococci, Clindamycin 300 to 600mg IV 8 hourly or gentamycin 80mg IM is given. Metronidazole is given in case of anaerobic flora in oral infections 400mg 8 hourly orally or intravenously.
5. **Supportive therapy:** it includes parenteral hydration, high protein diet and vitamin supplements and hydrotherapy.
   - Hydrotherapy: It is a method of cold application in order to reduce edema, inflammation and swelling.It is done by placing gauze pieces over the indurated area and wetting them with cold water.
   - Hydration: Intravenous fluids are given in order to overcome the diminished fluid intake associated with pain and discomfort during swallowing.
6. **Irrigation:** Irrigation of wound drains with bacitracin in mixture of

H2O2 and normal saline is done to control the infection within the spaces.

7. **Maintenance:** Regular follow-ups and re-evaluation of patient is necessary.

Complications:

1. Airway obstruction.
2. Septicemia.
3. Mediastinitis.
4. Pericarditis, meningitis.
5. Jugular vein thrombosis.
6. Brain abscess.
7. Cavernous sinus thrombosis.
8. Involvement of carotid sheath.
9. Death.

Suggested reading:

1. Anil Govindrao Ghom Textbook of oral medicine 2ND edition, Pg no 453-456.
2. Neelima Malik Textbook of oral and maxillofacial surgery Pg no 701-712

CHAPTER 20

Bacterial Infections

Introduction:

The oral cavity reflects the state of health of an individual more frequently than other parts of the body.Bacterial diseases such as syphillis, tuberculosis, myiasis, scarlet fever, actinomycosis, leprosy, noma, tetanus, diphtheria etc have oral manifestations and knowledge of bacterial infections is a must.

Q 1) Cancrum oris or noma:

RGUHS OCTOBER 2002 (5 Marks)

This term is taken from the Greek word nomein, which means to devour.

It is a gangrenous type of stomatitis which involves the mouth, and hard and soft tissues of the face especially in children of age between 2-16 years.

Etiololgy:

Though the exact cause of this condition is not known, certain factors like poor oral hygiene in children, poor nutritional status, weakened immune system, history of measles, typhoid, malaria, whooping cough, bacillary dysentry, scarlet fever, tuberculosis, malignancies and HIV, are considered as predisposing to noma.

The disease is not communicable but is bacterial in origin.

Causative organisms are Fusobacterium necrophorum, F necrophorum Prevotella, intermedia and Borellia vincenti.

Clinical manifestations:

- The mucous membranes, that is the gingiva, buccal mucosa become inflammed and followed by development of ulcer.
- There is spread of infection from the oral mucous membranes to the skin, which leads to necrosis of the tissues of the lips and cheeks.
- Sore mouth with focal edema and development of fetid odour and taste occurs.
- Oral discharge is foul smelling, purulent and associated with drooling, anorexia and palpable cervical lymphadenopathy.

- A bluish-black cone shaped mass is formed with the base in the oral mucosa.
- Within the next 4-72 hours there is rapid progress to gangrene.
- Any part of the face can be involved, and upper/or lower jaw can be affected and the involvement can be uni-or bilateral.
- There can be severe mutilation of the facial, intraoral structures and loss of function.
- There is continual, rapid breakdown of tissues and the gangrene can destroy the soft tissues including bone.
- There is degradation of the face of children within days.
- This condition causes, rapid, progressive destruction of tissues and occasionally genitals may be involved known as noma pudenda.
- Systemic symptoms include fever, tachychardia, tachypnea and anorexia. If untreated this condition can be fatal.

Treatment:

The treatment of this condition requires a multidisciplinary approach.

- In the early stages the child will need oral hydrogen peroxide and saline and 0.2% chlorhexidine irrigation. This will help the necrotic tissue to slough off.
- Proper hydration and maintenance of electrolyte balance, correction of vitamin deficiencies, and adequate nutritional support is vital even through nasogastric tube, if necessary.
- Chemotherapy consists of antibiotics, multivitamins and hematinics, metronidazole and penicillin for a week. Other drugs given are folic acid, iron supplements, and vitamin C.
- General patient management involves treating the existing diseases like measles, malaria, bronchopnemonia etc. Patients are given high protein diet.
- Surgical treatment is done to remove grade I and II teeth that are mobile and removal of sloughing tissue, sequestra to help in mouth opening. Sequestrectomy and release of ankylosis is advised under general anesthesia.

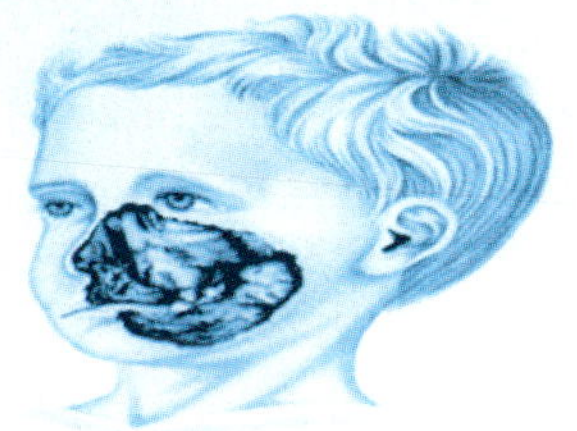

Fig. Illustrating Cancrum Oris

Suggested reading:

1. Anil Govindrao Ghom Textbook Of Oral Medicine, 3rd Edition, 366.
2. Burket's Oral Medicine, Diagnosis And Treatment, 12th Edition, 52-53.

Q 2) Describe in short etiology, clinical and oral manifestation of tuberculosis: (not specific to any university)

(5 Marks)

Tuberculosis is a granulomatous disease that runs a chronic course and is caused by acid fast bacilli Mycobacterium tuberculosis. Lungs are most commonly involved due to tuberculosis followed by others parts of the body.

Etiology:

Tuberculosis is mainly caused due the intracellular parasite namely M. Tuberculosis.It is anerobic, non motile, non sporing rod shaped bacilli. Other micro-organisms associated with tuberculosis include mycobacterium bovis, mycobacterium kanasasi, mycobacterium xenopi and mycobacterium malmoense.

Clinical Features:

1. The signs and symptoms of tuberculosis include episodes of fever and chills, malaise and easily fatigued. Patient complains of gradual weight loss and their is persistent cough with or without hemoptysis.
2. Tuberculosis is classified as pulmonary and extrapulmonary tuberculosis. Pulmonary TB involves the lungs while extrapulmonary TB includes tuberculosis of lymph nodes, bones and joints, pleura, genitourinary tract, peritoneum, pericardium, meninges.
3. Pulmonary tuberculosis may be classified as primary, secondary and miliary tuberculosis.
   Primary tuberculosis: It occurs in individuals unexposed to tuberculosis. It is most common in children but may also occur in adults. It is usually asymptomatic or there could be fever and cough. The lesion formed after the intial infection (Ghons focus) in the presence or absence of pleural reaction, thickening, regional lymphadenopathy together is referred as Ghons complex. Ghons complex is typical of primary pulmonary tuberculosis.
   Secondary tuberculosis: It occurs due to re-activation of bacteria due to compromised host defense. Symptoms of secondary tuberculosis includes, fever, cough, chest pain and hemoptysis. The lesion is usually located in the apical segments of upper lobe.
   Miliary tuberculosis: It occurs due to spread of infection through haematogenous route and involvement of organs such as kidney, liver etc.
4. Scrofula refers to a marked enlargement of cervical lymph nodes with caseation and breakdown. The involvement of skin in TB is known as Lupus vulgaris.
5. **Cold abscess :** It is typical feature of tuberculosis in which there is chronicity of infection and lack of pain or acute inflammatory symptoms. It is most commonly seen in the neck.

Oral Manifestations:

1. Tuberculosis in the oral cavity is relatively uncommon.
2. Predisposing factors for tuberculosis includes poor oral hygiene, trauma, fractures, pre-existing lesions such as leukoplakia, periapical granuloma, cyst, abscess, periodontitis, lowered resistance.
3. Primary lesion of tuberculosis in oral cavity occurs when the bacteria is directly inoculated in the oral tissue to the person who is not immune to the disease. Most common sites for primary tuberculosis includes gingiva, tooth extraction socket and buccal folds.
4. Secondary lesion occurs due to spread of tubercle bacilli by haematogenous route and deposit in the oral mucosa in case of extrapulmonary tuberculosis. Though the lesions of secondary tuberculosis can occur at any site of the oral mucosa, the tongue is the commonest, followed by palate, lips and buccal mucosa, gingiva and frenula.
5. The lesion of tuberculosis is preceded by vesicle or nodule which breaks down to ulcer which may be superficial or deep. The lesion is usually painful. Margins of ulcer is usually undermined and the base is yellowish and granular. The adjacent mucosa surrounding the ulcer is inflamed and edematous. The tuberculosis ulcers at the mucocutaneous junction are extremely shallow, painful and often oozing from the lesion is seen.
6. Sentinel tubercle refers to single or multiple nodules surrounding the tubercular ulcer.
7. Sometimes tuberculosis causes diffuse, nodular or hyperaemic papillary proliferation of gingival tissues.This condition is referred as tuberculosis gingivitis. It is mainly seen in primary tuberculosis where gingiva is most commonly involved.
8. Tuberculosis may involve maxilla or mandible. Patient experience difficulty in eating trismus, paresthesia of lower lip, regional lymphadenopathy, intraoral and extraoral fistulas. Jaw involvement mainly arises due to gingival lesion with deep extension, infected extraction of socket, extension of tuberculous granuloma at the apex of tooth or by means of haematological spread. In some cases involvement of temporomandibular joint may be present.

Suggested reading:

1. Anil Govindrao Ghom, Textbook of oral medicine by (2ND edition) Pg no 744-746.
2. Harrisons Principles of internal medicine (18th edition) Pg no 1341-1359.

CHAPTER **21**

Viral Infections

Q 1) Verruca Vulgaris:

RGUHS OCTOBER 2000 (5 Marks)

Verruca vulgaris is of the colour of flesh and is a firm nodule or papule which is because of infection of the epidermal cells by human papilloma virus. Also known as warts.Caused by HPV virus type 2, 4, 6 and 40.

Up to one in about 10 individuals will develop a wart at some point in their lives.Is most common in childhood and adolescence.Verruca and warts are usually harmless and may disappear by themselves.In children 9 out of 10 cases go away within 2 years but takes longer to fade away in adults.

Warts can vary in size and appearance and may range from 1mm-1 cm.Different types of warts are as follows:

(i) **Common wart or verruca vulgaris:** These growths are firm, raised and have rough surface and may resemble a cauliflower.They are frequently present on the backs of hands, fingers, knees and toes.

(ii) **Plantar warts:** They are commonly present on the soles of feet and may have dark spots in the center and could cause pain when weight is put on them.

(iii) **Verruca plana:** They are common on hands and face and are round, smooth, flat in shape and light brown in colour.

(iv) **Mosaic warts:** A cluster of verrucas placed close together usually on the hands and feet.

(v) **Filiform warts:** Common on the back region and face and are long and thin growths.

(vi) **Genital warts:** A different variety of HPV causes these warts and spread to other parts of the body usually through sexual contact. Can cause irritation or soreness around the area.

(vii) In case of oral lesions they occur commonly on the vermilion border of lips, labial mucosa and anterior part of tongue.

The cutaneous lesions are generally pink or yellow, or whitish in color, and oral lesions are generally white.

Surface is rough and pebbly and its base can be pedunculated or sessile.

In some cases extreme accumulation of keratin results in a hard surface projection. It is known as keratin horn.

Etiology:

HPV which are of over 100 types cause these lesions.They can be contagious and usually spread from direct skin contact or in moist places like the swimming pools and community showers.When scratched the viral particles can spread to the other areas of the person's skin.

Butchers who handle flesh a lot or work in an abattoir, are likely to develop warts more frequently although the reason is unclear.

Individuals with HIV/AIDS, or those on immunosuppressive medications having a weak immune system may be prone to develop these lesions.

Histopathology:

The verruca or wart shows papillomatous hyperplasia of the epidermis which is flower like, is hyperkeratotic and prominent granular cell layer, enlarged keratohyaline granules, and in some cases, intracytoplasmic eosinophilic viral inclusions.The reteridges are bent inwardly.

Treatment:

- Liquid nitrogen cryotherapy is the treatment of choice in this condition. It induces subepithelial blister which lifts the infected epithelium away from the connective tissue and allows its sloughing off.
- Surgical excision is done in cases of oral lesions.
- Creams containing an ingredient called imiquimod can be applied. Imiquimod stimulates immune system to recognise and attack the wart virus. Combination of salicylic acid and imiquimod is also used.
- Creams containing retinoids, often prescribed to treat acne, can also be useful at treating warts.
- Radiofrequency heat generators are used for localised heating and surgical excision with radiofrequency electrosurgical knives have been tried with moderate amount of success.
- Some success has been obtained by use of small patch which contains chemicals and produce heat by way of oxidation on exposure to air, have been applied to warts.
- As an alternative to CO2 laser treatment use of direct application of infrared contact coagulators have been found to be cheaper, safer and easier method to treat warts.
- A focused CO2 laser is generally used as a scalpel to excise the warts to the level of subcutaneous tissue and later the base of the wart is vapourised with help of defocused beam till a clean and clear surgical field is obtained.
- Selective microvascular destruction of the dilated capillaries in the warts is achieved by the pulsed dye laser.
- Common warts on the hands, flat warts and plantar warts have been tried to be treated with photodynamic therapy.
- Virucidal therapy includes use of glutaraldehyde, formaldehyde, formic acid, antiviral drugs like cidofovir.

- Antimitotic therapy includes use of bleomycin, retinoids, podophyllin, podophyllotoxin.

Suggested reading:

1. Michelle M. Lipke, An Armamentarium of Wart Treatments, Clin Med Res. 2006 Dec; 4(4): 273–293.

Q 2) Infectious Mononucleosis:

RGUHS OCTOBER 2000 (5 Marks)

Introduction:

A clinical entity which is characterised by pharyngitis, cervical lymphadenopathy, fatigue, fever, and is caused most often by the Epstein -Barr virus, is called Infectious mononucleosis. It is also called as 'glandular fever' or 'mono', 'kissing disease' because the virus spreads by intimate oral contact among the young adults.

In 1920 Sprunt and Evans first described this condition.

Etiology:

1. The most important risk factor in this EBV infectious disease is intimate contact with a person infected with EBV.
2. The oropharyngeal secretions harbor the EBV for months even after the resolution of the disease.
3. Individuals with congenital immunodeficiencies are prone to develop EBV induced infectious mononeucleosis.

Clinical Features:

1. Incubation period varies from 32 to 49 days.
2. Children and adolescents aged 4-15 years of age are prone to this condition. Children mostly acquire this disease by the virus from asymptomatic parents or siblings who give out low levels of EBV in their oral secretions and thus transmit smaller infectious inoculum.
3. The patient suffers from sore throat and is associated with fever malaise and fatiguability.
4. Other symptoms include, headache, nausea, vomiting, diarrhea, photophobia, erythematous macular rash .Palatal petechiae, periorbital and eyelid edema may also occur.
5. Enlarged palatine tonsils with cheesy yellow exudates flooding the crypts of tonsils, and presence of hepato and splenomegaly. Hepatitis occurs in 75% of patients but is usually subclinical. Superficial lymph nodes enlargement, especially the posterior cervical are involved and are, slightly tender on palpation.
6. **Chronic fatigue syndrome:** In this, patient notices, fever, severe fatigue, myalgia, headache, depression, cognitive defect.
7. **Complications:** Obstruction of the airway, rupture of spleen, hemolytic anemia and progressive neurological involvement.

Oral Manifestation:

1. Lesion commonly seen are on the soft palate, lip and buccal mucosa. Soft palate may show petechiae.

2. Ulcerative gingivitis, periodontitis, and stomatitis may be present and lesion normally persist for 3 to 11 days.
3. Tonsillitis with enlargement along with sore throat, difficulty in swallowing, and covering of tonsils with whitish or grayish pseudomembrane occur.
4. In one third of patients with a tendency towards hemorrhage, may exhibit oro-pharyngeal bleeding and, bleeding from gingiva.

Diagnosis:

1. **Clinical diagnosis:** Skin rash that is morbiliform, along with enlarged tonsils and associated fever.
2. **Laboratory diagnosis:** Patients will give positive Paul-Bunnel and mono-spot test.The most reliable and useful specific antibody tests are, VCA IgM, VCA IgG and EBNA-1 IgG which are mostly measured by enzyme immunoassay platform.

Management:

1. Researchers are giving priority to develop a prophylactic EBV vaccine since the idea was suggested by Epstein and Achong in 1973.
2. Hydrogen peroxide rinses can help in alleviating the fusospirochetal gingivitis and a topical anesthetic can be used to give respite from painful ulcers.
3. Antipyretic and anti-inflammatory therapy to control pain and fever.
4. Ganciclovir and alpha-interferon inhibits the replication of EBV in vitro. Valacyclovir 3 g day−1 for 2 weeks in a study showed significant improvement in symptoms.
5. Corticosteroid are indicated only in the presence of complications mentioned above.
6. Sports should be avoided as it can lead to splenic rupture.

Suggested reading:

1. Anil Govindrao Ghom, Textbook Of Oral Medicine, 3rd edition, 727.
2. Henry H Balfour, Samantha K Dunmire, Kristin A Hogquist, Infectious mononucleosis, Clin Transl Immunology. 2015 Feb;4(2).

Q 3) Hepatitis B

TNMGRU FEBURARY 2013 (5 Marks)

An infectious disease caused by hepatitis B virus (HBV) and which affects the liver is called hepatitis B.Both acute and chronic infections can occur. Many patients have no symptoms during the initial period of infection.In some cases, the onset can be rapid, with sickness, vomiting, development of yellowish colour of skin, fatigue and tiredness, dark urine, and pain in abdomen. These symptoms may last for few weeks and is rarely fatal.

Caused by the hepatitis B virus, is also called as serum hepatitis.

The hepatitis B virus:

It is a small, double-shelled virus in the family Hepadnaviridae.

The virus has a small circular DNA genome that is partially double-stranded.

Mode of transmission:

1. The virus is spread through the parenteral or mucosal exposure to HBsAg -positive body fluids from individuals having acute or chronic HBV infection.
2. The highest concentrations of virus are found in blood and serous fluids.
3. Lower concentrations are found in other fluids such as tears, saliva, urine and semen.
4. Semen is a vehicle for sexual transmission and saliva could be the medium of spread through bites.

Clinical Features:

1. The incubation period averages about 120 days and the clinical symptoms and signs are more frequently seen in adults than the children or infants who generally run an acute aymptomatic course.
2. The prodrome from the start of the symptoms to the onset of jaundice generally lasts from 3-10 days.The disease is typically characterised by insidious onset of malaise, nausea, vomiting, loss of apetite, abdominal pain in the upper right quadrant, fever. headache, myalgia, rashes on skin, pain in joints, arthritis, and dark urine which start 1-2 days prior to onset of jaundice.
3. The icteric phase generally lasts between 1-3 weeks and is typically characterised by jaundice, light or gray stools, tenderness and enlargement of liver.
4. During the healing and convalescent phase the malaise, tiredness may continue for weeks or months, but the jaundice, loss of appetite and other symptoms may fade away.
5. Usually the acute phase of HBV infection in adults result in complete recovery and there is elimination of HBsAg from the blood and there is production of anti-HBs resulting in immunity to further infection.
6. On the other hand a chronic hepatitis B infection could either be asymptomatic or could be associated with chronic hepatitis and may lead to cirrhosis over a period of time of about several years.This chronic type of infection increases the incidence of hepatocellular malignancy.
7. Apart from the symptoms of liver, in 1-10% of HBV patients there can be serum-sickness like syndrome, membranous glomerulonephritis, polyarteritis nodosa, and papular acrodermatitis of childhood.

Laboratory Diagnosis:

1. The most common test used to detect this condition is the HBsAg that can help diagnose acute phase of infection or the carriers. It can be either detected very early between 1-2 weeks or late between 11-12 weeks after exposure to HBV, in which case sensitive assays are used.
2. The presence of HBsAg suggests that the person has the infection which can be either acute or chronic.

3. Anti-HBc develops in all the cases of HBV infections and appears soon after HBsAg in case of acute conditions and suggests the presence of HBV infection at some point in the past.

Complications:

Chronic HBV infection can lead to cirrhosis and its complications including ascites, portal hypertension, hemorrhage, and hepatocellular carcinoma.

Treatment:

1. In case of acute hepatitis B infection, no specific treatment is required and generally the adults become free of the infection in due course of time.
2. Preventive measures include vaccination, screening, proper handling of donated blood and tissue.
3. For acute infection only supportive treatment is recommended.
4. For chronic hepatitis b infection following antiviral therapy is recommended:
   Adefovir, entecavir, tenofovir, lamivudine.
   However none of the drugs mentioned can get rid of the infection but can help the virus to stop replicating and helps in minimising damage to the liver.
5. Immunostimulator injectables: These help to stimulate the immune system to get rid of the liver cells infected with HBV.The treatment course is usually a 6-12 month.
   Following immunostimulator injection can be given:
   - Interferon alfa-2b - Administered subcutaneously 3-5 times/ week.
   - Peginterferon alpha-2a-It is given as a subcutaneous injection once a week.

Prognosis:

Infection with Hepatitis B virus can be acute and self-limiting or may run a chronic and long standing course. Patients with the acute and self limiting condition can spontaneously recover within weeks to months. Children however may not clear the infection like the adults. In 95% of cases infected with the HBV virus either adults or young adults will achieve full recovery and also develop immunity to the virus.But in younger children the chance drops to 30% and in new borns who acquire the infection through their mothers at birth only about 5% will be able to clear the infection.In such cases there is a 40% lifetime risk of death due to cirrhosis or hepatocellular carcinoma.The children between the age of 1-6 years about 70% can get rid of the infection.

Suggested reading:

1. Ascherio A, Zhang SM, Hernan MA, et al. Hepatitis B vaccination and the risk of multiple sclerosis. N Engl J Med 2001; 344:327–32.
2. Burket's Oral Medicine, Diagnosis and Treatment, 10th edition, chapter no22.pg no 549.

CHAPTER 22

Diseases of Cardiovascular System

Introduction:

A thorough knowledge about the disorders of the cardiovascular diseases is of great importance as it can have a major bearing on the treatment plan of dental disorders especially the dental surgical procedures.

The dental clinician needs to have extensive knowledge of how to appropriately handle cases who come with the cardiovascular problems.

Q 1) Angiography:

TNMGRU SEPTEMBER 2002 (5 Marks)

Definition:

Its an imaging technique used in the medical field to view the lumen of blood vessels and organs of the body, especially the arteries, veins and the heart chambers. It is performed by injecting radiopaque agents within the the blood vessel and imaging is done using X-ray based techniques like fluroscopy.The image thus obtained of the vessels is called angiograph or angiogram.

History:

This technique was first developed by a portuguese physician and neurologist Egas Moniz in 1927, so as to obtain a contrasted cerebral angiography so that various kinds of nervous diseases could be diagnosed.

Method:

The technique varies depending on the type of angiogram, but the access to the blood vessels is obtained usually through the femoral artery, to observe the left side of the heart and the arterial system.The medium is injected in the jugular or the femoral vein, to observe the right side of the heart and the venous system. Using a guide wire and catheters, a type of contrast agent is injected into the blood so that they can be seen on the X-ray images.

The images thus obtained could be still images displayed on an image intensifier or images in motion.Digital subtraction angiography is the method used to see all structures except the heart. The images are taken at the rate of 2-3 frames /second so that the interventional radiologist can evaluate the flow of blood through the vessels. In this method the bones and the organs are subtracted so that the contrast filled vessels only can be seen.The images of the heart are taken at 15-30 frames/second.In these techniques the interventional radiologist will be able to see any blockages or narrowing within the blood vessel that may be resulting in pain.

Uses:

1. **Angiography of coronary arteries:**
   This is the most common angiogram where in the blood in coronary arteries can be visualised.
   Coronary angiography is the name for a diagnostic x-ray procedure designed to visualize the small (1 to 3 millimeters in diameter) nutrient arteries of the heart.
2. A catheter which is a long thin flexible tube is used to inject the contrast agent in the area of interest. The catheter is introduced in to an artery of the forearm and then the tip is advanced through the arterial system in to the major coronary artery.
   The size of the arterial openings can be visualised by the X-ray images of the transient contrast medium distribution within the blood inside the coronary arteries allowing the visualisation.
   In order to detect the coronary artery disease, CT scan is better than MRI.
   Tiny blood vessels can be studied by micro-angiography.
3. **Neuro-vascular angiography:**
   Used for visualising the arterial and venous supply to the brain.
4. **Peripheral angiography:**
   This is performed to identify the narrowing of vessels in patients with pain or cramps in the legs due to reduced blood flow to the legs and feet. Can be used in patients with renal stenosis and also in the head to diagnose and repair stroke.
5. In medico-legal cases post mortem CT angiography.

Complications:

Complications can occur in cases of cerebral angiography which may include stroke, allergic reaction to anesthetic or other medications or to the contrast medium used, blockage or damage to one of the access veins, thrombosis or embolism formation. Minor complications include bleeding or bruising at the site where the contrast medium is injected.

When the contrast medium is injected, it produces a feeling of warmth, lasting only for few seconds, but could be felt to a greater degree in the region of injection. In case of allergy to the contrast medium, more serious side effects can occur. With the advent of new contrast mediums the risk of severe reactions is only 1 in 80, 000 examinations.

Suggested reading:

1. G.timothy jhonson MD, arteriogram, venograms, angiograms territory, 12 sep 2011.
2. O Aquilina, V Grech, H Felice, J Debono, and A Fenechmages, Paediatr Cardiol. 2006 Apr-Jun; 8(2): 1–16. Normal adult coronary angiography.

Q 2) Dental Consideration In patients with Ischemic Heart Disease:

TNMGRU FEBRUARY 2015 (5 Marks)

- In patients suffering from ischemic heart disease, for dental procedures, before performing any surgery a minimum safety period of 6 months has been established.
- At present, in the first 6 days after infarction the evaluation of exercise testing is considered important for assessment of risk and prognosis.If the test is well tolerated by the patients then the risk is considered to be low.
- During this period, the dental treatment should be done only in emergency cases just to give pain relief, unavoidable extractions, abscess drainage, pulpectomies, etc and should be carried out in the presence of hospital facilities.
- When the safety period is over, the decision of treatment should be based on the situation and the medical condition of the patient.
- Before initiating a dental treatment, consultation with treating physician is necessary, so as to know the type of heart disease present, the severity, amount of time elapsed after the cardiological event, the complications if any and the treatment received by the patient.
- The patient should continue the medications advised.
- In case the patient is advised nitrates, they should carry it along to each dental visit in case chest pain develops.

Preventive measures before proceeding for dental treatment:

1. Administration of nitrate which serves as a preventive measure before injecting local anesthesia.
2. For very anxious patients, some premedication to reduce anxiety and stress can be prescribed, like 5-10 mgs of diazepam the night before and 1-2 hours before treatment.
3. Sedation in inhalatory form like nitrous oxide/oxygen.
4. Time and duration of visit: The visits should be of less time, 30 minutes and should be scheduled during the day, avoiding the early mornings when heart attacks are frequent and late afternoon, when there is more of tiredness and stress.
5. **Local anesthesia:** The technique of anesthesia should be the best and care should be taken to avoid injecting directly into the blood vessel and the usage of maximum 2 carpules that too with a vasoconstrictor.In case anesthetic reinforcement is required then it should be given without vasoconstrictor.
6. **Position:** The patient should be placed in the most comfortable position usually a semi-supine one, and they should get up slowly and carefully to avoid orthostatic hypotension.
7. **Vital signs:** Pulse oxymetry and blood pressure monitoring may be required during dental procedure, depending on the patient.

Patient on anticoagulants:

In case the patient is receiving anti-coagulants, the international normalised ratio (INR) on the day of the procedure should be determined and the treatment should be provided within the recommended limits less than 3.5 and local hemostasis when surgery is to be done.

Three different protocols can be used to treat patients with significantly elevated INR:

A) *First protocol:*

- Warfarin is not discontinued. This minimizes adverse thrombo-embolic events but increases the risk for excessive bleeding after surgery.
- If localized antihemostatic measures are inadequate to stop bleeding after surgery, vitamin K injections and antifibrinolytic mouth rinses can be instituted.

B) *Second protocol:*

- Warfarin therapy is discontinued, and the patient is not placed on any alternative anticoagulation therapy.
- In order to diminish the anticoagulative effect of warfarin, the medication must be discontinued 2 to 3 days before surgery. It will take an additional 2 to 3 days after surgery to regain the therapeutic effect of the medication.

C) *Third protocol:*

- Warfarin therapy is discontinued, and the patient is placed on an alternative anticoagulation therapy.
- This protocol has both advantages and disadvantages. The greatest advantage is that the patient's risk for developing thromboembolic events is minimized.

Patient on antiplatelet medication:

In case the patient is being given anti-platelet medication it may become necessary to control excessive local bleeding.

The local bleeding control methods that can be used are bone wax, sutures, gelfoam, regenerated oxidized cellulose (Surgicel), platelet rich plasma, collagen, thrombin, fibrin sealants (Tissucol) electric or laser scalpels, anti-fibrinolytic agents like tranexamic acid, or epsilon-aminocaproic acid (Caproamin).

Patient who develop chest pain during dental treatment:

- The procedure should be stopped instantly, sublingual nitrate tablet, 0.4-0.8 mgs to be administered, along with nasal oxygen, 3 litres/minute.
- In case the pain alleviates, then the procedure can be resumed, or alternate appointment can be given on another day.
- If the pain doesnot subside, a second sublingual nitrate tablet should be given.

- In case the pain fails to subside, within 15 minutes of onset, acute case of myocardial infarction should be suspected and patient should be transferred immediately to hospital.

Suggested reading:

1. Burket's, Textbook of Oral Medicine Diagnosis & Treatment. Diseases of the Cardiovascular system, 10th edition, pg 363-88.
2. Marta Cruz-Pamplona et al. Dental considerations in patients with heart disease. J Clin Exp Dent.2011; 3 (2):97-105.

Q 3) Discuss the management of patient with prosthetic heart valve in dental clinic:

BFU MAY 2009 7$^{1/2}$ Marks.

- There are numerous types and models of prosthetic heart valves, each with their own characteristics. These valves are either mechanical or bioprosthetic.
- The risk of thrombo embolism is highest in the period following placement of the valve and decreases over time as the valve becomes endothelialized.
- Prosthetic heart valves increase the risk for infectious endocarditis, which typically manifests as fever and as other systemic symptoms. Although endocarditis within 60 days of surgery typically is caused by non-oral bacteria, the cause of endocarditis that occurs 60 days after valve surgery is similar to that of native-valve endocarditis.
- Antibiotic prophylaxis should be considered for all patients with valvular heart disease.
- Regular examinations, echocardiograms and antithrombotic therapy are a must in patients with prosthetic heart valves.
- According to the American Heart Association (AHA) while performing dental procedures, antibiotic prophylactic therapy is indicated in patients with heart disorders which are related to very high risk of developing endocarditis like the prosthetic heart valves and previous history of infectious endocarditis.
- The risk for thromboembolism increases in patients with prosthetic heart valves if anticoagulant therapy is discontinued. It is therefore prudent to continue anticoagulation therapy in patients who require intensive high INR (International normalized ratio) levels.
- In all dental procedures like manipulation of gingival tissue, periapical area of the teeth, perforations of the oral mucosa like extractions, endodontic treatment beyond the periapical limits, placement of retraction sutures, biopsies, suture removal, placement of brackets etc, prophylaxis is recommended.
- It is not recommended every time in cases of routine injection of anesthesia in non-infected tissues, during dental x-rays, removable denture placement, or orthodontic devices, or in case of bleeding secondary to lip or oral mucosa traumas.

Recommendations:

- AHA strongly recommends that best oral hygiene should be maintained in patients at risk of developing bacterial endocarditis. Maintaining the best oral hygiene is more important than prophylactic antibiotics for prevention of endocarditis, before certain dental procedures.
- Bacteremia has been observed to develop after a traumatic ulcer due to removable partial denture and hence periodic control is advised to prevent them from developing.
- 0.12% chlorhexidine mouth rinsing for 30 seconds is advisable prior to any dental treatment, since it remarkably reduces bacteremia of oral origin.
- In case the patient fails to follow the correct prophylactic regimen, antibiotics should be started immediately, because it has been shown to be effective when carried out, 2 hours following the dvelopment of bacteremia.

Table: AHA recommended prophylactic antibiotic protocol for infectious endocarditis

Situation	Agent	Single Dose 30-60 min Before Procedure		
Standard general prophylaxis (oral)		Amoxicillin	2gr	50 mg/kg maximum 2 gr)
Unable to take oral medication		Ampicillin Cefazolin or Ceftriaxone	2 gr im or iv 1 gr im or iv	50 mg/kg im or iv 50 mg/kg im or iv
Allergic to penicillins	Oral	Cephalexin* Clindamycin Azithromycin or Clarithromycin	2 gr 600 mg 500 mg	50 mg/kg 20 mg/kg 15 mg/kg
	Unable to take oral medication	Cefazolin or Ceftriaxone Clindamycin	1 g im or iv 600 mg im or iv	50 mg/kg im or iv 20 mg/kg

Suggested reading:

1. Marta Cruz-Pamplona, Yolanda Jimenez-Soriano, Maria Gracia Sarrión-Pérez. Dental considerations in patients with heart disease. J Clin Exp Dent. 2011; 3(2):e97-105.

Q 4) Management of cardiovascular patient in dental clinic:

BFU NOVEMBER 2007 5 Marks.

- Cardiovascular patients can be suffering from various problems like hypertension, coronary arterial disease, valvular heart disease, heart failure, arrhythmias and permanent pacemakers.
- Before embarking on dental procedures careful history has to be obtained and depending on the condition present modifications and precautions need to be taken while treating the patient for dental procedures.
- Patients with a suspect medical history, untreated cardiovascular disease, high blood pressure, high C-reactive protein levels, or any uncertain disease status can be referred to their physician.
- Depending upon the patient's medical history, risk factors, and vital signs, the physician and/or cardiologist should be consulted prior to treatment.
- CVD drug therapy and potential side effects, interactions, and oral adverse drug reactions are important for the dental office setting, and may have influence on the dental procedures.
- Patients with high BP(blood pressure) are at increased risk for adverse advents in a dental setting when target organ disease is present.
- In hypertensive patients, the dental treatment should be done cautiously because any stressful procedure may lead to increase in blood pressure and precipitate acute complications like cardiac arrest or stroke.
- In hypertensives, the initial evaluation should consist of detailed family history of any cardiovascular disorder and other related diseases, history of high blood pressure, medications, duration and history of antihypertensives, severity of the disease and any complications. The dentist has to carefully assess the presence of hypertension and determine associated organ disease and decide any changes in the dental treatment plan.
- In pregnant women the blood pressure should be accurately measured since it may alter the values, as more than 10% of such women have clinically relevant hypertension. The BP monitoring is also important in diabetics, patients with autonomous dysfunction, and in elderly patients for whom the orthostatic hypotension is a big problem.
- Other diseases treated with antihypertensives like headache, regional pain, renal failure, glaucoma and congestive heart failure should be known to the dentist.
- Local anesthetics with epinephrine result in a more long lasting and effective anesthesia than the simple LA and helps in avoiding an exaggerated response to stress.

- In patients taking non-selective beta-blockers or in patients with uncontrolled hypertension, local anesthesia with vasoconstrictors should be avoided or used in low dosages. In patients with cardiac risk the maximum dose of epinephrine is 0.04 mgs.
- Oral health care providers also need to be aware of medications that (1) may have systemic side effects that are of importance to the provision of care, (2) interact with medications used during dental care, and (3) cause intraoral changes.
- Several considerations need to be addressed when treating dental patients with CAD. The primary concern for the dental provider is to prevent the recurrence of ischemia or infarction.
- It is highly recommended that all dental providers treating patients who have a history of ischemic heart disease be versed in advanced cardiac life support (ACLS) or at least basic cardiac life support (BCLS).
- Various alternatives are suggested in treating CAD, including discontinuing all anticoagulation therapy before invasive procedures, changing the anticoagulation regimen, and making no changes.
- Antibiotic prophylaxis should be considered for all patients with valvular heart disease.
- According to AHA guidelines, antibiotic prophylaxis should be administered to patients who have undergone mitral or aortic valve repair or replacement, patients with a prior history of infective endocarditis, and patients with mitral or aortic regurgitation or stenosis.
- Patients with MVP(mitral valve prolapse) should receive prophylaxis only if there is valvular regurgitation or thickening of the mitral leaflets. Patients with MVP who do not have valvular regurgitation or thickening of the leaflets do not require antibiotic prophylaxis as the incidence of endocarditis among them is identical to that in the general population.
- For well-compensated patients with heart failure, no special dental modifications are necessary unless the underlying causes for the heart failure require modifications. However, when patients suffer from uncompensated CHF, it is prudent to inquire about the patient's ability to be placed in supine position because lying down flat in a dental chair my cause severe dyspnoea in such patients.
- It has been recommended that patients with a history of myocardial infarction in the previous six months should not be treated as outpatients, and that elective dental treatment should be postponed on patients with severe or uncontrolled high blood pressure.
- If a patient reports angina attacks at rest that are changing or increasing in severity, or that were diagnosed within the last 30 days, it has been recommended that they not receive elective dental care until their angina is stable, and patients with stable angina should be advised to bring their medication with them in

case it is needed during treatment.

- Minimizing stress: achieved through patient management, pain-free dentistry techniques, and, where appropriate, the use of sedatives and analgesics (taking into consideration potential drug interactions) is important.
- It has been recommended that appointments should be less than one hour to minimize stress, and traditionally in the morning, although research now suggests late morning or early afternoon may be better.
- Patients with congestive heart failure should not be placed in a supine position, and for other patients, the chair should be raised gently.
- Separate consideration is required for patients with valvular disease, heart transplants, prosthetic valves, previous bacterial endocarditis, pacemakers, or implanted defibrillators.
- CVD drug therapy and potential side effects, interactions, and oral adverse drug reactions are important for the dental office setting, with implications for treatment.
- Currently Available Drug Therapies for cardiovascular disease are complex and may involve combinations of drugs. Classes of drugs used in the treatment of cardiovascular disease include alpha and beta adrenergic blockers, calcium channel blockers, sodium channel blockers, potassium channel blockers, diuretics, ACE inhibitors, phenytoin, anticoagulants, angiotensin inhibitors, nitrates, platelet aggregation inhibitors, and recently statins. Many of these are used to treat several cardiovascular diseases.
- Combination drugs containing both diuretics and other antihypertensives have recently been introduced to treat hypertension.
- Combination of calcium channel blockers and angiotensin converting enzyme(ACE)inhibitors have also been introduced to treat CVD.
- In heart transplant patients, immunosuppressives are used to prevent rejection. Which classes of drugs and specific drugs patients are or were taking is essential information, as is when and for how long they were or are taking them, potential interactions and side effects for that class of drugs or specific drug, and potential oral adverse drug reactions.

Suggested reading:

1. Burket's, Oral Medicine Diagnosis and Treatment 10th edi, 364-384.
2. Sanda Mihaela Popescu, Monica Scrieciu, Veronica Mercuţ, Mihaela Ţuculina, and Ionela Dascălu, Hypertensive Patients and Their Management in Dentistry, ISRN Hypertension Volume 2013 (2013).

CHAPTER 23

Acquired Immunodeficiency Syndrome

Introduction:

Acquired Immunodeficiency Syndrome is a serious and fatal disease which has now become an epidemic through out the world.It is an incurable viral STD which is caused by Human Immunodeficiency Virus (HIV).

HIV attacks the immune system because of which the individual is not able to protect himself from potentially harmful organisms.

Oral and perioral lesions are common manifestations in AIDS. A dentist if well versed with the manifestations can help in diagnosing the disease. Hence the knowledge of this disorder is very important for the dental students.

Q 1) Oral Hairy Leukoplakia:

TNMGRU OCTOBER 1996 (5 Marks)
BFU MAY 2006 (5 Marks)

In some patients Oral hairy leukoplakia (OHL) could be the first sign of HIV infection. Greenspan first noticed it in a group of isolated patients in 1984 and described it as an asymptomatic, non-scrapable white patch, with vertically corrugated hyperkeratotic hair like projections which appeared on the lateral border of the tongue.

It is a corrugated white lesion that usually appears on the lateral or ventral surfaces of the tongue in patients with severe immunodeficiency.

The disease most commonly associated with hairy leukoplakia is HIV infection.

OHL is caused by the EBV. In rare cases it may occur in immunocompetent patients after getting local steroid therapy.

Clinical manifestations:

OHL most commonly affects the lateral border of tongue but may extend to the ventral or dorsal surfaces.

The lesions have a corrugated appearance and have shaggy or frayed appearance which may look like lesions caused by tongue chewing.

The lesion could have a plaque like appearance and is often bilateral.

These patches do not usually cause discomfort and generally do not affect the taste of foods or liquids.

In some cases, however, some times can cause mild pain and may cause alterations in taste and heightened sensitivity to food temperatures.

Histopathology:

The epithelium reveals severe hyperkeratosis with an irregular surface, acanthosis, superficial edema, and numerous koilocytic cells in the spinous layer.

A very typical feature is the presence of homogenous viral nuclear inclusions with a residual rim of normal chromatin. A definitive diagnosis can be achieved by demonstration of the presence of EBV by in-situ hybridisation, electron microscopy or the polymerase chain reaction.

Differential diagnosis:

(i) **Hyperplastic candidiasis:** The presence of candidal hypahe and location of the disease will help in differentiating.

(ii) idiopathic leukoplakia.

(iii) **Leukoplakia due to trauma of tongue chewing:** The history of this habit can be elicited.

(iv) **Tobacco associated leukoplakia:** The lesions have typical cracked mud like appearance and the location can be traced to the habit of keeping the quid.

(v) lichen planus, lupus erythemtosus, and verrucous leukoplakia.

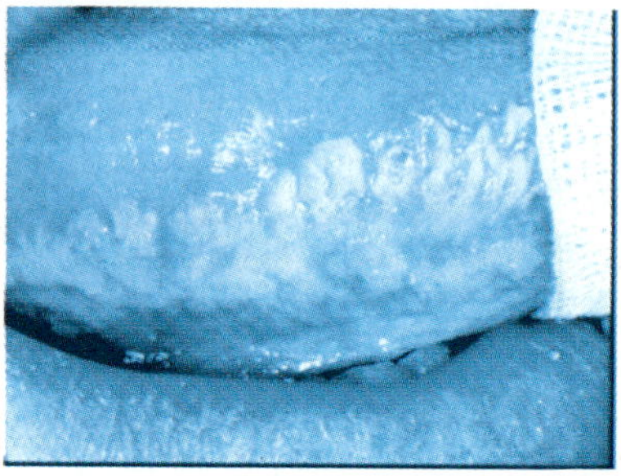

Fig. White folded leukoplakic lesions on the dorsolateral tongue, suggestive of OHL

Treatment and prognosis:

There is no treatment indicated.

The lesion disappears when antiviral medications like zidivudine, acyclovir, or gancyclovir are administered for the treatment of HIV infection and its complicating viral lesions.

Short term resolution of the lesions is seen with topical application of podophyllin resin or tretinoin, however relapse is often seen.

Suggested reading

1. Ajay Reginald, B. Sivapathasundharam Oral hairy leukoplakia: An exfoliative cytology study, Contemp Clin Dent. 2010 Jan-Mar; 1(1): 10–13.
2. Burket, Textbook of Oral Medicine.Edition 11th chapter 4; page. No. 84-85.

Q 2) Diagnostic test for HIV AIDS:

TNMGRU APRIL 2004 (5 Marks)

Diagnostic test for AIDS:

MUHS MAY 2003 (2 Marks)

Laboratory investigations of AIDS:

BFU NOVEMBER 2013 (4 Marks)

Identification of the HIV infection is done by detection of the HIV-specific antibodies in the serum or plasma of the patient by demonstrating the presence of virus by nucleic acid detection with the use of polymerase chain reaction (PCR), p24 antigen testing or by growing virus in cell culture.

The various tests used to diagnose AIDS are as follows:

1) **Elisa Test: (Enzyme Linked Immunosorbent Assay-ELISA**

   This is the most initial test to detect the HIV infection.

   If the test shows antibodies to the HIV then it is positive and usually repeated to confirm the diagnosis. If the ELISA is negative there is usually no need to carry out other tests. It has very low chances of false results, if the person is infected since a few weeks. The ELISA test uses components of the immune system and the chemicals to detect immune responses in the body.

   The types of ELISA:

   1. Indirect ELISA.
   2. Sandwich ELISA.
   3. Competitive ELISA.
   4. Capture ELISA.
   5. Immunometric ELISA.
   6. Cylinder or cassette ELISA.

2) **p 24 antigen:** Before antibody is detectable, in a small number of seroconverters, who are in the window period the p24 antigen may become positive.

   The p24 antigens test use antibody to capture the disrupted p24 antigen in the patient's serum and is EIA based. In some cases, the p24 antigen can be detected before the presence of HIV antibody.

3. **Western blot test:** In this test multiple proteins or antigens from a HIV infected person is placed in a line on a test strip and serum is added to check which antigen/antibody reaction occurs.

   The use of this as a confirmatory test for ELISA is questionable, because it is an antibody test and is not fully independent.

   The Western blot assay is thus a method where in the individual proteins of an HIV-1 lysate are separated according to size by polyacrylamide gel electrophoresis.

   The proteins of the virus are then transferred to the nitrocellulose paper and a reaction is brought about with the patient's serum.

4. **Polymerase Chain Reaction:** This test requires expensive equipments and technical skill and is done to find the genetic material DNA of HIV.It is very helpful to find very recent infection.

5. **HIV DNA PCR test:** This test is a qualitative molecular assay which

is done to determine whether the HIV is present in peripheral blood mononuclear cells.It is a gold standard for early diagnosis of definitive HIV-infection.

6. **Rapid Test:** One-step rapid HIV test that can be performed with whole blood either in the laboratory or at the point of care. With this test, it is possible to obtain results in as little as 20 minutes from the time the specimen is collected. It should be noted that rapid HIV tests are also serologic tests that use technology similar to that of standard ELISA antibody tests. Hence, the results of a rapid HIV test should be treated in the same fashion as the result of a standard (nonrapid) test.
7. **HIV Viral Load:** The HIV viral load represents another laboratory test commonly performed in individuals with chronic HIV infection. This test simply measures the quantity of HIV virus in a single micro litre (mL) of serum. Like the CD4 count, this test can be a useful marker of disease progression and of response to antiretroviral therapy.
8. **Other Serologic Tests:**
   Oral Fluid Tests: An oral fluid-based HIV serology test is now available for testing in public health departments, physicians' clinics, and AIDS service organizations. This is not a saliva test. This is not a home test either. Studies indicate that oral sample for HIV antibody test is as sensitive and specific as a blood sample for testing of HIV infection. The test uses a specially treated pad that is kept between the lower buccal mucosa and the gingiva for two minutes. The pad is then placed in a vial and submitted to the laboratory. The result must be confirmed with a Western blot.
   - Home Test System: There are a number of home collection test systems and kits available in the market. The consumer obtains blood using a sterile lancet and the blood sample is placed on a filter strip which is then mailed to a reading center. Results are generally available in 10 days.
   - Indirect Fluorescent Anti-body test: This test helps in detecting HIV antibodies. It is used to confirm the results of an ELISA test.

Suggested reading:

1. J B Jackson and H H Balfour.Jr, Practical diagnostic testing for human immunodeficiency virus, Clin Microbiol Rev. 1988 Jan; 1(1): 124–138.
2. Margaret Fearon, The laboratory diagnosis of HIV infections, Can J Infect Dis Med Microbiol. 2005 Jan-Feb; 16(1): 26–30.

Q 3) Oral manifestations of AIDS:

MUHS NOVEMBER 2009 2 Marks

Discuss the oral manifestations of AIDS:

BFU MAY 2009 (7½ Marks)

1) Fungal infections:

(i) Oral candidiasis: Oral candidiasis is often the first manifestation of HIV disease. Four forms of oral candidiasis have been identified with HIV infection. They are:

- **Pseudomembranous candidiasis (thrush):**
  Most common form of candidiasis in HIV infected persons. Lesions are characterized by yellow-white, curd-like loosely adherent (wipeable) plaques, located anywhere in the mouth.
  Removal of lesions leave erythematous areas with or without pin point bleeding.
- **Erythematous candidiasis:**
  Erythematous (atrophic) macular patches on mucosal surfaces.
  Dorsum of the tongue often shows depapillation and palatal mucosa is usually affected at the same time.
- **Angular cheilitis:**
  It is characterized by linear ulcers or fissures at the angles of the mouth unilaterally or bilaterally.Opening of mouth may become restricted and painful.
- **Hyperplastic candidiasis:**
  This form of candidiasis is also known as candidal leukoplakia and is the least common form of candidal infections in HIV patients.
  It is characterised by white patches that are firmly adherent to the underlying mucosa.It is more resistant to anti-fungal therapy.

(ii) **Histoplasmosis:** Its caused by the fungus histoplasma capsulatum. Oral involvement by histoplasmosis is secondary to pulmonary infections.
The oral lesions may appear as papules, nodules, ulcers or vegetations.
Cervical lymph nodes are enlarged and firm.
In HIV infections oral histoplasmosis could be the initial sign.

(iii) **Cryptococcosis:** It is a sub acute or chronic infection caused by Cryptococcus neoformans.Pulmonary cryptococcosis may lead to mild pneumonitis.Oral manifestations are rare and consist of ulcerative lesions.

2) Viral infections:

(i) Hairy leukoplakia: Oral hairy leukoplakia is a corrugated white lesion that usually occurs on the lateral or ventral surfaces of the tongue in patients with severe immunodeficiency.
Epstein-Barr virus has been reported as the causative agent in oral hairy leukoplakia.

(ii) Herpes simplex virus infection: Small vesicles occur on the oral mucosa.
The vesicles are thin walled and surrounded by an inflammatory base. They rupture rapidly forming shallow round ulcers.

(iii) Varicella-zoster virus infection: Unilateral vesicles are seen. Opthalmic, maxillary and mandibular branch of trigeminal nerve are involved.

(iv) Oral kaposi's sarcoma: Kaposis's sarcoma is a lesion malignant and multifocal systemic disease that arises from the vascular endothelium and is known to be caused by the human herpes virus 8 (HHV 8).

It appears as red or purplish macules, papules or nodules and may ulcerate and cause destruction of tissues. The palate and the gingiva are most commonly affected.

(v) **Cytomegalovirus infection:** This infection related ulcers are not very frequent but is a recognised complication of HIV infection. These lesions have been described as exanthema, plaques, nodules, ulcerations, or keratotic lesions.

(vi) **Human papilloma virus infection:** HPV is a cause of a multiform group of oral lesions that have been described as oral papillomas, verruca vulgaris, focal epithelial hyperplasia and condyloma acuminatum.

Clinically, they show a variegated aspect that includes nodular or papular lesions, single cauliflower like growths or multiple papilliferous projections.

(vii) **Molluscum contagiosum:** The lesions of this condition occur as single or multiple papules on the skin of the face, back, arms and buttocks. Usually occurs in children and young adults. Few cases of perioral lesions have been reported in patients with AIDS.

3) Bacterial infections:

(i) Gingivitis And Periodontitis: HIV associated gingivitis is an early lesion in HIV-infected patients and presents a distinct linear marginal erythema of the free gingiva, or focal enlargement of the gingiva.

The hallmark of HIV gingivitis is its resistance to conventional therapy.

HIV associated necrotizing gingivitis is characterized by localized or diffuse ulceration, necrosis and/or destruction of the interdental papillae covered with a fibrinous slough.

Periodontitis shows soft tissue necrosis and rapid destruction of the periodontal attachment and bone.

(ii) **Linear gingival erythema:** Called as red band gingivitis, presents as red band along the gingival margins and may or may not be accompanied by occasional bleeding and discomfort. Seen commonly in the anterior teeth region.

(iii) **Epitheloid Angiomatosis (Cat Scratch Disease):** Lesions are proliferation of vascular papules that simulates the pyogenic granuloma.Oral mucosal lesions in patients with AIDS have been reported.

(iv) **Mycobacterium Avium Intracellulare:** Oral lesions might appear as necrotic ulcers of the palate and gingiva.

(v) **Actinomycosis Israelli:**

(vi) **Oral infection with enteric organisms:** A small number of cases of oral infections with enteric bacteria have been reported in patients with AIDS.

4) HIV related salivary gland disease:

(i) **Salivary gland enlargement:** Occurs in about 0-3% of adults infected with AIDS and higher frequency is seen in children. Typically the parotid gland is involved usually bilaterally and may be cystic in some cases.

(ii) **Xerostomia:** In HIV infected patients xerostomia is a common symptom.

5) Neoplastic tumors:

Non-Hodgkin's lymphoma: In patients with HIV this is the second most common tumour that occurs. It includes soft tissue masses with or without ulceration.There is tissue necrosis involving the gingival, palatal and alveolar mucosa.

6) Aphthous ulcerations

Lesions occur on non-keratinised mucosa and are very painful. In patients with AIDS these lesions tend to persist for a longer duration.

7) Dental caries

In patients with HIV disease, as a result of xerostomia and lack of oral hygiene maintenance, the, risk for dental caries is high.

8) Hypersensitivity and lichenoid reactions:

Acquired allergies, autoimmune reactions, adverse drug reactions are seen in form of irregular ulceration, vesicles, bullae, sloughing.

9) Thrombocytopenia:

Seen in 10% of AIDS patients. Seen as ecchymosis, petechiae or spontaneous hemorrhage.

10) Hyperpigmentations:

Seen as brownish black spots, striations, focal melanosis.

Suggested reading:

1. Neville, Textbook of Oral & Maxillofacial pathology.2nd Ed.

Q 4) Kaposi's sarcoma:

RGUHS APRIL 1999 (5 Marks)

Kaposi's sarcoma is a low-grade vascular tumor associated with herpes virus/human herpes virus 8 (KSHV/HHV8) infection. Kaposi sarcoma lesions are predominantly present at mucocutaneous sites, but may involve all organs and anatomic locations.

It is accurately described as a multifocal angioproliferative neoplasm that primarily involves the skin in non-HIV infected patients.It is most commonly a manifestation of infection with HIV, that frequently involves the oral cavity.

The epidemic occurrence of this neoplasm in patients with AIDS suggests a causal relationship between the immune deficiency and the appearance of this neoplasm.

Clinical features:

- Age and sex distribution: It is most common in fifth, sixth and seventh decades. There is a marked male predilection with a gender ratio of 20:1.
- Appearance: The tumour begins as a multicentric neoplastic process which manifests as multiple red or purplish macules and in more advanced types, nodules, occurring on skin and mucosal surfaces.
- Progression: The lesion tends to enlarge and become darker and may coalesce or form clusters of single nodules.
- AIDS associated: Occurrence of this lesion in AIDS patients in the head and neck area is common.The tip of the nose is a frequent location.Facial, scalp area, periorbital and conjunctival involvement are also typical.The neoplasm can involve the lymph nodes, soft tissue of the extremities and gastrointestinal tract.
- Clinical presentation: Four types are recognised.
  - (i) **Classic type:** Most common in men and occurs in late adult life Multiple bluish purplish macules and plaques that are present on the skin of lower extremities.
  - (ii) **Endemic:** There are four sub types:
    - Benign nodular type.
    - Aggressive type.
    - A florid form.
    - A unique lymph adenopathic type.

(iii) **Iatrogenic type:** Iatrogenic immunosuppression associated Kaposi's sarcoma most often occurs in recipient's organ transplants.

(iv) **AIDS related kaposi's sarcoma:** Frequently involves the head and neck.

Oral manifestations:

- **Location:** The appearance is similar to those of the cutaneous nodules. May involve any oral site but is common on the palate, gingiva and dorsum of the tongue.
- **Appearance:** Oral lesions occur as red to purple nodules and macules with ulceration in more mature cases.
- **Symptoms:** There is pain, dysphagia, difficulty in mastication, bleeding and may cause poor esthetic appearance.
- **Palpation:** The lesion does not blanch with pressure.Early lesion may appear similar to ecchymosis or hemangioma.

Differential diagnosis:

- Hemangioma-Blanches on pressure.
- Purpura-It is presented as multiple papules on the soft palate.
- Nevus-Not such a aggressive lesion.
- Melanoma-It is not multicentric.

Management:

- **Radiation therapy:** Radiotherapy is given in fractionated dose of 25-30 gray over 1 week.
- **Surgical eradication:** Because of the multiplicity of lesions of the lesion surgical treatment is difficult.Carbon dioxide or argon laser can be effective in the treatment of lesions in the upper aerodigestive tract.
- **Systemic chemotherapy:** The most commonly used regimen is the alternating weekly vinblastin and vincristine. Other effective agents include doxorubicin in low doses, bleomycin and methotrexate. Recombinant interferon alpha -2A and alpha 2B have been identified as efficacious agents in treatment of Kaposi's sarcoma.
- **Intralesional injection:** the intralesional use of vinblastine, in doses varying from 0.01-0.04 mgs, may be effective in the treatment of small lesion in the mouth.
- Combination therapy for AIDS associated Kaposi's Sarcoma: A great variety of treatment regimens such as single agents, combined chemotherapy, or zidovudine with interferon alpha and radiotherapy have been tried. Circumscribed lesions within the mouth may be treated with surgical excision, cryotherapy, or even sclerotherapy, to which these lesions rapidly respond.

Suggested reading:

1. Anil Govindrao Ghom, Text Book Of Oral Medicine, Third Edition, 459-460.

CHAPTER 24

Endocrine Disorders

Introduction:

Hormones are substances released from cells that circulate and affect distant organs. The main physiologic function of the hormones are growth, maintenance of homeostasis, and reproduction. They vary in chemical composition and biologic activity. Disorders of the endocrine system has effects on the skeletal system and rest of the body due to altered metabolism. The major endocrine glands are pituitary, thyroid, parathyroid, adrenal glands, and pancreas.

Q 1) Oral manifestations of diabetes mellitus:

RGUHS APRIL 2006 (4 Marks)

Diabetes mellitus is a chronic disease affecting all age groups.

It is a metabolic disorder in which there is hyperglycemia which results from defective insulin secretion, action or both.

It is one of the leading causes of mortality and morbidity worldwide.

Many chronic macrovascular and microvascular complications of diabetes have been reported and there are often chances of oral complications and hence it is important for the dentists to know about them.

In the oral cavity a variety of soft tissue abnormalities have been observed associated with this condition. They are:

(a) **Periodontal diseases (periodontitis and gingivitis):** Periodontal disease has shown an increased rate of occurrence and severity in patients having type 1 and type 2 diabetes. In patients with diabetes the chances of developing periodontitis has been reported to be thrice higher than in general population.
The reduced salivary flow leads to dryness and more chances of plaque formation making the oral cavity more prone to periodontal diseases.

(b) **Dysfunction of saliva:** Leads to a decrease in salivary flow and alterations in saliva composition and also taste dysfunction.
Saliva has a major role in maintaining a healthy oral cavity.The salivary hypo-secretion and xerostomia leading to various complications in oral cavity has been reported in patients with diabetes.

Sialosis has been found to be more prevalent in patients with diabetes mellitus.

(c) **Oral fungal and bacterial infections:** Diabetic patients having complications and poor metabolic control are more likely to recurrent bacterial infection that has the tendency to spread.
In diabetics the local and systemic predisposing factors increase the risk of oral candidiasis.

(d) **Other complications include**: Stomatitis, geographic tongue, fissures on tongue, traumatic ulcers, lichen planus, angular cheilitis and lichenoid reactions.

(e) **Delayed mucosal healing of wound:** During oral surgical procedures, the diabetics suffer from complications of poor soft tissue regeneration and delayed osseous healing.Hence the treatment and management of diabetics who require to undergo oral surgery is more complex.

(f) **Mucosal neuro-sensory disorders:** Burning mouth syndrome and other abnormal oral sensations like numbness, tingling and dryness or sore mouth may exist at the same time in diabetics.

(g) **Dental caries and loss of teeth:** In diabetics there is susceptibility to oral infections that can cause caries and tooth loss.

Suggested reading:

1. Sandberg GE, Wikblad KF: Oral dryness and peripheral neuropathy in subjects with type 2 diabetes. J Diabetes Complications. 2003 Jul-Aug; 17(4):192-8.

Q 2) Hyperparathyroidism:

TNMGRU AUGUST 2014 (5 Marks)

Overactivity of the parathyroid glands is called hyperparathyroidism and results in excess production of the parathyroid hormones (PTH). The calcium and phosphate levels are regulated by this hormone and helps to maintain their levels. When the excess secretion is due to the glands it is referred to as primary hyperparathyroidism and this leads to raised calcium levels.When the excess secretion occurs in response to low calcium levels, such as in case of vitamin D deficiency or chronic disease of the kidney, it is called secondary hyperparathyroidism.The raised PTH levels is harmful to the bone and requires treatment.

Hyperparathyroidism can be:

1. **Primary hyperparathyroidism:** When the excess secretion is due to an adenoma of the gland, hyperplasia or a carcinoma. This condition is characterised by four signs, stones, bones, groans, and psychic overtones(moans), referring to the presence of kidney stones, hypercalcemia, peptic ulcers, constipation, as well as depression, respectively.
2. **Secondary hyperparathyroidism:** It occurs due to the physiologic secretion of the PTH by the glands in response to low levels of calcium in blood. The most common cause of this is vitamin D

deficiency due to lack of sunlight, malabsorption, or diet and chronic failure of kidneys.

Deficiency of vitamin D causes reduction in calcium absorption by the intestines leading to hypocalcemia and increased secretion of PTH. This results in resorption of bone.In case of kidney failure the problem is failure to convert the vitamin D to its active form in the kidney.In secondary hyperparthyroidism due to renal failure the bone disease caused is called renal osteodystrophy.

3. **Tertiary hyperparathyroidism:** In patients with long term secondary hyperparathyroidism, Tertiary hyperparathyroidism is seen. It finally leads to hyperplasia of the gland and causes loss of response to serum calcium levels. This condition is mostly seen in patients with chronic renal failure.
4. **Quaternary and quintary hyperparathyroidism:** These are rare and seen after the surgical removal of the glands in primary hyperparathyroidism when it leads to kidney damage and now causes another form of secondary (quaternary) hyperparathyroidism, that may result in quintary form. After the parathyroidectomy, quaternary hyperparathyroidism may occur due to hungry bone syndrome.

Clinical Features:

- Women are twice to thrice more prone to get affected than men by primary hyperparathyroidism.
- The condition occurs mainly in those, 30 to 60 years of age.
- Gastro-intestinal problems: Symptoms such as anorexia, nausea, vomiting, abdominal cramps may be present.
- Bone and joint pain: Pathologic fractures, bone pain and deformities may occur.
- Psychological problems: Patients may suffer from emotional instability.
- Hypercalcemia: Associated with muscle weakness, fatigue, weight loss, insomnia, headache, polydypsia and polyurea.
- The clinical feature is thus a combination of moans, groans, aches and pains.
- There is a wide range of clinical features like renal calculi, peptic ulcers, psychiatric problems or bone and joint pains.
- The clinical manifestations are mainly due to hypercalcemia.
- There may be slow but progressive loosening, drifting and exfoliation of teeth.
- Definite consistent hypercalcemia is virtually pathognomonic of primary hyperparathyroidism.
- Serum calcium levels should be checked at different intervals because of the tendency for daily fluctuations.
- A reliable indicator of the turnover of bone, the serum alkaline phosphatase levels will show increase in levels in hyper-parathyroidism.

Radiographic features:

- General changes include erosions of bone, demineralisation of the skeleton, osteitis fibrosa cystica, brown tumors, pathologic calcifications in soft tissues, granular appearance of the entire calvarium.
- Radiographic features of the jaws: There is often demineralisation and thinning of the cortex of jaws, like in inferior border of mandible, mandibular canal, and the cortical lining of the maxillary sinuses.
- There is decreased bone density of the jaws and appears radiolucent in contrast to the dense teeth that stand out.
- There can be a change in the pattern of trabeculae giving a ground glass appearance of several, small randomly oriented trabeculae.
- The Brown tumours of this condition may affect any bone, but often involve the facial bone and the jaws especially in long-standing cases of the disease.
- There can be multiple lesions within a single bone.
- The lesions have variable defined margins and can cause cortical expansion.
- The solitary appearing lesions may mimic a central giant cell granuloma or an aneurysmal bone cyst.
- It is interesting to note that the histo-pathologic features of the brown tumours is similar to that of giant cell granuloma.
- Therefore, it is important that when a giant cell granuloma occurs after the 2nd decade, the patient should be screened for increased serum calcium levels, PTH and alkaline phosphatase.
- Skull bones: Entire calvarium has granular appearance due to loss of trabeculae and thinning of cortical tables.

Radiographic features of the teeth and associated structures:

- Periapical radiographs of these patients may reveal loss of lamina dura.
- Loss of lamina dura may affect only one or almost all the teeth depending on the severity and duration of the disease.
- The loss could be partial or total around the tooth.
- The roots of the teeth give a tapered appearance due to loss of lamina dura as a result of decreased image contrast.
- Although the parathyroid hormone mobilises the minerals from the skeleton, the mature teeth are immune to this process.

Diagnosis:

Clinical diagnosis is by typical symptoms like bone pains, aches, moans and groans due to peptic ulcers, and renal calculi.

Radiologically diagnosis is done by features of generalised demineralisation of bone, pepperpot skull, osteitis fibrosa cystica, brown tumours.

Laboratory diagnosis reveals raised serum calcium levels and alkaline phosphatase levels.Increase in circulating parathyroid hormone can be demonstrated by radioisotopic studies.

Radiographic differential diagnosis:

- **Unilocular:**
  Post extraction tooth sockets, surgical defects, primordial cysts, traumatic bone cysts, odontogenic cysts-History, serum chemistry will help in differentiation.
- **Multilocular:**
  - Pagets disease: Serum calcium is normal.
  - Ameloblastoma: Honey comb appearance and normal serum chemistry.
  - Central giant cell granuloma: normal serum chemistry.
  - Cherubism: Bilateral multilocular radiolucencies and more common in children.
  - Aneurysmal bone cyst, osteomalacia, fibrous dysplasia, multiple myeloma.

Treatment:

- Once the parathyroid adenoma is surgically removed, almost all the radiographic changes revert back to normal.
- Only the site of brown tumour which heals with bone may appear radiographically more sclerotic than normal.
- Oral administration of vitamin D in secondary hyperparathyroidism can prevent skeletal demineralisation.
- Restriction of dietary phosphate, phosphate binding agents and aluminium salts should be advocated.

Calcimimetics:

A calcimimetic is a type of therapy for patients with severe hypercalcemia and primary hyperparathyroidism who cannot undergo removal of the parathyroid and those patients with secondary hyperparthyroidism on dialysis.

Suggested reading:

1. McConnell, Thomas H. (2007). The Nature of Disease: Pathology for the Health Professions. Lippincott Williams &Wilkins .p. 466.
2. Oltmann, Sarah C.; Maalouf, N. M.; Holt, S. (March 2011). "Significance of Elevated Parathyroid Hormone after Parathyroidectomy for Primary Hyperparathyroidism". Endocrine Practice **17** (S1): 57–73
3. Ott, SM (April 1998). "Calcimimetics–new drugs with the potential to control hyperparathyroidism".J. Clin. Endocrinol. Metab. **83** (4): 1080–2.

CHAPTER 25

Blood Disorders

Introduction:

The cellular elements of blood and its plasma proteins play an important role in many physiologic mechanisms of the body.The circulating blood plays an important role in the maintenance of normal oral mucosa and especially the mucosa of tongue.

Several disorders of blood have manifestations in the oral mucosa and many times an astute dentist could be the first to diagnose blood disorders.It is therefore important to know the blood disorders and their oral manifestations.

Q 1) Cyclic Neutropenia

TNMGRU FEB 2006 (5 Marks)
RGUHS OCT 1999 RGUHS (5 Marks)

Definition:

Cyclic (periodic) neutropenia is a rare hematological disorder which is benign and has typical cyclical depression of the peripheral blood polymorphonuclear leukocyte (PMNL) count at 21- day intervals which occurs due to periodic failure of the stem cells in the bone marrow.This failure occurs due to an abnormality in the regulation of precursor cells of the bone marrow release of inhibitors of neutrophils released by monocytes. Between the neutropenic episodes the patient is healthy. However at some regular intervals the neutropenic count falls to as low as 500/mm3 and in some cases may fall to 0.

Although cyclic neutropenia usually manifests initially in infancy or childhood, it may also appear in adulthood. There may be a familial tendency.

Though the exact cause is not known in about 1/3rd of cases it appears to be inherited in an autosomal dominant pattern. It is also thought that it could be due to abnormality in the regulation of early precursors of the hematopoietic cells.

Hormonal causes have been suggested but are not stated with certainty.

Clinical Features:

This condition is characterised by fever, malaise, oral ulcerations associated with scarring, gingivitis, periodontitis, and the disappearance of neutrophils from the blood and bone marrow at regular 21 days intervals.

Patients with this disease have most commonly pharyngitis, and skin abscesses. stomatitis, cervical lymphadenopathy during the recurrent episodes of neutropenia.

The severity of neutropenia decides the severity of the infections eg.in some patients with severe periodic neutropenia suffer from few infections due to compensatory monocytic increase which then act as phagocytes to prevent the spread of bacterial infections.In some cases, patients suffer from lung and urinary tract infections and ulcers of the rectum and vagina. The expectancy of life is good if carefully monitored.

It is thus:

1. An unusual form of agranulocytosis.
2. Characterized by a periodic or cyclic dimunition in circulating polymorphonuclear leukocytes as a result of bone marrow maturation arrest.
3. Accompanied by mild clinical manifestations, which regresses only to recur subsequently in a rhythmic pattern.
4. Exact etiology is unknown.

Oral manifestations:

(i) In this condition oral lesions are common and could be a major and important clinical manifestation of the disease.

(ii) Mucosal ulcers and periodontal disease are the two most important features.

(iii) With every new episode of the neutropenia, the ulcers recur and may look like the large, deep and scarring ulcers, seen in major aphthous stomatitis.

(iv) Bacterial infections of the dental supporting structures can cause manifestations ranging from marginal gingivitis to rapidly progressing periodontal bone loss.

(v) This is generally due to bacterial invasion, chiefly from gingival sulcus.

(vi) With return of neutrophil count to normal, the gingiva acquires a almost normal clinical appearance.

(vii) In cases when there are major aphthous ulcers or rapidly progressing generalised periodontitis that cannot be justified by local factors, cyclic neutropenia should be ruled out as a possible cause.

(viii) When these conditions are seen in children it could be highly suspicious of cyclic neutropenia.

(ix) Total of three TLC and DLC/week for 4-6 weeks is essential to rule out this disorder.

(x) In patients who are known cases of this condition, dental treatment should be done frequently and dilligently to minimise the effects of progressive, rapid periodontitis.

(xi) When the neutrophil count is above 2000/mm3 the routine treatments should be scheduled.

(xii) Neutrophil counts should be taken on the day of the dental procedure, which can be a wise precaution as the counts can change rapidly.

(xiii) Meticulous oral hygiene maintenance is a must and patients should be recalled every 2-3 months for prophylaxis.

(xiv) The reduction in oral ulcerations and periodontal diseases has been brought about by the use of colony-stimulating factor in these patients.

Treatment:

The patients with this condition require local and symptomatic treatment for the recurring oral ulcers and pharyngitis and antibiotics for treatment of sinusitis, pneumonia, peritonitis and bacteremia.

Glucocorticoids, plasmapheresis and androgens therapy have proven to be effective in some adult patients, but there is no therapy that could alter the cyclical phases of blood counts in children.

The best antibiotic is the oral sulfamethoxazole/ trimethoprim combination at a daily dose of 50 mg/kg.

Despite the cyclical episodes of illnesses the patients suffering from this condition develop and grow normally.

Its important to note that an alert physician or dentist can help diagnose this condition and can help improve the quality and life expectancy of the patient.

Suggested reading:

1. Dale D C.Hammond W P, 4th: Cyclic neutropenia: A clinical review.Blood Rev.1988 Sep; 2(3):178-85.
2. Robert J.Gorlin, Anand P .Chaudhary, Neutropenia:Does Periadenitis Mucosa Necrotica Recurrence(Sutton)Exist?A Need For Revaluation, Dermatol.1960;82(3):344-348.
3. R. Ebru Tirali, Zeynep Yalçınkaya-Erdemci, S. Burçak Çehreli Department of Pediatric Dentistry, Başkent University Faculty of Dentistry, Ankara, Turkey, Review Oral findings and clinical implications of patients with congenital neutropenia: a literature review, The Turkish Journal of Pediatrics 2013; 55: 241-245 .

Q 2) Plummer Vinson Syndrome:

TNMGRU AUGUST 2010 6 Marks
BFU MAY 2007 5 Marks
MUHS MAY 2008 2 Marks

This rare condition is also known as Paterson-Brown -Kelly syndrome and is characterized by classical triad:

I) Difficulty in swallowing.(dysphagia)
II) Iron deficiency anemia.
III) Oesophageal webs.

This disease has become rare in this era and if it occurs it affects post menopausal women. It is important to diagnose and treat this disease because it involves an increased risk of developing squamous cell carcinoma of the oesophagus and pharynx.

Etiology:

The most important cause is iron deficiency.Other factors could include malnutrition, autoimmune process or genetic perdisposition.

Clinical features:

(i) Occurs most commonly in white middle aged women usually in 4th to 7th decade.
(ii) It has also been seen in children and adolescents.
(iii) The chief clinical manifestation is the post cricoid dysplasia, webs of the upper esophagus and iron deficiency anemia.
(iv) Dysphagia is usually painless and progresses slowly over many years, and is usually associated with solid food and may be accompanied with weight loss.
(v) Symptoms result from anemia and are weakness, pallor, fatigue.
(vi) Tachycardia is common and may be dominatingly present.
(vii) Other features are glossitis, angular cheilitis, and koilonychias(spoon shaped nails).
(viii) Enlargement of the spleen and thyroid may be present.
(ix) About 3 to 15% of the patients with this syndrome are known to develop esophagial or pharyngeal cancer.
(x) The prevalence of this condition is however reduced over the years.

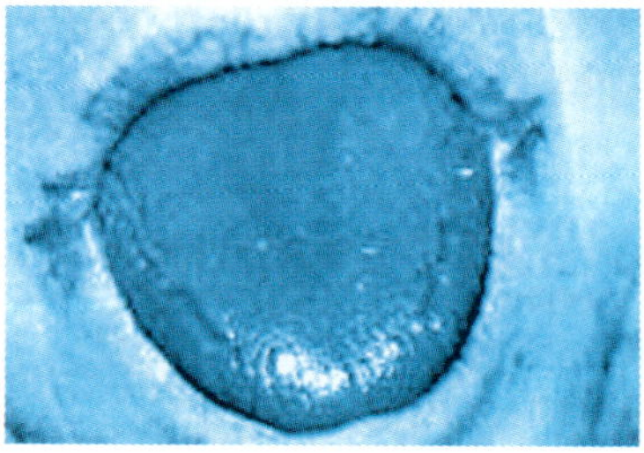

Fig. Glossitis and angular cheilitis in plummer Vinson syndrome

Diagnosis:

Its given on the basis of evidence of iron deficiency anemia, esophagial webs which can be detected by barium swallow test and x-ray, and by upper gastrointestinal endoscopy.

Laboratory tests:

Usually show iron deficiency anemia and reduced hemoglobin, hematocrit, mean corpuscular volume, serum iron and ferritin and an increase in iron binding capacity.

Any other laboratory abnormalities are not seen.

Differential diagnosis:

All other conditions that can cause dysphagia like, malignant tumours, benign strictures or esophageal rings should be ruled out.

Some other causes of dysphagia like diabetes mellitus, diverticuli, achalasia, spastic motility disorders, scleroderma, gastroesophageal reflux disease neuromuscular and skeletal muscle disorders should be differentiated.

Management:

(i) The most important step in managing this condition is to ascertain the cause of iron deficiency in order to exclude, active hemorrhage, malignancy or celiac disease.

(ii) Supplementation of iron itself can help resolve the problem of dysphagia in many cases, otherwise mechanical dilation is done .

(iii) If there is significant destruction of the lumen of the esophagus by the web and there is persistent dysphagia even with iron supplementation, then rupture and dilation of the web can be done.

(iv) Generally dilation done once can relieve the dysphagia but sometimes multiple interventions may be required.Baloon dilation has also given successful results.

(v) This syndrome has been associated with an increased risk of malignancy of the pharynx and esophagus and hence the patients should be followed up regularly and the upper gastro-intestinal endoscopy is recommended every year.

Suggested reading:

1. Chung S, Roberts-Thomson IC, Gastrointestinal: upper oesophageal web. JGastroenterol Hepatol. 1999 Jun; 14(6):611.
2. Hoffman RM, Jaffe PE Plummer-Vinson syndrome. A case report and literature review, Arch Intern Med. 1995 Oct 9; 155(18):2008-11.

Q 3) Hemoglobinopathies:

TNMGRU APRIL 1996 (4 Marks)

The normal function and total amount of hemoglobin (Hb) depends on its adequate synthesis and precise structure. When these conditions are not met, the red cells of the carrier contain either a decreased amount of Hb or a Hb variant that may have abnormal properties. These conditions are collectively described as haemoglobinopathies.

A normal hemoglobin molecule consists of two pairs of amino acid chains, the alpha and beta chains.

In hemoglobinopathies, abnormal hemoglobins are produced either in the form of abnormal chains (gamma or delta chains) or due to alterations in the alpha or beta chains.

Definition:

The hemoglobinopathies are inherited disorders of haemoglobin synthesis (thalassemia) or structure (sickle cell disorders) that are responsible for significant morbidity or mortality all over the world.

They are more commonly seen in individuals who originate from Africa, the middle east, the Mediterranean, Asia and the Far east.

These disorders result in errors in oxygen carrying capacity of haemoglobin.

Sickle cell and thalassemia are inherited disorders that are passed on from parents to children through unusual hemoglobin genes.

This disorder is present in persons in case two unusual hemoglobin genes are inherited, one from mother, and one from father.

When only one unusual gene is inherited, those persons are called carriers who are healthy and devoid of this disorder.

1) Thalassemia:

In this disorder there is deficient synthesis of either alpha or beta chains of globin in the hemoglobin molecule.

Beta thalassemia major or cooley's anemia is the most severe form of congenital haemolytic anemia.

Clinical features:

(i) The hematocrit can reach to less than 20 and the haemoglobin levels may fall to below 2-3 gms /dl.

(ii) Slow growth and development in children and in adolescents secondary sexual characteristics are delayed.

(iii) The skin color may become ashen due to pallor, jaundice and hemosiderosis.

Oral manifestations:

(a) Bimaxillary protrusion and other abnormalities.

(b) Short roots and taurodontism.

(c) Marked open bite, malar bone prominence and saddle nose.

(d) Child may have typical chipmunk facies.

Radiological features:

The jaws may exhibit generalised rarefaction of the alveolar bone, thinning of the cortex, absent inferior alveolar canal, enlarged marrow spaces, and coarse trabeculae.

Bones may show typical hair on end appearance.

Treatment:

In thalassemia major cases the patient survives on blood transfusions. This may lead to iron overload which is generally treated with continuous injections of a chelator, deferiprone which mobilises and excretes the excess iron.

Folic acid supplements are of some benefit.

Hematopoietic stem cell transplantation may be a future hope for treatment of thalassemia.

2) Sickle cell disease:

In this condition there is an abnormality at the beta chain of haemoglobin. As a result the normal discoid shape of the RBC is changed to sickle shape.

This condition leads to:

- Stasis and hemolysis of the red cells.
- This results in very low oxygen tension, increased pH and further sickling.
- This reduces their plasticity and life span from 120 to 14 days.

Thus anemia and hypertrophy of bone marrow occurs.

Clinical features:

- There is marked underdevelopment and patients often die before 40 years of age.
- Clinical features seen are due to:
  - (i) Anemia
  - (ii) Jaundice, pallor and cardiac failure.
  - (iii) Necrosis following stasis of blood which leads to blindness, chronic leg ulcers, strokes, abdominal and bone pains, splenic infarction.
- Acute chest syndrome: Includes fever, cough, dyspnoea, hypoxia.
- Infarcts and necrosis in long bones.
- Aplastic crises may develop due to infections or hypersensitivity reactions. The patients may become acutely sick, and the red cells production literally stops and haemoglobin levels drop to acutely low levels.

Oral manifestations:

- Jaundice and pallor of oral mucosa.
- Delayed eruption and hypoplasia of the dentition.
- Interruption of blood supply causes anesthesia of inferior alveolar nerve and pulpal necrosis of otherwise healthy premolar and molar teeth.
- In dental radiographs increasing radiolucency and typical step ladder appearance of the trabeculae of alveolar bone between roots of teeth.
- Patients with this disorder are prone to develop osteomyelitis.

Treatment:

- Treating the symptoms.
- Antibiotics and analgesics for infection and pain control.
- Folic acid dietary supplements.
- Cytotoxic agents like hydroxyurea is given to increase hemoglobin F and reduce the painful episodes.
- Allogenic stem cell transplantation is being suggested as a curative for severely affected young patients.

Dental considerations:

- Elective dental procedures which involve the soft tissues should be postponed in patients with poorly controlled disease unless very urgent as there may be delayed wound healing and complications due to anemia.

- Oral sources of infection should be eliminated as infections can precipitate an aplastic crisis.
- General anesthesia to be used with caution.

Preoperative transfusions to be given to prevent sickle cell crisis.

Suggested reading:

1. H R Umarji, Concise Oral Medicine, page 156-160.
2. M. H. Steinberg and J. G. Adams. Thalassemic hemoglobinopathies. Am J Pathol. 1983 Dec; 113(3): 396–409.

Q 4) Chronic lymhocytic leukemia:

RGUHS OCTOBER 2002 (4 Marks)

Chronic lymphocytic leukemia (CLL) results from a slowly progressing malignancy involving the lymphocytes.

More than 90% of cases involve the B lymphocytes, which are responsible for immunoglobulin synthesis and antibody response, rather than T lymphocytes, which account for only 5% of cases.

The chronic lymphocytic leukemia B lymphocytes do not carry out their normal immunologic function and do not differentiate into normal immunoglobulin-producing plasma cells when exposed to antigen.

One reason the disease progresses slowly is that, unlike the cells in other forms of leukemia, the CLL cells do not turn off normal marrow cells until late in the course of the disease.

Occasional cases of T-lymphocytic CLL have been reported.

Clinical Manifestations:

(i) CLL occurs most frequently in males older than 40 years, with 60 years being the most common age of onset.

(ii) As a result of the slow natural history, it is not uncommon for the disease to be detected incidentally by routine hematology before any signs or symptoms are apparent.

(iii) The peripheral blood shows many small well differentiated lymphocytes, hundreds of thousands, even millions, of cells per cubic millimeter may be present in the peripheral blood.

(iv) The asymptomatic phase of the disease may last for years, but eventually signs and symptoms of infiltration of leukemic cells in the bone marrow, lymph nodes, or other tissues appear.

(v) Bone marrow infiltration causes anemia and thrombocytopenia, resulting in pallor, weakness, dyspnoea, and purpura.

(vi) There is a feeling of tiredness and ill being and proneness to develop infections.

(vii) There is a tendency to bruise and bleed easily.

(viii) Night sweats and weight loss are commonly seen.

(ix) Infiltration of other tissues causes leukemic infiltrates of skin or mucosa.

(x) Lymphadenopathy, splenomegaly, hepatomegaly, may occur and cervical lymphadenopathy and tonsillar enlargement are frequent signs in the head and neck region.

(xi) Patients with CLL exhibit some degree of hypogammaglobulinemia, with an increased susceptibility to bacterial infection.

(xii) Infection with varicella-zoster virus also is common.

(xiii) Late in the disease, massive lymphadenopathy may cause intestinal or urethral obstruction and obstructive jaundice.

(xiv) Leukemic infiltrates result in skin masses, liver dysfunction, intestinal malabsorption, pulmonary obstruction, or compression of the central or peripheral nervous system.

(xv) Abnormal immunoglobulins may cause hemolytic anemia or thrombocytopenia.

Oral and Dental Consideration:

As there are many oral complications occurring in this condition, and oral infections are a source of morbidity and mortality, the dentists should be aware of the signs and symptoms of chronic lymphocytic leukemia. Dentist could be the first to suspect this disease.

Signs in the head and neck regions are seen because of leukemic infiltrates or failure of the marrow.

The signs consist of cervical lymhadenopathy, bleeding from oral cavity, oral infections and ulcers and gingival infiltrates.

There is pallor of the oral mucosa due to thrombocytopenia and anemia caused due to bone marrow suppression from the disease and chemotherapy, petechiae, ecchymosis and also gingival bleeding.

The severity of the gingival bleeding depends on the extent of thrombocytopenia and local irritants.In cases where the platelet count falls below 20, 000/mm3; severe gingival bleeding can occur.

Oral ulcerations:

They are common in leukemic patients undergoing chemotherapy and are the result of direct and indirect effects of the drugs on the oral mucosa.

Ulcers secondary to chemotherapy begin approximately 7 days following the start of treatment.

Oral ulcerations are common due to bacterial invasion due to severe neutropenia and could be the early sign of this disease.

The ulcers are large in size, irregular and emitting foul smell and lack the inflammatory halo due to anemia and lack of normal inflammatory response.

Leukemic patients receiving chemotherapy develop ulcers in the oral cavity mainly due to recurrent HSV infection. These infections involve the oral mucosa and lips. However they respond well to the parenteral acyclovir given by mouth or intravenously.

Topical antibacterial treatment consists of use of povidone-iodine solutions, bacitracin-neomycin ointments or chlorhexidine mouth rinses.

Intra-oral infections:

These infections are serious and potentially fatal complications in the leukemic patients with neutropenia.

The diagnosis of the periodontal and pericoronal dental infections is difficult in neutropenic leukemic patients as the normal inflammatory response is absent.

However, it is important to diagnose the oral infection in early stages because it has been shown that the oral flora can be an important source of potentially life threatening infections due to gram-positive and negative bacilli.

It is a dentist's obligation to carry out screening examinations and eliminate obvious sources of potential acute infection or bacteremia before chemotherapy is instituted although platelet transfusions and intravenous combinations of antibiotics may be required before dental treatment.

Diagnosis:

It is established using the blood counts, blood smears, and immunophenotyping of the circulating B-lymhocytes, that can identify a clonal B-cell population carrying the CD5 antigen along with B-cell marker.

Treatment.

Most oncologists do not treat asymptomatic CLL patients with chemotherapy because there is no convincing evidence that early treatment enhances survival.

Treatment is indicated in cases of severe and progressive fatigue, lymhadenopathy that can be troublesome, or the presence of anemia and thrombocytopenia.

In cases of patients who are physically fit, the use of chemoimmunotherapy using cyclophosphamide, fludarabine, and rituximab is considered a standard therapy.

In case of physically unfit patients, treatment with anti-CD20 antibody like obinutuzumab, rituximabor ofatumumab along with a mild chemotherapeutic like chlorambucil may be given.

The standard treatment for CLL used to be chlorambucil; however, fludarabine has been shown to produce a higher response rate.

Suggested reading:

1. Burket's, Oral Medicine Diagnosis and Treatment 10th edi. 446-448.
2. Hallek M. Chronic lymphocytic leukemia: 2015 Update on diagnosis, risk stratification, and treatment. Am J Hematol.2015 May; 90(5):446-60.

Q 5) Agranulocytosis:

TNMGRU FEBRUARY 2010 6 Marks

It is also called as agranulocytopenia, neutropenia, and granulocytopenia. It is a serious disease characterized by marked leukopenia with reduction and absence of neutrophilic leukocytes. Neutropenia is decrease in number of neutrophils and agranulocytopenia is absence of neutrophils.

Types:

- Primary agranulocytosis: In this, etiology is unknown.
- Secondary agranulocytosis: In it, cause is recognized.

- Mild neutropenia: when 1000 / mm3 to 2000 /mm3 neutrophils are present.
- Moderate neutropenia: when 500 / mm3 to 1000 / mm3 neutrophils are present.
- Severe neutropenia: when 500 / mm3 neutrophils are present.
- Agranulocytosis: when no neutrophils are seen in peripheral blood smear.

Etiology:

- **Idiosyncrasy:** idiosyncrasy or sensitization to certain drugs like aminophylline, chlorpromazine and phenylbutazone, benzene, bismuth, chloramphenicol, sulfonamides and use of cytotoxic drugs or antimetabolics, valproic acid, carbamazepine, diuretics, antihistamins, hypoglycemic agents, anti-inflammatory drugs, analgesics, antibiotics and cardiovascular drugs.
- **Deficiency:** Deficiency of vitamin B12 and folic acid.
- **Infections:** Infection with Hepatitis A and Varicella zoster virus are commonly associated with neutropenia. Overwhelming bacterial infection, particularly septicemia can be accomplished by neutropenia because cells are used at rapid rate to overcome infection.
- **Diseases:** Systemic lupus erythematosus and Felty's syndrome cause sequestration of neutrophils. It can be associated with leukemia, pancytopenia and hypersplenism.
- **Hemodialysis:** Hemodialysis patient experience decrease in neutrophils due to destruction by complement, activated by the dialysis membrane.
- **Irradiation:** Excessive irradiation can cause neutropenia due to direct toxic effects on division of bone marrow cells.

Clinical features:

- It can occur at any age but is somewhat more common in adults, particularly in women. Congenital forms are more common in childhood and acquired forms in elderly.
- It is also common in professionals and in hospital as they have easy access of the offending drugs and often use drug sample injudiciously.
- Patients often report a new drug being introduced or a recent change in medication.
- The onset may be sudden or gradual. The condition begins with sore throat and difficulty in swallowing, high fever and often rigors, which may be followed by prostration.
- The skin appears pale and anemic. In some cases jaundiced.
- There is rapidly advancing necrotic ulceration of throat and mouth with little evidence of pus formation. In case of agranulocytopenia patient dies within 3-5 days due to toxemia and septicemia.

Oral manifestations:

- **Sites:** The most common sites are gingiva, palate, tonsil and pharynx.
- **Symptoms:** There may be associated pain, excessive salivation and spontaneous oral hemorrhage.
- **Appearance:** The oral lesions appear as necrotizing ulcerations of oral mucosa, tonsils or/and pharynx.
- Painful aphthous ulcers may be present in oral cavity.
- Swollen and painful gums are common.
- **Surface of the lesion:** The lesions appear as ragged and necrotic tissue and is often associated with foul smell.
- **Margins of the lesion:** There is lack of inflammation at the margin of lesion.
- **Supporting structures:** The disease spreads quickly in gingival tissues causing destruction of supporting structures and inevitable loss of deciduous and permanent teeth. Stomatitis and periodontitis accompanied with pain.

Radiological findings

- **Destruction of alveolar bone:** Supporting alveolar bone is rapidly destroyed, so that teeth are denuded of bone and are supported only by soft tissues.
- **Osteomyelitis:** Very rarely, infection spreads deep into the marrow to cause osteomyelitis.

Diagnosis:

- **Clinical diagnosis:** Gingival ulceration, infection and anemic patient may give clue to the diagnosis.
- **Laboratory diagnosis:** Majority of patients show a leukocyte count below 2000 cells per mm3 and granulocyte count below 100 cells per mm3. Hemoglobin and platelet counts are normal.

Differential diagnosis:

- **Leukemia:** Anemia, purpura and WBC leukocyte above 1000, 000/ mm3 with prolonged bleeding and clotting time.
- **Cyclic neutropenia:** Marked cyclic appearance every 20 to 25days.
- Wegener's granulomatous: Kidney and lung involvement.
- **ANUG:** Necrosis starts on the tip of papilla and in the interdental papilla and grayish pseudomembrane is present and the lesions are punched out and, not necessarily associated with leucopenia.
- **Necrotizing sialometaplasia:** Large ulcerations occur with induration on hard and soft palate, with flat border and is painless. General condition is not affected.
- **Erythema multiforme:** Target lesions are typical and no specific blood picture.

Management:

- **Removal of causative agent:** The most important measure is removal of the offending agent if it can be identified.

- **Transfusion:** If hemoglobin is less than 10 gm/dl, transfusion of red cell concentrate is given. In some cases, white blood cell transfusion can be given.
- **Antibiotics:** Septicemia can be controlled by parenteral antibiotic therapy along with corticosteroid therapy. A combination of carbenicillin, methicillin and gentamycin is commonly used because of broad coverage against most organisms.
- **Granulocyte macrophage colony stimulating factors (GM-CSF):** This is given if agranulocytosis is related to cancer treatment.

Oral and dental considerations:

- Antibacterial mouth rinse may be helpful for ulcers.
- The soft splint which covers entire maxillary area and carries a medication is used in palatal lesions.
- The pain of oral ulcer is reduced by use of topical anesthetic mouth rinses. A solution containing 5% dyclonine and 5% diphenhydramine hydrochloride (benadryl) mixed with magnesium hydroxide (milk of magnesia) or kaolin with pectin is useful for this purpose.
    - **Splenectomy and other surgical procedures:** In patients having recurrent bacterial infections that can be life threatening, splenectomy is the treatment of choice. Surgical drainage of abscesses having pus or watery exudates may prove to be life saving.
    - **Dietary education:** avoid raw uncooked food, outdated and moldy products. In patients with periodontitis and stomatitis, soft liquid diet is indicated.

Suggested reading:

1. Andrès E, Maloisel F. Idiosyncratic drug-induced agranulocytosis or acute neutropenia, Curr Opin Hematol. 2008 Jan;15(1):15-21.
2. Anil G. Ghom, Textbook of Oral Medicine; Third edition, Page no. 870 – 8

Q 6) Answer on polycythemia vera:

MUHS MAY 2015 (3 Marks)

It is a myeloproliferative disorder characterized by excessive proliferation of erythroid elements along with granulocytic and megakaryocytic cells.

Possible cause is acquired genetic changes in the stem cell leading to disturbances of normal cellular growth.

The red blood cell (RBC) volume increases to an erythrocyte count of 6 to 12 million/mm3 with a hemoglobin concentration of 18 to 24 g/dL, leading to increased blood viscosity and thrombosis.

Clinical features:

- Cyanosis of face and extremities.
- Headache, dizziness, tinnitus, fullness of the head and face and

pruritus are common features.
- Physical examination reveals splenomegaly.
- Coronary thrombosis and hemorrhage may develop in later stages of the disease.
- Erythromelalgia a frequent complication may manifest as paresthesias involving the cranial nerves.

Oral manifestations:

- Purplish red discolorations can be seen on tongue, buccal mucosa and lips.
- Gingival inflammation and bleeding is common.
- Petechiae and ecchymosis could be seen in the oral cavity.
- Varicosities on the ventral surface of the tongue is very prominent in patients with polycythemia vera.

Treatment:

- Major therapy involves repeated phlebotomy.
- Myelosuppressive agents to reduce the hematocrit to its upper limit of 50%.
- Treatment with hydroxyurea decreases the thrombotic complications.
- Chemotherapy with agents such as busulfan, chlorambucil, cyclophosphamide and melphalan may be beneficial.

Oral and dental considerations:

- Complete blood count before treatment.
- While treatment the possibility of bleeding or thrombosis should be kept in mind.
- Special attention to local hemostasis is required.
- Preoperative myelosuppressive treatment should be considered prior to dental treatment when the blood counts cannot be controlled by phlebotomy alone.

Suggested reading:

1. Burket's Oral Medicine Diagnosis And Treatment, 10th edition, 430.

Q 7) Describe the oral manifestations of leukemia:

MUHS NOVEMBER 2014 (3 Marks)

Acute leukemia:

Oral manifestations:

- Oral mucous membrane shows pallor, ulceration and necrosis, petechiae, ecchymosis, and tendency to bleed.Severe necrosis of the lingual mucosa with sloughing is commonly seen.
- Gingiva is hypertrophic, boggy, edematous, deep red and bleeds easily due to ulceration of sulcus epithelium and necrosis of underlying tissue.
- Mobility of teeth.

- Crusting on the lips.
- Oral cavity is prone to candidal, viral and bacterial infections and pose serious and fatal complication in leukemic patients.
- Paresthesia of the lower lip and chin may be present.There may be toothache due to leukemic cell infiltration.
- Submental, cervical, and pre and post auricular lymph nodes may be involved.

Chronic leukemia:

Oral manifestations:

- Most common finding is the hypertrophy of the gingiva.There may be ulceration and necrosis with gangrenous degeneration.There may be fetid odour from mouth and dark brown exudates is often present.
- Swelling and enlargement of the tongue is common.
- There is regional lymhadenopathy.
- Mobility of teeth due to necrosis of periodontal ligament.
- Destruction of alveolar bone occurs in some cases.

Suggested reading:

1. Anil govindrao ghom, textbook of oral medicine 3rd edition, 341-343.

Q 8) Oral changes in Anemia:

MUHS MAY 2010 (2 Marks)

Anemia is the abnormal reduction in the number of circulating RBCS, the quantity of haemoglobin, and the volume of packed red cells in a given quantity of blood.

Oral changes:

- Pallor of the oral mucosa is the major manifestation.Normal pink colour is lost. In sickle cell anemia jaundice is also seen. In cooley's anemia a lemon yellow tint is seen due to chronic jaundice. The colour is best seen at the termination of hard palate and in the floor of the mouth. In pernicious anemia the oral mucosa may show a greenish -yellow colour.
- Generalised atrophy of the oral mucosa involving tongue and buccal mucosa.
- Atrophy of the tongue causing a bald look, burning and painful tongue with soreness is a common feature. Beefy red tongue is seen in pernicious anemia. Fiery red tongue is seen in megaloblastic anemia.
- Angular cheilitis is a common feature especially in iron deficiency and megaloblastic anemia.
- The oral mucosa is prone to ulceration and sloughing. These could be painful and bleeding. In aplastic anemia there is petechiae present on the soft palate and in severe cases there is submucosal ecchymosis. Ragged large ulcers which are covered by grayish,

black necrotic membrane is typical feature.

- Gingival enlargement may be present.
- Teeth: In hemolytic anemias teeth may show deposition of blood pigments in enamel and dentin imparting a green, brown or blue hue.
- In sickle cell anemia teeth may show delayed eruption and hypoplasia.
- Maxillary teeth have spacing and protrusion in cooley's anemia.
- In pernicious anemia, osteomyelitis may occur.
- Jaw bones: In sickle cell anemia there is mongoloid facies with high cheek bones and bimaxillary prognathism.
- In cooley's anemia there is rodent facies due to over development of maxilla associated with hyperplasia of alveolar process. Chipmunk facies is also seen in this kind of anemia.
- Nerves: In sickle cell anemia, patient may present with paresthesia of mental nerve which may be secondary to occlusion involving the nerves and blood supply.
- In almost all types of anemia the healing is poor after dental treatment especially so in cooley's anemia.

Suggested reading:

1. Anil govindrao ghom, text book of oral medicine, 3rd edition, 857-868.

Q 9) Bence jones proteins:

RGUHS OCTOBER 2004 (2 Marks)

It is a monoclonal globulin protein found in the blood or urine. They are antibody immunoglobulin free light chains which are produced by the neoplastic plasma cells.They are made of plasma cells which is a type of white blood cell.Henry Bence Jones in 1847 described the Bence Jones protein and published in 1848.

- Malignancy of the plasma cells is associated with the presence of these proteins in the urine of the patient.The disease most often associated with these proteins is multiple myeloma which is a tumour of the plasma cells.
- The severity of the tumour is indicated by the amount of the Bence Jones proteins in the urine. Bence Jones proteins testing is used for diagnosis of this disorder and also to check, how well the tumour is responding to the treatment.
- It is also present in urine in patients of Waldenström's macroglobulinemia, certain lymphomas and leukemias, cycloglobulinemia, osteogenic sarcoma, amyloidosis, light chain disease, malignant B-cell disease and cancer that has involved the bone.

Method:

The classic reaction includes heating of urine to 60 degrees c. At this temperature the bence jones proteins show clumping which disappear if the urine is more heated and reappear when the urine is cooled. The other procedures to observe the clumping of these proteins are, using salts, acid and other chemicals these tests will reveal the presence or absence of the bence jones proteins but not the amount.

Suggested reading:

1. Frank W. Putnam And Peter Stelos; Proteins in Multiple Myeloma II. Bence-Jones Proteins; Department Of Biochemistry, University Of Chicago, Chicago, Illinois January 29, 1953.

Q 10) Multiple myeloma:

TNMGRU APRIL 1997 (4 Marks)

Also called as 'myelomatosis', is a malignant neoplasm of the plasma cells of the bone marrow with widespread involvement of the skull, jaws and the entire skeletal system. Thought to be immunosuppressive, multicentric in origin. It originates by the proliferation of a single clone of plasma cells that are abnormal, in the bone marrow and in some cases only light chains are produced and they appear in urine as Bence jones protein.

Clinical features:

- Seen in age group of 40 & 70 years, male predilection is 4:1, usually involves skull, clavicle, vertebrae, ribs, pelvis, femur and jaws.
- Symptoms such as skeletal pain associated with pressure or motion, which aggravates on exercise and relieved on rest. Vomiting, pathological fractures, bleeding such as bruising on skin, anemia, thrombocytopenia are present.
- Swelling over the involved bone, hypercalcemia resulting in nephrocalcinosis, lethargy, drowsiness and if not treated results in coma.
- Cause of death is renal failure, due to accumulation of abnormal proteins in the renal tissue.

Oral manifestations:

- Orally the mandible is affected more commonly than the maxilla particularly at the angle region, and TMJ is also involved in some cases.
- Patient experiences pain, swelling and numbness of the jaw, epulis formation and unexplained mobility of teeth is also detectable.
- Intraoral swelling tends to be ulcerated, rounded and bluish red and sometimes may erode the buccal plate and produce the rubbery expansion of jaw. On palpation swelling is tender and elicits eggshell crackling. Pallor of the oral tissues, intraoral hemorrhage due to thrombocytopenia, secondary to plasma cell proliferation in the marrow.
- Tongue becomes enlarged and studded with small garnet colored enlargements, including nodules on lip and cheeks and thus impairing speech, mastication and deglutition.
- Oral hairy leukoplakia can be present in rare case of multiple

myeloma.

Radiographic features:

They are usually bilateral, seen in mandibular posterior region and ramus, appears as multiple, small rounded, oval and discrete radiolucency having punched out appearance, with well defined margins, that lacks the circumferential osteosclerotic activity, size few millimetres to centimetres in diameter or more, teeth appears more opaque, lamina dura and follicle of the impacted tooth shows loss of cortication and in mandible may cause thinning of cortical lower border or endosteal scalloping.

Diagnosis:

- Clinically skeletal pain, oral amyloidosis with bleeding tendency may give clue to the diagnosis.
- Radiological features such as punched out lesions in the skull is typical of multiple myeloma.
- Laboratory diagnosis:
    - Round, ovoid plasma cells with eccentrically placed nuclei exhibits chromatin clumping in 'cartwheel' or check board pattern.
    - Russels body are common findings in multiple myeloma.
    - Bence jones proteins, which coagulates at 40 degree Celcius, can be demonstrated in the urine of patients suffering from multiple myeloma.

Differential diagnosis:

1. Metastatic carcinoma-absence of definitive treatment & history of treatment of earlier tumour indicates metastatic carcinoma.
2. Histiocytosis X-common in children, lesions have ragged and vague margins.
3. Cherubism-seen in 1st and 2nd decades, lesions may be uni or multi locular, elliptical without well circumscribed hyperostotic borders.
4. Advanced osteomyelitis-presence of visible cause.
5. Simple bone cyst- seen in much younger population, may be bilateral but are corticated and characteristically interdigitate between roots of teeth.

Management:

1. Chemotherapy: chemotherapeutic agents like melphalan and cyclophosphamide.
2. Management of anemia –alkalization of urine with oral bicarbonates, high fluid intake, corticosteroids.
3. Hypercalcemia – mithramycin.
4. Hb less than 10g/dl –blood transfusion.
5. Stem cell autotransplant for improving quality of life and survival.
6. Radiotherapy for localised pain not responding to analgesics and

for pathological fractures.

7. B_{15}-therapy.
8. Other drugs such as alpha interferon, inorganic fluoride phosphate to reduce bone pain.

Suggested reading:

1. Anil Govindrao Ghom. 'Textbook Of Oral Medicine' ch 13; pg no -344-354

Q 11) Define purpura and petechiae:

MUHS DECEMBER 2005 2 Marks

(i) **Purpura:** It is a reddish or purple lesions that are flat and caused by extravasation of blood from the vessels and which leaks into the subcutaneous tissue.

- According to size they are classified as petechiae or ecchymosis and these lesions donot blanch on pressure.

(ii) **Petechiae:**

- These are purpuric lesions that are 1-2 mms in diameter.
- Petechiae are minute pin point hemorrhages.
- These are common on lips and face, and occur soon after a traumatic event with extravasation of erythrocytes in to the submucosa.

Suggested reading:

1. Burket, Text book of Oral Medicine, 10th edition, pg on-51

Q 12) Cooley's anemia:

TNMGRU OCTOBER 1995 (5 Marks)

Also known as thalassemia, Mediterranean anemia and erythroblastic anemia.

It is an inherited impairment of hemoglobin synthesis in which there is complete or partial failure to synthesise a special type of globin chain.

Types:

(i) Alpha thalassemia: In this condition there is reduction or absence of the alpha chain synthesis.

(ii) Beta thalassemia: In this case there is reduction or absence of the beta chains.

(iii) Thallasemia major: Also known as cooley's anemia.

(iv) Thalassemia intermedia: Clinical manifestation are moderate.

(v) Thalassemia minor.

Clinical features:

- Depends on the severity of the disease and may range from none to life threatening.
- These patients develop signs and symptoms between 6 and 24 months and may include pallor of skin, weakness, jaundice, protruding abdomen, splenomegaly and hepatomegaly, abnormal facial bones, growth retardation, failure to thrive and dark urine.

- Compensatory hypertrophy of erythroid marrow with extramedullary erythropoiesis may result in deformities of the long bones and typical craniofacial changes.
- There is frontal head bossing, marked overdevelopment of malar bone, short nose and depressed bridge, giving a mongoloid appearance.
- Due to multiple transfusions and excessive iron deposition there can be multiple organ failure.
- In most cases the patients die in child hood itself because of anemia and cardiac failure.

Oral manifestations:

- There is excessive growth of maxilla resulting in excessive lacrimation and stuffiness of the nose.
- There is reduced posterior facial height, increased anterior facial proportion leading to chipmunk facies.
- Over development of maxilla and hyperplasia of alveolar process leading anterior open bite and prominence of cheek bones leading to rodent facies.
- There is protrusion of maxillary teeth and spacing and short upper lip. Due to deposition of iron discoloration of dentin and enamel may occur.
- There is poor healing after dental treatment and pigmentations of oral cavity may be present.

Radiographic features:

- Tooth roots are spiky and short. There is thinning of lamina dura.
- Alveolar bone shows osteoporosis and blurring of trabeculae.
- Skull shows thickening.
- Antra are small due to excessive bone formation and encroachment and may sometimes be completely obliterated.
- The premaxilla is prominent resulting in malocclusion.
- There is generalised thinning of the cortical bone.
- The skull shows typical hair on end kind of trabecular pattern.

Diagnosis:

- Mongoloid appearance, chipmunk and rodent facies with discoloration of dentin can give clue to clinical diagnosis.
- Radiologically the typical hair on end appearance and the spiky and short roots of teeth are typical.
- Laboratory diagnosis will show hypochromic microcytic anemia. Peripheral smear will show abnormal RBCs.
- There is lowered hemoglobin and defects in alpha and beta chains of haemoglobin.

Management:

- The prognosis has improved dramatically in the past few decades.
- Patients with mild HbH may require intermittent transfusions.

- Those with more severely affected HbH may require frequent transfusions.
- Sometimes splenectomy may be required.
- Regularly transfused patients may require iron chelation to resolve the excessive iron accumulation in the organs. There are 3 FDA approved iron chelators used, deferoxamine, deferasiroxand deferiprone.
- Bone marrow transplantation is the only cure for thalassemia.
- Cord blood transplantation may be used successfully.
- Future therapeutic strategies which involve normal gene transfer via a suitable vector are being investigated.

Complications:

Infections are the major complications and common cause of mortality and morbidity in patients with cooley's anemia.

The most common causative organisms of the bacterial infections are the Klebsiella spp in Asia and in the western countries, Yersinia enterocolitica.

It is important to recognise and treat these infections as quickly as possible.

There are no contraindications for doing routine dental treatment for these patients under proper medical care.

Antimicrobial prophylaxis for manipulative dental care is recommended.

Suggested reading:

1. Burket's Oral Medicine, 12th edition, 446-448.

CHAPTER 26

Metabolic Disorders

Introduction:

Metabolism is a sum of total tissue activity as considered in terms of physiochemical changes associated with and regulated by availability, utilisation, and disposal of protein, fat, carbohydrates, vitamins, minerals and water and the influence which the endocrine exerts on this processes. Alteration from these normal metabolic process constitutes the disturbances in metabolism.

Q 1) Eosinophilic granuloma:

RGUHS APRIL 2001 (5 Marks)

Its a variety of histiocytosis X of unknown etiology. It occurs as a single or multiple lesions causing bone destruction. It may be found in all ages but more common in children or young adults. Other regions like the lungs or the gastro-intestinal tract may be involved.

It is a benign Langerhans cell histiocytosis. This term was introduced first by Jaffe in the year 1940.

Etiology:

Though the etiology is unknown, it is thought that, uncontrolled proliferation of Langerhan's cells, previous inflammations or tumours and auto-immune disorders could be the cause. The auto-immune theory is thought because of the co-existence of psoriatic arthritis and eosinophilic granuloma in patients.

Clinical Features:

- **Age and sex:** Occurs primarily in older children and young adults. Male to female ratio is 2:1.
- **Site:** Skull and mandible are commonly affected but femur, humerous, ribs and flat bones may be affected.
- This condition is generally asymptomatic or there may be palpable, tender mass on the affected bone.
- **Symptoms:** There may be local pain which may be dull and steady, swelling and tenderness may be present. Generalised malaise and fever may accompany the eosinophilic granuloma of bone.

- According to the location of the lesion the symptoms can vary, like neurological symptoms such as numbness, limping, fractures, loosening of teeth, otitis media or exophthalmos.
- **Signs:** The lesion is destructive and well demarcated, roughly round or ovoid in shape.The destroyed area is replaced by soft tissue. Tissue of early lesion is soft and brown and not friable. Later on it can become fibrous and grayish.

Oral manifestations:

- **Site:** It may occur in jaws and overlying soft tissues.
- **Juvenile periodontitis:** There is loss of superficial alveolar bone often mimicking juvenile periodontitis.
- Symptoms; Gingivitis, bleeding gums, pain or ulceration.
- **Signs:** Loosening and sloughing of teeth occurs when there is destruction of alveolar bone. Sockets fail to heal normally.

Radiological features:

- **Site:** Mandible is more commonly affected than maxilla; posteriorly it is more common than anterior. Plasma cells, lymphocytes, and multinucleated giant cells.
- **Shape:** Eosinophillic granuloma may be solitary or multiple and the lesions are circular or elliptical in shape.
- **Margins:** It is moderately well defined at its radiographic periphery.
- **Punched out appearance:** the lesions in the jaw have fairly discrete borders, which are rarely hyper-ostotic. Thus they have punched out appearance.
- **Floating teeth appearance:** Jaw lesions are usually seen as areas of pure osteolytic activity in close vicinity to the alveolar process.
- **Periosteal new bone:** Periosteal new bone formation is observed in some cases.
- **Bone sclerosis:** Sclerosis is a common observation in inflammatory lesion of jaws and the fact that it appears frequently in the oral cavity that results in superimposed infection.

Diagnosis:

- **Clinical diagnosis:** Punched out destruction of skull, diabetes insipidus, ulcerative lesion, skin lesion with exophthalmos will give clue to diagnosis.
- **Laboratory diagnosis:** Biopsy shows Langerhan's cells which contain rod shaped cytoplasmic structures known as Birbeck granules. Plasma cells, lymphocytes and multinucleated giant cells are also seen. Patients also suffer from anemia and less frequently leukopenia and thrombocytopenia. Serum cholesterol level is normal but tissue cholesterol level is raised.

Differential Diagnosis:

- **Oral carcinoma:** found in older age.
- **Primordial cyst / dentigerous cyst:** they are more or less rounded

while eosinophilic granuloma is not likely to be round.

- **Benign giant cell tumor:** they usually contain some bone within the cavity while eosinophilic granuloma does not. They also cause expansion of bone while in eosinophilic granuloma there is no expansion as such.
- **Traumatic bone cyst:** they have got well defined borders as compared to eosinophilic granuloma.
- **Fibrous dysplasia:** they have got clearly marked and corticated borders.
- **Apical infection:** In this case, pulp is non-vital.
- **Cherubism:** Limited to jaw, and it is bilateral.
- **Metastatic carcinoma:** Incidence of histiocytosis is higher in children. A history of primary tumor helps to distinguish multiple punched out lesions of histiocytosis and metastatic carcinoma.
- **Leukemia:** Jaw bone lesions of eosinophilic granuloma are most common at crest of the alveolar ridge. But in contrast, those of leukemia characteristically originate in the deeper medullary portion.
- **Multiple myeloma:** It has to be differentiated by laboratory tests. The ratio of albumin to globulin is reserved and Bence Jones proteins are present in the urine in multiple myeloma.

Management:

- **Curettage:** it is usually treated by curettage and excision of lesion.
- **Radiation:** The lesions which are inaccessible are treated by radiation.
- **Corticosteroids:** Intralesional injection of corticosteroids may be effective in local lesions.
- **Chemotherapy:** drugs like prednisolone, vinblastine, etoposide and cyclophosphamide may be given.

Suggested reading:

1. Rashmi Kaul, Neelam Gupta, Sourav Gupta, and Manish Gupta Eosinophilic granuloma of skull bone J Cytol. 2009 Oct-Dec; 26(4): 156–157.

CHAPTER 27

Neuromuscular Disorders

Q 1) Bell's Palsy:

RGUHS OCTOBER 2005 (2 Marks)

This condition is so called, after the Scottish anatomist Sir. Charles. Bell and is a very common disorder affecting a single nerve. It is the most common diagnosis that is associated with facial nerve weakness /paralysis. This condition is characterised by very rapid unilateral facial nerve weakness or paralysis and usually the cause is not known. This causes either partial or complete inability of the facial muscles to move voluntarily, of the affected side. Although its a self limiting disease the facial paresis/paralysis can cause significant though temporary incompetence of the oral region and also inability to close the eyelids, which can cause potential injury to the eyes.Some other ill outcomes can occur in the long term and can be devastating for the patient.

It is also known as 7th nerve paralysis.

Etiology:

(i) **Cold:** Many a times associated with sudden exposure to cold draft of air, but according to some it is just coincidence.

(ii) **Trauma:** May follow extraction of teeth especially due to local anesthesia.

(iii) **Surgeries:** Especially of parotid gland tumor where facial nerve damage could be possible.

(iv) **Ischemia:** Can be caused by ischemia of the nerve near the stylomastoid foramen.

(v) **Familial:** Hereditary and familial causes have been indicated.

(vi) **Tumors:** Tumors of cranial base, parapharyngeal space, and infratemporal fossa may cause 7th nerve paralysis.

(vii) Other causes: Multiple sclerosis, changes in atmospheric pressure, and pregnancy can be triggering factors for Bell's palsy.

Clinical Features:

- Women are more commonly affected and in the middle age. More commonly in spring and fall seasons.
- Begins abruptly and unilaterally.

- There could be prodromal pain on the side of the face especially in the ear, temporal region, jaw, and mastoid area.
- Speech and eating becomes difficult and there could be altered taste sensation on anterior part of tongue.
- Eye of the affected side cannot be closed and there is watering and is prone to infection.
- On smiling the affected side lips and corner of the mouth does not move or rise and the forehead and the eyebrows also remain static.
- All these conditions give the patient a mask like expression on the face.
- There is drooling of saliva from affected side corner of the mouth.
- Bell's palsy is also a feature of Melkersson-rosenthal syndrome.

Diagnosis:

The mask like face, drooling of saliva and slurred speech can help in clinical diagnosis.

Management:

- The main aim of the treatment in the acute phase of this condition is to bring about speedy recovery and prevent the corneal complications to as great an extent as possible.
- The care of eyes includes using an eye patch and lubrication and the drops should be used frequently during the day and use of an ointment for the eyes at night is recommended.
- Strategies to fast and speedy recovery consist of physical therapy, corticosteroids and anti-viral agents.

Prednisolone:

In the acute phase of Bell's palsy there is inflammation and edema of the facial nerve and the cortico- steroids have a potent anti-inflammatory action which can reduce the damage to the nerve and improve the out come.

Anti-viral agents:

There is evidence that the inflammation of the nerve in Bell's palsy could be related to the HSV and hence the importance of using antiviral drugs.

The benefits of using acyclovir or valacyclovir either singly or in combination with prednisolone in the treatment of this condition is not fully established.

Physical therapy:

Various physical therapies like exercise, bio-feedback, laser, massage and thermotherapy, electrotherapy have been used to fasten the process of recovery. However the evidence of efficacy of these treatments is not very convincing.

- Use of a vasodilator like histamine has been beneficial in some cases.

- Decompression and anastomosis with facial and hypoglossal nerves have restored partial function in some cases.
- Nicotinic acid, systemic steroids or ACTH injections have shown some positive results.

Suggested reading:

1. Anil Govindrao Ghom, Text Book Of Oral Medicine, third edition, 759-760.
2. Baugh RF, Basura GJ, Ishii LE, Schwartz SR, Drumheller CM, Burkholder R, Deckard NA, Dawson C, Driscoll C, Gillespie MB, Gurgel RK, Halperin J, Khalid AN, Kumar KA, Micco A, Munsell D, Rosenbaum S, Vaughan W. Clinical practice guideline: Bell's palsy. Otolaryngol Head Neck Surg. 2013 Nov; 149(3 Suppl):S1-27.
3. J. M. K. Murthy and Amrit B. Saxena Bell's palsy: Treatment guidelines, Ann Indian Acad Neurol, 2011 Jul; 14(Suppl1): S70–S72.

CHAPTER 28

Miscellaneous

Q 1) Anaphylactic shock:

RGUHS APRIL 2005 (4 Marks)

Ana (without), phylaxis (protection)

Definitions:

(i) Acute multisystemic allergic reaction that involves the skin, airway, vascular and GIT system.It is a severe immediate (type I) hypersensitivity reaction.

(ii) Its a life threatening syndrome which occurs due to sudden release of mast cell and basophile-derived mediators in to the blood system. Anaphylaxis is caused by medications and food and the cause and effect can be established, however possibly any agent that can directly or indirectly activate the mast-cells or the basophils can lead to this condition.

(iii) This condition is an immediate, systemic, hypersensitivity type of reaction to an allergen that could be injected, injested or inhaled which can include bites/stings or medical treatment. The symptoms can occur, 5-30 minute within exposure.

- The onset can be life threatening and fulminant. The typical case of anaphylaxis results from IgE mediated degranulation of mast cell causing release of histamine and other mediators.
- Some cases have been reported following exercise or sudden exposure to cold. Quite a few cases can be idiopathic. Anaphylactoid or non-IgE mediated reactions can be identical clinically and occur due to direct mast cell stimulation.

Etiology:

- Food-causes anaphylactic shock in about 34% of cases. (eg. peanuts, seafood, wheat)
- Idiopathic-About 37% of cases cause cannot be defined.
- Drugs-In 20% cases drugs can induce it. (eg. antibiotics like penicillin, NSAIDs, like aspirin.)

- Exercise-In approximately 7% cases exercising can precipitate an attack of anaphylactic shock.
- Latex, hormones and insect bites-About 2% cases can occur due to these factors. (latex rarely causes it, and stings of bees, ants, wasps and hornets and yellow jacket can lead to it.)

Signs and symptoms:

(i) Skin-Itching, flushing, hives, or swelling.

(ii) **Eyes:** Itching, excessive secretion of tears, redness and swelling around the eyes.

(iii) **Nose and mouth:** Sneezing, rhinitis, nose congestion, swelling of tongue or metallic taste.

(iv) **Lungs and throat:** Coughing, tightness in the chest, difficulty in breathing, wheezing etc, increase in mucous production, swelling in the throat, feeling of choking or itching, change in voice.

(v) **Heart and circulation;** There can be dizziness, fainting, weakness, rapid, slow or irregular heart beats or low blood pressure.

(vi) **Digestive system:** Nausea, vomiting diarrhoea and cramps.

Differential diagnosis:

- Severe attack of asthma.
- Heart attack.
- Panic attack.
- Food poisoning.
- First aid:
- Place patient in Trendelenburg position.
- Maintenance and establishment of airway.
- Oxygen to be given through the nasal cannula.
- A tourniquet to be placed above the reaction site.
- Administration of epinephrin at the site of antigen injection.
- Begin the IV to raise the blood pressure.

Suggested reading:

1. A.F.T. BROWN, Anaphylactic shock: mechanisms and treatment-Journal of Accident and Emergency Medicine 1995 12, 89-100.
2. Jasmeet Soar. Emergency treatment of anaphylaxis in adultsClinical Medicine Vol 9 No 2 April 2009.

Q 2) Halitosis

TNMGRU AUGUST 2005 5 Marks

It is a term used to describe a disagreeable or bad odour in the expired air, regardless of the fact whether the odorous substances originated from oral or non-oral sources. In 80-90% of the cases originates within the oral cavity, where anaerobic bacteria degrade sulphur that contain amino-acids to foul smelling volatile sulphur compounds namely, hydrogen sulphide and methyl mercaptan. Non oral causes accounts for 10-20%.

Types of Halitosis:

1. **Genuine halitosis** - where halitosis is a real problem that can

easily be diagnosed by Organoleptic methods or by measurement of the responsible compounds. It is subclassified as:
   (a) Physiologic-morning breath, smoking tobacco, and some foods and medications.
   (b) Pathologic intra-oral or extra-oral origin.
2. **Pseudo-halitosis** - where the malodour does not exist, but patient believes that he or she has it.
3. **Halitophobia** - where the patient "believes" that he or she has halitosis even after successful treatment of the same and is a recognized psychiatric condition.

Sr. no.	Odours	Diseases responsible for it
1	Sour odour	Hyperacidity, digestive dysfunction, peptic ulcers.
2	Foetid odor	ANUG, bronchiectasis.
3	Urinals odor	Kidney dysfunction or uremia
4	Acetone breath	Diabetes mellitus
5	Stench breath	Gangrene, necrotic lesions or malignant lesion
6	Mousy (dead rat smell)	Liver cirrhosis
7	Bloody odour	Intestinal hemorrhage
8	Fruity odour	After use of general anesthesia

Common causes of halitosis:

The Microrganisms that are associated with halitosis are Fusobacterium periodonticum, Porphyromonas endodontalis, Porphyromonas gingivalis, Prevotella (Bacteroides) melaninogenica, Prevotella intermedia.

1) Local causes:

A. Food impaction, ANUG, acute gingivitis, adult and aggressive periodontitis, pericoronitis, dry socket, xerostomia, oral ulceration and malignancy.
B. Respiratory diseases such as sinusitis, tonsillitis, malignancy, bronchiectasis etc.
C. Volatile food stuffs such as Garlic, Onions, Spiced foods etc.

2) Systemic causes:

- Acute febrile illnesses, leukemias, upper respiratory tract infection, helicobacter pylori infection, pharyngo-esophgeal diverticulum, duodenal obstruction.
- Hepatic failure, renal failure (last stage), diabetic ketoacidosis.
- Trimethyl aminuria, hypermethioninemia.
- Menstrual breath in menstruation.
- Gastro-oesophageal reflux disease.

Diagnosis:

Assessment of halitosis is usually subjective. Various methods are:

1. Direct methods like osmoscope, cryoscope measurement, gas chromatography, portable sulfide monitor, electronic nose have been utilized to determine the intensity of odors.
2. Indirect methods like, Bacterial culture, BANA hydrolysis- a microbiological investigations (benzoyl argininen aphthylamide)
3. Halimeter: Equally sensitive to H2S and CH3SH.

Treatment:

1. Treatment of the cause.
2. Regular meals.
3. Abstinence from smoking and foods such as onions and garlic.
4. Reduction of micro-organisms and intra-oral nutrients mechanically- By cleaning of tongue, use of tooth brush, interdental flossing, professional therapy for the periodontal conditions.
5. Reduction of the oral microbial load by use of chemicals: Chlorhexidine mouth wash, essential oils, triclosan, stannous fluoride, hydrogen peroxide, oxidising lozenges.
6. Mouth rinses, sprays, lozenges containing volatiles, chewing gums.
7. Herbs and essential oils, fennel, cardamom tea, thymol, is contained in antiseptic mouthwashes, Tea tree oil drops, lemon or peppermint essential oils can be added to warm water as an effective mouth wash freshner.

Suggested reading:

1. J lindhe. Clinical periodontology and implant dentistry; vol 1: 5th edition
2. Newman, Takei, Carranza. Clinical periodontology; 10th and 11th editionCH-29; Pg-463-473.

Q 3) Sebaceous Nevi:

OCTOBER. 2002 RGUHS (5 Marks)

Sebaceous nevus is a rare condition that affects most commonly the face and scalp and comprises mainly of sebaceous glands, abortive hair follicles and ectopic apocrine glands.

Its a benign hamartoma of the skin which is characterised by hyperplasia of the epidermis, immature hair follicles, sebaceous and apocrine glands. It is also known as nevus sebaceous of Jadassohn.

Often present at birth and in childhood it may appear as a circumscribed slightly elevated, hairless plaque which is often linear in form. The lesions become more nodular and verrucous at puberty and acquires its diagnostic histologic appearance.

Epidemiology:

- This condition occurs in about 0.3% of new borns and has no sex predilection.
- Though generally sporadic, some familial cases have been reported.
- Neoplastic changes may occur in about 10-30% of cases and the commonest are, basal cell carcinoma and syringocystadenoma papilliferum.

Pathogenesis:

- This condition and its associated syndrome, Schimmel penning syndrome is thought to be caused post zygotic mutations in the HRAS or KRAS genes.
- The cell growth is promoted by RAS by activation of multiple pathways, that include the mitogen activated protein kinase (MPAK) signal-transduction pathway.
- In this gene family the mutation activation leads to pathogenesis of several inherited malformations like the Costello, and Noonan's syndrome, neurofibromatosis 1, and out of these some are associated with an increased cancer risk.

Associated Syndrome:

- Nevus sebaceous syndrome, also called Schimmel penning syndrome.
- There are symptoms like seizure, intellectual disability, Jadassohn nevus, eye abnormalities, hemimegaloencephaly, skeletal abnormalities, defects in heart and increased risk of cancer.

The sebaceous nevi pass through 3 clinically distinct stages:

- At birth or in the early infancy stage, it appears as a solitary, hairless, round or linear, pinkish, yellowish orange, slightly raised plaque having a smooth or velvety surface. They are often located on the scalp near the vertex or on the face. Extensive lesions apart from the region of head have been reported.
- At the arrival of adolescence it becomes nodular and verrucous, round, oval or linear in shape and can be of size, 1-10 cms. Though they usually occur as a single lesion, multiple and extensive lesions could be present.
- In the later part of life it can be associated with certain tumours like the trichoblastoma, basal cell carcinoma, etc and less commonly, squamous cell carcinoma, sebaceous epithelioma, keratoacanthoma, sebaceous epithelioma etc.

Clinical Features:

- These lesions are usually present at birth and appear typically like waxy, yellowish-orange or light-brown hairless plaques with smooth and velvety surface.
- The lesions most commonly occur on the scalp and face and are circumscribed.
- They have a tendency to become raised, thickened, nodular and become more verrucous towards the beginning of puberty.

Oral manifestations:

Oral involvement is rare but when affected, occurs as papillomatous growths on the tongue, gingiva, palate and may be associated with dental abnormalities like anodontia and dysodontia.

Differential diagnosis:

- Congenital nevi.
- Aplasia cutis congenita.
- Epidermal nevus syndrome.
- Non-genital warts.
- Seborrheic keratosis.

Treatment:

- Surgical excision of the lesion.
- Laser surgery.

Suggested reading:

1. Fearfield LA, Bunker CB. Familial naevus sebaceous of Jadassohn. Br J Dermatol. 1998 Dec; 139(6):1119-20.
2. Vidya Baliga, V P K Gopinath, Sudhindra Baliga, and Umesh Chandra, Oral findings in a patient with Sebaceous Nevi - A Case Report, J Int Oral Health. 2013 Oct; 5(5): 139–142.

Q 4) Hamartomas:

TNMGRU AUGUST 2005 (5 Marks)

This term has been derived from the Greek word hamartia which refers to a defect or an error.

The term hamartoma is derived from the Greek word "hamartia" which refers to a defect or an error. It was originally coined by Albrecht in 1904 to denote developmental tumour-like malformations.

Definition:

It can be defined as a non-neoplastic, uni or multifocal, developmental malformation, which consists of a mixture of cytologically normal mature cells and tissues, indegenous to the anatomic location, exhibiting disorganised architectural pattern and predominance of one of its components.

Classification of oral hamartomas:

They are classified as:

A. Odontogenic Origin:

- Those involving teeth:
- **Dens invaginatus:** Its a developmental variation and is thought to arise because of invagination in the surface of the crown of the tooth before the occurrence of calcification.
- **Dens evaginatus:** Occurs as a developmental condition that appears as globule of enamel or accessory cusp on the occlusal surface between lingual and buccal cusps of premolars. They are rarely seen on molars, cuspids or incisors.
- **Talons cusp:** It is an anomalous structure resembling an eagles talon.

Those not involving teeth:

- **Peripheral odontogenic fibroma:** It is an uncommon lesion of gingiva and is slow growing.It is painless, hemmorhegic, and often lobulated mass of gingival or alveolar mucosa often with areas of surface ulceration.

- **Ameloblastic fibro odontoma:** It is a rare odontogenic tumour composed of morphologic features characteristic of ameloblastic fibromas on one hand and complex odontomas on the other. It is a well circumscribed, painless, slow growing and expanding tumour with no inclination for bony invasion. Radiographically they are well circumscribed and usually surrounded with a sclerotic margin.
- **Odontoma:** i) Complex odontomas are slow growing, expanding and painless lesions.

(ii) Compound odontomas are painless, benign with limited growth potential than complex odontomas.

- **Adenomatoid odontogenic tumor:** It is known to be a non-neoplastic lesion with slow but progressive growth. Most commonly seen in second decades of life. Radiographically it is well circumscribed, unilocular lesion usually around the crown of an impacted tooth. They may have radiopaque foci distributed throughout the lesion.
- **Squamous odontogenic tumour:** It is slow growing and may cause mobility of teeth, swelling of alveolar processes, and there may be moderate pain. Mandible is more commonly affected and the premolar –molar region is often involved.
- **Dental lamina cyst of new born:** It is commonly seen in newborn and rarely after 3 months of age. Most of them disappear, rupture through the surface epithelium and exfoliate.

B. Non Odontogenic Origin:

1. **Vascular origin:**
   - **Hemangioma:** They are noticed in the first month of life and show a rapid proliferative phase and may gradually become non-existent. More common in head and neck region.
   - **Lymphangioma:** Its a benign hamartomatous hyperplasia involving the lymphatic vessels.Common sites are tongue, palate, buccal mucosa, gingiva and lips.
   - **Glomus tumor:** Arise from modified smooth muscles located in the walls of specialized anastomoses which are involved in temperature regulation. Occur predominantly in the subcutaneous tissues of extremeties. May occur on nose, skin of neck, cheek and face.
2. **Osseous origin:**
   - **Fibrous dysplasia:** Its a developmental condition that resembles a tumour and is associated by replacement of the normal bone by excessive proliferation by the cellular fibrous connective tissue which is mixed with irregular trabeculae of bone. It can be monostotic, poyostotic and craniofacial.
3. **Oral & labial melanotic macule:** These are focal pigmented

lesions that may represent intraoral freckle, pigmentation, post inflammation, and macules that are associtaed with Addison's disease and Peutz-Jegher's syndrome.

4. **Pigmented cellular nevus:** Nevi are benign proliferations of nevus cells in either epithelium or connective tissue.They may be congenital or acquired.
5. **Neural origin:**
   - Neurofibromatosis: The condition is characterized by numerous neurofibromas of the skin, oral mucosa, nerves, central nervous system and occasionally the jaws.
6. **Multiple hamartoma syndrome:** It is a rare condition that has malignancies and benign hamartomatous lesions as components of syndrome. Cutaneous lesions appear by second decade of life. Multiple small papules, on facial skin, around mouth, nose and ears are seen.

   Oral lesions vary in severity from patient to patient and consist of multiple papules affecting gingivae, dorsal surface of tongue and buccal mucosa.
7. **Adenomatoid hyperplasia of mucous glands:** These are unusual lesions of oral mucous glands and are idiopathic though chronic, local trauma may be an important cause.

Clinical features of hamartomas:

- They are rare in the head and neck region but commonly seen in lungs, pancreas, spleen, liver and kidneys.
- They are usually congenital and have their major period of growth when the rest of the body is growing. Once they have achieved their adult dimensions, they do not extend to involve more tissue and rarely increase in size unless trauma, thrombosis, or infection cause edema, inflammatory infiltration, and filling of new vascular channels.
- Age ranging from infancy to 5th decade, but the developmental malformations could be present at birth and manifest later.
- The growth is self-limited and in co-ordination with that of the surrounding tissues.
- They usually manifest as single polypoid, sessile or pedunculated mass or multiple masses.
- Usually present along the tongue and rarely palate (associated with cleft palate) in the oral cavity.They have no capsules and have ill-defined margins.
- These are not true neoplasms, but neoplastic transformations may occur in hamartomas and may regress spontaneously.
- May be associated with chromosomal abnormalities and syndromes.

Differential diagnosis:

- Supernumerary teeth.
- Ectopic salivary gland tissue.

- True benign tumors - relatively unlimited capacity for expansive growth.

Management :

- The treatment of hamartomas is essentially a cosmetic problem.
- The complete removal of these lesions is often neither desirable nor possible.
- Surgical resection remains the most important treatment for patients with hamartomas in oral and maxillofacial region.
- Complete surgical resection reduces recurrence and improves prognosis.

Suggested reading:

1. Burket's Oral Medicine Diagnosis & Treatment; Edition: 10th.

Q 5) Write a short answer on intrinsic staining of teeth:

MUHS MAY 2012 (3 Marks)

Intrinsic staining of teeth occurs during development of teeth and causes alteration in the properties of light transmission of the tooth structure.

Causes:

1. **Alkaptonuria:** This is an inborn error of metabolism where in there is incomplete metabolism of tyrosine and phenylalanine, that helps to build up the homogenistic acid.This affects the permanent dentition and causes a brownish discoloration.
2. **Congenital erythropoietic porphyria:** Error in porphyrin metabolism leads to deposition of porphyrin giving a red-brown discolouration.
3. **Congenital hyperbillirubinemia:** The hemolysis and its breakdown products cause yellowish-green dicoloration of the teeth.
4. **Amelogenesis imperfecta:** Enamel formation is disturbed and it leads to yellow to yellow-brown discolouration.
5. **Dentinogenesis imperfecta:** Defects in the dentine can occur genetically or due to environmental factors.The teeth are bluish or brown in colour.
6. **Systemic syndromes:** Several syndromes like vitamin D dependant rickets, pseudohypoparathyroidism, epidermolysis bullosa, Ehler's Danlos syndrome may cause intrinsic discoloration of teeth.
7. **Dentinal dysplasias:** The teeth may have amber translucency, and also show brown discoloration.
8. **Tetracycline staining:** During the developmental phase of teeth, systemic administration of tetracycline can result in deposition within the teeth and bones and may give a yellowish or grey-brown appearance which is the worst on eruption and decreases with time. Chlortetracycline may give slate gray colour and oxy tetracycline will give a creamy yellow colour to the teeth.

9. **Fluorosis:** In this condition the enamel appears chalky white to dark brown or blackish in appearance.
10. **Enamel hypoplasia:** This condition could be localised or generalised and the appearance could be pitting, or grooving predisposing to external stains of the enamel in the region of the teeth affected and may often become internalised.
11. **Pulpal hemorrhagic products:** Staining of teeth after trauma is common and is because of pulpal hemorrhage. Hemolysis of the RBCs release the haem which combine with the putrefying pulpal components to form iron sulphide that is black. The teeth may have a pinkish hue soon after trauma and later develop a greyish black discolouration.
12. **Resorption of roots:** It is a clinically asymptomatic condition and the initial clinical presentation could be the pink appearance at the amelo-cemental junction.
13. **Ageing:** The physiologic deposition of secondary dentine can affect the properties of light transmission of the teeth and can result in gradual darkening of the teeth with age.

Suggested reading:

1. A Watts, M Addy, British Dental Journal 190, 309 - 316 (2001)
2. Vogel R I. Intrinsic and extrinsic discolouration of the dentition. A review. J Oral Med 1975; 30: 99–104.

Q 6) Pink tooth:

RGUHS APRIL 1997 (5 Marks)

Internal resorption is insidious in onset, rare and resorptive pathological process, that begins in the pulpal space and then extends into the surrounding dentine. The diagnosis and management of this condition is quite challenging for the dentist. As it is insidious the internal resorption can progress to a large extent before it is detected. It is usually asymptomatic and is seen as a pink spot on the tooth crown.

It can some times occur after dental trauma. In such case the dentine is resorbed and replaced by vascular and hyperplastic pulp tissue. Chronic pulpitis can some times cause internal resorption. As the internal resorption starts to approach the external tooth surface, a pink hue is visible because of the replacement pulp tissue that become visible through the remaining tooth substance. This appearance is called the pink tooth of Mummery. The internal resorption of teeth was described initially by Bell in 1830 and in 1920 anatomist Mummery described the pink spot on the tooth and hence is so called.

Classification of internal resorption:

(i) Inflammatory:
(ii) Transient:
(iii) Progressive.
(iv) Replacement:

- Inflammatory resorption is more likely to occur due to damage to the pre-dentine as a result of bacterial infection or trauma.
- The transient type of this condition is again a trauma induced infective, self-limiting resorption and it will usually follow luxation injury.
- The progressive type occurs due to stimulation by continual inflammation that follows infection.
- Root canal replacement type of internal resorption includes deposition of tissue that is mineralised and resembles bone and cementum but not dentine.

Clinical features:

1. It is more common in males.
2. It is commonly seen in central incisor, lateral incisor, premolar and canine and third molar.
3. It is asymptomatic.
4. There can however be pain in cases of severe resorption causing perforation of the crown.
5. There is appearance of a light pink colored area on the crown of the tooth that represents the hyperplastic pulpal tissue, filling the area that is resorbed and which shows through the overlying tooth substance that is remaining. It is called as pink tooth of mummery.
6. The resorption can involve only the crown or root or sometimes both.
7. The duration can vary with rapid progression in a month or two or can be slow and carry on for one to two years.
8. It may perforate the crown with hemorrhagic tissue projecting from the perforation, results in infectious pulpitis.

Radiographically:

1. The lesion appears as round to oval, uniform radiolucent area of the enlarged pulpal space.
2. The margins are uniform and smooth and well defined and showing distortion of the original outline of the root canal.
3. There are no bone changes seen until when the perforation occurs.

Management:

1. Extirpation of pulp with routine endodontic treatment.
2. If in some cases the condition still progresses to causing perforation of the root, calcium hydroxide paste is used to seal and repair that area, so that a calcific barrier is formed. After this gutta percha that is plasticised is used to obturate the canals.
3. Extraction of tooth, if perforation occurs.

Suggested reading:

1. Mummery JH. The pathology of "pink-spots" on teeth. British Dental Journal. 1920;41:301–311.

Q 7) Chemical Mediators Of Inflammation:

TNMGRU APRIL 1995 (5 Marks)

Inflammation is a reaction of a living tissue and its microcirculation to a pathogenic insult.

- It's a defense mechanism for survival.
- Inflammation is response of the body tissues to harmful stimuli such as pathogens, damaged cells or irritants and which is a complex biological response.
- It involves, immune cells, blood vessels and molecular mediators and is a type of protective response. The main function of the inflammation is the elimination of the initial cause of injury to the cell, clearing out of the necrotic cells and tissues damaged due to the original insult and the inflammatory process and to begin the repair of the tissues.

Chemical Mediators:

Definition: Any messenger that acts on the blood vessels, inflammatory cells or other cells to contribute to an inflammatory response.

The biochemical mediators that are released during the inflammation cause intensification and propogation of the inflammatory response.These mediators are soluble and diffuse molecules.

Classification:

1. Released by cells.
2. Released by plasma.

Actions of chemical mediators:

- Serotinin, histamine, bradykinin, activated hageman factor, C3a, C5a, LTC4, LTD4, kinongen fragments, fibrinopeptides causes vasodilation, increased vascular permeability.
- Prostaglandins cause fever and pain.
- Bradykinins cause pain.
- LTB4, txa2, LTC4, LTD4 C5a causes vasoconstriction.
- Smooth muscle contraction and mast cell degranulation is caused by bradykinin, serotonin, C3a, C5a, LTB4.LTC4.TXA2
- Stem cell proliferation is caused by IL-3, G-CSF, M-CSF, G-CSF.
- Histamine PAF, 5-HETE, C5a, LTB4, IL-8 causes chemotaxis.
- C5a, IL-8, PAF causes Lysosomal granule release.
- C3b, iC3b causes Phagocytosis.
- TXA2, PAF cause Platelet aggregation.
- Endothelial cell stickiness is caused by IL-1, TNF-alpha, ltb4.
- IL-1, TNF-alpha cause Granuloma formation.
- PGE2, bradykinin, histamine, serotonin cause Pain.
- Fever is caused by IL-1, IL-6.TNF-alpha, PGE2

The other mediators of inflammation are obtained from the cells of injured tissue or leukocytes assigned to the area of inflammation.

The vasoactive amines serotinin and histamine are produced by the mast cells, platelets and basophils.

Arteriolar dilation, increased capillary permeability, contraction of the non-vascular smooth muscles and eosinophil chemotaxis are caused by histamine and they can stimulate the nociceptors responsible for the response of pain.

A vasoactive mediator that is similar to histamine is serotinin and are found in the mast cells and platelets in the GI tract and the CNS.

The vascular permeability, dilation of the capillaries and the contraction of the non-vascular smooth muscles are increased by serotinin.

The macrophages and lymphocytes produce the cytokines including, interleukins 1-10, tumor necrosis factor alpha and interferon gamma, however they can be synthesised by other types of cells as well.

The role of these factors in inflammation is complex and these polypetides help in modulation of the activity and function of the other cells so that they can co-ordinate and control the response of inflammation.

By the action of PLA2 the platelet activating factor (PAF) is derived from the cell membrane phopholipids.

Platelets, mast cells, neutrophils and eosinophils synthesise PAF which induces platelet aggregation and causes stimulation of the platelets which release the vasoactive amines and synthesise thromboxanes.

The vascular permeability is increased by the PAF and it causes the aggregation and degranulation of the neutrophils.

The role of nitric oxide is also well established in the process of inflammation.

Nitric oxide in small amounts plays a role in the maintenance of resting vascular tone, vasodilatation and anti-aggregation of platelets.

Relatively large amounts of nitric oxide production is stimulated in response to certain cytokines like TNF-alpha and IL-1 and other mediators of inflammation.

Nitric oxide in larger quantities acts as a potent vasodilator and facilitates macrophage induced cytotoxicity and may be a contributor to the destruction of joints in some types of arthritis.

Suggested reading:

1. Harsh Mohan Text Book Of Pathology, Page No103.

Q 8) Dysgeusia

TNMGRU OCTOBER 1995 (5 Marks)

Dysgeusia is defined as an altered taste sensation in which a foul, rancid, salty or metallic taste may persist in the mouth.

Long standing, severe dysgeusia could be clinically significant as it can lead to loss of interest in food that can hamper the dietary intake and result in nutritional deficiencies and exacerbation of pre-existing disease.

Causes:

1. **Local factors:** Oral candidiasis, dental abscess, oral galvanism, periodontitis, oral lichen planus & xerostomia.

2. **Systemic factors:**
    - Vitamin deficiency.
    - Nutritional deficiency.
    - Food allergy.
    - Sjogrens syndrome.
    - Liver diseases.
    - Crohn's disease.
    - Depression .
    - Alcoholism.
    - Temporal arteritis.
    - Migraine.
    - Upper respiratory tract infection.
    - Chronic gastritis.
    - Radiation therapy to head &neck.
    - Taste disturbances could be due to tumours at the cerbellopontine angle, such as shwannoma or meningioma.
    - Central neurological causes such as hemorrhage, ischemia or demyelination affecting the gustatory pathway in the brain, or epilepsy of the temporal lobe, also need to be excluded.
3. **Pharmacological agents: Drugs such as:**
    - Anti-inflammatory agents.
    - Anticoagulants.
    - Antihistaminics.
    - Antihypertensive.
    - Antimicrobial.
    - Antipsychotic .

Clinical features:

- Onset is sudden and noticed promptly by the patient.
- The cause generally decides the duration of symptoms of dysgeusia.
- Symptoms such as altered, metallic, foul, rancid taste.
- If the alteration in the sense of taste is due to gingivitis, periodontitis, dental plaque, temporary medication or conditions like cold, dysgeusia might disappear once the cause is eliminated.
- However in some cases, if the nerves are damaged due to lesions present in the taste pathway this condition could become permanent.

Diagnosis:

- A thorough history and questions regarding salivation, swallowing patterns, oral pain, oral hygiene, any GIT associated disturbances and ear infections is obtained.
- Diseases such as diabetes mellitus, hypothyroidism and malignancies have to be ruled out.
- A thorough clinical examination of oral cavity and tongue should be carried out.

- Gustatory testing is done as regional or whole mouth procedure and natural or electrical stimuli are used.
- Threshold test for sucrose, citric acid, sodium chloride and quinine are many times performed with natural stimuli.
- Topical anesthesia of the tongue is used as diagnostic aid as it relieves the symptoms of dysgeusia temporarily.

Management:

- o Removal of the underlying cause.
- o If the cause is xerostomia artificial saliva and pilocarpine can be advised. Pilocarpine helps stimulating the salivary glands to produce saliva actively and may help in remission of symptoms.
- o Zinc supplementation has shown to improve the taste sensation in patients with this condition.
- o Zinc has also been infused with chemotherapy to reduce the chances of dysgeusia.
- o Alterations in drug therapy that leads to bad taste sensation.
- o Alpha Lipoic Acid which is an antioxidant has shown to cause improvement in taste sensation.
- o Avoiding metallic or bitter tasting food, eating food flavoured with spices and seasoning can help.
- o Eating cold food, frequent brushing of teeth, use of mouth wash, sugar-free chewing gums, and sour tasting drops might help fight this condition of bad taste.
- o In one of the studies bad metallic taste was completely resolved with Mirtazapine given in 7.5 mg / night and increased to 15mg/ night within a month.
- o In patients with idiopathic dysgeusia, there will generally be a resolution of the symptoms, quite often spontaneously, but in some cases there may be requirement of clinical psychology or psychiatric management.

Suggested reading:

1. Emma Brown and Konrad Staines Vestibular Schwannoma Presenting as Oral Dysgeusia: An Easily Missed Diagnosis, Case Rep Dent. 2016; 2016.
2. Kalpana P. Padala, Cheryl K. Hinners, and Prasad R. Padala, Mirtazapine Therapy for Dysgeusia in an Elderly Patient Prim Care Companion J Clin Psychiatry. 2006; 8(3): 178–180.
3. Norman M. Mann, MD, “Management of Smell and Taste Problems, ” Cleveland Clinic Journal of Medicine Apr. 2002: 334.

Q 9) Pulp polyp

TNMGRU SEPTEMBER 2002 (5 Marks)

An irritant that causes an inflammatory response of the connective tissue of pulp is called pulp polyp. There is absence of pain because of reduced inflammatory exudate and hence there is reduced intrapulpal pressure that is below the threshold limits of pain receptors.

Etiology:

- Slow and progressive exposure of the pulp due to caries.
- Nature of the pulp response is decided by the strength and the duration of the irritant, extent of tissue affected and the previous status of health of the pulp.

Signs and symptoms:

- Due to low activity of the forces of exudates the pain is absent. Here proliferative granulomatous forces dominate.
- Symptoms develop only when there is interference with drainage of exudates.
- In children and adolescents the teeth show a hyperplastic form of chronic pulpitis in which case the pupal tissue has high resistance and the carious lesions that are large and allow free proliferation of the hyperplastic tissue.
- It contain few nerve fibres, it is non-painful but bleeding is frequent because of a rich network of blood vessels.

Histopathology:

- There is formation of sclerotic and irritation dentine.
- There is initially minimal amount of vasodilation and infiltration of cell, but after the exposure of pulp, it increases.
- Stratified squamous epithelium covers the surface of the pulp which could be derived from the gingiva, desquamated epithelial cells of the mucosa and tongue.

Diagnosis:

- There is absence of pain.
- Pulp polyp exhibits a fleshy, reddish pulpal mass that almost fills the chamber of the pulp. The sensitivity is lesser than that of the normal pulp but bleed easily when probed.

Radiographic features:

- Chronic apical periodontitis is present in long standing cases.
- This low grade but long standing irritation, stimulates the deposition of periapical bone that is condensing osteitis in young patients. Radiography reveals dense radiopaque bone surrounding the apices of the involved teeth.

Vitality tests:

- The tooth usually responds weakly or not at all to the heat test, but could respond to a very cold stimulus.
- More than normal current is required to elicit the response by normal pulp tester.

Differential diagnosis:

- Proliferating gingival tissues should be differentiated from Pulp polyp and this can be achieved by raising the tissue and tracing the stalk of the tissue to its origin, that is the pulp chamber.

Management:

- It is done by complete removal of the pulp which is followed by its restoration.
- There should be complete removal of the polypoid tissue with the help of periodontal curette or spoon excavator and should be followed by extirpation of the pulp.
- In case the tooth cannot be restored, it should be extracted.

Suggested reading:

1. Nisha Garg, Textbook of Endodontics, Third Edition, chapter 3, page no. 30, 31.

Q 10) Dental hypersensitivity:

TNMGRU OCTOBER 1998 (5 Marks)

Definition:

Dental hypersensitivity is a short, sharp pain that arises from the exposed portion of dentin that appears in response to tactile, thermal, evaporative, osmotic or chemical stimuli, and which cannot be explained to be arising from any other dental disease or defect.

Etiology:

- It arises in the cervical aspect of the teeth on the facial surfaces and commonly involves the premolars and canines and commonly involves the patients ranging from 20-50 years of age.
- Recession of cementum which follows non-surgical periodontal therapy, leads to this condition.
- Improper brushing habits and diseases of the periodontium can cause gingival recession and this condition of sensitivity.
- Gingival recession is the most common reason for exposed dentinal tubules.
- Most commonly caused by abrasion due to improper brushing, chronic exposue to bacterial plaque, lacerations of gingiva due to habits like tooth picking, excessive flossing, inadequacy of the attached gingiva, inadequate labial plate of the alveolar bone, and loss of gingiva due to disease or surgery.
- Loss of enamel, attrition, abrasion, dietary erosion, parafuntional habit, loss of cementum, denudation of root surface, malalignment of tooth, tooth preparation.
- Irreversible loss of enamel is most commonly caused by erosion.
- Eating disorders such as bulimia.

Theories:

- Transducer theory.
- Modulation theory.
- Odontoblastic transduction theory.
- Gate control theory.
- Hydrodynamic theory.

Diagnosis:

During the visual examination of teeth, the reasons for open or exposed tubules should be ascertained. History should be obtained in detail. Certain useful diagnostic tools include, air/water syringe, dental explorer, percussion test, thermal tests like use of ice cubes, assessment of occlusion and bite stress tests.

Treatment:

- Removal of factors that cause risk of this condition by educating the patient.
- Recommend different brushing methods.
- Desensitizing agents:

Desensitising tooth pastes contain potassium nitrate which is known to interfere with the impulses of nerves.

Indirect treatment includes use of stannous fluoride which is effective in preventing dental caries, reduction of plaque formation, and control of gingivitis.

Tooth pastes and powders containing arginine are proved to be effective. Mouth washes containing potassium nitrate and fluoride reduce dentinal hypersensitivity.

Potassium chloride containing chewing gums have been found to be effective.

- Therapy given at the clinic:

  Application of potassium nitrate, sodium fluoride 2% concentration, application of 28% potassium oxalate, Fluoride varnishes.

  Adhesive resins, that include repairing resin composites varnishes, bonding agents. The composites are known to seal the dentinal tubules effectively by forming a hybrid layer.

  According to some reports use of bio glass in mineralisation and infiltration of the dentinal tubules is effective.The main component in it is the silicate that acts as nucleus for precipitation of calcium and phosphate.

  In the management of dentinal hypersensitivity, silicate cement that is derived from portland cement has been found to be effective and helps in the occlusion of tubules by remineralisation.

  Lasers have been found to be effective in the treatment of dentinal hypersensitivity.

Suggested reading:

1. AR Davari, E Ataei, and H Assarzadeh, Dentin Hypersensitivity: Etiology, Diagnosis and Treatment; A Literature Review J Dent (Shiraz). 2013 Sep; 14(3): 136–145.

Q 11) Cause of perforation of palate:

MUHS MAY 2010 (2 Marks)

1. **Developmental:** The palatal shelves coalesce to form the hard palate in the 6th week of prenatal period. When there is failure

in integration it results in cleft palate.Certain syndromes, use of alcohol by mothers, smoking, folic acid deficiency, use of corticosteroids and anticonvulsant therapy are some of the causes for this abnormality.

2. Sometimes an elderly complete denture wearer complains of a perforation in his/her Palate, could be due to complete maxillary denture with suction cup used for better retention.
3. A previously impacted canine may emerge in the form of palatal perforation due to bone resorption.An OPG can easily reveal the tooth.
4. **Infections:** Certain infections that can cause palatal perforation are leprosy, tertiary syphilis, tuberculosis, rhinoscleroderma, leishmaniasis, actinomycosis, coccidiomycosis, histoplasmosis and diphtheria. They may cause perforation of the palatal roof.
5. **Autoimmune:** Certain autoimmune disorders that can cause this condition are lupus erythematosus, sarcoidosis, crohn's disease, and wegner's granulomatosis.
6. **Neoplastic:** Different tumors may result in extension from the maxillary sinus or nasal cavity and may cause palatal perforation. These tumours generally extend as a mass but in severe cases can cause perforation during the course of the disease or treatment.
7. **Drug related:** Palatal perforation due to cocaine consumption is quite well known and other drugs like heroine and narcotics can also lead to this condition.
8. **Iatrogenic:** After extraction of maxillary molars an oroantral fistula can develop.Some other surgical procedures such as maxillectomy for treatment of carcinomas, corrective surgeries or intubation can cause palatal perforation.
9. **Rare causes:** Rhinolith can result in palatal perforation.
10. Patients with psychologic problems can present with a fictitious palatal perforation.

Suggested reading:

1. Yogesh Rao, Pankaj Yadav, Jagjeet Singh, Divyang Patel, and Amit Aggarwal, Surgical and Prosthetic Management of Suction Cup Induced Palatal Perforation: Case Report, J Clin Diagn Res. 2013 Sep; 7(9): 2086–2087.

Q 12) Midpalatal swellings:

RGUHS APRIL 2000 (5 Marks)

1. **Torus Palatinus:** It is a slowly growing flat bony protuberance or excrescence located in the midline of the palate.
   The palatal tori mostly are less than 2 cms in diameter but their size can change through out life. They are more common in Asians and native Americans and are twice more common in females. They are common in the early adult life and may keep on increasing in size. In some older patients, the size may decrease due to bone reorption. These tori appear as flat growths located in the midline

of the palate and extending on both sides, and have a broad base and smooth surface. Tori called as spindle tori have a ridge on their midline. Nodular tori consist of multiple growths and each nodule has its own base. Lobular tori also have multiple growths but have a common base. They are usually found on routine clinical examination and require no treatment. Sometimes due to repeated trauma, ulcers could form on the surface .The presence of tori however can complicate denture fabrication and removal may be necessary where in surgery is done to reduce the bulk.

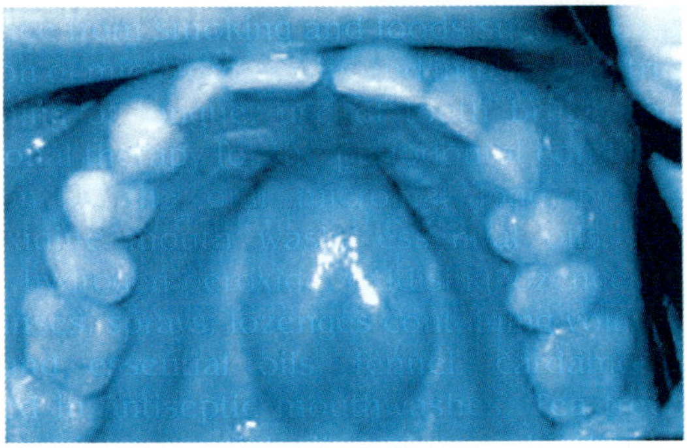

Fig. Torus Palatinus

2. **Palatal Abscess:** Accumulation of pus between the bony palatal plate & the periosteum. The abscess on the palate represents the palatally directed drainage of pulpal or periodontal origin. It is quite often seen in the pre molar-molar region and appears as a compressible swelling generaly lateral to the midline.
3. **Median palatine cyst:** They are rare odontogenic lesions of the hard palate and are not known to affect the palatine papilla or the incisive canal and are usually asymptomatic and fluctuant swellings. The nasal floor could be involved and is located on the midline and posterior to the palatine papilla.
4. **Nasopalatine duct or incisive canal cyst:** Nasopalatine duct cysts are the developmental, epithelial and non-neoplastic cysts that are considered to be the most common of non-odontogenic cyst. Its uniqueness is their development in only one location that is the anterior maxilla.
5. **Palatal cysts of the new born:** They are also called as Epstein pearls and are small whitish or yellowish cystic vesicles often appearing on the median palatine raphe of the new born. Their main etiology is the trapped epithelium during palatal development. No treatment is required as they disappear on their own in first few weeks of life.
6. **Palatal papillary hyperplasia:** Inflammatory hyperplasia of the palate is non-neoplastic lesion that is caused by an ill fitting denture of the maxilla associated with candidal infection.When associated with severe inflammation it gives a ripe mulberry like appearance.

7. **Necrotising sialometaplasia:** It may present as a palatal swelling which can occur in the midpalatal region.Though it is a swelling initially, later ulceration might develop and look like a menacing neoplasm quite like squamous cell carcinoma. Though the exact cause is not known, it generally gets resolved spontaneously within 2-3 months without any treatment.
8. A case of a mid-palatal swelling which was caused by a dentigerous cyst, which was associated with an impacted canine has also been reported.
9. **Pleomorphic Adenoma:** It is a benign neoplasm which is commonly encountered in the parotid gland. At times they can also develop in minor salivary glands of the palate and cause midline swelling.
10. **Monomorphic Adenoma:** This tumor of the minor salivary glands represents about 15% of all salivary gland tumours.

    It can cause a mid palatal swelling.
11. **Ductal Papilloma:** It is a group of relatively rare and benign, papillary salivary gland tumour which is also known as inverted ductal papilloma or intraductal papilloma. They represent adenomas with unique papillary features with a common relationship to the excretory salivary duct system, a nonaggressive biologic behavior and a predilection for the minor salivary glands. May occur in mid palatal region.
12. **Low grade mucoepidermoid tumour:** It is a very common tumour which is malignant involving the minor salivary glands (12– 29%). When mucoepidermoid carcinoma arises in minor salivary glands it can be located on the palate and may present as midpalatal swelling.
13. **Mucous adenocarcinoma:** It is a low grade rare malignant neoplasm. The incidence is unknown but submandibular gland is the most common site. A few cases with minor salivary gland have also been reported. The tumor could be associated with dull pain and tenderness. It can involve the minor salivary glands on the palate and may be located midpalatally.
14. **Papillary cystadenoma lymphomatosum or Warthins tumor:** It is the 2nd most common tumour of the salivary glands occurring exclusively in the parotid gland. The intra-oral accessory salivary gland are rarely affected and may occur as a midpalatine swelling.

Suggested reading:

1. Cicciù M, Grossi GB, Borgonovo A, Santoro G, Pallotti F, Maiorana C. Rare bilateral nasopalatine duct cysts: a case report. Open Dent J. 2010. 4:8-12.
2. Gingell JC, Levy BA, DePaola LG. Median palatine cyst. J Oral Maxillofac Surg. 1985 Jan; 43(1):47-51
3. Grossmann SM, Machado VC, Xavier GM, et al. Demographic profile of odontogenic and selected nonodontogenic cysts in a Brazilian population. Oral Surg Oral Med Oral Pathol Oral Radiol Endod. 2007 Dec. 104(6):e35-41.

Q 13) Systemic Lupus Erythematosus:

TNMGRU AUGUST 2005 (5 Marks)

Its a recurrent, chronic potentially fatal, inflammatory disorder, that involves multiple systems, that is autoimmune in nature and often affects the kidneys, joints, heart, lungs, blood or brain.

Etiology:

- The occurrence of this lesion in identical twins, and its increased frequency in the first degree relatives and the increased chances of developing in siblings of SLE patients, suggests a genetic suceptibility and reflects polygenic inheritance of the disease.
- B cell activation leading to increased autoantibody formation mainly IgG.
- Deposition of immune complexes in tissues leading to vasculitis and various organ disorders.
- Impaired T-cell regulation of the immune response.
- Abnormal metabolism of estrogen has been known to occur in patients with SLE of both the sexes.
- Regular use of permanent hair colouring agents are known to trigger SLE.
- Dietary factors like ingestion of Alfa-Alfa sprouts have been linked to development of this condition.
- The consumption of meat and milk products of live stock that are fed with synthetic estrogen is believed to increase the exposures of humans to the environmental estrogens.
- Environmental factors: Ultraviolet light exposure, certain drugs like trimethoprim and sulphamethoxozole, procainamide and hydralazine, viral infections and smoking.

Clinical features:

1. Occurs in 3rd decade in (female) &4th decade in (male) and shows female predilection.
2. It affects women 8 times more than men.
   Symptoms appear between 15-25 years of age.
3. Episodes of repeated remissions and exacerbations in the common sites being the face, neck, upper arm, shoulders & fingers.
4. Symptoms of fever, pain in the muscles & the joints are common findings. It can be associated with itching or burning sensation and areas of hyperpigmentation which can get intensified severely after exposure to sunlight.
5. The cutaneous lesions represent patches of erythema on the face that coalesce in forming almost symmetrical pattern over the cheeks and across the nose and is called as butterfly distribution.
6. Skin lesions are widespread, bilateral and associated with signs of acute inflammation.
7. Kidney &Heart involvement seen.

Oral manifestations:

- Common sites are buccal mucosa, lip & palate.
- Symptoms such as burning sensation, xerostomia or soreness of mouth.
- Lesions are similar to those of DLE except for the fact that edema, hyperemia and extension of lesions are more pronounced, and greater tendency to bleed and petechiae, suspected ulcerations surrounded by erythematous halo.
- The intraoral lesion is made of a central area that is depressed, red and atrophic which is surrounded by 2-4 mm elevated keratotic zone surrounded with small white lines.
- Lesions on the lip appear as areas of central atrophy with small white dots and surrounded by border that is keratinised which is composed of radiating small white striae with ocassional ulceration in the center.

Diagnosis:

1. Atrophic and erythematous lesion involving the skin and the oral mucosa will suggest SLE and the oral and nasopharyngeal ulceration is diagnostic of SLE.
2. LE cell inclusion phenomenon with surrounding pale nuclear mass which is devoid of lymphocytes.
3. Anemia, leucopenia, thrombocytopenia and increase in the sedimentation rate, increased serum gammaglobulin and positive coomb's test.
4. Positive lupus band test showing deposition of IgG & IgM or complement component in the skin.

Differential diagnosis:

1. **Lichen planus:** homogenous picture, no dark erythema and no telengectasia.
2. **Lichenoid reaction:** drug history is present.
3. **Ectopic geographic tongue:** systemic manifestations present in SLE is absent in ectopic geographic tongue.
4. Leukoplakia and erythroplakia lesions maintain the same appearance and there are no skin changes.
5. **Electrocoagulation lesion:** dissimilar restorations present in oral cavity.
6. **Beningn mucous membrane pemphigoid:** no systemic complaint & serological test to be done.

Management:

1. **Prevention:** avoid excessive alcohol consumption, smoking, and overexposure to the sun.
2. Corticosteroids such as prednisone.
3. Antimalarial medications such as hyrdoxychloroquine combined with NSAIDS.

4. Immunosuppressants such as mycophenolate, cyclophosphamide, azathioprine, leflunomide, leflunomide, methotrexate, and belimumab.

Suggested reading:

1. C C Mok and C S Lau Pathogenesis of systemic lupus erythematosus J Clin Pathol. 2003 Jul; 56(7): 481–490.
2. Ramos-Casals M, Font J, Garcia-Carrasco M, Cervera, R, Jimenez, S, Trejo, O, De La Red, G, Sanchez-Tapias, J, and Ingelmo M. Hepatitis C Virus infection mimicking systemic lupus erythematosus. Arthritis Rheum. 2000; 43(12):2801-2806.

Q 14) Alkaline Phosphatase:

TNMGRU FEBRUARY 2013 (5 Marks)

It is a hydrolase enzyme that is mainly responsible for removing the phophate groups fom various types of molecules, which includes, proteins, nucleotides, and alkaloids.

The process that involves the removal of the phosphate group is known as dephosphorylation. Alkaline phosphatases as per its name are most effective in the alkaline environment. It is also sometimes referred to as basic phophatase.This test measures the amount of the enzyme alkaline phophatase (ALP) in the blood.

Alkaline phosphatase occurs in many tissues of body in humans but is most commonly concentrated in the liver, bile duct, bone, kidneys, mucosa and the placenta. The liver manufactures the most ALP than the other organs or bones.

Increase in its serum concentration occurs as a result of increased osteoblastic activity which occurs due to obsructive liver diseases, abscess of liver, leukemia, sarcoidosis, rickets, osteomalacia, hyperparathyroidism, Paget's disease etc.

Normal level of serum alkaline phosphatase is 20 to 140 IU/L, in adults. Their levels are much higher in the pregnant women and children. Interpretation of the blood test should be done by using the reference range from the laboratory that it has been performed in. If the bile ducts are obstructed the ALP levels can be high. It is also high during the process of active bone formation, because it is a by-product of the osteoblastic activity eg.paget's disease. In coeliac disease patients also the levels are elevated. The ALP test is used for detecting diseases of liver or bone.

Diagnostic Use:

This test is often performed to detect blockages in the bile ducts, as the ALP is particularly high in the edges of cells that join to form the bile ducts. In case one or more of them are obstructed, eg by a tumour then the ALP levels in blood will be high. Moreover any condition that affects the growth of bone or results in increased activity of bone can affect the levels of ALP in blood.

ALP test can be used to detect the following:

- Malignancies that have involved the bones.

- To diagnose paget's disease, that can lead to malformed bones.
- To monitor conditions like vitamin D deficiency and treatment of paget's diease or other conditions of bone.
- Increased ALP levels are seen in coeliac disease patients.
- The source of elevated levels of ALP can be inferred from obtaining the serum levels of gamma glutamyl transferase (GGT).
- Increase in levels of ALP and GGT can help in suspecting hepatobiliary disease.
- In case of increased levels of ALP more tests can be prescribed to find out the cause.
- The amounts of various types of ALP can be measured in blood and used to determine whether the high levels are due to liver or bones. This test is called the phosphatase isoenzyme test.

(i) **Causes of elevated alkaline phosphates levels:** Obstruction of the bile ducts, bone conditions, osteomalacia, liver disease or hepatitis, osteoblastic bone tumours, leukemia, lymphoma, paget's disease, hyperthyroidism and, pregnancy.

(ii) **Causes of decreased alkaline phosphatase:** Autosomal recessive disease, hypophosphatasia, postmenopausal women on estrogen therapy to combat osteoporosis, men with recent heart surgery, magnesium deficiency, malnutrition, hypothyroidism, severe anemia, children suffering from cretinism or achondroplasia, children after a severe episode of enteritis, pernicious anemia, aplastic anemia, chronic myelogenous leukemia, Wilson's disease.

Suggested reading:

1. Tamás L, Huttová J, Mistrk I, Kogan G (2002). "Effect of Carboxymethyl Chitin-Glucan on the Activity of Some Hydrolytic Enzymes in Maize Plants" (PDF). Chem. Pap. **56** (5): 326–329.
2. Vroon, David. "Clinical Methods: The History, Physical, and Laboratory Examinations. 3rd edition".

Q 15) Epileptic patient and the dentist:

CSVTU APRIL 1995 (4 Marks)

Epilepsy has direct negative effects on patients suffering from this condition and also affects the dentition and oral health, both are then further affected due to poor oral hygiene. The bad oral hygiene results from epilepsy associated bad health. As a result it can lead to loss of teeth, periodontal disease and caries and require more careful dental treatment. The dentist thus needs to be aware of this condition and should be well prepared to treat them.

The medicines prescribed by the dental clinician interact with the anti-epilepsy drugs (AED) and reduce the effect of the same. The NSAIDs and certain antifungals such as fluconazole, miconazole and even metronidazole affect the metabolism of carbamazepine and phenytoin negatively. It is thus advised that combination of these medications should be avoided.

Points to be considered while treatment:

- The number of times seizures occurs.
- The last date of seizure.
- The status of consciousness and the condition of respiratory system during the seizures.
- The condition of patient physically after the seizure has subsided.
- The presence of aura before the seizures.
- Whether the presence of aura always leads to a seizure.
- Whether there is existence of status epilepticus.
- Stress being an important predisposing factor to cause seizure, elimination of these factors before starting the dental treatment.
- Appointments should be scheduled during the morning hours and each session should be short and sudden stimulation like very bright lights and loud noise should be avoided.
- In case there is history of about one seizure /month then treatment should be deferred if not urgent.
- Local anesthetics during treatment are safe but overdoses should be avoided.
- General anesthesia should be considered in cases where it is difficult to control the seizures.However local anesthesia is generally preferred over general anesthesia.
- While carrying out the dental treatment it is advised to control the seizure by sedation with inhalation of nitrous oxide or benzodiazapine intravenously.
- Inspite of conscious sedation if seizure develops then the treatment should be postponed.
- It is observed that during the seizures there are chances of injuries to the soft tissues, tongue, fractures of the maxillofacial region, subluxation of the TMJ, fractures of tooth, or avulsion.
- Fractured teeth can be treated with normal procedure but the reimplantation of avulsed tooth should be avoided.
- In case of maxillo-facial fractures in patients who have uncontrolled seizures, it is important to make sure that the airway is not blocked.
- In these cases, open reduction should be preferred and bimaxillary fixation should be avoided.
- It is important for the dentist to note that tooth ache and oral infections can cause pain and make the patient uncomfortable and can provoke a seizure.
- It is therefore advised to eliminate these stimuli and treat the conditions during periodic dental checkups before these complications arise.
- In epileptic patients poor oral hygiene and dental condition exists.
- It is thus very important to to use protective methods such as use of chlorhexidine and fluorides, and proper education of the patient to maintain good oral hygiene, regular check ups, and instructions to avoid sugars and confectionaries and drinks.

- Restorative treatment: Temporary metal crowns and implant supported bridges are preferred over amalgam and porcelain restorations as there is risk of damage during episodes of seizures. Use of rubber dam is very important.
- Prosthetic treatment: In patients requiring dentures no special treatment is required, in case the patient is free of seizures for prolonged periods.
- Special treatment is required for patients suffering from tonic-clonic seizures with involuntary muscle contractions including those of the masticatory muscles.
- In these patients fixed prosthesis is preferred over removable ones.
- A good denture with accurate fit along with good oral hygiene measures reduces the chances of phenytoin induced hyperplasia of gingiva.
- Orthodontic treatment can be done in these patients without any problems and fixed appliances are preferred over removable ones.

Action plan if a patient experiences seizure during dental treatment:

- The dental treatment should be ceased, and dental tampons, instruments and prosthesis should be removed.
- The position should be changed to supine.
- The prevention of any injury is the prime concern and the patient should be assisted accordingly.
- Loosening of tight clothing to be done.
- In case the patient can sense an aura, thick gauze tampons should be put in the mouth of patient to avoid any injury or damage to the teeth.
- When the patient goes into deep sleep after a seizure, they should be carefully monitored.
- In case of a seizure lasting for more than 3 minutes, admininstration of drugs is advisable.
- Care should be taken to ensure that the air-way is unobstructed.If the seizure continues for a longer period inspite of medication the patient should be transferred to a hospital.
- After gaining consciousness the patient should be sent home to rest and the treatment should be postponed till a better time.

Suggested reading:

1. Yaltırık Mehmet, Özer Senem, Tonguç Sülün, Kocaelli Hümeyra, Management of Epileptic Patients in Dentistry, Surgical Science, 2012, 3, 47-52.

CHAPTER 29

Forensic Odontology

Q 1) Wound Certificate:

RGUHS APRIL 2006 (2 Marks)

There is a standardised system that exists to classify wounds in the hospitals that grade the condition of wounds that pre-exist and those that occur after surgery. Classifying the healing wounds into categories for analysis helps the surgeons and the medical staff to determine as to what extent there is infection or contamination in the wound and what treatment is required to help in healing. It also can predict the likely outcome of the surgical procedure.

There are four classes in the wound classification system:

Class I or Clean Wounds: A surgical wound that shows no infection or inflammation after surgery and are primarily closed.

Class II Clean-contaminated wounds: A wound due to surgery where the alimentary, respiratory, genital or urinary tracts are entered under surgical conditions but without any contamination or infection.

Class III or contaminated wounds: Fresh wounds and open accidental wounds that are present before surgery and those that are made during surgery when a major breakdown of the sterile technique occurs during the surgery.

Class IV or dirty and infected wounds: Wounds that are old and traumatic with retention of devitalised tissue, having existing purulent infection before surgery. A patient is hence under bigger risk of post-operative infection and poor outcome for healing after surgery compared to the other wounds.

Suggested reading:

1. Jacqueline Lynch BNET website, e Medicine - WebMD, Access My Library - AORN journal.

Q 2) Bitemarks:

TNMGRU AUGUST 2014 (5 Marks)
RGUHS APRIL 2003 (4 Marks)

It is defined by McDonald as a mark that is created by the teeth either alone or in combination with other parts of the mouth.

It is a patterned injury produced by teeth on animate or inanimate objects.

It can be caused by either humans or animals on tissue, food items, or other objects.

Causes:

(i) Sexual assault.
(ii) Child abuse.
(iii) Homicide.
(iv) Domestic violence.
(v) Sports.
(vi) Self inflicted.

Importance of bite mark:

Precise identification is possible because the alignment of teeth are typical each individual. Distinct traits of specific types of teeth can be identified and accurately recorded eg, the central and lateral incisors produce a rectangular, where as the canines create a triangular pattern of injury .How ever recording in the bitemark of individual characteristics are importantly needed so as to be able to identify positively the cause of bitemark. The process of comparing bitemarks with the dentition of the suspects includes the measurement and analysis of the size, shape and the position of the teeth. Almost all comparison methods include the fabrication of the overlays.

The forensic odontologist plays an important role of recording the impressions of the bite, make dental impressions of the suspects and be ready to show the comparisons and if deemed necessary, so that the evidence can be presented in the court as an expert witness. It is now realised that bitemarks can provide details about an individual almost comparable to finger prints.

Classification:

(a) Non-human.
(b) Human.
- In food stuffs.
- On non-biological object (pencils, pipe stems, and detonators)
- On human skin:
  - Non-criminal (erotic bite)
  - Criminal-can be during sexual assault, homicide and other offences.

Types of bitemarks:

- Definite bite mark.
- Amorous bitemark.
- Moderately aggressive bitemark.
- Aggressive bite marks.
- Very aggressive bitemarks.

Typical Bitemark Presentations:

- Bite-marks that have been caused slowly exhibit a suck mark with abrasion pattern that simulates a sun burst.
- Circular or elliptical injury that can record the typical characteristics of the teeth.
- The shape of the injury could resemble a doughnut with the typical characteristics along the perimeter of the mark.
- Two horse-shoes shaped arches that are separated by an open space at their bases. The injury diameter can range from 25-40mm.
- Central area of bruising within the marks of teeth.

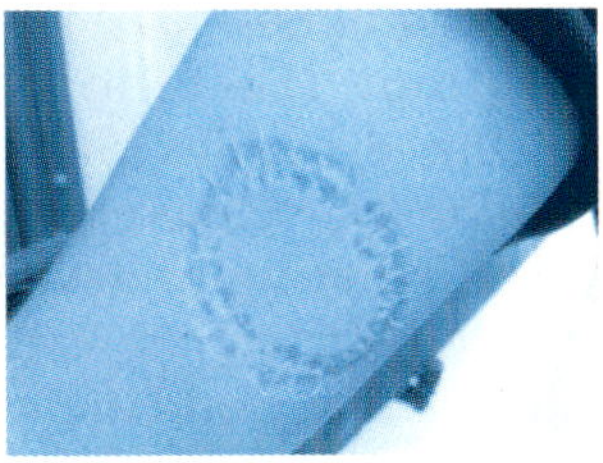

Fig. Bite marks on skin

As mentioned above the incisors and canines produce typical pattern of injuries that can be identified and the traits can be recorded accurately. However individual characteristics need to be properly recorded in the bitemarks so as to identify positively the causer of bitemark.

Characters such as rotations, fractures, abrasions, attritions, congenital malformations etc when recorded properly in the injury may help to compare them to identify the specific tooth of a person that caused the injury.

There are also restorations, fillings, rotations, teeth loss, breakages and injuries that can make one persons teeth different from any other individual. Sometimes a bitemark has to be studied and charted from many angles and sometimes only one tooth can help in identification.

The skill of comparing the dental impressions taken from a person's mouth to the bite mark impressions on the skin of victims is possessed by the Forensic odontologists. There are about thirty seven to seventy six comparison factors that can help in identification like matching the whorls, striations, pitting and abrasions which is most often done by using computer enhanced photography.

The typical physical characteristics of the bite mark wound and the suspects dentition include:

- The distance from canine to canine.
- The shape of the arch of the mouth.
- The evidence of out of alignment of tooth.
- Width and thickness of teeth and the spacing between teeth.
- Missing teeth.
- The biting edges curve.
- Unique dentistry.
- Patterns of wear such as chips or grindings.

Analysis of Bitemarks:

To standardise the analysis of bitemarks the American Board Of Forensic Odontologists have laid down certain guidelines:

1. **History:** To obtain a thorough history of any dental treatment carried out after the suspected date of the bitemark.
2. **Photography:** Extraoral photographs of the full face and profile views.The intra-oral photographs should include the frontal view, two lateral views, and occlusal views of each arch. Including a photograph of maximal mouth opening can be useful.If materials like food stuff are used for test bites the results should be captured and preserved by photographs.
3. **Extra-Oral Examination:** The factors of soft and hard tissues that may influence the dynamics of biting should be observed and recorded meticulously. Measurements should be taken of the maximal mouth opening and any deviations during opening and closing.
4. Salivary swabs should be taken and the tongue should be examined to assess the size and function. The status of periodontium should be noted and any mobility of teeth should be recorded. A dental chart should be prepared.
5. As per the recommendations of the American Dental Association materials should be used to take two Impressions of each arch and the occlusal relationship should be noted.
6. Where ever possible sample bites should be taken into an appropriate material that will simulate the type of bite under study.
7. Type II stone should be used to prepare casts and additional casts should be made by duplication of the master casts.

Q 3) Importance Of Incremental Lines In Forensic Odontology:

RGUHS OCTOBER 1999 (5 Marks)

Dental age estimation is important not only for identification of the deceased victims but also in connection with crimes, accidents, legal matters, school attendance, social benefits, records, employment and marriage. The estimation of age by the counting of incremental lines of cementum is considered an acceptable method by some authors. According to the recent research it is said that the tooth cementum annulations (TCA) can be used more reliably than the morphological or histological traits of the skeleton of adults in the estimation of age.

Before the tooth erupts, the first layer of acellular cementum is produced. The further layers are then added during and after eruption. Lieberman and Schroder gave a biological explanation for these alternating layers suggesting that the dark lines are the stop phases of mineralisation as the fibroblasts continue to grow, that leads to a change in the orientation of mineral crystal. This alternating pattern is visible as alternating light and dark line under the microscope. The dark lines are called as the incremental

7. There should be signature or initials of the treating clinician only on all entries.
8. It is important to have informed consent forms with signature of the patient to carry out invasive procedures, sedation etc.
9. If the patient refuses to undergo treatment inspite of the fact that the clinician feels it is important, signature of the patient is important as it is in the consent form.
10. The records should be objective in nature and should contain facts related to the case.
11. Mistakes in the record should be corrected with a single line drawn across the incorrect material and there should be no deliberate tampering with the written record after the facts are noted.
12. All the communications with the patient including the emergency telephonic consultations should be recorded.
13. When the patient is dissatisfied the communications to that effect should be recorded including the problem, the attempts to deal with it and the solutions.
14. In case the patient wishes to discontinue the treatment, it should be noted and reason mentioned.
15. All files of the patients should be classified as active, in which case it holds the records of patient taking treatment from the clinician and inactive where in the patient has not reported for more than 24 months.

B. Business records:

It should contain all the details of billing, with date and amount, copies of claim forms given by the patient, information related to name, address, nature of the services of laboratory used, its charges, scheduling of appointments etc.This should be maintained separately.

C. Record of drugs prescribed:

Certain drugs are prescribed by the dentist to treat certain conditions and though limited, there can be serious implications and extreme care should be taken while prescribing to make the best use and avoid any side effects.

The drug record should include:

1. The date and method of prescription/administration/dispensation.
2. Name, strength and quantity and the form of drug.
3. Directions for use of drug.
4. Condition being treated.
5. The prescription pads should never be presigned and should be out of reach of patient lest it is misused.

Suggested reading:

1. Arishka Devadiga, What's the deal with dental records for practicing dentists? Importance in general and forensic dentistry, Journal Of Forensic Dental Sciences Year: 2014 | Volume : 6 | Issue : 1 | Page : 9-15
2. Lawney M N Y State Dent J. 1998 May; 64(5):34-43.

ORAL AND MAXILLOFACIAL RADIOLOGY

SHORT ANSWERS QUESTIONS

CHAPTER 1

Radiation Physics

Introduction:

X-ray radiography has become an important diagnostic procedure in dentistry.

Basic knowledge about the production of x-rays, their properties, and interactions which result in formation of the radiographic image is required.

Q 1) X-ray tube:

OCTOBER 1997 RGUHS (5 Marks)

X-ray tube:

- It is the main component of x-generation system.
- It is made up of glass leaded tube, which is situated inside a lead metal housing.
- The glass leaded tube of x-ray contains two electrodes, anode and cathode.
- Metal housing is filled with insulating oil. It prevents over heating by that is created by the production of x-rays.
- The step up and step down transformers are located inside the metallic housing.
- Metal housing also consist of tube head seal made up of aluminum which allows the exit of x-rays from the head of the tube.

Components of tube of x-rays:

It is composed of:

(a) A leaded glass housing
(b) A negative cathode
(c) A positive anode.

A leaded glass housing:

- The glass tube is evacuated i.e. all the air from the tube has been removed.
- It consists of two electrodes, anode and cathode.
- The leakage of radiation is prevented by the leaded glass tube which contains vaccum.

- There is an area in the center that has a window which allows the x-ray beams to come out of the tube and it helps direct the beam towards the aluminum disk. Collimator made of lead and the position indicating device.

Cathode:

- The electrons that move towards the anode come out of the cathode.
- The cathode lies within an evacuated glass tube.
- When electrons from the cathode strike the target located on the anode, x-rays are produced.
- The cathode consists of a focusing cup and a filament.
- When the filament is heated it emits electrons within the tube.
- The filament is made of coil of tungsten wire that is about 2 mm in diameter and 1 cms or less in length.
- It is mounted with the help of two stiff wires which support it and carry the electric curent.
- These two wires help in connecting to high and low voltage electric sources through the tube envelop.
- When the filament is heated to incandescence by the current from low voltage source it emits electrons at the rate which is proportional to the temperature of the filament.

Focusing cup:

- It is made up of molybdenum and is concave reflector and negatively charged.
- The focusing cup directs the electrons emitted by the filament with a narrow beam that is directed at the rectangular anode called the focal spot.
- The electrons are so directed due to the negatively charged cathode from which they get attracted to the positive anode.
- The tube is vaccumised to allow smooth unobstructed transit of electrons towards the anode so as to maintain their speed.

Anode:

- It consists of a copper stem with tungsten target embedded in it.
- The function of the anode is to convert the kinetic energy of the electrons in to photons of x-ray.
- In this process about 99% of the kinetic energy is converted to heat.
- The target is made of tungsten.

  Properties of tungsten:

  The tungsten possesses high atomic number (74), high melting point and high thermal conductivity, low vapour pressure at the temperatures of an x-ray tube.

- The target with high atomic melting point and number produces x-rays efficiently.
- A target has a high melting, it is necessary because heat is generated at the anode.
- The tungsten also has high thermal conductivity that helps in dissipating heat into the copper stem.
- The low vapour pressure at high temperatures help to maintain the vaccum at high tube temperatures.
- The tungsten is embedded in the copper stem for the dissipation of heat.
- As copper dissipates the heat perfectly, it reduces the chances of melting the target.
- The circulating oil between the glass envelop of the tube further helps in dissipation of heat arising from the copper stem.
- There are two types of anode, Stationary anode and Rotating anode.
- Above mentioned anode is stationary anode.
- There is also a rotating anode that is a beveled disc and rotates when the tube is in operation. The electrons strike hence at different areas and help in dissipation of the heat from a small focal spot by providing a wider area.

Focal spot:

- It is an area on the target made of tungsten on which the electrons from the focusing cup are directed.
- The image sharpness increases as the focal spot size decreases but the heat generated per unit area becomes greater.
- To have a smaller focal spot and yet get a larger area for distribution of electrons, the the target is placed at an angle to the electron beam and hence it is placed at an angle of 20 degrees to the central beam of the electrons. This helps to reduce the effective focal spot to 1mm x1mm as compared to the actual size of 1mm × 3mm.

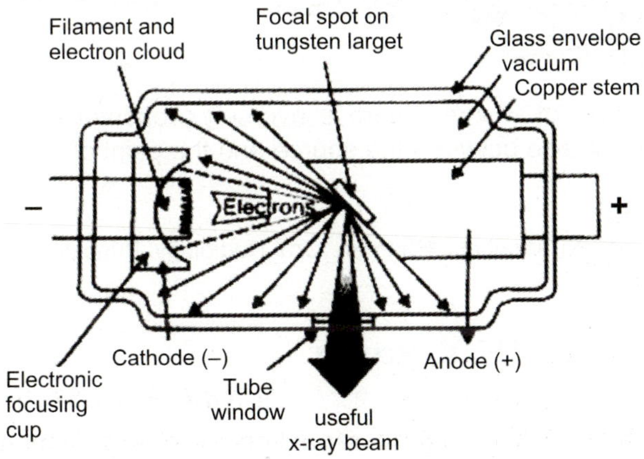

Fig. Diagrammatic representation of components of x-ray tube

Suggested reading:

1. Freny R. Karjodkar. Textbook of Dental and Maxillofaciall Radiology, 2nd edition. Page no. 36-41.
2. Stuart C White, Michael J Pharoah, Oral Radiology, Principles and Interpretation 6th Edition, page no. 7-9.

Q 2) Describe inverse square law and its application.

MUHS MAY 2011 (2 Marks)

- The x-ray beam intensity depends on the distance of measuring device from the focal spot.
- The intensity of a beam is inversely proportional to the square of the distance from the source.
- The reason for this decrease in intensity is because the x-ray beam spreads out as it moves from the source. The relationship is as follows: I1/ I2 = (D2)2 / (D1)2
  Where; I = intensity and D= distance.
- Hence if given dose of 1 gray is measured at distance of 2 m, a dose of 4 gray will be found at 1m and 0.25 grays at 4m.
- Hence the altering of the distance between the x-ray tube and the patient markedly affects the beam intensity.
- But this change should be followed by a corresponding modification of the KVp and the MAs if the exposure parameter of the film has to be kept constant.

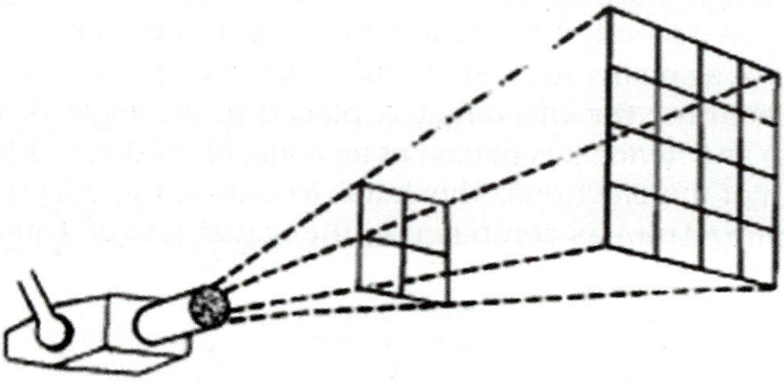

Fig. The intensity of an x-ray beam is inversely proportional to the square of the distance between the source and the point of measure

Suggested reading:

1. Stuart C White, Michael J Pharoah, Oral Radiology, Principles and Interpretation 5th Edition, 12.

Q 3) Properties Of X-Rays:

TMNGRU AUGUST 2014 (5 Marks)

X-rays are defined as weightless packets of energy which is pure and without any electrical charge and travel in wave along a straight line and has specific frequency and speed.

Properties of x- rays can be broadly classified in to four categories:

A. Physical
B. Chemical
C. Biological
D. Physiochemical.

Properties that are physical:

1. X-rays belong to the electromagnetic radiation family and have wave lengths ranging from 10 Å -0.01Å.
2. They travel in a wave motion through space.
3. They travel in a straight line in free space.
4. They travel at the same speed as that of light. (1,86,000 miles / seconds)
5. They produce electrical field at right angle to the path of their propagation in the space and the magnetic field is at right angle to the electric field.
6. They cannot be seen by the eyes and cannot be heard or smelt.
7. An electric or magnetic field cannot reflect, delect or cause refraction of x-rays as they don't have charge.
8. They show the properties of interference, diffraction and polarization, as that of visible light.
9. They don't require a medium for propagation.
10. The x-rays consist of pure energy, no mass and the energy is transferred in the form of photons (quanta).
11. They follow the principle of inverse square law in free space which states that for a point source of radiation intensity (I) at a particular place is proportional inversely to the square of the distance from the point source to the area at which the intensity is being considered. $I \alpha\ 1/d^2$ or I= kd where k is constant.
12. The collision of electrons with tungsten atoms produce the x-rays. The collision of two types giving rise to two types of x-ray spectra:
    (i) The continuous spectra or /Bremsstrahlung or braking radiation.
    (ii) Characteristic / Line radiation/spectrum.
13. **Penetration:** The x-rays can penetrate solids, gases and liquids and the degree of penetration depends upon the quality, intensity and the wavelength of the beam of x-rays.
14. **Property of fluorescence:** When the x-ray beam falls on certain materials, they will emit visible light.
15. X-rays also possess properties of production of heat.
16. They have the capacity to ionise the materials that they penetrate and interact with.
17. They possess the property of attenuation, absorption and scattering.
18. X-ray Interact with matter:
    (i) Classical or Coherent Scattering
    (ii) Photoelectric Effect
    (iii) Compton Scattering

(i) **Coherent / Classical / Elastic /Thompson Scattering:** In this process the radiation gets deflected without the loss of their energy.

(ii) **Photoelectric effect:** It is the interaction of an incident photon with a bound electron of inner shells of an atom leading to emission of characteristic radiation.

The absorption of about 30% of photons from a dental x-ray beam are so done by the photoelectric process.

(iii) **Compton Scattering / Inelastic scattering:** It is an interaction of photon with the free outer shell electrons that are loosely bound.

Chemical properties:

1. The x-rays possess the property of inducing change in colour of several substances or their solutions.
   (a) Methylene Blue gets Bleached.
   (b) Sodium platinocyanide that is apple green in colour turns into darker shades, then into light brown and then dark brown.
2. They can bring about chemical changes in the solutions as they produce a highly reactive OH radical in water, which react with the solutes. This brings about molecular changes in biological molecules.
3. They can cause the destruction of the fermenting powers of the enzymes. (enzymes are the vital substances for the metabolism of the cells of living organisms)

Biological Properties:

When x-rays are incident on an atom, it causes excitation of an atom causes biological damage to the cells.

1. The property of excitation of the x-rays is used in the treatment of malignant lesions.
2. They also possess bactericidal and germicidal effects.

   Biological properties of x-rays can be classified as:

   (i) **Somatic effect:** It can range from a simple sun-burn, to severe dermatitis or a change in blood supply to the malignancies.

   (ii) **Genetic effect:** It is due to the mutation of genes and chromosomes induced by radiation. These changes can be seen in the off-springs of the parents who have been irradiated.

Physiochemical Properties:

1. **Photographic effect:** Photographic paper or film exposed to x-ray radiation and then developed causes blackening, due to release of metallic silver. This blackening of the film is called film density.

X-rays are defined as weightless packets of pure energy photons that are without electrical charge and travel in wave along a straight line with a specific frequency and speed.

Suggested reading:

1. Freny R. Karjodkar. Textbook of dental and maxillofaciall radiology, . 2nd edition. Page no. 27-35.

Q 4) Compton effect:

TNMGRU AUGUST 2007 (5 Marks)
RGUHS OCTOBER 1998 (5 Marks)

- When a photon interacts with an outer orbital electron Compton scattering occurs.
- About 62% of the photons that are absorbed from a dental x-ray beam are absorbed by this process.
- In this interaction the incident photon collides with an outer electron which then acquires the kinetic energy and recoils from the point of impact.
- From the site of collision the path of the incident photon is deflected by the interaction and gets scattered.
- The scattered photon possess energy that is equal to the energy of the incident photon from which the sum of the kinetic energy gained by the recoil electron and its binding energy is subtracted.

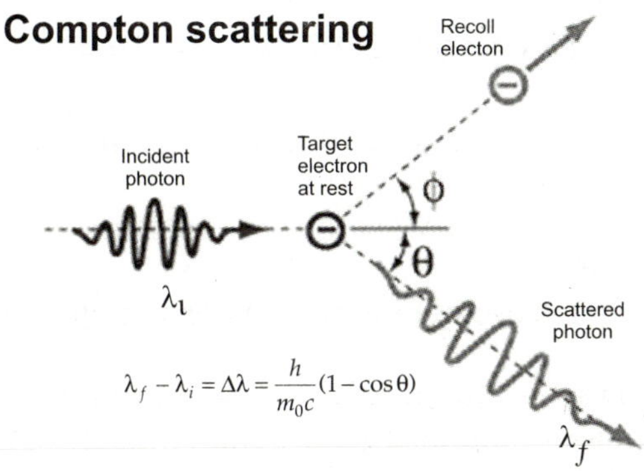

Fig. Mechanism of Compton scattering

- Similar to the case of photoelectric absorption the compton scattering results in loss of an electron, and also causing ionisation of the atom that absorbs.
- The photons that are scattered continue on their new paths, causing further ionizations.
- Similarly, the recoil electrons give up their energy by ionizing other atoms.

- The probability of a Compton interaction is directly proportional to the electron density of the absorber.
- The number of electrons in bone is greater than in soft tissue and hence the probability of the compton scattering is greater in bone than other tissues.
- About 62% of the photons coming out of dental x-ray beam undergo compton scattering.
- The scattered photons can travel in any direction.
- In the incident photon possessing higher energy there is greater probability that the angle of scatter of the secondary photon will be small and the direction will be forward.
- From the scattered photons formed during dental exposure about 30% exit through the head of the patient.
- The advantage is that some of the energy of the incident x-ray beam can escape the tissue and disadvantage is the non-specific darkening of the film.
- In the hard tissues the number of compton and photoelectric interactions are greater than in the soft tissues and as a result more number of photons in the beam come out of the patient through the soft than the hard tissues.
- In hard tissue the number of compton and photoelectric interactions are greater than the soft tissues.

Suggested reading:

1. Stuart S White, Michael J Pharaoh, Text book of Oral Radiology, Principles And Interpretation, 5th Edition, 17-19.

Q 5) What represents the particulate radiation?

MUHS MAY 2005 (2 Marks)

Particulate radiation consists of atomic nuclei or subatomic particles moving at high velocity.

Alpha particles, beta particles, and cathode rays are examples of particulate radiation.

- Alpha particles are helium nuclei consisting of two protons and two neutrons.
- They result from the radioactive decay of many elements.
- Due to their double charge and heavy mass alpha particles densely ionize matter through which they pass.
- As a result they tend to rapidly give up their energies and penetrate only a few microns of the tissues of the body.
- The beta particles are the electrons which are emitted by the radioactive nuclei.
- Beta particles with high speed are able to penetrate the matter to greater depth than the alpha particles, to a maximum of 1.5em in tissue.
- The penetration to a greater depth by the beta particles is because they are smaller and lighter and carry a single negative charge and

have lesser chances of interacting with the matter than the alpha particles.

- Accordingly, they ionize matter much less densely than alpha particles.
- Cathode rays are also high speed electrons but are produced by devices that are manufactured eg. x-ray tube.
- Linear energy transfer (LET) is the rate of loss of energy from a particle as it moves along its track through the matter.
- Alpha particles have high charge and lower velocity and hence high LET. Beta particles are less densely ionising because they have lighter mass and lower charge and hence have lower LET.

Suggested reading:

1. Stuart C White, Michael J Pharoah, Oral Radiology, Principles and Interpretation 5th Edition, 4-5.

Q 6) Electromagnetic Spectrum:

MUHS MAY 2005 (2 Marks)

Introduction:

The distribution of the electromagnetic radiation depending on the energy, frequency or wave length is called the electro magnetic spectrum. The electromagnetic radiation can be defined as a stream of photons that are travelling in a wave like motion and moving at the speed of light.

The gamma-rays, x-rays, ultraviolet rays, visible light, infrared radiation, microwaves, and radiowaves are example of electromagnetic radiation.

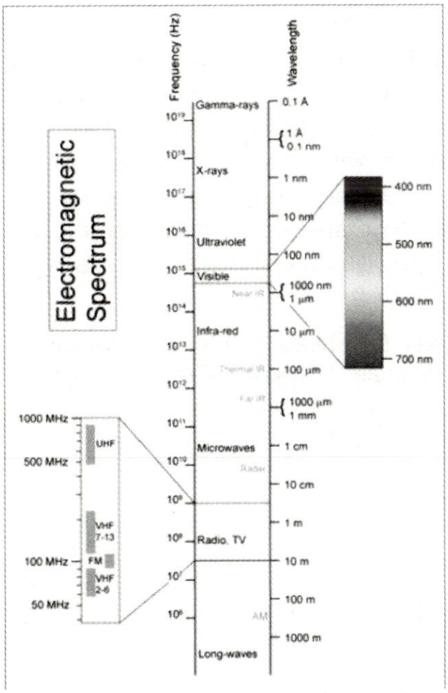

Fig. The Electromagnetic spectrum

1. **Radio Waves:** Their wavelengths range from 100 micrometer to 100 kilometers. They possess the lowest energy levels Radiowaves that are artificially generated are used for fixed and mobile radio communication, broadcasting, radar and other navigational systems.
2. **Microwaves:** It can be measured in centimeters. They have wave lengths that range from one meter to one millimeter. Microwaves of short wavelengths are sometimes used in doppler radars for predicting the weather forecasts.
3. **Infrared Radiation:** They have longer wavelengths than that of the visible light, ranging from 700 nanometers to 1 mm.The energy can be released as heat or thermal energy. It can be bounced back and is called infra red because its similar to visible light energy.
4. **Visible light:** The only part of the electromagnetic spectrum that the humans can see with naked eyes. In this part of the spectrum there is inclusion of a range of colours that have a particular wave lengths ranging from 400-700 nanometers and the range of colours vary from violet to red.
5. **UV radiation:** They have wavelength ranging from 10 nm to 380 nm and are shorter than the visible light but longer than the x-rays.This radiation is present in sunlight, and can be produced by electric arcs, and other types of specialised lights such as mercury vapour lamps, tanning lamps and black lights. Its known for its bad effect on the skin from the sun, sometimes leading to cancer.
6. **X-ray:** Are used to image parts of the body for diagnostic purpose. They have wavelengths ranging from 0.01 -10 nm and their energies vary from 100eV-100KeV. Their wavelengths are shorter than the ultraviolet rays and longer than the gamma rays. The x-rays with energy of photons in the range of above 5-10KeV are called hard x-rays and those with lower energies are called soft x-rays. The x-rays that are hard are used for imaging.
7. **Gamma Rays:** The shortest waves, which are approximately 10-12 m in wavelength. It is used in radiotherapy to treat cancer.

Suggested reading:

1. Freny. R Karjodkar, Essentials of Oral and Maxillofacial Radiology, page no 21.
2. Stuart C White, Michael J Pharoah, Oral Radiology, Principles and Interpretation 5th Edition, page no 3.

CHAPTER 2

Radiation Biology

Q 1) Acute radiation syndrome:

TNMGRU FEBRUARY 2011 6 Marks

After an acute exposure of whole body to radiation, a collection of signs and symptoms are experienced by individuals called as the acute radiation syndrome.

It consists of following stages:

1. **Prodromal stage:** After an exposure of the entire body to radiation of about 1.5 Gy, within first few minutes to hours, the patients may develop symptoms characteristic of the gastrointestinal tract disturbances may develop which could be, nausea, vomiting, diarrhea, weakness and fatigue.
2. **The latent period:** After the prodromal phase there is an onset of the latent phase in which there is apparent feeling of well being and there are no signs of radiation sickness. The extent of this period depends on the dose of radiation. It can at supralethal exposures extend from hours to days or to a few weeks at sublethal exposures.

   If the individuals are exposed to lethal or supra lethal dosages, then symptoms will follow the latent period.
3. **Hematopoietic syndrome:** When an individual is exposed to whole body radiation of 2-7 Gy, it can lead to injury of the hematopoietic stem cells of the bone marrow and spleen.

   The changes in the differential blood count donot occur at the same time.

   The life span of a particular cell in the peripheral blood will decide the rate of fall in the circulating levels of that cell.

   Infection, hemorrhage, and anemia are some of the clinical signs involving the hematopoietic syndrome.

   The probability of death is low after exposures at the low end of this range but much higher at the high end.
4. **Gastro-intestinal syndrome:** The radiation exposure to the whole body in the range of 7-15 Gy can lead to extensive damage of the gastro-intestinal system.

This damage along with damage of the hematopoietic system, causes signs and symptoms called the gastrointestinal syndrome.
In the GIT syndrome electrolytes and plasma are lost and efficient absorption in the intestine fails to occur. There is development of ulcerations and hemorrhagic bleeding from intestines.
Because of these changes there is presence of diarrhea, dehydration and loss of weight. Septicemia occurs due to the endogenous bacteria in the intestine causing invasion of the denuded surface.
The body's defense mechanism against the bacterial infection falls down and the effectiveness of the clotting mechanism decreases.
Death occurs within 2 weeks due to due to combined effects on the stem cell systems from a combination of factors which include loss of fluids and electrolytes, infections and nutritional impairment.

5. **The cardiovascular and the central nervous system syndrome:** If the radiation exposure exceeds 50 Gy then death can occur in 1-2 days.
   Those exposed can show collapse of the circulatory system with a steep drop in blood pressure in the hours preceeding death.
   The individuals who are exposed to such high radiations can exhibit intermittent stupor, disorientation, in -coordination, and convulsions suggestive of severe damage to the nervous system.
   The serious radiation induced damage to the neurons and the fine vasculature of the brain most likely cause the symptoms.
   The clinical course may last from only a few minutes to about 48 hours as this syndrome is irreversible and death may occur.
   The syndromes involving the cardiovascular and the central nervous system run such a rapid course that the person exposed to such high radiation dies even before the effects of damage to the bone marrow and gastrointestinal system can develop.
   The acute radiation syndrome is a collection of signs and symptoms experienced by persons after acute whole-body exposure to radiation.

It consists of following stages:

1. **Prodromal period:** Within the first minutes to hours after exposure to whole-body irradiation of about 1.5 Gy, symptoms characteristic of gastrointestinal tract disturbances may occur.
   The individual may develop anorexia, nausea, vomiting, diarrhea, weakness, and fatigue.
2. **Latent period:** After this prodromal reaction comes a latent period of apparent well-being, during which no signs or symptoms of radiation sickness occur.
   The extent of the latent period is also dose-related.
   It extends from hours or days at supralethal exposures to a few weeks at sublethal exposures.
   Symptoms follow the latent period when the individuals are exposed to lethal or supra lethal dosages.

3. **Hematopoietic syndrome:** Whole-body exposures of 2 to 7 Gy cause injury to the hematopoietic stem cells of the bone marrow and spleen.
   The changes in the differential blood count donot occur at the same time.
   The rate of fall in the circulating levels of a cell depends on the life span of that cell in the peripheral blood.
   The clinical signs of the hematopoietic syndrome include infection hemorrhage, and anemia.
   The probability of death is low after exposures at the low end of this range but much higher at the high end.
4. **Gastro-intestinal syndrome:** Whole-body exposures in the range of 7 to 15 Gy cause extensive damage to the gastrointestinal system.
   This damage, in addition to the hematopoietic damage described previously, causes signs and symptoms called the gastrointestinal syndrome.
   In the GIT syndrome plasma and electrolytes are lost, efficient intestinal absorption cannot occur.
   Ulceration also occurs, with hemorrhaging of the intestines.
   All these changes are responsible for the diarrhea, dehydration, and loss of weight that are observed.
   Endogenous intestinal bacteria readily invade the denuded surface, producing septicemia.
   There is marked lowering of the body's defence against bacterial infection and a decrease in effectiveness of the clotting mechanism.
   The combined effects on these stem cell systems cause death within 2 weeks from a combination of factors that include fluid and electrolyte 'loss,' infection, and possibly nutritional impairment.
5. **Cardiovascular and Central nervous system syndrome:** Exposures in excess of 50 Gy usually cause death in 1 to 2 days.
   Those exposed can show collapse of the circulatory system with a steep fall in blood pressure in the hours preceding death.

Victims also may show intermittent stupor, incoordination, disorientation, and convulsions suggestive of extensive damage to the nervous system.

Symptoms most likely result from radiation induced damage to the neurons and fine vasculature of the brain.

The syndrome is irreversible, and the clinical course may run from only a few minutes to about 48 hours before death occurs.

The cardiovascular and central nervous system syndromes have such a rapid course that the irradiated individual dies before the effects of damage to the bone marrow and can develop gastrointestinal symptoms.

Suggested reading:

1. Stuart C White, Michael J Pharoah, Oral Radiology, Principles and Interpretation 5th Edition, 37-39.

CHAPTER 3

Production of X-Rays

Q 1) Bremsstrahlung Radiation:

TNMGRU FEBRUARY 2005 (2 Marks)

(i) 'Braking rays is a german term that means Bremsstrahlung. Its a very important phenomenon in the generation of x-rays.

(ii) Also called as continuous spectra or braking radiation.

(iii) The Bremsstrahlung's interactions are the main source of x-ray photons arising from a x-ray tube and are caused by sudden slowing or stopping or deflection of high-speed electrons at the target.

(iv) The process entails slowing or complete stopping of the travelling of high speed electrons by the forces of tungsten (target) atom that it encounters.

(v) If a high-speed electron directly hits the nucleus of the tungsten target then the entire kinetic energy of that electron is converted into a photon of x-ray.

(vi) In case the electron misses the direct hit of the nucleus, it is slowed down and will produce a photon of x-ray with lesser energy.

(vii) The energy required by the atom to slow down the electron is excessive to the atom and this energy will be radiated as x-ray of equal energy.

(viii) In case the electron hits the nucleus directly and is stopped completely by the strong force of the same, then the x-ray photon that is generated will have energy equal to the kinetic energy of the electron.

(ix) This x-ray generated has the energy equal to the potential difference applied across the anode and the cathode of the x-ray tube at the instance of its passage.

(x) Generally the trend of the high speed electrons is of near or wide misses with the nuclei of the tungsten atom.

(xi) In these interactions the negatively charged electrons are attracted to the positively charged nuclei and loses some of its velocity.

(xii) This deceleration of the electrons cause them to lose some of their kinetic energy which is radiated in the form of several new photons.

(xiii) As the high speed electron approaches the nuclei, there is a greater electrostatic attraction on the electron and the braking effect and the energy of the resulting bremsstrahlung photons.

(xiv) Final kinetic energy of the electron=the initial kinetic energy of the electron-the energy of the photon of x-ray.

(xv) The energy that is lost is emitted as photons of x-rays.

(xvi) The bremsstrahlung radiation intensity is proportional to the square of the target's atomic number (Z), the number of unit charges of the particles that are bombarding (z) and inversely with the mass of the particles that are bombarding (m):Z^2z/m.

(xvii) X-ray photons with a continuous spectrum of energy are generated with bremsstrahlungs interactions.

There are three reasons for this continuous spectrum:

- The constant variation of the voltage difference between the target and the filament that results in the electrons striking the target to possess varying levels of kinetic energy.
- The electrons that are bombarding at the target pass at varying distances about the tungsten nuclei and their deflection varies. Because of this effect they give up varying amounts of energy in the form of bremsstrahlungs photons.

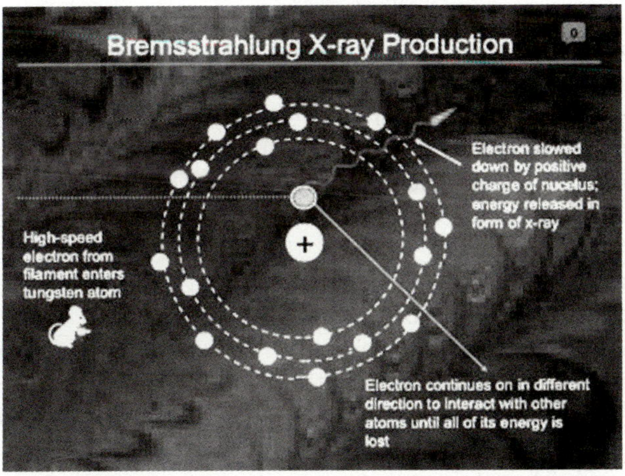

Fig. Interactions of electrons with nucleus of tungsten target

- There are many interactions in which the electrons participate before they lose all their kinetic energy. Because of these factors the electrons carry different amounts of energy while they interact each time with the tungsten nucleus which results in the x-ray photon generation.

(xviii) The highest energy the x-ray beam may possess can be described by the peak operating voltage that is KVp.

(xix) Eg a dental x-ray machine operating at 70 KVp will release photon of maximum energy of 70KVp.

Suggested reading:

1. Freny R. Karjodkar, Essentials Of Oral and Maxillofacial Radiology, 2nd Edition, 15.
2. Stuart C White, Michael J Pharoah, Oral Radiology, Principles and Interpretation 5th Edition, pg 12.

Q 2) What is Benson's Line Focus principle? Write a short answer on Line-focus principle:

MUHS MAY 2012 (3 Marks)
MUHS MAY 2009 (2 Marks)

In the year 1918 Benson's line focus principle was introduced

The radiographic image quality is dependent on the geometry of the target. Sharpness of the image increases as the size of the focal spot decreases.

Focal spot is the area on the target onto which the focusing cup directs the electrons from the filament.

As the focal spot becomes smaller the generation of heat /unit area of the target is greater.

Hence in order to derive benefit from a small focal spot and to effectively distribute the bombarding electrons over a greater surface of a large target, the target is placed at an angle to the electron beam. This reduces the effective focal spot size.

The target is inclined at an angle of 20° to the central ray of the electron.

This helps the effective focal spot size to be 1mm × 1mm, as opposed to 1mm × 3mm, which is the actual focal spot size.

This results in smaller focal spot size with resultant sharper image but with actual focal spot size which is larger for effective dissipation of heat.

This phenomenon is known as the line – focus –principle and the 20^0 angle is called the angle of truncation.

Thus the line focus principle is the use of an anode with the target material angulated in such a way that the effective focal spot appears smaller than the actual focal spot. The use of this principle allows the x-ray to be generated over a large area on the target, and hence less heat per unit area is produced. Therefore greater number of electrons can be used and more number of photons of x-ray are generated.

Effective focal spot can be decreased and sharpness increased.However in practice, extent to which the focal spot can be decreased is limited to 20^0.

If further reduction is done the useful beam is non uniform and the angulation of the target on the anode is limited by Heel effect.

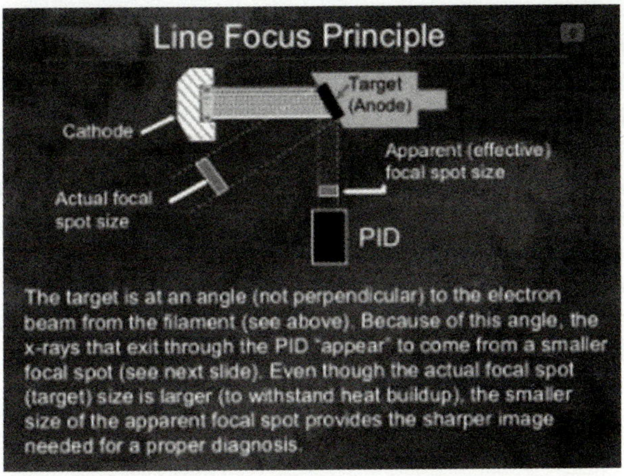

Fig. The principle of Benson's line focus principle

Suggested reading:

1. Freny R.Karjodkar, Essentials of Dental And Maxillofacial Radiology 2nd Edition. Chapter4, Page no 41-42.

Q 3) Characteristic radiation:

TNMGRU AUGUST 2014 (5 Marks)
RGUHS APRIL 1999 (5 Marks)

- Charles Glover Barkla in 1909 discovered the characteristic radiations. In 1917 he received a Nobel prize in physics for this discovery.
- They occur when an electron from the filament displaces an electron from the shell of the tungsten target atom causing ionisation of the atom.
- The emission of Characteristic x-rays occur when an electron of the outer shell fills the vacancy in the inner shell of the tungsten atom, thereby causing the release of x-rays in a pattern that is characteristic to each element.
- The striking of a high energy electron or the incident electron on a bound electron of the tungsten target electron in an atom, there is ejection of the target electron from its inner shell of the atom.
- After the ejection of the electron, the atom is left with a vacancy of energy level which is also known as the core hole. The electrons of the outer shell jump into the inner shell and emit quantized photons which possess energy that is equivalent to the difference between the binding energies of the two orbits.
- Unique set of energy levels are possessed by each element and hence the transition from higher levels to lower levels of energy produce x-rays having frequencies which are characteristic to each element.
- The photons are named as K or L depending upon which shell they have been emitted from.

- The x-ray emitted is called K-alpha when the electron falls from the L shell to the K shell.
- And the x-rays are called K-beta when the electrons fall from the M shell to the K shell.
- In some cases however instead of the release of energy in the form of x-rays the energy is transferred to another electron which then gets ejected from the atom. This known as the Auger effect, and the electron that is ejected is called the Auger electron.
- Compared to the bremsstrahlungs radiation, the characteristic radiation from the shell K occurs only above 70KVp with the tungsten target and occurs as discrete increments.
- The characteristic photons possess energies that are a function of various levels of the orbital electrons and are thus characteristic of the target atoms.
- Characteristic radiation is a minor source of radiation from an x-ray tube.

Summary:

As the L lines have very little energy, only the K lines are of diagnostic importance.

There should be sufficient energy of the bombarding electrons with high speed (69.5 KV) so as to displace an electron from the tungsten K shell to produce K line on the spectrum.

Characteristic K-line photons are not produced by the x-ray tubes with the tungsten targets which are operating at less than 69.5 KV which is referred as the critical voltage. The dental x-ray equipments usually operate in the range of 50 KV and 90 KV.

Suggested reading:

1. Eric Whaites, Essentials Of Dental Radiography and Radiology, 3rd edition, page 19-20.
2. Stuart C White, Michael J Pharoah, Oral Radiology, Principles and Interpretation 5th Edition, page 13.

Q 4) Generation of X-rays:

RGUHS APRIL 2005 (4 Marks)

- Electrons that travel from the cathode filament to the target anode, results in conversion of some of their kinetic energy into photons of x-rays.
- X-rays are produced by the collision of electron with the tungsten atoms. The collisions which occur are of two types, thus giving rise to two types of spectra.
- X-rays are produced by formation of bremsstrahlung's or characteristic radiations.

I) Bremsstrahlung's radiation:

- The primary source of x-ray photons from a x-ray tube are the bremsstrahlung's interactions.

- The sudden slowing or stopping of the high speed electrons at the tungsten target are responsible for these type of photons.
- Bremsstrahlung in german means braking radiation.
- X-ray photons are generated when the electrons from the filament strike the target atoms and they can either hit the nucleus directly or there can be near misses and may pass away from close to the nucleus.
- If a high-speed electron directly hits the nucleus of the tungsten atom, its entire kinetic energy will be transformed in to a photon of x-ray energy.
- The energy of the electron matches the energy of the resultant photon.
- The energy is in turn equivalent to the kilovoltage applied across the x-ray tube during its passage.
- In most of the cases the electrons have near or wide misses with the nuclei of the atoms.
- In these interactions, a negatively charged high-speed electron is attracted towards the positively charged nuclei of the target atom and it loses some of its speed.
- This slowing down of the electron results in loss of some of its kinetic energy which is emitted in the form of many new photons.
- The nearer the high speed electron approaches the nuclei, the greater is the electrostatic attraction on the electron, the braking effect, and the energy of the resulting bremsstrahlung photons.
- A continuous spectrum of x-ray photons are generated by the bremsstrahlung's type of interactions.
- The energy of the x-ray photon depends on the peak kilovoltage of that machine.
- If a dental x-ray machine has a peak kilovoltage of 70 then the highest energy of the x-ray photon of that machine will be 70 KeV.

The reasons for the continuous spectrum of x-rays are:

1. A continuous variation of voltage difference between the cathode and the anode which is characteristic of half-wave rectification which causes the electrons to strike the target at varying levels of kinetic energy.
2. The electrons that bombard the target nucleus pass at varying distances around them and get deflected to varying extents and hence give up varying amounts of energy in the form of bremsstrahlung photons.
3. Most electrons have their participation in production of many bremsstrahlung's interactions in the target before losing all their kinetic energy.

II) Characteristic radiation:

- These radiations result when the electrons emitted from the filament displace an electron from the shell of the tungsten target thereby ionising the atom. Thus an electron of higher energy in an outer shell of the tungsten atom is rapidly attracted to the void created in the deficient inner shell.

- When the outer shell electron replaces the displaced electrons, a photon of x-ray energy is released which possess energy which is equivalent to the difference between the binding energies of the two orbits. K-shell characteristic radiations occur at kilovoltages above 70 with the tungsten target and occurs as discrete increments as compared to the bremsstrahlung's radiations.
- The characteristic radiations possess energies that are a function of the levels of energy of various electron orbital levels and hence are characteristic of the target atoms.
- Characteristic radiation is only a minor source of radiation from an x-ray tube.

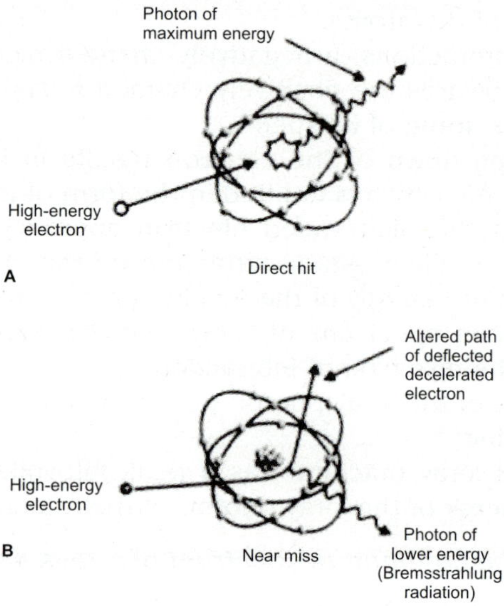

Fig. Production of Bremsstrahlung radiation

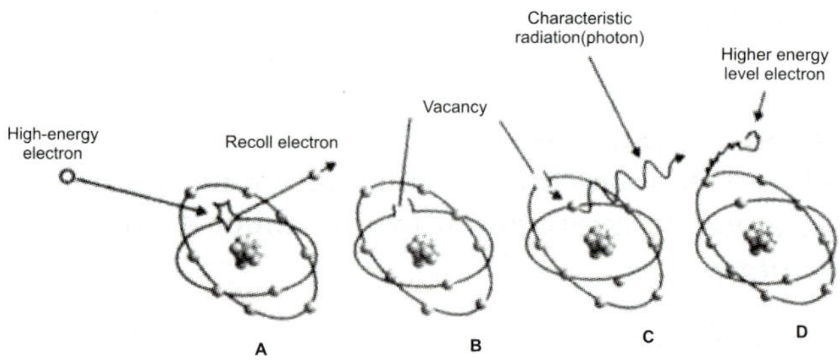

Fig. Production of Characteristic radiation

Suggested reading:

1. Stuart C White, Michael J Pharoah, Oral Radiology, Principles and Interpretation 5th Edition, 12-13.

Q 5) Why is tungsten used as target material in an x-ray tube:

MUHS OCTOBER 2002 (2 Marks)

The anode consists of a copper stem in which the tungsten target is embedded. The kinetic energy of the electrons generated from the filaments are directed at the tungsten target and its function is to convert their energy to x-ray photons.

The use of tungsten as a target material in an x-ray tube is because:

- It possesses a high atomic number (74): This is beneficial as it helps in most efficient production of x-rays.
- **High melting point:** Because of the heat generated at the anode, there is important requirement that the target should have high melting point.
- **High thermal conductivity:** This helps in efficient dissipation of heat into the copper stem.
- **Low vapour pressure:** The low vapour pressure of the target at high temperatures helps in maintaining the vaccum in the tube despite high temperatures.

Suggested reading:

1. Stuart C White, Michael J Pharoah, Oral Radiology, Principles and Interpretation 5th edition, pg no.8.

CHAPTER 4

Properties of X-Rays

Introduction

For a radiographer to get good quality radiographs it is important to know the properties of x-radiation and thus their behaviour.It will help not only to get good quality radiographs but also help in protecting themselves, environment and the patient from the hazardous effects of radiation.

Q 1) Name four diagnostic properties of x-rays:

MUHS NOVEMBER 2011 (2 Marks)

Diagnostic radiography includes both the ionising and nonionising radiations for image creation for medical diagnosis.After the laboratory tests the x-rays are most commonly used for diagnosis.

The diagnostic properties of x-rays are as follows:

(i) X-rays have a wide range of wavelengths ranging from 0.01-o.05mm in length.
Because of their extremely short wave-lengths they are able to penetrate materials that absorb or reflect visible light.
This ability to penetrate and come out of objects and on to the films that form image of the objects through which they pass is useful for diagnostic radiography.

(ii) X-rays are absorbed differentially by the matter and this depends upon the atomic structure of the matter and the wave-length of the x-rays.
This property of x-ray helps to produce image on a photographic film, which in turn can be made visible by chemical development.

(iii) Chemical changes occur due to x-rays in the radiographic and photographic films which is helpful to create diagnostic radiographs.

(iv) Certain substances are fluoresced when exposed to x-rays and thus allows to emit radiation of higher wave-length (eg visible and ultraviolet radiation).
With this property it is possible to use intensifying screens in radiography, as they emit visible light to expose the film when x-rays fall on them. They help to reduce the x-ray exposure to half.

Suggested reading:

1. Freny R Karjodkar, Text Book of Dental and Maxillofacial Radiology, 2nd Edition, 27.

Q 2) Uses of X-RAYS: (Not specific to any university)

1. **Radiology:** X-rays are used in diagnosis of various pathological lesions in the field of medicine and dentistry. It is mainly used for
   (a) Differentiation between normal and pathologic tissues.
   (b) Study of effects of diseases on the structure of tissues eg bone structure changes in rickets, cancer and other bone diseases.
   (c) Study of structure of living tissues such as nerve and muscles on body tissues.
   (d) Identification of mineral deposits in organs such as calcifications, gall stones and siliceous deposits.
2. **Radiotherapy:** X-rays are beneficial for curing malignant tumours and skin diseases. Radiotherapy may be used in combination with the surgical therapy.
3. **Pharmaceutical industry:** X-ray powder diffraction is mainly used to characterize composition of pharmaceuticals. It is used to identify the ingredients or understand the effectiveness of a drug coating and packing material. It is also used to determine the shelf life of pharmaceutical agents.
4. **Forensic science:** X-rays are used in forensic science for chemical analysis of forensic specimens their identification and comparison. They are also used in contact trace analysis of trace elements for eg. flakes of paints, hair, glass fragments, soil, stains of any description and loose materials in powdered form. Determining the trace quantities of element can help in detecting the person suspected in the involved crime.
5. **Geological industry:** X-rays are key tool in mineral exploration. The surface of soil consists of mixture of minerals and organic matter. X-ray diffraction has been known for identification and quantification of minerals present in the soil. Geologists can also determine degree of clay mineralization, measure specimen purity and measure the hydration properties.
6. **Glass industry:** They are used in glass industry for detection of crystalline particles that create minute faults in the bulk glass and measurement of crystalline coatings for texture, crystallinity and crystal size.
7. **Corrosion analysis:** X-rays are beneficial to locate the origin of corrosion and for the quantification & identification of the compounds present in the deposit.
8. **Sterlization:** X-rays have been used as an alternative to gamma and E-beam methods for sterilization purposes.
9. **Radiobiology:** X-rays can be used for locating alteration of cells

and tissues in case of experimental purposes.

10. **Applications in metallurgy:** It is mainly used for identification of alloy and determining the structure and composition of alloy.
11. **Applications in general and physical chemistry:** It is used for determination of crystal structure, lattice types, unit cell dimensions and atomic positions of various substances. It is also beneficial for calculating crystal size in microscopic and sub-microscopic ranges.

Suggested reading:

1. Freny R Karjokar Textbook of dental and maxillofacial radiology (2nd edition) Pg no. 34-35.
2. Current applications of x-ray powder diffraction – a review. Rev. Adv. Mater.Sci.38 (2014)95-109.
3. X-ray diffraction: Instrumentation and Applications. Critical reviews in analytical chemistry. April 2015.

CHAPTER 5

Radiation Protection

Introduction:

An intelligent dental practitioner must understand the benefits and possible hazards of radiation. Radiographs should be advised judiciously and where it is an important diagnostic tool the dentist should be aware of exposing the patient, himself and the surrounding with minimum radiation exposure and hence should be well aware of radiation protection techniques.

Q 1) Collimation and Filtration:

RGUHS OCTOBER/NOVEMBER 2005 4 Marks

Collimation:

Its a metallic barrier that has an aperture in the middle which is used for reduction in the size of the x-ray beam and thus reduce the volume of tissue irradiated in the patient.

The tissues absorb about 90% of the x-ray photons when the x-ray beam is directed at the patient and only about 10% of the photons pass through the patients and reach the film.

Use of collimators prevents this and reduces patient exposure. Use of collimation helps achieve better contrast and thus better image quality.

X-ray beams used in dentistry are usually collimated to circle of 23/4 inches (7 cm) in diameter.

There are three types of collimator:

1. Round collimators
2. Rectangular collimators.
3. Slit type collimator.

Round collimators:

- Its a thick plate made of radiopaque material usually lead and has a circular opening which is centered over the port in the x-ray tube head from which the x-ray beam emerges.
- These are built into open ended aiming cylinders.

Rectangular collimators:

- These collimators limit the size of the x-ray beam to just about little larger than the size of the x-ray film.
- It is important to reduce the beam to the size of the film to further reduce the unnecessary exposure to the patient.
- Some film holding devices may also provide rectangular collimation of the x-ray beam.

Slit type collimator:

- Slit type collimator is used in ortho pantomography.

Filtration:

A beam of x-rays contains a spectrum of x-ray photons of different energies.

The photons that possess sufficient energy have the ability to penetrate through the structures and reach the film and only those are useful for diagnostic radiology.

The photons with low energy contribute only to patient exposure rather than in diagnostic value as they donot have enough energy to reach the film.

It is therefore important to remove the less penetrating photons and reduce the patient exposure.

This can be achieved by introducing a filter in the path of the x-ray beam. Aluminum filters are generally used.

This aluminum filter removes preferentially many of the low energy photons and have lesser effect on the photons with high energy that can reach the film. The filtration commonly used in dental radiology are aluminum disks of minimum 0.5 mm thick which are placed in the path of the x-ray beam. The longer wavelength, non-penetrating x-rays are filtered out resulting in a higher energy and most penetrating useful beam, which is less harmful to patient.

There are mainly two types and additional third types of filtration:

1. Inherent filtration
2. Added filtration
3. Wedge filtration

1. **Inherent filtration:**

   When the primary beam exits through the glass window of the x-ray tube, the insulating oil and the tube head seal act as filters.

   In dental x-ray machine the inherent filtration is approximately equivalent to 0.5-1mm of aluminum.

   This amount of filtration usually fails to meet the standards regulated by the state and federal law (in USA) and therefore added filtration is required.

2. **Added filtration:**

   It refers to the placement of aluminum disks in the path of the x-ray beam between the collimator and the tube head seal in the tube head of the x-ray aluminum disk may be added in 0.5mm increments.

The amount of filtration should be in accordance with the machines operating range:

- Below 50 kvp: 0.3-0.5mm of aluminum
- 50-70 kvp: 1.2-1.5mm of aluminum
- Above 70 kvp: 2.1- 4.1mm of aluminum

3. **Wedge filter:**
   - It is occasionally used in diagnostic radiology to obtain film of more uniform density when the part being examined is very thin than other side, within the field.
   - Filter is like a wedge.

Suggested reading:

1. Freny R karjodkar, Essentials of Dental and Maxillofacial Radiology; page.no. 68-69.
2. Stuart C White, Michael J Pharoah, Oral Radiology, Principles and Interpretation 5th Edition, page no. 15-16.

Q 2) Thermoluminescent Dosimeter/ film badge:

MUHS OCTOBER 2004 2 Marks

A radiation dose measuring device is called as thermoluminescent dosimeter or TLD.

It helps in monitoring environmental and also staff personnel in facilities which involve radiation exposure.

Used for measurement of actual dose received by the operator / patient as a result of radiography or radiotherapy exposures.

It is the most common type of personnel monitoring device.

TLD BADGE:

The TLD badge in India consists of a TLD card holder cassette of high plastic impact.

The TLD card consists of nickel plated aluminum plate having three symmetrical holes over which 3 identical $CaSO_4$ Teflon disks are dipped. These disks are clipped on an aluminum card loaded in the cassette having three filters:

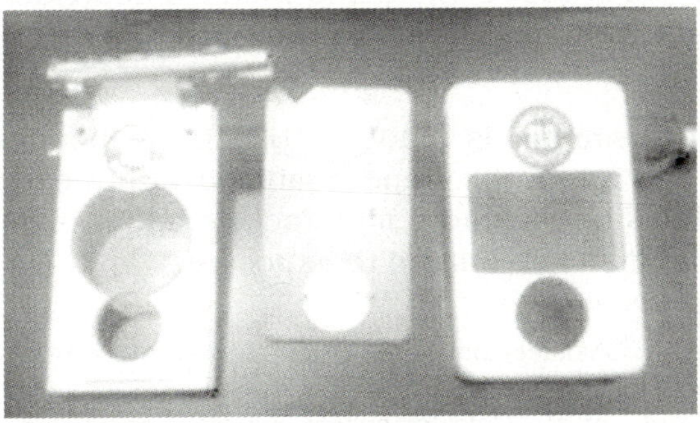

Fig. TLD Badge

1. Open region.
2. Copper.
3. Aluminum.

TLD Reader:

The equipment used to heat the exposed material and measure the emitted light is called the TLD reader.The reading given by this equipment is used as a measure of the absorbed dose to which the material was subjected and consists of 3 main parts, the heater, photomultiplier tube and electronic system.

The ionising radiation exposure is measured by the TLD badge by measuring the intensity of the visible light which is emitted by a crystal in the detector when it is heated. The amount of radiation exposure defines the intensity of the light emitted. Some of the materials that show thermoluminescence when exposed to ionising radiation are calcium fluoride, calcium sulphate, lithium fluoride, lithium borate, calcium borate, potassium bromide and feldspar.

Types of TLD:

The two types that are commonly used are:

1. Calcium Fluoride.
2. Lithium fluoride, that has one or more impurities to produce trap states for the energetic electrons.

The calcium fluoride variety is used to record gamma exposure.

The lithium fluoride type is used for gamma and neutron exposure.

The other varieties are that use berryliun oxide, and calcium sulfate doped with thulium.

When the ionising radiation interacts with the crystal in the TLD, it causes the electrons in the crystals to jump to a higher states of energy.They remain trapped because of intentionally added impurities like manganese or magnesium in the crystal till it is heated.

When the crystal is heated, the electrons drop back to their ground state and release a photon of energy that is equal to the difference in energy between the trapped state and the ground state.

The electrons can also go back to their ground state after prolonged time, and this effect is called the fading which is dependent on the energy of incident radiation and the intrinsic properties of the TLD material.

Film Badge:

This type of dosimeter is made of plastic or metal, and is typically 50 mm square by 12 mm thick and equipped with a clip for attaching to clothing. It contains one or more film packets and it is developed and its density is measured and co-related to exposure.

Suggested reading:

1. Tochilin, E., N. Goldstein, and W. G. Miller. "Beryllium oxide as a thermoluminescent dosimeter." Health physics 16.1 (1969): 1-7.
2. Yamashita, T., et al. "Calcium sulfate activated by thulium or dysprosium for thermoluminescence dosimetry." Health physics 21.2 (1971): 295-300.

Q 3) What is ALARA principle?

MUHS MAY 2012 (2 Marks)

Research studies measuring the risk of x-ray exposure in the increase in occurrence of diseases like cancer, cataracts, defects at birth, and life span shortening have been controversial and are not conclusive, while cases of radiation damage from dental x-rays have not yet been reported. However it still cannot be proved that there is no possibility of a hazard to the patient.

This situation has produced the concept of keeping the exposure to radiation to As Low As Reasonably Achievable (ALARA).

Federal and state regulations have been established to limit occupational exposures. There are limits to the whole body dose, dose to lens and eyes, and the dose to any other organ of the body.

The limitation on whole body dose for a worker in the radiation field is 50 mSv (5 Rem or 5000mrems) per year. The dose limits/quarter is 12.5mSv. There is also a limit on the total dose that can be accumulated in a life time, which is called cumulative limit. The cumulative effective dose limit (E) is the age in years (N) times 10mSv.

Although most x-ray technologists never receive even a small fraction of the annual dose limit, they are still issued personnel radiation monitors.

For members of the general public, the recommended dose limits are one tenth of the effective dose limit for the worker of radiation.

Hence the bottom line is that all unnecessary radiation exposure should be avoided. This is a philosophy of radiation protection and it should be followed by everyone. All radiation protection programmes must operate under the principle of keeping the radiation exposure to staff, patients, and public As Low As Reasonably Achievable (ALARA). Thus this principle recognizes the possibility that no matter how small the dose, some stochastic effect may result.

It is the responsibility of the radiographer that steps must be taken to reduce radiation exposure well below maximum regulatory limits. Technological factors such as kvp, mA, length of exposure, distance, shielding, filtration, collimation, beam area and type of image receptor all influence the radiation levels to the public and staff. Industrial workers in radiation industries appear to be acting in accordance with this philosophy, in so far as their average annual individual effective dose is 1.56mSv, 3% of the annual limit.

The dosage for individuals occupationally exposed in the operation of dental x-ray equipment is even less, that is 0.2 mSv, or 0.4% of the allowable limit.

Radiation dose for women of reproductive age and pregnancy is supposed to not exceed 10 mSv (0.1 rem).

Annual effective dose for the public should not exceed 1 mSv.

When performing radiographic procedures the radiographer must apply the three methods or cardinal rules for radiation protection. They are:

(i) Reduce the time spent in the vicinity of radiation.

(ii) Increase distance from the radiation source.

(iii) Wear appropriate shielding to attenuate radiation.

Suggested reading:

1. Robert Fosbinder, Denise Orth, Essentials of Radiologic Science, Lippincott Williams & Wilkins, page 322.
2. Freny R Karjodkar, Essentials of Oral And Maxillofacial radiology, edition 1st, page 60.

Q 4) Dosimetry:

TNMGRU SEPTEMBER 2002 (5 Marks)
RGUHS NOVEMBER 2005 (2 Marks)

Dosimetry is a term used to determine the quantity of exposure of radiation or dose.

Radiation dosimetry: It is related to the measurement of absorbed dose or dose rate that results from the interaction of the ionising radiation with matter.

Dose: It is a term used to describe the amount of energy absorbed/unit mass at the area of interest.

Exposure: The ability of radiation to produce ionisation in air under standard conditions of temperature and pressure (STP) and its measure is called exposure.

The SI unit of exposure is KERMA which is an acronym for kinetic energy released in matter.

It is a measure of kinetic energy transferred from the photons to electrons which is expressed in dosage units of Gy, where 1 Gy is equal to 1 joule/kg.

Kerma is the total of the initial kinetic energies of all liberated charged particles by uncharged ionising radiation (neutrons and photons) in a sample of matter, that is divided by the mass of the sample.

It has replaced the roentgen(R).

Roentgen (R):

Is defined as a traditional unit of radiation exposure equals to the quantity of ionizing radiation that will produce one electrostatic unit of electricity in one cc of dry air at 0°C and standard atmospheric pressure.

Absorbed dose:

The absorbed dose is a measure of the energy absorbed by any type of ionising radiation/unit mass of type of matter.

Absorbed dose = ED / m, Ed: Energy imparted by radiation that is ionising to the matter in a volume of element; m: mass of matter in a volume of element.

Rad is the traditional unit of absorbed dose.

Rad (r) it is the production of 100 ergs of energy in one gram of tissue by any form of ionizing radiation.

1 rad = 100 ergs/g of absorber.

The SI unit is the gray (Gy) where 1 Gy=1 joule/kg.1 Gy =100Rads.

Dose equivalent:

The dose equivalent (HT) is used for comparing the biologic effects of different types of radiation to a tissue or organ.

It is total of the products of the absorbed dose (DT) which is averaged over a tissue or organ and the radiation weighting factor (WR):

$$HT = \sum WR \times DT$$

Equivalent dose is expressed as a sum to allow for the possibility that the tissue or organ has been exposed to more than one variety of radiation.

Thus high LET-radiations which can cause more damage to the tissues than the low LET radiations have correspondingly higher WR.

The standard unit of equivalent dose is Sievert (Sv).

1 Sievert = 1 Gray

The traditional unit of equivalent dose was the rem.

Rem (Rad Equivalent Man) it is the unit of dose equivalent. This unit is used to facilitate comparison between biological effect of exposure and various types of radiations.

1 Sievert = 100 rem

Effective dose (E):

The risk to humans can be detected by this.

It is the sum total of the products of equivalent dose to each tissue or organ (HT) and the tissue weighing factor (WT).

$$E = \sum HT \times WT$$

The unit of Effective dose is the Sievert.

Quality factor (QF)

It relates all radiation to biologic systems in terms of its biological effects relative to standard exposure of x-rays.

Eg: In some systems a dose of 0.1 rad caused by fast neutrons has the biological effect as 1.0 rad of X-rays.

Therefore QF =10(1.0/0.1) =10(10).

For radiations used in dental radiology, it is sufficiently accurate for protection calculation to assume that an exposure of 1 R will result in an absorbed dose of 1 Rad which will produce a dose equivalent of 1 Rem. Thus,

In diagnostic radiology: 1R = 1r = 1 rem.

Radioactivity:

The measurement of radioactivity (A) describes the rate of decay of a sample of radioactive material.

The traditional unit of radioactivity is the curie (Ci) which is corresponding to the activity of 1 g of radium (3.7 × 1010 disintegrations/second)

1 mCi = 37 megaBq;

1 Bq = 2.7 × 10-11Ci.

TABLE showing Summary of Radiation Quantities and Units:

QUANTITY	SI UNIT	TRADITIONAL UNIT	CONVERSION
Exposure	Air kerma (Gy)	Roentgen (R)	1 Gy = 100 rad 1 rad = 0.01 Gy (1 cGy)
Absorbed dose	Gray (Gy)	Rad	1 Gy - 100 rad 1 rad = 0.01Gy (1cGy)
Equivalent dose	Sievert (Sv)	Rem	1 Sv= 100rem 1 rem = 0.01 Sv (1 cSv)
Effective dose	Sievert (Sv)	-	-

Maximum Permissible Dose (MPD) = 0.05 Sv/ yr

(i) Average weekly exposure for patient or operator, is 0.001Sv

(ii) maximum of 13 week is 0.05 Sv

(iii) for the general public MPD is limited to 1/10th or 0.005 Sv/ year.

Operator accumulated dose (OAD) / maximum accumulated dose (MAD):

OAD = 5(N-18), where N is equal to age of patient.

This indicates that higher limit permitted for occupationally exposed persons do not pertain to individuals under the age of 18, for them the same exposure limit as the general public is considered that is 0.005 Sv/ yrs.

The recommendation of NCRP and ICRP on the amount of radiation received by public and occupationally exposed individuals.

Occupational dose limit: 50mSv / yr

Nonoccupational / public dose limit:

5 mSv / yr ---- NCRP

1 mSv / yr ----- ICRP

Suggested reading:

1. Freny R Karjodkar, Text book of Dental and Maxillofacial Radiology, 2nd edition, 61-64.

Q 5) Dosimeter

TNMGRU FEBRUARY 2013 (5 Marks)

- Dosimeter is a device called an electrometer, which has two electrodes charged from external connections. As these electrodes have similar charges and hence they repel each other.
- When ionising radiation passes through these electrodes, charge on the electrode is neutralized. When the charge is reduced the electrodes move away from the zero calibration. The display of this motion against a scale is done by a magnifier.

- The charge is a small box, that is usually powered by a battery.The battery voltage is stepped up by an electronic circuit to several thousand volts. The box consists of a fixture that has to be pressed at the end of the dosimeter on the charging electron.
- Some charges have a light for illumination of the measurement electrode, so that the measurement, logging and recharging can happen with one routine motion.
- The dosimeters are made in different ranges: During the peace time the ranges of exposure due to occupation usually measure up to 500 rems (5mSv), which exceeds the normal US yearly dose of 360 mrems (3.6 mSv). The wartime fall out meters measures upto 500rem (5Sv) which is the lethal dose.

Personal monitoring devices:

1. Pocket dosimeter
2. Digital electronic dosimeter
3. Film badge
4. Thermoluminescent dosimeter (TLD)

1. Pocket dosimeter:

- Provides an instant reading of the exposures to the x-rays and the gamma-rays.
- Commonly worn in the pocket.
- Dosimeter should be recharged and recorded at the start of each working shift.
- Leakage can affect the reading. Leakage should not be greater than 2% of full scale in 24 hr period.
- It is reusable.
- It is unable to provide a record that is permanent and has the potential for discharging and loss of reading due to dropping or bumping of dosimeter.

Types

(i) **Minometer / Condensor type / Indirect reading type:**

It is an ion chamber which has a voltage potential placed on it by insertion into a charger. Radiation penetrating the chamber causes the current to leak off in proportion to radiation exposure. By reinserting the dosimeter into the charge reader at the end of the day, the resulting voltage drop is calibrated in milliroentgen. Usually two dosimeters are worn at the time with the lower of the two readings are taken as more accurate. It is necessary to recharge the indirect reading pocket dosimeters after every reading.

(ii) **Direct read pocket dosimeter:**

Its size and shape resembles a fountain pen. The volume of an ionization chamber is approximately 2 mm. Ionization chamber contains a central wire anode and a metal coated quartz fiber. When the anode is charged to a positive potential, the charge is distributed between the wire anode and the quartz fiber. The quartz fiber is repulsed by the electrostatic charge and higher the charge greater is the deflection of the quartz fiber. Inside the ionisation chamber is a central wire anode, and attached to this wire anode is a metal coated quartz fiber. When a anode charged to a positive potential, the charge is distributed between wire anode and a quartz fiber. Electrostatic repulsion deflects the quartz fiber, greater the charge the greater the deflection of quartz fiber. Radiation incident on the chamber produce electrons by ionization and the produced electrons are attracted to, and collected by the positively charged central anode. The collection of electrons reduce the net positive charge and allows the quartz fiber to come back to its original position. The amount of ionisation that occurs proportionately causes the movement. It gives immediate readings and it is re-useable.

***2.* Digital electronic dosimeter:**

- They record the information of dose and dose rate.
- Most often use Geiger-Muller counters.
- Include an audible alarm, which beep or chirp with each recorded increment of exposure. Some models can give continuous audible signal when preset exposure is reached.
- Five to two hundred times more sensitive than TLD.

Types:

(i) **Arrow –Tech dosimeters (pocket fountain pen sized):**
A metal chip is used to attach the dosimeter to the pocket of an individual or to a object that is available in the area to be monitored for total exposure of radiation.

(ii) **Personal alarm dosimeter:**
The active element of a track etch dosimeter is a piece of CR–39 plastic. When a high energy charged proton recoiling from the fast neutron transfers the material, it gives up energy and leaves chemical damage. The material subsequently exposed to a suitable etchant such as sodium hydroxide and damage sites are preferentially etched, leaving pits which can be observed and counted under the microscope.

(iii) **Bubble detector dosimeter:**
It is based on the change of gas bubbles of super heated liquid triggered by fast neutron interactions. A commercial bubble detector dosimeter consists of a clear plastic tube with an aluminum filter at one end. On exposure to fast neutrons, small uniform- sized bubbles form. The bubbles are counted visually and a fast neutron dose calculated using a calibration-factor determined for that dosimeter.

3. Film badge:

- Housing is of plastic or metal, typically 2 by 0.5 inch dimensions, and equipped with a clip for attaching to clothing.

- It contains one or more standard dental x-ray film packets.
- The side of badge housing is equipped with one or more filters of 6 quadrants; open, lead, aluminum, copper, silver, cadmium, cupric, which covers the different parts of the film.
- The phenomenon that x-ray blackens the film is applied here.
- The blackening of film alone is not reliable indicator of exposure. So the film is sandwiched between two thin sheets of tin, each about 1mm thick.
- The tin has practically no effect on high energy radiation, thus the blackening per unit exposure is practically unaffected. However, low energy radiations are attenuated by the tin so that blackening it produces is reduced.
- The degree of blackening produced on the film by radiation is measured by densitometer then adequately calibrated, gives the amount of radiation exposure.
- The uncovered part of film is important, if the blackening of the open part is four times greater as that of under the tin then low energy x-rays must be involved. If both portions are almost equally blackened then hard gamma rays & high energy x-rays are involved.
- **Advantages:**
  - Good for measuring any type and energy of radiation.
  - Continuous assessment is possible
  - Accumulated dose can be calculated
  - Provides a permanent record of dose received.
  - Simple, robust and relatively inexpensive.
- **Disadvantages:**
  - Accuracy is only 10-50%.
  - Range of exposure is less.
  - No immediate indication of exposure, all information is retrospective.
  - The darkening is not necessarily linear to the dose, due to the presence of scattered radiations.
  - Badges are prone to filter loss.

4. *Thermo-luminescent dosimeter (TLD):*

- This is used to measure the actual dose received by the operator as a result of radiography or radiotherapy exposures.
- Most common personnel monitoring device.
- It is of small size.
- The TLD badge in India, consist of a TLD cardholder cassette of high impact plastic.
- The TLD card consist of nickel plated aluminum having three symmetrical holes, each of diameter 12mm. on which three identical $CaSO_4$ embedded Teflon disks are dipped. These disks are clipped on an aluminum card loaded in the cassette, having three filters:

- ❖ Open region
- ❖ Copper
- ❖ Aluminum

- ✪ Thermoluminescence is the property of a substance i.e. lithium fluoride to emit light or energy which it has stored when it is heated.
- ✪ TLD Principle:
  When the phosphor is irradiated, the X-ray energy is absorbed and secondary electrons are produced. The secondary electrons cause holes in the field zones by lifting the electrons to the conduction band. These fall back into traps in metastable state, where they are held. When the phosphor is heated to 200-300°C, the trapped acquire energy to escape back to the conduction band. From the conduction band they fall back to fill holes in the filled zone and when they recombine, visible light is produced called thermoluminescence.
- ✪ TLD Reader:
  1. Heater
  2. Photomultiplier tube
  3. Electronic system

Suggested reading:

1. Freny R. Karjodkar, Textbook of dental and maxillofacial radiology, 2nd edition, Page no. 74 – 80.

Q 6) Enumerate the methods of radiation protection for the patient

MUHS NOVEMBER 2014 (3 Marks)

Protection of patient includes:

(i) **Patient selection:** Only those patients to be selected where the x-ray will contribute to proper diagnosis and treatment outcome.

(ii) **Conduct of examination:**

(a) **Selection of image receptor:**
- o Use of high speed films-E speed films are recommended.
- o Screen films-Are recommended.

(b) **Use of intensifying screens:** For reduction of exposure.

(c) **Focal spot-film distance:** Longer F-S-F-D results in 31% less exposure.

(d) **Collimation of the beam:** Helps to control size and shape of beam and allows only useful x-rays to emerge.

(e) **Filtration:** Absorbs undesirable photons of low energy that are undesirable as they only add to the patient dose and do not contribute to image formation.

(f) **Use of high KVp:** Allows the incident skin dose to be acceptable.

(g) **Use of position indicating device:** Allows to minimise the volume of tissue irradiated.

(h) **Film holding device:** Use of this reduces chances of retakes.

(i) **Timers:** They should be properly maintained and use of electronic timers permits exposure as low as 1/20 to 1/30 seconds, which is not possible with traditional mechanical timer.

(j) **Use of protective barriers:** Leaded aprons, gonadal shields, leaded thyroid shields, and use of film holders with facial shields can provide protection to patient.

(k) **Use of proper technique:** This will help to reduce radiation exposure.

(l) **Processing of image:** It should be accurately done to prevent retakes and extra exposure to patients.

(m) **Interpretation of the image:** Radiographs should be viewed under proper conditions with an illuminated viewer. This will remove the necessity to retake radiographs and prevent un-necessary exposure to patients.

Suggested reading:

1. Freny. R Karjodkar, Textbook of Dental And Maxillofacial Radiology, 2nd edition, 66-71.

CHAPTER 6

Projection Geometry

Introduction:

A conventional radiograph is a two dimensional image of a three dimensional structure.

To get the best radiographs a dentist should have a thorough knowledge of the principles of projection geometry so as to get as accurate a radiograph as possible. Proper basic knowledge of these principles will help to obtain high quality radiographs.

Q 1) Millers technique:

TNMGRU AUGUST 2004 (2 Marks)

Millers technique or the right angle technique is a simple, easy low cost technique used for orientation or localisation of structures or objects in a radiograph in the oral and maxillofacial region. Indications of this technique are localisation of:

1. Foreign bodies.
2. Impacted teeth.
3. Unerupted teeth.
4. Retained roots.
5. salivary stones.
6. Determine displacement of jaw fractures.
7. Localising broken needle and instruments.
8. To determine root position.
9. for differentiating buccal and palatal roots as well as additional root canals in endodontic practice.
10. Evaluation of restorative materials.
11. Localising displaced roots in the maxillary sinus.
12. Establish position of structures in the buccolingual plane.

A radiograph is a two dimensional representation of a three dimensional structure in the superio-inferior and antero-posterior plane. In many clinical situations proper localisation of the object becomes necessary for proper diagnosis and management.

The localisation technique is very useful in obtaining the three dimensional information from two dimensional images.This is achieved by taking two radiographs. Thus when two radiographs are taken which are at right angles to each other it is called as Miller's technique.

(a) A periapical film is first exposed using a proper technique to show the position of the object in superio-inferior and antero-posterior relationship.

(b) Next an occlusal film is taken with central ray perpendicular to the film. This film represents the object in bucco-lingual and antero-posterior relationship.

(c) The two radiographs are compared for locating the object in three dimension.

This technique is effectively used in locating maxillary impacted canine, with periapiacal and maxillary occlusal projection, and in case of fracture mandible to locate any displacement, with orthopantomogram or lateral oblique and mandibular occlusal projection.

In extraoral radiographs used for localisation of objects one radiograph is the true lateral which will give the location of object in anteroposterior plane and the second one is posteroanterior view which will give the location in a mesio-distal plane.

Suggested reading:

1. Pramod John R.Essentials of radiology, Jaypee brothers, page 111-112.

Q 2) Write about various object localisation techniques:

MUHS MAY 2012 (3 Marks)

There are four techniques for object localisation:

1. **Right angle technique or the Miller's technique:** This technique uses two radiographs taken at right angles to each other. First a periapical radiograph is taken to show the position of the object in the superio-inferior and antero-posterior relationship. Then an occlusal radiograph is taken with central x-ray beam perpendicular to the film and this depicts the object in buccolingual and antero-posterior relationship. The two radiographs are compared to show the location of object in three dimensions.
2. **Tube-shift principle:** This technique uses a different horizontal angulation to show whether the object is placed buccally or lingually. First radiograph is taken using standard parameters.Then a second radiograph is taken with the tube shifted 20 degrees either mesially or distally. The point of entry, vertical angulation and film position is the same as that of the first film.
   When the two radiographs are compared the object present on the buccal aspect seems to be moving in the opposite direction of the projection angle in the second radiograph and the object on the lingual side moves in the same direction as that of the changed projection.
   This technique is also called as Clarke's technique or SLOB (same lingual opposite buccal).
3. **Definition and Evaluation technique:** This technique uses the fact that structures that are placed close to the film are more well defined than those away from the film. Since in the intra-oral radiographic technique the film is placed lingually, the object in

question, if clearly defined is assumed to be placed lingually in relation to the other structures. This is not a very reliable method.

4. **Pantomography:** In some older pantomographic units, the structures in the anterior region may be repeated twice. The technique of localisation involves comparing the relative movement of the object with the adjacent structures from one side of the film to the other, with the direction that the clinician views the film (eg. left to right). If the object is present lingually, it seems to be moving in the same direction as the clinician's viewing movement and in the opposite direction if it is present on the buccal side.

Suggested reading:

1. Pramod John R.Essentials Of Radiology. Jaypee Brothers. Page 111-114.

Q 3) Enumerate the factors affecting sharpness of an x-ray film:

MUHS NOVEMBER 2012 (2 Marks)

Sharpness is defined as a measure of how well the boundaries between two areas of different radiodensities are depicted.

It is thus the ability of a radiograph to define edge of an object.

Factors affecting sharpness are:

1. **Effective size of the focal spot:** Dental x-ray machines should have a nominal focal spot size of 1.0mm or less. Some tubes used in extraoral radiography have effective focal spots measuring 0.3 mm, which greatly adds to image clarity.
   X-ray tube manufacturers uses an effective focal spot as small a size as is consistent with the requirements for heat dissipation.
   The angle of the target with respect to the long axis of the electron beam, dictates the size of the effective focal spot.
   Smaller the angle, smaller is the effective focal spot, decreased un- sharpness, and increased image sharpness and resolution, but greater wearing effect on the target.
2. **Distance between the focal spot and the film:** Increasing the distance between the focal spot and the object decreases the blurring of the image by reducing the divergence of the x-ray beam. When the focal spot to object distance is longer the rays of x-ray photons are almost parallel and the blurring is minimal. To achieve this long open ended cylinders are used as aiming devices on the dental xray machines. It reduces the blurring of the image by reducing the divergence of the x-ray beam.
3. **Distance between the object and the film:** Reducing the distance between the object and the image receptor maximises the sharpness by minimizing the x-ray photons divergence.

Suggested reading:

1. Stuart C White, Michael J Pharoah, Oral Radiology, Principles and Interpretation 5th Edition, 86-87.

CHAPTER 7

Imaging Principles

Q 1) Name five principles of shadow casting:

MUHS NOVEMBER 2011 (2 Marks)

The principles are as follows:

1. The focal spot, that is the source of radiation should be as small as possible.
   Smallest source of radiation as possible should be used for emission of x-rays because smaller the focal spot, sharper is the image.
   If the focal spot is larger the penumbra increases and, and less sharp is the image.
2. The object to x-ray source distance should be as long as possible. Longer the Position Indicating Device and the target to film distance less is the magnification of an image.
3. The object to film distance should be as less as possible.
   As the object-to-film distance is reduced, the unsharpness decreases, resulting in enhanced image clarity and increased sharpness.
   Closer the proximity of the object to the film, lesser is the magnification of the image.
4. The object and the film should be parallel to each other. When the long axis of the tooth and the film are parallel to each other the image shape distortion is minimised.
   When the object and the film fail to be parallel to each other, an angular relationship is formed and image distortion occurs.
5. The central ray of the x-ray beam should be perpendicular to the object and the film both. In case it is not perpendicular to either one of them it can result in elongation or shortening of the image.
6. There should be almost no movement of the film, tube and the patient during x-ray exposure. In case either of the things happen, it can cause blurring and image unsharpness due to penumbra formation.

In panoramic radiography however there is deliberate movement of x-ray tube and the film to blur the images of unwanted layer of the object.

Suggested reading:

1. Freny R Karjodkar, Essentials Of Oral And Maxillofacial radiology, edition 2nd, page 124.

CHAPTER 8

X-Ray Films and Accessories

Introduction:

X-ray films are used to capture the image of objects after the x-rays pass through them. Its a medium which changes x-ray beam into visible image.

Q 1) Moving Grid:

TNMGRU OCTOBER 1995 (5 Marks)

Enumerate types of grid:

MUHS OCTOBER 2002 (2 Marks)

What is a grid? Where is it used?

MUHS OCTOBER 2003 (2 Marks)

Grids:

When x-ray's strike a patient, many of the incident photons undergo compton interaction and produce scattered photons.

The number of scattered photons in the remnant beam that reach the film is two-three times the number of primary photons that do not undergo absorption.

Scattered radiation increases with increased subject thickness, field size, and kVp.

Scattered photons produce fog and reduce subject contrast.

Grid is a device that reduces this scattered radiation and improves image quality.

Q 2) Definition:

MUHS OCTOBER 2003 (2 Marks)

Grids are thus the devices used in radiography that reduce the scattered radiation from reaching the film, while allowing the primary beam to reach the film. It is placed between the subject and the film.

Composition:

Grid is a thin flat rectangular device that consists of alternating strips of radiopaque and radiolucent materials.

- The radiopaque material is usually lead foil. They are easy to shape and relatively inexpensive. Due to this factor and high atomic number it becomes the best material to clean up the scatter.
  A grid absorbs scatter from the exit radiation before it reaches the film.
  It is located between the patient and the film.
  X-ray photons scatter in various angles as they leave the patient and are preferentially attenuated by the lead foil strips, because they are not parallel to the grid interspaces.
- The interspace material, which is the radiolucent space between the lead strips, is made of plastic fiber or aluminum.
  Aluminium has a higher atomic number and produces less visible lines on the image.
  The use of aluminum increases the absorption of primary x-ray photons in the interspace, especially at low k_{vp}.
  They increase patient exposure by 20%.
  Plastic fiber interspace materials are preferred to aluminum because there is no need to increase the patient dose.
  As there are positive and negative aspects to both the interspace materials, both types are used in manufacturing of grids.

Functions of grids:

(i) Grids are device used to absorb scattered radiation before it can reach the image receptor and fog the film.

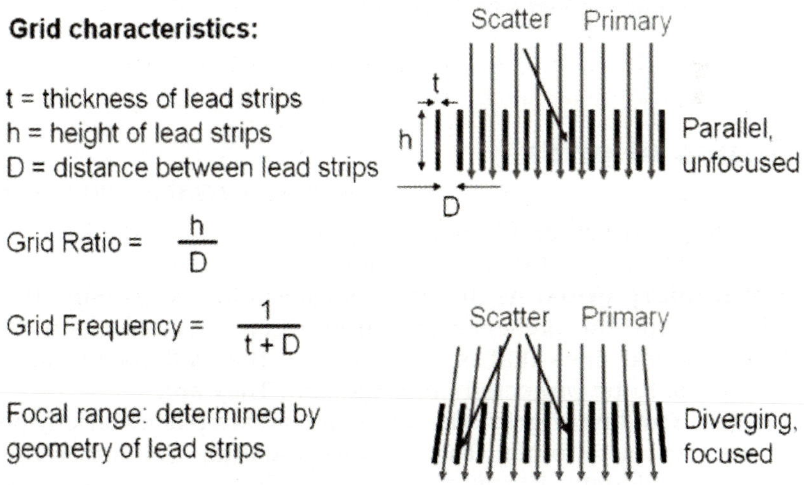

Fig. Grid characteristics

(ii) They are used in radiographic exams which require a high kvp setting. High kvp settings cause high intensity beams and results in more compton interactions.

(iii) As the grids reduce scattered radiation from reaching the film, it controls and improves contrast of the image.

(iv) Thus the grids clean up scatter, which improves image contrast, and makes the manifest image visible.

(vi) It is generally used where the object thickness is more than ten cms.

(vii) Its also used where the kvp is more than 60.

(viii) Used in case of radiography of soft tissue structures to increase contrast.

(ix) Structures affected by pathological condition that would increase scatter production.

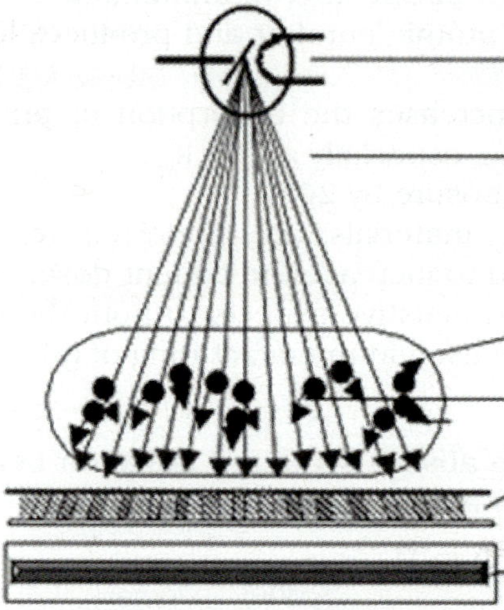

Fig. Grid mechanism

Q 3) Types of grids

MUHS OCTOBER 2002 (2 Marks)

A) Focussed and nonfocused grids.

B) Moving and stationary grids.

1. **Stationary grids:** As the name suggests it is stationary. However in this type the presence of grid between the object and the film causes grid lines that is the image of the radiopaque absorbing material to be projected on to the film. They are:
   - **(a) The linear grid:** The strips of lead are placed strictly parallel to each other. The primary radiation will meet the grid obliquely. The grid line on the film will appear wider. The central beam should be in a plane parallel to the grid lines.
   - **(b) The focussed grid:** In this the grid strips of lead are angled progressively from the center towards the edge so that the inter spaces point at the focal spot. Thus their direction coincides with the direction of diverging photons in the

primary x-ray beam and helps to accommodate their passage through the grid.

They are manufactured with varying number of line pairs of absorbers and radiolucent spaces per inch. 80 or more do not cause much objectionable grid lines on the image.

(c) **The pseudo-focused grid:** In this type the height of the strips is reduced progressively from the center resulting in a reduced grid ratio from the center to the edge.

(d) **The crossed grid:** The crossed grids overcome the limitations of the linear grid which clean up the scatter in only one direction. These grids are made by placing two linear grids on top of each other with the grid lines perpendicular to each other. Crossed grids are more efficient at removing scattered radiation than linear grids. These can remove at least twice the amount of scatter than the linear or parallel grids.

Q 4) Moving grids

TNMGRU OCTOBER 1995 5 marks

Stationary grids with low grid frequencies produce noticeable grid line on the final image.

One of the ways to eliminate this is to move the grid during exposure. The motion of the grid blurs the grid lines, and hence not noticeable on the image.

The image of the radiopaque grid lines on the film can be deleted by mechanically moving the grid in a direction of 90^0 to the grid lines, but not the object, during exposure.

This results in evening or blurring out the radiolucent lines and resulting in a more uniform exposure. It doesnot interfere with the absorption of scattered photons.

Moving grids are called bucky grids named after the inventor, Dr. Gustave Bucky.

Dr.Bucky's grid design was modified by Dr. Hollis Potter a Chicago radiologist, in 1920 when he placed the strips in one direction, made the strips thinner, and designed a device that allowed the grid to move during exposure.

The device is called the Potter-Bucky Diaphragm, Bucky diaphragm and Bucky grid.

The Potter-Bucky diaphragm is mounted underneath the table top, directly above the image receptor.

The grid in the Bucky must move side to side or in a circular fashion perpendicular to the lead strips to blur out the grid lines effectively. If the Bucky were to move in the same direction as that of the lead strips, the grid lines would be visible.

There are two types of moving grids:

- Reciprocating grid.

- Oscillating grid.

1. **Reciprocating grid:** This type of grid is driven by a motor.During exposure it moves back and forth multiple times.
   The grid moves not more than a 2-3 cms at a time.
   A selector at the control panel activates the grid motor. If the motor is not activated, the grid remains stationary during exposure, and the grid lines will appear on the image.
2. **Oscillating grid:** The oscillating grid is suspended in the center of a frame by four spring like devices.

At the time of the exposure, an electromagnet pulls the grid to one side and then releases it. The grid will oscillate in a circular motion within the grid frame for approximately 20-30 seconds before stopping the motion.

Advantages of a moving grid:

Moving grids have greatly improved the overall image quality and the disadvantages are out weighed.

- **Motion blur:** The grid mechanisms which are operating properly will completely blur out the grid lines, making the overall image more diagnostic.
- **Usage in radiography:** The moving grid is consistently used in radiography for body parts that measure more than 10 cms.

Disadvantages of a moving grid:

The early use of grids demonstrated grid lines or the checkerboard pattern due to large thick strips and interspace material. Although the grids cleaned up the scatter, and improved the contrast of the images, the grid lines were not acceptable as they distracted from the image. The moving grid was designed to remove the grid lines, but there were some disadvantages with the design and placement of moving grids.

- **Grid mechanism:** Mechanical mechanism that was subject to failure.
- **Increased object to film distance:** There was an increase in the object to film distance due to the size of the grid mechanism. The increased object to film distance tended to create magnification and blurring of the image.
- **Motion:** The nature of the moving grid increased the motion of the film holder, and if not operated properly, the result would be additional image blur.
- **Longer exposure time:** The exposure time must be lengthened to allow the motion of the moving grid to have the intended effect of removing the grid lines.

For some patients this could be problematic due to their inability to hold still or to hold their breath during the entire exposure.

Suggested reading:

1. Robert Fosbinder, Denise Orth, Essentials of radiologic science, 2011, Lippincott Williams & Wilkins, page 165-172.

2. Freny R Karjodkar, Text Book Of Dental And Maxillofacial Radiography, IInd edition, page no 122-124.

Q 5) Composition of Intra-oral films:

MUHS NOVEMBER 2010 (2 Marks)

Composition:

There are two principal components of an x-ray film:

Base and Emulsion:

The emulsion is sensitive to the x-rays and visible light and the radiographic image is recorded on it.

1. **Base:** The emulsion is supported by the base which is its primary function.
   There should be a proper degree of flexibility of the base so that it allows easy handling of the film.
   The base of the x-ray film used for dental purposes is made of polyester, polyethylene terephthalate and is 0.18 mm in thickness.
   The base of the film is translucent uniformly and produces no patterns on the final radiograph.
   According to some a slight bluish tint of the base can help in improving the viewing of diagnostic details.
   The base of the film should have properties to withstand exposure to processing solutions with out becoming distorted.
2. **Emulsion:** The emulsion consists of two main components which are grains of silver halide that are sensitive to visible light and x-rays and the matrix made of gelatin in which these crystals are suspended.

The grains of silver halide are basically composed of silver bromide.

In ultra-speed films, iodide is added because its large diameter as compared to bromine causes disruption of the regularity of the crystal of the silver halide and increases the sensitivity to x-radiation.

Trace amounts of sulfur containing compounds also alters the photosensitivity of the crystals of silver halide. Trace amounts of gold also may be added to improve the sensitivity of the silver halide crystals.

When the film is being manufactured, the grains of silver halide are suspended in a vehicle which is applied to both sides of the supporting base.

The gelatinous and non-gelatinous materials that form the vehicle helps in keeping the grains of silver halide dispersed evenly.

A layer of adhesive material that is thin is added to the base before applying the emulsion so as to ensure its proper adhesion that is good to the base of the film.

During film processing, the vehicle tends to absorb the processing solutions and allows the chemicals to react with the grains of silver halide.

Supercoat:

It is a protective, transparent, non-abrasive layer over the emulsion.

This is an additional layer of gelatin which is applied to the surface to serve as a protective coat and prevents damage to the film during mechanical handling.

This barrier helps in protecting the film from damage due to scratching, contamination or pressure from rollers in automatic processors.

The films are made as double emulsion films, that is the coating of emulsion is on both sides of the base.

When a film is of double emulsion, it requires less amount of radiation to expose the film and to produce an image.

For intra-oral examination, direct exposure films are used, because it results in higher resolution images than in the screen-film combination. In contrast to screen films direct exposure films are used for intraoral examination as it provides higher resolution of images.

For certain conditions like incipient carious lesions and early periapical disease, their detection requires higher resolution.

For proper orientation of the film, there is a raised small dot on one corner of the film used for dental radiography.

The side with the raised dot is placed facing the x-ray tube when the dental film is placed in the mouth.

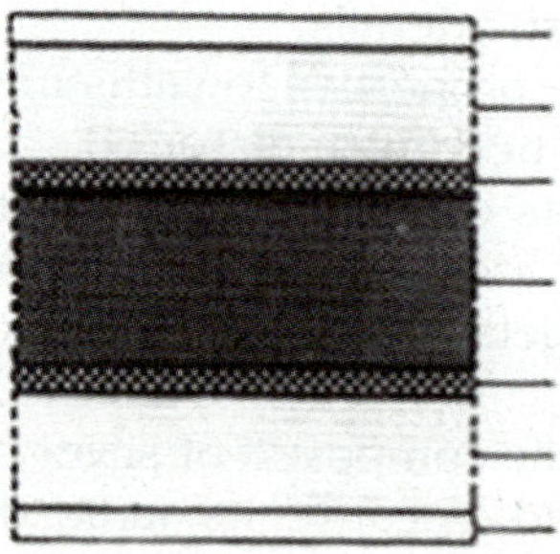

Fig. Different layers of IOPA film

Suggested reading:

1. Stuart C White, Michael J Pharoah, Oral Radiology, Principles and Interpretation, 5th edition, 72-73.

Q 6) Intensifying screens:

TNMGRU AUGUST 2011 6 Marks

A plastic sheet coated with a fluorescent material called phosphors is known as an intensifying screen. The phosphor materials fluoresce that is emit visible light when exposed to x-rays.

The intensity of this fluorescence is proportional to the x-ray energy absorbed.

The sum of the effects of the x-rays and the visible light emitted by the screen phosphors exposes the film in an intensifying cassette.

These are used in extra oral radiography to reduce the dose of x radiation. It makes the x-ray film 10-60 times more sensitive to x-rays than the films used alone.

Characteristic features of an intensifying screen:

1. It consists of a base made up of polyester or cellulose triacetate which is similar to a radiographic film.
2. This base must be radioparent.
3. Should be chemically inert.
4. It should possess both, toughness and flexibility.
5. There should be no curling.
6. It should not discolour with age.
7. A reflective layer of titanium dioxide is coated on the base so that it can bounce back the light onto the film. However divergence of the light rays leads to image unsharpness.
8. It has a phosphor layer that is homogenous that is standard or rare earth.

   There is thin transparent protective super coating of gelatin. The purpose of this supercoating is to protect the screen and it is very thin and care should be taken while handling the screen to avoid abrading it.
9. The material needs to be flexible so that the screen does not crack on bending and such types of screen are used with panoramic radiography.

The standard screens used calcium tungstate phosphors, while the rare earth screens use gadolinium or lanthanum phosphors.

In conversion of x-rays to visible light, the rare earth screens are more efficient and help in reduction of patient exposure to radiation.

The intensifying screens are placed in close contact with the x-ray films in the cassette.

The function of these screens is to enhance the effect of x-rays by subjecting the emulsion to the effect of light as well as the ionising radiation.

The ultimate benefit is the reduction in dose of ionising radiation to the patient.

Composition:

Intensifying screens are made of a base supporting material, a phosphor layer, and a protective polymeric coat.

In all dental radiographic examinations, the intensifying screens are used in pairs, one on either side of the film and they are placed inside a cassette. The purpose of a cassette is to hold each intensifying screen in close contact with the x-ray film in order to enhance the sharpness of the image.

Most cassettes are rigid, but they maybe flexible.

Base:

Some form of polyester plastic that is about 0.25mm thick forms the base material of the intensifying screen.

The base provides the mechanical support for the other layers of the screen.

In some intensifying screens the base also is reflective, thus it reflects light emitted from the phosphor layer back towards the x-ray film.

This has the effect of increasing the light emission of the intensifying screen.

However, it also results in unsharpness of the image because of the divergence of the light rays which are reflected back to the film.

Some fine detail intensifying screens omit the reflecting layer to improve image sharpness.

In other intensifying screens the base is not reflective, and a separate coating of titanium dioxide is applied to the base material to serve as a reflecting layer.

Reflecting layer:

- Consists of thin layer of white material (i.e. magnesium oxide and titanium dioxide) between the base and luminescent layer.
- It serves to redirect to the film a large fraction of emitted visible light which is moving away from film.
- Thus it increases sensitivity but some degree of unsharpness is created because of divergence of light reflected back to the film.

Phosphor Layer:

- The phosphor layer is composed of radiation-sensitive phosphorescent crystals suspended in a plastic material.
- When the crystals are struck by photons, they fluoresce and emit visible light photons that expose the X-ray film.
- Speed of the screen increases as the crystal size increases but the overall image quality may be degraded.

Types of Phosphors used:

(i) Crystalline Calcium Tungstate, that fluoresces in blue portion of the spectrum.
Conventional Screens used with blue sensitive films (Kodac X-Omati screen films)

(ii) Rare Earth Intensifying Screens using terbium activated gadolinium oxysulphide and thulium activated lanthanum oxybromide, which fluoresce in green portion. Their fluorescence can be increased by the addition of small amounts of thulium, niobium, or terbium.

- A pair of rare earth intensifying screens absorbs about 60% of the photons that reach the cassette after passing through a patient.
- These phosphors are about 18% efficient in converting this x-ray energy to visible light.
- Rare earth screens convert each absorbed x-ray photon into about 4000 lower-energy, visible light (green or blue) photons which then expose the film.
- The speed of the screen depends on crystal size and the thickness of the phosphor layer (larger crystals and thicker

layer increase speed). But these produce images with low resolution.

Phosphorescent crystals suspended in a polymeric binder compose the phosphor layer.

Protective layer:

Over the phosphor layer a protective polymer coat is placed to protect it and to provide a surface that can be cleaned.

The intensifying screens should be kept clean because any debris, spots, or scratches may cause light spots on the resultant radiographs.

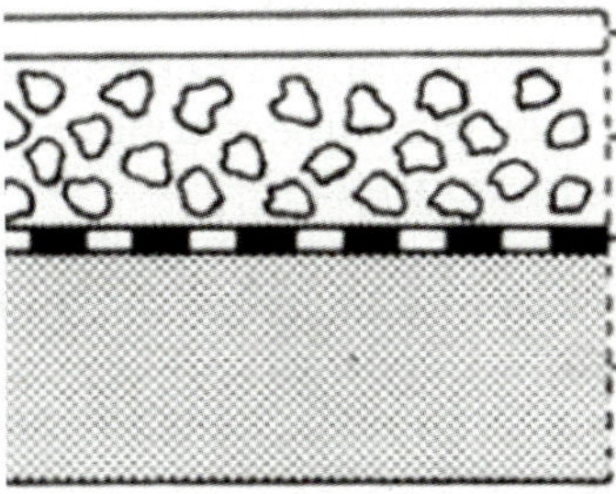

Fig. Cross section of typical intensifying screen

The speed and resolution of a screen depends on many factors including:

- Phosphor type and phosphor conversion efficiency.
- Thickness of phosphor layer and coating weight. (amount of phosphor/unit volume)
- Presence of reflective layer.
- Presence of light-absorbing dye in phosphor binder or protective coating.
- Phosphor grain size.

Care of Intensifying Screens:

Screens are delicate and can be damaged easily.

If the active surface is soiled even slightly the fluorescent emission is affected. Hence the screens must be kept clean, otherwise the light photons will be prevented from reaching the film to create an image.

Dirt can produce high spots that can create wear.

Antistatic solutions are used to clean the screens.

A damp cloth is used to rub gently.

It is ensured that the screen is dry before closing the cassette, to prevent the gelatin on the surface to cause sticking of the screens.

The cassette should never be left open as it can accumulate dust on the screen.

Suggested reading:

1. Stuart C White, Michael J Pharoah, Oral Radiology, Principles And Interpretation, 5th edition, page 75-77.
2. Freny R Karjodkar, Essentials of Oral and Maxillofacial Radiology, 2nd edition. pg no.119-121.

Q 7) Define radiographic contrast and state factors influencing contrast:

MUHS MAY 2009 (2 Marks)

Radiographic contrast is defined as the difference in densities between light and dark regions on a radiograph.Thus it is a general term that describes the range of densities on a radiograph.

Factors that influence contrast are:

- **Subject contrast:** It is influenced largely by the thickness, density and atomic number of the subject. The energy and intensity of the x-ray beam also influences the image contrast.
  As the kvp of the x-ray beam increases subject contrast decreases. And conversely when low kvp is used the subject contrast increases. Most commonly between 70-80 kvp is used.
  Changing the time mA of exposure also influences subject contrast.
- **Film contrast:** It is defined as the capacity of the radiographic films to display differences in subject contrast. A high contrast film reveals areas of small difference in subject contrast more clearly than does the low contrast film.
  Film contrast also depends on the range of density being examined. Properly exposed films have more contrast than the under exposed film.
  Film contrast is maximised by optimal processing conditions. Excessive or incomplete developing diminishes contrast. Storage of films at very high temperatures, exposure to very bright sunlight, or light leakage in darkrooms can degrade the contrast. Film fog also reduces contrast.
- **Scattered radiation:** These can cause fogging of a film resulting in loss of radiographic contrast. Using a relatively low kvp, collimation of the beam and use of grids in extra oral radiography can reduce scattered radiation and improve contrast.

Suggested reading:

1. Stuart C White, Michael J Pharoah, Oral Radiology, Principles and Interpretation 5th Edition, 59-61.

CHAPTER 9

Processing of X-Ray Films

Introduction:

Once the film is exposed to radiation, some chemical changes occur in the film emulsion and a latent image is formed. To make this image visible the radiographs are taken through a process of developing and fixing which is called processing.

Q 1) Composition & functions of Developing solution:

MUHS NOVEMBER 2010 (2 Marks)
MUHS MAY 2012 (3 Marks)

Developing solution contains the following chemicals:

1. **Developer:** The primary function of the developing solution is to convert the exposed silver halide crystals into metallic silver grains. This process begins at the latent image sites, where electrons from the developing agents are conducted into the silver halide crystal and reduce the constituent silver ions to solid grains of metallic silver.
   Two developing agents are used in dental radiology:
2. **Pyrazilodone type compound usually Phenidone:**
   Phenidone serves as the first electron donor that converts silver ions to metallic silver at the latent image site. 'This electron transfer generates the oxidized form of Phenidone.
   Hydroquinone:
   Hydroquinone provides an electron to reduce the oxidized Phenidone back to its original active state so that it can continue to reduce silver halide grains to metallic silver.
3. **Activator:** The developers are active only at alkaline pH values, usually around 10.
   This is achieved with the addition of alkali compounds (activators) such as sodium or potassium hydroxide.
   Buffers are used to maintain this condition-usually sodium bicarbonate. The activators also cause the gelatin to swell so that the developing agents can diffuse more rapidly into the emulsion and reach the suspended silver bromide. Activators also cause the

gelatin to swell so that the developing agents can diffuse more rapidly into the emulsion and reach the suspended silver bromide crystals.
Sodium hydroxide in conjunction with sodium carbonate may be used to give higher contrast.

4. **Preservative:** The developing solution contains an antioxidant or preservative, usually sodium sulfite.
It protects the developer from oxidation by atmospheric oxygen and thus extends their useful life and also combines with the brown oxidized developer to produce a colorless soluble compound. If not removed, oxidation products interfere with the developing reaction and stain the film.
5. **Restrainer:** Bromide, usually as potassium bromide, and benzotriazole are added to the developing solution to restrain development of unexposed silver halide crystals. The restrainers act as antifog agents and increase contrast.
Although bromide and benzotriazole depress the reduction of both exposed and unexposed crystals, they are much more effective in depressing the reduction of unexposed crystals.
Consequently, the restrainers act as antifog agents and increase contrast.
6. **Developer Replenisher:** In the normal course of film processing, Phenidone and hydroquinone are consumed, and bromide ions and other by-products are released into solution.
Developer also becomes inactivated by exposure to oxygen.
These actions produce a seasoned solution, and the film speed and contrast stabilize.
The developing solution of both manual and automatic developers should be replenished with fresh solution each morning to prolong the life of the developer.
7. **Hardener:** Glutaraldehyde is added especially in automatic processing to prevent the emulsion from softening and sticking to the roller.
8. **Fungicide:** To prevent bacterial growth.
9. **Buffer:** To maintain pH (+7). Sodium bicarbonate is usually used.
10. **Solvent:** Water is used as solvent of the chemicals and as a medium in which they react with the silver bromide of the film emulsion.

Suggested reading:

1. Freny R Karjodkar, Essentials Of Oral and Maxillofacial radiology, chapter 10, pg no.131-132.
2. Stuart C White, Michael J Pharaoh, Oral Radiology, Principles And Interpretation, 5th edition, 96-97.

Q 2) Automatic film processors:

TMNGRU FEBRUARY 2011 6 Marks

Automatic film processors automate the film processing steps.

There are two types:

(a) Automatic dunking models that produce a washed film which has to be dried.

(b) Miniature roller type that produces dried films.

Depending on the equipment and temperature of operation it takes only 4-6 minutes to develop, fix, wash and dry the films.

Many automatic processors have light shielded compartments where the intra-oral film can be unwrapped even in day light, however for the extra-oral films this shield can be removed to provide enough room to feed the larger films.

The density and contrast of the film processed by this method remains consistent, but the higher temperature of the developer and artefacts caused by rollers reduce the quality of films.

Advantages:

- Rapidity of the process which requires less than 4-7 minutes.
- Uniformity of results.
- Less floor space is required and loading can be done in daylight.
- No need of film hangers and dryers.
- Density and contrast of the films are consistent.

Disadvantages:

- The quality of radiographs is not as high as that of manually processed films.The resultant image is more grainy.
- High cost of equipment and maintenance.

Mechanism:

(i) Consists of a transport mechanism that picks up the unwrapped film and passes it through the developing, fixing, washing and drying sections.

(ii) The transport system consists of series of rollers driven by a constant speed motor that operates through gears, belts and chains.
The rollers often consist of independent assemblies of multiple rollers in a rack, with one rack for each step in the operation.

(iii) The primary function of the rollers is to move the films through the developing solutions. It however has three other functions:

- Their motion causes agitation of the solutions and hence contributes to uniformity of the processing.
- The rollers press on the emulsion resulting in promotion of exchange of solution.
- The top rollers at the crossover points between the developer and the fixer, removes the developing solution preventing carrying over of the developing solution into the fixer tank. This feature helps to maintain the uniformity of the processing chemicals.
- The chemical composition of the developer and fixer are modified to operate at higher temperatures than those of the

manual method, and also for more rapid developing, fixing, washing and drying requirements of the automatic method.

- The fixer also has a special hardener to help the emulsion withstand the rigorous transport system.

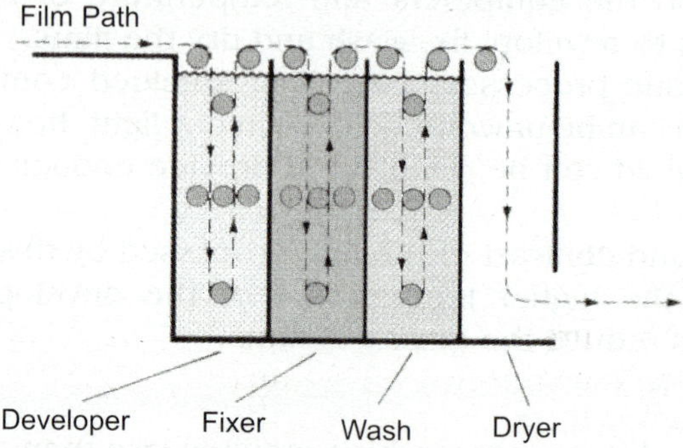

Fig. The inside components of automatic film processor

- **Replenishment:** To maintain quality of developer and fixer, replenishment is necessary. Some automatic processors have have automatic replenishment system. About 8 ounces of fresh developer and fixer should be added per gallon of solution / day.

Suggested reading:

1. Freny R Karjodkar, Textbook Of Dental And Maxillofacial Radiology, 2nd edition, 247-248.
2. Stuart, C White, Michael, J Pharaoh, Oral Radiology Principles And Interpretation, 5th edition, 103-104.

Q 3) Processing of x-ray films:

RGUHS OCTOBER 2002 (4 Marks)

This process makes visible the latent image that is produced in the film emulsion that is exposed to radiation.

Under special darkroom conditions when the film with latent image is immersed in a series of chemical solutions a chemical reaction takes place.

Thus the latent image is made visible by following a processing process.

Film processing involves the following procedures:

1. The exposed film is immersed in a developer.
2. The film is rinsed in a water bath.
3. Then the film is immersed in a fixer.
4. The film then is washed in the water bath.
5. Film is then dried and mounted for viewing.

Two types of processing methods are used:

1. Manual method.

2. Automatic film processing method.

This procedure is carried out in the dark room.

Manual processing:

Involves the following steps:

(i) **Replenish solution:** The first step in manual processing is to replenish the developer and the fixer solutions.

(ii) The developer and fixer solution are then stirred to mix the chemicals and to equalise the temperature through out the tanks.

(iii) The films are clipped to hangers using only the safety lights in the darkroom by removing them from their light proof packets or cassettes.

(iv) The temperature of the developer solution is checked and the timer is set according to the manufacturer's instructions.

(v) The timer is started and the films are immediately immersed in the developing solution. The hanger is agitated gently to remove any air bubbles sticking to the film. The film is allowed to remain for the predetermined time in the developer.

(vi) After developing the hanger is removed and kept under running water for thirty seconds.

(vii) The hanger is then placed in the fixer solution for 10 minutes and it is agitated every 5 seconds for 30 seconds.

(viii) After the fixing the films are again washed under running water for several minutes to remove the residual processing solutions and then kept for drying.

1. Developing:

As mentioned above the film is placed first in the developing solution at certain temperature for a fixed time.

The developing solution contains: Reducing agents that are hydroquinone, phenidone and elon.

Activator as sodium hydroxide.

Restrainer is potassium bromide and preservative as sodium sulphite.

The developing solution can distinguish between the exposed and unexposed silver halide crystals and it initiates a chemical reaction which reduces the exposed silver halide into particles of metallic silver and is responsible for creating the dark areas on the radiograph.

If developer is allowed to remain in prolonged contact with silver bromide crystals that do not contain a latent image it will slowly reduce them also and thereby over develop the film. Reduction of unexposed crystals results in production of chemical fog and not a dark radiograph.

Following the developing process, the film is rinsed in water to remove the developing solution remaining on the film. After the development of the film, the emulsion swells and becomes saturated with the developer and hence the film should be rinsed with gentle agitation for 30 seconds. Rinsing dilutes the developer slowing down the developing process.

After rinsing, the film is placed in the fixer for a specific amount of time.

The fixer solution contains: Ammonium thiosulfate or sodium thiosulfate is used as a clearing agent.

Acetic acid is used as acidifier. Hardener is aluminum sulphate and preservative is ammonium sulphate.

This solution is responsible for removing all the unexposed silver halide crystals from the film and creates white or clear areas on the radiograph. The undeveloped silver bromide gives the film a dense opalescent appearance and if exposed to light in this state the film will darken slowly. A second function of fixer solution is to cause hardening of the film emulsion so as to prevent any damage to it by handling and also shrinks the emulsion.

After the fixing of the film it is washed under water to remove any remaining solution. Warm water should not be used as the emulsion can get damaged. If any silver compound or thiosulfate remains on the film, due to inadequate washing, it can lead to discolouring and stains that are most visible on the radiopaque areas. Washing time longer than 30 minutes should be avoided as this can cause damage to the emulsion.

Drying: after thoroughly rinsing, the film is dried. The films can be kept in a drying cabinet or hung up in a well ventilated dust free room. Care should be taken that wet emulsion is not touched or damaged films should not be splashed with water during drying cycle as this will produce spots.

After films have been removed hangers should be cleaned in running water to remove any traces of residual chemicals.

Automatic processing:

Automatic processors have a in built arrangement and consists of a transport mechanism which picks up the unwrapped film and passes it through developing, fixing, washing and drying process.

Suggested reading:

1. Stuart C White, Michael J Pharoah, Oral Radiology, Principles and Interpretation 5th Edition, 96-104.

Q 4) Discuss in detail processing of Radiographs and formation of latent image:

BFU MAY 2006(15 Marks)

Processing is a collective title given to a series of operations carried out in the dark room, which cause chemical changes in the exposed radiographic film, making the invisible latent image, contained in the sensitized film emulsion into a visible, permanent radiographic image.

Processing of radiographs can be classified as:

Manual: There are three types:

(i) Time temperature.
(ii) Modified time-temperature.
(iii) Visual.

II) Automatic processing.

III) Daylight processing.

IV) Self developing films.

Film processing involves the following procedures:

1. Immerse exposed film in developer.
2. Rinse developer off film in water bath.
3. Immerse film in fixer.
4. Wash film in water bath to remove fixer.
5. Dry film and mount for viewing.

Following exposure, each grain of silver halide in film emulsion contains neutral silver atoms at their latent image sites. These latent image sites render the crystal sensitive to development and image formation.

Developer converts silver bromide crystals with neutral silver atoms deposited at the latent image sites into black, solid silver metallic grains. Fixer removes unexposed, undeveloped silver bromide crystals on the film in unexposed areas.

Thus the radiographic image is composed of light (radiopaque) areas, where few photons have reached the film, and dark (radiolucent) areas of the film that were struck by many photons.

Developing solution:

The developing solution contains four basic components all dissolved in water.

Reducing agents Phenidone Hydroquinone Metol or elon	Phenidone serves as the first electron donor that converts silver ions to metallic silver at latent image site.
Phenidone is used in automatic processing	Hydroquionone provides an electron to reduce the oxidized phenidone back to its original active state so that it can continue to reduce silver halide grains to metallic silver.
	Metol or elon helps develop the shadow areas or shades of gray on the film and brings out the details. It does not produce a high contrast. It is less sensitive to temperature changes.
Activator Sodium hydroxide Potassium hydroxide Potassium carbonate/ sodium carbonate.	Developers are active only at pH values around 10; and this pH is achieved only by addition of activators and they are also called the accelerator. The activators also cause the gelatin to swell so that the developing agents can diffuse more rapidly into emulsion to reach silver bromide crystals
Preservative Sodium sulfite	It extends the useful life of solution. Preservative combines with oxidized developer to produce a compound that subsequently stains images brown if not washed out.

Restrainer Potassium bromide or benzotriazole	Prevents excessive fogging of film and increases the contrast
Hardener Glutaraldehyde	This is added to automatic processing to prevent the emulsion from softening and sticking to rollers.
Fungicide	To prevent bacterial growth

Rinsing:

After development the film emulsion swells and becomes saturated with developer. At this point the films are rinsed in water for 30 seconds with continuous, gentle agitation before they are placed in fixer.

Rinsing dilutes the developer slowing the development process.

It also removes the alkali activator preventing neutralization of the acid fixer. This rinsing process is typical for manual processing but is not used with most automatic processors.

Fixing solution:

Fixing solution also contains four components all dissolved in water

Clearing agent Ammonium thiosulfate or sodium thiosulfate	It removes the unsensitized silver halide crystals. It forms stable water soluble complexes with silver ions, which diffuse from the emulsion.
Acidifier Acetic acid	It contains an acetic acid buffer system (pH 4 to 4.5) to keep the fixer pH constant the acid fixing solution also inactivates and residual developing agents in the film emulsion
Preservative Ammonium sulfate	Prevents oxidation of thiosulfate clearing agent.
Hardener Aluminum sulfate	It complexes with gelatin during fixing and prevents damage to gelatine.

Washing:

After fixing the processed film is washed in water to remove all thiosulfate ions and silver thiosulfate complexes.

Washing efficiency is declined rapidly when the water temperature decreases to less than 60 F.

Formation of latent image:

1. latent image is invisible image that is produced in film emulsion by light or x-ray and is converted into visible image by processing.
2. The sulfur compounds play an important role in image formation

along with physical irregularities in crystal produced by iodide ions. Sulfur compounds create sensitivity site, the sites in the crystal that are sensitive to radiation.

3. Exposure to radiation chemically alters the photosensitive silver halide crystals to produce latent image.
4. When the silver halide crystals are irradiated x-ray photons interact primarily with bromide ions by compton and photoelectric interactions.
5. These interactions result in removal of an electron from bromide ions by loss of an electron, bromide ions are converted into neutral bromine atom. The free electrons move through crystal until they reach sensitivity site, where they become trapped and impart negative charge to site.
6. The negatively charged sensitivity site then attracts positively charged free interstitial silver ions. When silver ion reaches negatively charged sensitivity site, it is reduced and forms a neutral atom of metallic silver. The sites containing these neutral silver atoms are now called latent image sites.
7. The process occurs numerous times within a crystal. The overall distribution of crystals with latent image sites in a film after exposure constitutes the latent image. Processing the exposed film in developer and fixer converts the latent image into the visible radiographic image.

Suggested reading:

1. Stuart C White, Michael J Pharoah, Oral Radiology, Principles and Interpretation 5th Edition, 94-104.

CHAPTER 10

Intra Oral Radiographic Techniques

Introduction:

The radiographic procedures for taking images of teeth and its associated structures is called intra oral imaging. The radiographs should include images of the crown, root and the surrounding periapical area, adjacent teeth, interdental bone, alveolar bone, periodontal ligament space and the nearby structures. The film is placed in close proximity of the tooth quadrant of interest and exposed to radiation.

It includes three basic techniques:

- Intraoral periapical.
- Bitewing technique.
- Occlusal radiography.

Q 1) Advantages of paralleling technique:

MAY 2003 MUHS (2 Marks)

Paralleling technique is a type of intra oral periapical radiographic procedure where in the film and the object that is teeth are parallel to each other which is achieved by using a film holder.

They can be Rinn -XCP holders or according to choice of the operator it also has a position indicating device because of which the central x-ray can be directed through the precise point of entry for the particular tooth or teeth quadrant.

This however increases the distance between the teeth and the film and this is compensated by increasing the distance between the target and film which is about 16 inches as opposed to about 8 inches in short cone technique.

The central ray thus can be directed perpendicular to the object as well as the film. This technique hence satisfies almost all the principles of shadow casting and the radiographs produced have optimum features of an ideal intra oral radiograph.

The advantages can be summarised as follows:

1. **Accuracy:** The size and shape of the image is representative of the actual tooth. The distortion is minimum and detail and definition is maximum.
2. **Simplicity:** The use of a film holder helps to standardise and

accurately position the film and central ray alignment device helps to reduce the manual error and vagueness of positioning and hence the accurate vertical and horizontal angulations are correctly applied reducing chances of distortion.

3. **Duplication:** This technique is easy to standardise and can be duplicated or repeated when serial radiographs are indicated. Because of which the comparisons of serial radiographs made using this technique have great validity.

Suggested reading:

1. Eric Whaites, Essentials of Dental Radiography and Radiology, Third Edition, Churchill Livingstone, 76-77.

Q 2) Advantages and disadvantages of paralleling angle technique:

MUHS NOVEMBER 2009 (2 Marks)

Advantages:

(i) **Accuracy:** With this technique an image that has dimensional accuracy can be produced and is very much representative of the actual tooth.

The image is free of distortion and exhibits maximum detail and definition.

There is no overlap of related structures and all shadows of anatomical structures are cast in their appropriate anatomic positions.

This accuracy is due to:

- Increased target to film distance.
- Object and the film are parallel to each other.
- Central ray is perpendicular to the tooth and the film.
- Though the object to film distance is increased, it is compensated by increase in target to film distance.

(ii) **Simplicity:** The technique is easy to learn and also use.

The film holder and the position and the beam alignment indicating device helps to determine the vertical and horizontal angulations and eliminates chances of dimensional distortions and cone cuts.

(iii) **Duplication:** This technique is easy to standardise and can be accurately duplicated or repeated. Hence comparison of serial radiographs exposed using this technique have great validity.

(iv) The periapical tissues are well delineated with minimum elongation and shortening.

(v) There is decreased secondary radiation.

(vi) Crowns of teeth are well seen without overlap and hence proximal caries can be well detected.

(vii) Periodontal bone levels are well represented.

(viii) The positions of the film, the teeth and the x-ray beam can be maintained irrespective of head position and hence helpful in handicapped and compromised patients.

Disadvantages:

(i) **Film placement:** The film holding device is difficult to place and adjust especially in children and adults with a small mouth or shallow palates.

(ii) Positioning of the film holders in the mouth especially if narrow opening can be difficult.

Advantages:

1. Very little magnification is present and the images are geometrically accurate.
2. Superimposition of the zygomatic buttress is avoided and it is projected above the apices of molars.
3. The levels of the periodontal bone are well seen.
4. There is accurate depiction of the periapical tissues with minimal elongation and shortening.
5. The vertical and horizontal angulations are properly aligned due to the position indicating device and are automatically determined with little or no chances of cone cutting.
6. The radiographs can be reproducible at different visits with different operators.
7. As the position of the film, patient and the beam is always fixed, accurate radiographs are always possible and especially helpful in patients with disabilities.

Disadvantages:

1. Placing the film holder can be uncomfortable especially in the posterior teeth region also causing gagging sometimes.
2. Positioning the film holders can be difficult for inexperienced operators.
3. The anatomy of the mouth like the shallow, flat palate can some times make the technique difficult.
4. The apices of the teeth can sometimes be projected very near to the edge of the film.
5. The technique will be difficult to perform using a short F-S-F-D. as it can result in magnification.
6. The film holders have to be autoclavable or disposable.

Suggested reading:

1. Freny R Karjodkar page, Essentials of Dental and Maxillofacial Radiology, 2nd edition, 126.

Q 3) Bitewing Radiograph:

TNMGRU SEPTEMBER 2002 (5 Marks)

Give the indications of bitewing x-ray:

MUHS OCTOBER 2004 (2 Marks)

Advantages of bitewing radiograph:

MUHS MAY 2008 (2 Marks)

Bitewing examinations were introduced by Dr. Raper in 1925. Bitewing images focus on the clinical crowns of the maxillary and mandibular teeth. Bitewings do not show the apices of the tooth and cannot be used to diagnose in this area. It is also known as interproximal radiographs and include the crowns of the maxillary and mandibular teeth including the crest of the alveoli in the same film.

This technique is so called because of the tab used on which the patient bites to hold the film in place.

A pre-molar and molar film are taken on each side and thus total of four posterior radiographs are taken.

Indications:

MUHS OCTOBER 2004 (2 Marks)

- For detecting interproximal caries in the early stages of development.
- Secondary caries below restorations.
- Monitoring progression of dental caries.
- Evaluating periodontal conditions.
- They provide a good perspective of the crest of the alveolar bone and the changes in height can be accurately assessed through comparison with the adjacent teeth.
- Calculus deposit between teeth.

Principles:

- The film is placed in the mouth which is parallel to the crowns of the upper and lower teeth.
- The patient bites on the tab of the film holder to stabilise the film.
- The central x-ray beam is directed through the contact points of the teeth with a+10 vertical angulation.

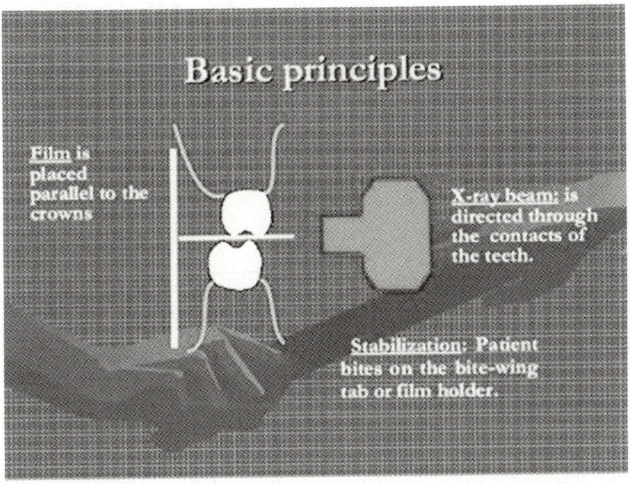

Fig. Basic principles of bitewing radiography

Film holder and bite wing tabs:

- The Rinn XCP bitewing instrument has a plastic bite block, aiming ring and a metal indicator arm.

- A snap ring collimator may be added to reduce the exposure to the patient.
- These holders are reusable.
- **Bite wing tab:** It is an alternative to a film holding device. A film can be fitted with a bite tab or bite loop. It is a very heavy paper board tab or loop with adhesive which may be attached to the white side of the periapical film. Readymade bitewing films with attached tabs are also available.

Bitewing films: Four sizes of the films are available.

- **Size 0:** It is used to x-ray the posterior teeth of children and are placed horizontally.
- **Size 1:** Its useful for examining posterior teeth in the cases of mixed dentition or anterior teeth of adults. It has to be placed horizontally for the former and vertically for the latter.
- **Size 2:** It is used to examine the posterior teeth of the adults and is always placed horizontally.
- **Size 4:** It is a longer and narrower film used only for the bite wing radiographs and spans horizontally the premolar to molar region.

Technique:

- The head is positioned normally in such a way that the maxillary arch is parallel to the floor and the mid-saggital plane is perpendicular to the floor.

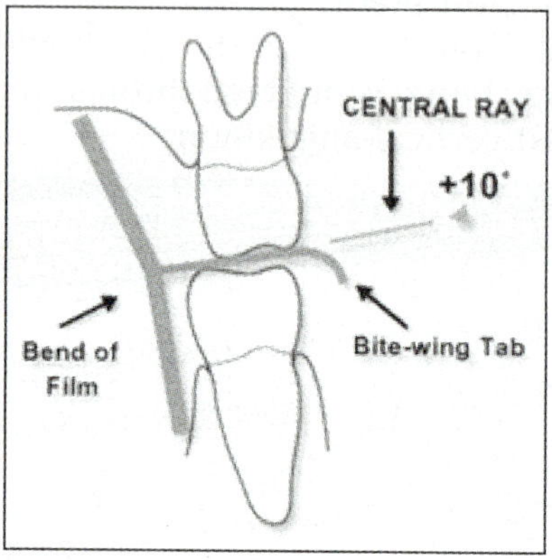

Fig. Placement of film and direction of central ray in bitewing radiography

Premolar bitewing technique:

(i) The film is placed so that it is centered on the second premolar and the front edge of the film should reach at least upto the middle of canine.
(ii) Hold the film in place until the patient's mouth is completely closed.
(iii) Holding the film while closing prevents it from being displaced distally.
(iv) The horizontal angulation is such that the central ray is directed to the centre of the film through the premolar contact areas.

(v) To compensate for the slight inclination of the film against the mucosa of the palate, the vertical angulation should be about +10 when using the bitewing tabs.

(vi) The central ray should penetrate at the level of the line of occlusion at the point of contact of the second premolar and the first molar.

Molar technique of bitewing:

(i) The distal margin of the film should extend about 1-2 mm beyond the most posterior erupted molar.

(ii) Project the central ray to the centre of the film and through the contact of the first and second maxillary molars.

(iii) A vertical angulation of +10 degrees is given.

(iv) The central ray should be directed through the cheek below the lateral canthus of the eye at the level of the occlusal plane.

Advantages:

MUHS MAY 2008 (2 Marks)

- Its a simple procedure to follow.
- Its inexpensive.
- As the tabs are disposable, no sterilisation protocol to be adopted.
- Easy to use in children.
- Good amount of information about the posterior teeth is obtained in just four radiographs.

Suggested reading:

1. Freny R Karjodkar, Essentials of Oral and Maxillofacial radiology, edition 1st, page 114-116.

Q 4) Indications for occlusal radiography:

RGUHS APRIL 2006 (4 Marks)

- Its a radiographic technique that is deviced in such a way that the film is placed between the occlusal surfaces of the teeth and the central x-ray beam is directed at 90 degree or at about 50-60 degrees to the plane of the film which depends upon the area to be radiographed.
- By this technique, larger areas of the maxillary and mandibular arches can be examined. The floor of the mouth and the palate can also be examined.
- This technique is used in coordination with periapical or bitewing radiographs.
- These films are available as D or E speed films or Insight 41 or 42 and the package and the contents are similar to the intra-oral films, but are 2.25 × 3 inches in size.

Indications:

- To examine the patients with trismus due to various causes, where in the patient can open the mouth only few millimetres, and intra-oral periapical radiography poses a difficulty.

- To locate the roots, supernumerary teeth, unerupted and impacted teeth and especially the impacted canines and the third molars.
- Location of roots of extracted teeth.
- The true occlusal view is used to locate teeth and other structures, tori, as well as foreign bodies in the maxilla and mandible, as it gives the location in bucco-lingual direction.
- Used in conjunction with other radiographic views for object localisation.
- To localise sialoliths in the submandibular or sublingual salivary glands.
- It can help in determining, demonstrating and evaluation of the anterior, medial and the lateral walls of the maxillary sinus and their integrity.
- To find out about the nature, location, displacement and its extent of the fractures of the mandible and the maxilla.
- To assess the medial and lateral extent of the diseases like the cysts, benign tumors, osteomyelitis, malignancies, and their extension on to the palate.
- To examine the region of the cleft palate.
- To assess and measure the changes in the size and shape of the maxilla.
- For detection of diseases involving the palate and the floor of the mouth.
- As a midline view for assessing the bucco-palatal or lingual positions of the unerupted canines.

Suggested reading:

1. Freny R Karjodkar, Essentials Of Oral And Maxillofacial Radiography, 2nd edition, page 193.

Q 5) How will you manage the problem of gagging in a patient during the periapical technique:

MUHS OCTOBER 2004 (2 Marks)

Quite a few times during intra-oral radiographic procedures a patient may experience a gag reflex on slightest provocation. Following protocol can be followed to manage this problem:

(i) An effort should be made to relax and reassure the patient.
(ii) procedure should be explained and described properly.
(iii) It can be controlled if the operator boosts the patient's confidence by way of technical competence, showing authority and compassion.
(iv) Patients, especially children if well rested can help control the gag reflex.
(v) The dorsum of the tongue and the soft palate are very sensitive and causes the gag reflex. Hence the tongue should be well relaxed and towards the floor of the mouth and can be accomplished by asking the patient to swallow deeply just before opening the mouth for film placement.

(vi) Film placement should be attempted with minimum stimulation of the sensitive structures.
(vii) The technique should be perfect and fast to reduce the chances of gagging.
(viii) This can be achieved by adjusting the patient position, the exposure parameters, placement of position indicating device, before the film is placed in the mouth so that exposure can be done fast and reduce the chances of gagging.
(ix) Breathing rapidly through the nose reduces the gag reflex and reverse is true for mouth breathing.
(x) Distracting the patient from the procedure without affecting the procedure can be helpful.
(xi) Patient can be asked to hold the breath and suspending a foot or arm during film placement can create a distraction.
(xii) In very severe cases, anesthetic spray can be used to produce numbness of tongue and palate.
(xiii) Best approach is to minimise tissue irritation, reduce apprehension, and encourage rapid breathing through the nose.
(xiv) As a last resort extra oral radiograph can be taken.

Suggested reading:

1. Stuart C White, Michael J Pharoah, Oral Radiology, Principles and Interpretation Fifth Edition, 163.

Q 6) Occlusal radiographs:

TNMGRU FEBRUARY 2014 (5 Marks)

It is a radiographic technique that shows larger areas of the maxillary and mandibular dental arches.

It may include the palate or floor of the mouth and a reasonable extent of the contiguous lateral structures.

The film is placed sandwiched between the occlusal surfaces and held in place by the patients teeth.

Film size is 7.7 × 5.8cm.

Indications:

(i) To locate accuartely the roots and supernumerary, unerupted and the impacted teeth.
(ii) To locate the foreign bodies in the jaws and the sialoliths in the ducts of the submandibular and sublingual glands.
(iii) Demonstrate and evaluate the integrity of walls of maxillary sinus.
(iii) To aid in the examination of patients with trismus.
(iv) To evaluate displacement of fractures of the mandible and maxilla.
(v) To assess the medial and the lateral extensions of the diseases like cysts, osteomyelitis, malignancies and also to detect the diseases of the palate and the floor of the mouth

Types of occlusal radiographs:

I) Anterior Maxillary Occlusal Projection:

- Patient's head is adjusted in such a way that the saggital plane is perpendicular to the floor and the occlusal plane is horizontal.
- Film is placed in the mouth with the exposure side toward the maxilla, the posterior border touching the rami, and the long dimension of the film perpendicular to the saggital plane.
- Central ray is directed from the nose tip towards the centre of the film with an angulation of +45 degrees vertical and 0 degree horizontal.

II) Cross-Sectional Maxillary Occlusal Projection:

- The patient sits upright with the sagittal plane perpendicular to the floor and the plane of occlusion horizontal.
- the film is placed, with its long dimension perpendicular to the sagittal plane, crosswise in the mouth and pushed backwards till it touches the anterior border of mandibular rami.
- The central ray is directed at a vertical angulation of +65 degrees and 0 degree horizontal angulation, toward the bridge of the nose below the nasion at the center of the film.

III) Lateral Maxillary Occlusal Projection:

- The film is placed with its long axis parallel to the sagittal plane and on the side of interest, with the tube side toward the side of the maxilla in question.
- Position the lateral border of the film parallel with the buccal surfaces of the posterior teeth, extending laterally approximately 1 cm past the buccal cusps. Patient holds the film by gently closing the mouth.
- The central ray is oriented with a vertical angulation of +60 degrees, to a point 2cms below the lateral canthus of the eye, and directed to the center of the film.

IV) Anterior Mandibular Occlusal Projection:

- The patient is seated tilted backwards so as to keep the occlusal plane at 45 degrees above the horizontal.
- The placement in the mouth is such that the long axis is perpendicular to the sagittal plane and is pushed posteriorly till it touches the rami.
- The film with the pebbled side is placed down and the patient is asked to bite gently to hold the film in position.
- Central ray is directed with a - 10 degree angulation from the point of the chin towards the center of the film.

V) Cross sectional mandibular occlusal projection:

- The patient is seated in a semireclining position with head tilted backwards so that the ala-tragus line is almost perpendicular to the floor.
- The film is placed in the mouth such that its long axis is perpendicular to the sagittal plane and the tube side facing the mandible.

- The anterior border of the film should project about 1cm beyond the mandibular incisors.
- The central ray is directed in the midline through the floor of the mouth about 3cm below the chin.

VI) Lateral Mandibular Occlusal Projection:

- Patient is seated in a semireclining position with the head thrown back so that the ala-tragus line is perpendicular to the floor
- The placement of film in the mouth is such that its long axis is parallel to the sagittal plane and with the pebbled side down toward the mandible.
- The lateral border of the film is parallel in relation to the buccal surfaces of the posterior teeth and it extends laterally about 1cm.
- Central ray is directed perpendicular to the middle of the film through a point under the chin, about 3cms posterior to the and 3cm lateral to the midline.

Suggested reading:

1. Stuart. C White, Michael. J. Pharaoh, Oral Radiology Principles And Interpretation, 5th edition, 154-160.

Q 7) Describe the radiographic technique of making a bite wing radiograph of molar region:

MUHS NOVEMBER 2013 (3 Marks)

Bitewing technique is so called because a 'bitewing' or a 'bitetab' is attached to the film on which the patient is made to bite.

Bitewing radiographs have been used in dental practice for many decades.

The central ray is targeted interocclusally with the mouth closed.

These radiographs can be used to answer many questions concerning health and/ or disease in the posterior regions of mandible and maxilla.

Most frequently, however, bitewing images are used for the early detection/diagnosis of proximal carious lesions, because the roentgen rays target the proximal surfaces tangentially and loss of hard substance can be noted early as a radiolucency (or subtraction effect) in dental enamel.

Patient positioning: The patient sits upright with the head straight and not inclined to any one side.

Image field: This projection should show the distal surface of the most posterior erupted molar and equally the crowns of the maxillary and mandibular molars. Because the maxillary and mandibular molar contact areas may not be open from the same horizontal angulation, they may not be visible on one film. In this case it may be desirable to open the maxillary molar contacts because the mandibular molar contacts usually are open on the periapical films.

Placement of image receptor: Image receptor is placed on the lingual side of the maxillary and mandibular teeth such that it is parallel to the long axes of the teeth. Further, the receptor should be kept very close to the teeth to be examined.

For the molar projection, the anterior edge of the receptor should cover the distal half of the second mandibular premolar.

The distal margin of the film should extend 1 to 2 mm beyond the most posterior erupted molar.

Direction of Central Ray: The central ray is directed perpendicular (in both vertical and horizontal planes) to the film. A slight positive angulation (+5) may be given if maxillary teeth are the prime concern.

Centering Point:

For the molar projection, the central ray should enter the proximal contact between the 1st and the 2nd molars at the level of the occlusal plane.

The central ray should be projected to the center of the film and through the contact of the first and second maxillary molars. The central ray should be angled slightly from the anterior because the molar contacts usually are not oriented at right angles to the buccal surfaces of these teeth. A vertical angulation of +10 degrees is recommended.

Exposure Parameters:

- Tube voltage = 65 kVp
- Tube Current = 10 mA
- Exposure time = 0.3 S for molars.
- TID = 20 cms
- Type & Size of film = Non-screen film, size 2 for molar projections.

Suggested reading:

1. Stuart C White, Michael J Pharoah, Oral Radiology, Principles and Interpretation 5th Edition, 150-153.

CHAPTER **11**

Radiographic Anatomy

Introduction:

The radiographic recognition of disease requires a sound knowledge of the radiographic appearance of normal structures. Intelligent diagnosis mandates an appreciation of the wide range of variation in the appearance of normal anatomic structures.

Similarly, most patients demonstrate many of the normal radiographic landmarks, but it is a rare patient who shows them all.

Accordingly, the absence of one or even several such landmarks in any individual should not necessarily be considered abnormal.

Q 1) Lamina Dura:

TNMGRU AUGUST 2014 (5 Marks)

Normal radiograph of a sound tooth would demonstrate presence of thin layer of dense bone surrounding the roots which is termed lamina dura. The name lamina dura or hard layer is so termed as it appears more radiopaque than the adjacent bone.

This layer is in continuity with the shadow of the bony cortex at the level of the crest of the alveolus.

It is just a little more thicker and similarly mineralised as the trabeculae of the cancellous bone in the area.

The radiopaque appearance radiographically is due to the x-ray beam that passes tangentially through the thin bony wall many times its thickness which results in the attenuation that is observed.

The lamina dura, developmentally is an extension of the thin bony crypt lining that surrounds the teeth during development.

There could be varied appearance of the lamina dura on the radiographs.

A statistical evaluation of the full mouth radiographs of about 300 individuals revealed that the appearance, the structural characteristics, and the degree of radiopacity of the lamina dura, depends on the rate of eruption of teeth and changes with each stage of eruption.

The radiopacity of the lamina dura around the actively erupting tooth is as great as the much thicker and more highly calcified dentin in the same film.

As the tooth comes into full clinical occlusion and the rate of eruption slows down, the lamina dura becomes thinner and much less radiopaque.

The lamina dura appears well defined and radiopaque when the x-rays are directed through a relatively long expanse of the structure.

It is less prominent in the upper incisor region than in the bicuspid and molar regions in the same arch, probably because the proper angulation is more difficult in the incisor area.

However when the x-ray beam is directed obliquely, the lamina dura may appear more diffuse and may not be visible to the eye.

Though the bone surrounding the root socket could be intact in a healthy arch, the lamina dura surrounding completely every root, may be difficult to identify on exact film but is evident to a certain extent about the roots on each film.

Superimpositions of the trabecular pattern and small nutrient canals passing from the mandibular bone to the periodontal ligament, may cause small variations and disruptions in the continuity of the lamina dura.

The occlusal stress to which, each tooth is subjected to, can cause variations in the thickness and density of the lamina dura on the radiograph.

The teeth subjected to greater occlusal stress will show lamina dura that is wider and more dense than on the teeth subjected to lesser occlusal stress.

The image of a double lamina dura is not uncommon in case the mesial or the distal surfaces of the roots present two elevations in the path of the x-ray beam.

This is commonly seen with the mandibular first molar, due to the buccal and lingual eminences on the mesial surface.

The removal of an antagonistic tooth leads to supra eruption of a tooth and in such cases the lamina dura becomes markedly accentuated in thickness and radiopacity during the period of occlusal movement.

The lamina dura is absent about teeth which are embedded or so ankylosed that they cannot migrate.

The presence of lamina dura in the radiographs is an important diagnostic feature. In case of an intact lamina dura around the apex of the tooth, suggests positively the presence of a vital pulp.

As the appearance of lamina dura on the radiograph can be variable its absence in some cases, can be considered normal.

In some cases even in the absence of disease the lamina dura could be absent around the apex of a molar tooth seeming to extend in to the maxillary sinus.

Hence its important for a clinician to take other signs and symptoms, along with the integrity of the lamina dura, while establishing a diagnosis and treatment plan.

The absence or diminution of lamina dura may suggest presence of pathosis like hyperparathyroidism, osteoporosis, paget's disease and periapical or periodontal infection.

Various studies indicate that lamina dura is affected very early in nutritional deficiencies.

An early sign of a diffuse alveolar atrophy or a generalised alveloclasia is the disappearance of lamina dura.

Whereas the density increase in lamina dura could be suggestive of occlusal traumatism.

Suggested reading:

1. Stuart C White And Michael .J Pharaoh, Oral Radiology, Principles And Interpretation, 5th edition, 168-169.
2. Tanwar Renu, Panwar Rajneesh, Lamina Dura In Health And Disease, Journal of Oral SignYear: 2012, Volume: 4, Issue: 1, page 21-22.

Q 2) Normal anatomical landmarks in maxillary anterior region on intraoral x- ray film:

MUHS MAY 2012 (2 Marks)

Normal anatomical structures:

Enamel: appears most radiopaque.

Dentin: appears less radiopaque than enamel.

Lamina dura: Appears as a radiopaque line surrounding the tooth sockets.

Alveolar crest: appears as a thin opaque layer of bone around teeth as it is composed of dense cortical bone.

Trabeculae: thin radiopaque rods and plates that surround several small radiolucent pockets of marrow.

Pulp: composed of soft tissue and consequently appears radiolucent.

Periodontal ligament space: appears as a space that is radiolucent space between the tooth root and the lamina dura.

Anterior radiolucent land marks of the maxilla:

- **Intermaxillary suture:** It appears as a thin line that is radiolucent in the midline between two parts of the premaxilla.
- **Incisive foramen:** seen as oval radiolucency between maxillary central incisors and is the terminus in the oral cavity of the nasopalatine canal.
  - Lateral fossa: Its a shallow depression in the maxilla near the apex of the lateral incisor.
- **Nasal cavity:** Radiolucent cavity above the central incisors.
  - Nasopalatine canal: can be recognized as two areas of radiolucency above the apices of the central incisors in the region of the floor of the nasal cavity near its border and on both sides of the septum.

Anterior radiopaque landmarks of maxilla:

- **Anterior nasal spine:** It is radiopaque because of its bony composition and is usually V-shaped.
- **Floor of the nasal fossa:** appears as line of radiopacity which extends bilaterally away from the base of the anterior nasal spine.
- **Median nasal septum:** arises directly above the anterior nasal spine.

- **Inferior nasal choncha:** seen as radiopaque structure in the nasal fossa in anterior maxillary radiograph.

Suggested reading:

1. Stuart C White, Michael J Pharoah, Oral Radiology, Principles and Interpretation, Fifth Edition, 166-176.

Q 3) Enumerate normal anatomical landmarks in mandibular anterior area as seen in IOPA:

MUHS NOVEMBER 2013 (3 Marks)

Normal anatomical structures:

Enamel: appears most radiopaque.

Dentin: appears less radioopaque than enamel.

Lamina dura: Appears as radiopaque line surrounding the root socket.

Alveolar crest: appears as a thin opaque layer of bone around teeth as it is composed of dense cortical bone.

Trabeculae: They are thin plates and rods surrounding several small pockets of radiolucent bone marrow.

Pulp: It is composed of soft tissue and hence is radiolucent.

Periodontal ligament space: Its a thin radiolucent space which appears between the root of the tooth and the lamina dura.

Anatomical landmarks:

I) Anterior radiopaque landmarks:

- **Genial Tubercles:** The genial tubercles (also called the mental spine) are located on the lingual surface of the mandible slightly above the inferior border and in the midline.
- **Mental Ridge:** On periapical radiographs of the mandibular central incisors, the mental ridge (protuberance) may occasionally be seen as two lines of radiopacity which extends bilaterally forward and upward toward the midline.

II) Anterior radiolucent landmarks:

- **Symphysis:**
  A thin radiolucent line through the midline of the jaws between the images of the developing deciduous central incisors.
  This suture generally closes by the end of the first year of life.
- **The lingual foramen:**
  Its a small radiolucent dot like appearance that is located below the apices of the mandibular incisors.
- **Nutrient canals:**
  These are slender vertical lines of radiolucency which is more prominent in the anterior region.
- **Mental fossa:**
  A radiolucent region that appears above the mental ridge.

Suggested reading:

1. Stuart. C White, Michael. J. Pharaoh, Oral Radiology Principles and Interpretation, 181-183.

CHAPTER 12

Faulty Radiographs

Introduction:

Faulty radiographs can result either due to faulty technique or improper processing. It can hamper the diagnostic quality of a radiograph. It is necessary to know the errors in radiography and their causes so that they can be avoided in future.

Q 1) Faulty radiographs:

TNMGRU AUGUST 2015 (5 Marks)

Faulty radiographs can be either due to improper radiographic procedure, improper processing, or artefacts. In either case their diagnostic value is lessened and knowledge of faulty radiographs is essential because certain artifacts if not known about can lead to misdiagnosis.

Following are some errors in radiography:

(i) **Foreshortening of the image:** It refers to shortening of the images of objects. In intraoral radiography the teeth will appear shorter than normal. This occurs due to excessive vertical angulation.

(ii) **Elongated images:** The image appears elongated. In intraoral radiographs the teeth appear too long. It occurs due to decreased vertical angulation.
Elongation of few teeth can occur due to too much bending of the film while attempting to place in the mouth.In the bent portion the image appears elongated.

(iii) **Overlapping of crowns:** Overlapping of crowns can occur due to improper horizontal angulation. This especially hampers proper diagnosis of proximal caries.

(iv) **Slanting of occlusal plane:** When the film is not placed properly parallel to the occlusal plane, it gives a slanting appearance in the film.

(v) **Partial image:** The image on the film is partly seen and either the crown portion is cut off or the periapical region is not completely visualised due to improper placement of the film. Partial image can also be seen due to the film sticking to the tank during developing. The developer is prevented from coming in contact with the film and hence image is seen partly.

(vi) **Light film:** The film may appear light due to inadequate exposure time or less milliamperage and kVp and also due to lesser time in the developer or keeping it too long in the fixer.

(vii) **Dark radiographs:** These may result due to over exposure, and excessive milliamperage and kVp. It can also occur due to keeping for a longer time in developing solution.
This can also occur due to accidental exposure of the film to light before processing.

(viii) **Blurred image:** Blurred and ill defined images can occur due to movement of the film, x-ray tube, or patient, during shooting of radiographs.

(ix) **Herring bone, car-tyre or tyre track appearance:** When the film is kept reverse, that is the lead side facing the x-ray tube, the films appear lighter and also show patterns embossed on lead on that particular type of intraoral film.

(x) **Film creasing:** Excessive pressure on film while placement can result in a crack in the emulsion causing a radiolucent line on the film.

(xi) **Nail marks:** Curved dark marks can be seen on some radiographs due to excess pressure of nails which cause the emulsion to break in that area.

(xii) **Double image:** Some radiographs may show double image due to exposing the film which has already been exposed once.

(xiii) **Film fog:** Fogging of film refers to a film which appears dark grayish and lacks image detail and contrast. This occurs due to improper safe lighting conditions, light leakage, improper storage of films, expired or out dated films, contaminated processing solutions, or high temperature of developing solution.

(xiv) **Insufficient contrast:** Occurs due to underdevelopment, underexposure, excessive kVp, excessive film fog.

(xv) **Yellowish or Brown stains:** These can occur on films due to inadequate washing with water after fixing, depleted developer or depleted fixer, or contaminated solutions.
Brownish discoloration of the film can also occur due to inadequate fixing due to which there is reaction of the unexposed silver halide crystals remaining on the film with light. Hence for longer radiographic life the film should be kept in the fixer solution for optimum time.

(xvi) **Light spots:** Film contaminated with drops of fixer before processing. Can occur also due to film in contact with tank or another film during processing.

(xvii) **Emulsion peel:** Can occur due to abrasion of image during processing and excess time in wash water.

(xviii) **Dark spots or lines:** Could occur due to fingerprint contamination, black wrapping paper sticking to film surface, film in contact with tank or another film during fixing.

(xix) **Phalange image:** While taking intraoral radiograph the image of the finger that holds the film can be visible on the radiograph and should be recognised as such, also called as phalangioma.

(xx) **Static electricity:** Rapid removal of films from the packet or cassette can result in dark leafless branches like appearance on the film which is due to exposure of the film by production of static electricity produced due to friction.

(xxi) **Images of clips, earrings, necklaces:** It is important to recognise these images, especially in extraoral radiography, which can occur due to failure to remove the accessories before taking the radiograph.

Suggested reading:

1. Pramod John R, Essentials Of Dental Radiology, page 69-71.
2. Stuart. C. white & Michael J. Pharaoh, oral radiology, principles and interpretation, fifth edition, 105-107.

Q 2) Enumerate various radiographic artefacts.

MUHS MAY 2012 (3 Marks)

An artifact is an appearance or a structure on the radiograph which is not present normally on a radiograph and is produced by artificial means.

Following are various radiographic artifacts:

1. Pressure from incisal edges and cusp of teeth gives pressure marks and may appear as black or white.
2. **Double image:** When the film is exposed twice the reexposure results in superimposed images.
3. **Tyre track pattern / herring bone pattern:** It can occur when the x-rays are passed through the lead foil side of the film.
4. **Embossed dot artifact:** It produces a circular radiolucent artifact on radiograph.
5. **Black line:** Excessive bending of film.
6. **Reticulation:** Cracked appearance on film- due to sudden changes in temperature of developer and fixer.
7. **Black spot:** When the film gets contaminated by a developer before immersing into the developer.
8. **Brown Stains of fixer:** Due to improper fixing.
9. **White spot or patch:** when the film gets contaminated by a fixer before processing.
10. **Yellowish brown discoloration:** Due to insufficient rinsing.
11. **Writing lines:** Due to writing on film packets.
12. **Finger nail artifacts:** Black / white crescent shaped mark which occurs due to rough and careless handling of films.
13. **Developer cut off:** A straight blank or white border on the film due to either undeveloped or under developed part. It happens when the film is not completely immersed in the developer.
14. **Fixer cut off:** When the film is not completely immersed in the fixer solution.

15. **Overlapping of films:** Films which overlap in developer are white, while those overlapping in fixer are black.
16. **Finger print or smudge marks:** When the film is touched by fingers that are contaminated by fixer or developer.
17. **Scratched film:** White lines appear on the film due to scratches as a result of careless handling of films. In case of automatic processors due to foreign objects on roller.
18. **Static electricity:** due to films forcibly unwrapped. These are seen in dry or hot environment and appear as black branchless tree like appearance. Due to rapid removal of the film especially the screen films.
19. Images of body piercing like nose ring, ear rings, clips, jewellery more commonly seen in extraoral radiographs.
20. In panoramic radiographs ghost images of objects that are in the line of x-rays but out of focal trough are seen.
21. Roller marks seen on films when automatic processors are used.
22. Drying pattern on the film surface due to high temperature of dryer in automatic film processors.
23. **Dark flow marks:** occur due to vigorous agitation of film in the solutions.
24. Emulsion peel can occur due to abrasion of the image during processing and in automatic processors due to high temperature of developer.
25. **Phalangioma:** Image of patient's finger on the film due to holding of the film.
26. In computed tomography images, Ring artefact caused by miscalibrated or defective detector element, noise, seen as thin bright and dark streaks, metal artifacts and out of field artefact due to suboptimal algorithm can be seen.

Suggested reading:

1. Pramod John R, Essentials of dental radiology, 68-74.

Q 3) What Do You Mean By Cone Cutting In Intraoral Periapical Radiography?

MUHS NOVEMBER 2013 3Marks

For taking an ideal radiograph the object of interest has to be placed on the centre of the film and the direction of the central ray has to be towards the center of the receptor, with the x-ray beam directed perpendicular to the film.

When proper care is not taken to direct the central ray, and the placement of the object in the center of the film a cone cut occurs. After processing of such films it appears as a clear zone on the traditional radiographs because of the lack of exposure in the area of cone cut.

When the digital radiographs are made the cone cut occurs as a white or opaque area. The type of collimator used while exposing the film decides the shape of the cone cut.In case a round collimator is used, the cone cut will appear curved and will appear square when a rectangular collimator is used.

In order to correct a cone cut, the x-ray beam should be re-centered towards the center of the film. When the film holding devices are not placed properly, cone cuts can occur.

When placing the devices, it should be ensured that the entire film shall be visible while looking through the indicator ring.

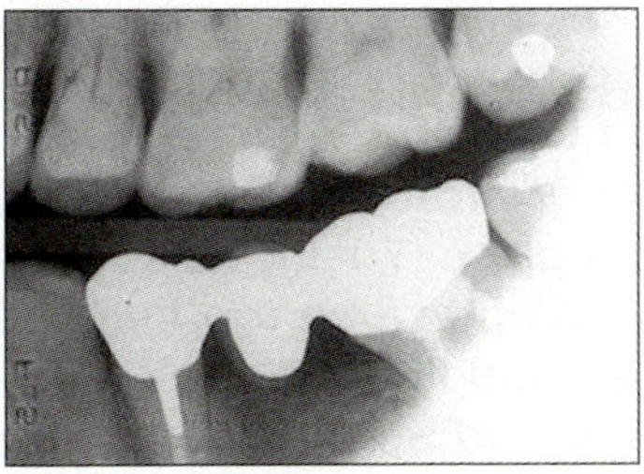

Fig. White area of cone cut

Suggested reading:

1. Freny R Karjodkar, Textbook Of Dental And Maxillofacial Radiology, 2nd Edition, 94-95.

Q 4) What are the causes of fog on radiograph:

MUHS DECEMBER 2005 2 Marks

Fog on an X-ray film results in increased film density arising from causes other than exposure to the resultant film.

Causes of film fogging are:

1. **Light**
   - Light leaks in the dark room.
     Check vents, doors, walls for leaks, cracked safe light filter.
   - *Improper safe light:* Reduce wattage of the bulb, keep adequate distance of 4 feet between safe light and working area.
   - *Turning over head (white) light on too soon:* The film should be fixed for 1-2 min before turning on the light.
   - *Prolonged exposure of film to the safe light:* Reduce exposure time of film to the safe light.
   - *Improper safe light filter:* Filters for safe lights should be used as per recommendations. They should be checked from time to time for any cracks which can lead to film fog. If need be they should be replaced.
2. **Radiation:**
   - Insufficient protection of films from radiation.
     Scattered radiation can cause fogging of film if not stored properly. Unexposed films should be stored in lead boxes.

3. **Chemical:**
   - *Developer temperature too high:* Reduce temperature of developer to manufacturer's optimum temperature (70° F).
   - *Strength of developer:* Check tank capacity and mixing directions.
   - *Prolonged development:* Developing by time temperature method will reduce the chances of film fog.
   - *Contaminated developer:* Developer tank should be cleaned periodically to help prevent contamination of the solution and thus reduce chances of film fog.
4. **Deterioration of the film:**
   - *Temperature of storage area too high:* The films should be stored at cool place (70° F).
   - *Humidity of storage area too high:* Store the film in dry place (50% relative humidity).
   - *Strong fumes and smoke:* Films should be kept away from fumes like those of ammonia, fresh paint and smoking.
   - *Exposed to radiations:* Unexposed film should be stored away from source of radiation in a protective compartment. Preferably should be stored in lead container.
   - *Outdated films:* Films should be used before expiry date mentioned on the packet. If not used before that should be discarded. Films supply should be according to need so that they are utilized properly and within time.
5. **Improper film screen combination:**
   Specially when using high speed film the manufacturer's recommended combination should be followed.

Suggested reading:

1. Freny R Karjodkar, Text book of dental and maxillofacial radiology, chapter 8, pg no.101-102.

CHAPTER 13

Panoramic Radiography

Q 1) Image layer or focal trough:

MUHS NOVEMBER 2006 (2 Marks)

Can be defined as a three dimensional curved zone, the structures when placed in the centre of this zone are clearly demonstrated on panoramic radiograph.

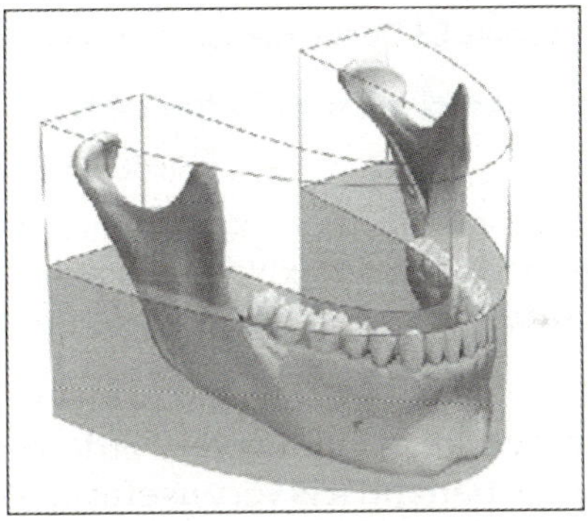

Fig. Focal trough

It is a horse shoe shaped imaginary zone.

While taking an orthopantomograph the mandible and the maxilla should be placed within the focal trough, if not the image will be blurred or indistinct.

If the jaws are placed within the focal trough the image will be clear.

Image layer thickness depends upon the effective radius of projection and width of the x-ray beam.

Knowledge about focal trough is important as many technical errors can occur due improper positioning of jaws within the focal trough.

(i) When the object is in front of the focal trough it will become narrow and elongated.

(ii) When the object is placed behind the focal trough it becomes magnified mesiolaterally.

(iii) Object within the focal trough is depicted correctly.

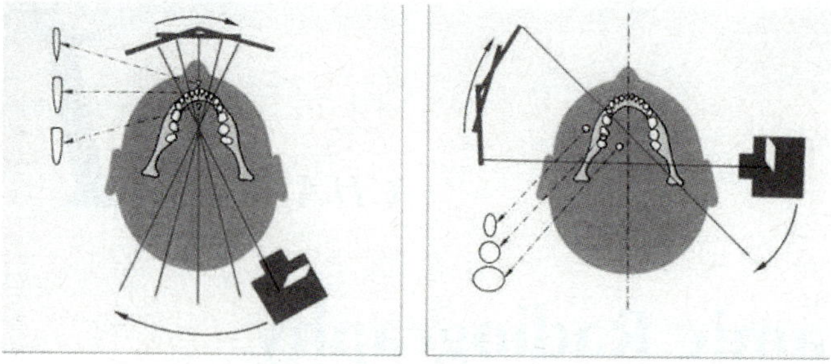

Fig. Distortion of images when objects are placed ahead or behind the focal trough

Thickness of the focal trough varies with different machines and manufacturers. In most cases it is narrower in the anterior than the posterior arch region.

The closer the center of rotation to teeth, narrower the focal trough.

The focal trough is also referred as focal corridor many a times.

Objects that lie in the line of x-rays but are outside the focal trough cause ghost images.

Suggested reading:

1. Eric Whaites, Essentials Of Dental Radiography and Radiology.3rd edition, 168.

Q 2) Advantages and disadvantages of OPG:

TNMGRU AUGUST 2011 6 Marks

Ortho pantomography is a form of rotational tomography that produces a single tomographic image of the maxillo facial structures that includes the maxilla and mandible and their supporting structures.

Advantages:

- Its a simple procedure requiring very little patient compliance.
- Convenient for the patient. It is very useful in patients having difficulty in opening the mouth and those who have a severe gag reflex.
- It consumes less time and is more convenient than the full mouth radiography.
- The exposure is much less almost 10 times than the full mouth radiography.
- The maxilla and mandible portions lying within the focal trough can be visualised on a single film.
- Patient's x ray dose is relatively low.
- Diagnostic panoramic radiographs can act as very good visual aid for the patient education.
- There is broad anatomic coverage, and along with the teeth and its supporting structures, the entire maxillary, mandibular along with the temporomandibular joint region is visualised.
- On the same film, styloid process, hyoid bone and pharyngeal airspace can be visualised.
- The anatomical structures are clearly identifiable and the teeth are

oriented in their correct relationship to the adjacent structures and to each other.

- Multiple lesions when present can be seen on a single film.
- The position of unerupted teeth can be assessed for orthodontic treatment.
- Generalised periodontal disease and bone loss can be assessed on one film.
- As all parameters are standardised, it helps in comparing the films especially to assess treatment outcomes.
- Useful for mass screening. Helpful for localisation of the objects/ pathology with the help of occlusal or intraoral films.

Disadvantages:

- Areas of diagnostic interest outside the focal trough may be poorly visualised.
- Due to inherent magnification, geometric distortion, poor definition, and loss of detail, the film may lack high diagnostic quality.
- Overlapping of teeth in the maxillary and mandibular bicuspid area is seen.
- Severe proclination of anterior teeth may result in poor images of this region.
- The overlapping of the spine can result in lack of clear image in the central portion of the film.
- Confusing radiopaque and radiolucent shadows may be present due to superimposition of real/double or ghost images and also due to the shadows of the soft tissues and the air spaces.
- In patients with facial asymmetry the image may not be satisfactory.
- Artifacts are more commonly seen and are misinterpreted easily on an OPG film.
- The joint spaces of TMJ cannot be accurately assessed.
- Cost and maintenance of machine is high.
- The ease of obtaining the the OPG may lead to carelessness in evaluation of the patients specific needs.

Suggested reading:

1. Freny. R Karjodkar, Text Book Of Dental And Maxillofacial Radiology, 2nd edition, 247-248.

Q 3) Ghost Images:

TNMGRU FEBRUARY 2013 (5 Marks)

Ghost Image:

A ghost image occurs when the object of interest is placed between the source of x-ray and the center of rotation.

They have the following six characteristics:

1. The image has the similar shape as that of its real counterpart.

2. It appears on the opposite side of the x-ray film from the real counterpart.
3. Appears higher up on the radiograph than its real counterpart.
4. The image is more blurred than that of the real counterpart.
5. The vertical component of the image is more blurred than the horizontal component.
6. The vertical component of the image is almost always larger than its counterpart, whereas the horizontal component may or may not be severely magnified.

Structures that generally appear as ghost images:

The anatomical structures:

- The hyoid bone.
- Cervical spine.
- The inferior border of the mandible.
- Posterior border of the mandible,
- Auditive canal / meatuses,
- Turbinates,
- Mastoid apophysis.

The non-anatomical structures:

- Chin rest,
- Right and left edges / markers of some apparatuses.
- Earrings, pins, necklaces and napkin chains.
- Hearing prostheses.
- Shoulder straps of lead aprons.

The Formation Of Ghost Images:

- It is formed of objects that are in the line of the x-ray beam but out of focal trough.

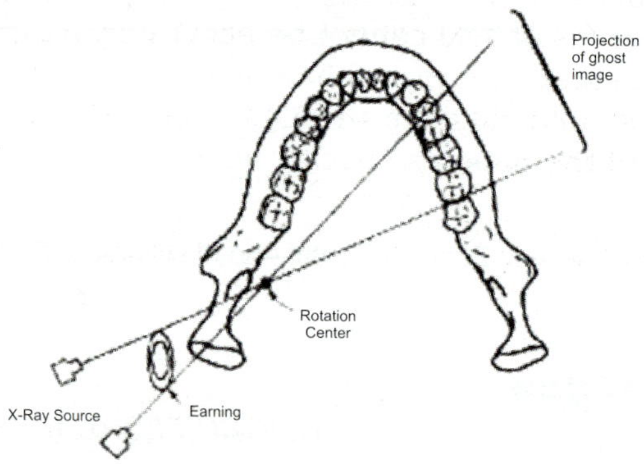

Fig. Formation of ghost image

- Structures like the spine, and horns of the hyoid usually produce ghost images. Though with advanced techniques these can be minimized but are inevitable in some cases. Eg in case of an edentulous patient who have relatively thin soft tissues, it is quite common for the formation of ghost image of the mandibular ramus to be seen clearly in a magnified form on the contralateral side of the body of the mandible.

- The projection geometry of most panoramic machines is such that the ghost images are not seen in an image of a properly positioned patient. Non anatomic structures include those of earrings, coat zippers, necklaces, hairpins etc.
- The ghost images of the earrings are often magnified and appear over the region of the maxillary sinus and the mandibular body on the side opposite to the radiographic image. Orientation decides their actual appearance.
- In case the earring is on one side only and solid, its ghost image might be confused with an odontoma or other conditions with radiopacity.
- Ghost images can also be formed due to bullets or shrapnels in the soft tissues and they appear magnified and in the contralateral position in the panoramic image. Knowledge about this is important.
- There can be tongue piercings and rings in the center of the tongue and their ghost image can be projected upwards in the nasal passageway. The position of the ghost image depends on the position of the tongue.

Precautions To Avoid Error of Ghost Image:

- Generally, the presence of ghost images is the result of technique errors. Recognition of these undesirable ghost images helps to identify and eliminate technique errors.
- In edentulous patients as the soft tissue is thin, the mandibular rami can be projected as ghost images over the contralateral body of the mandible in a magnified form.
- The formation of ghost images is usual in panoramic radiography and may not be considered as an error in technique.
- Though the ghost images of some anatomic structures cannot always be avoided, quite a few of them can be excluded or reduced with proper technique.
- The ghost image of the cervical spine can be undesirable and is cast in the mandibular incisor teeth region, which can be avoided by asking the patient to stand or sit straight with out slouching and the neck straight and extended. In case the neck is slouched, the x-rays traverse several vertebrae while recording the image of mandibular incisors and obscure them with their opaque shadow.
- The best way to prevent ghost images of non-anatomical structures is to remove them before exposure.

Suggested reading:

1. Allan G. Farman, Panoramic imaging news, volume2, issue 1.
2. Kaugars GE, Collet WK. Panoramic ghosts. Oral Surg Oral Med Oral Pathol 1987; 63:103–108.

CHAPTER 14

Extraoral Radiographic Techniques

Introduction:

In extraoral radiographic examinations both the x-ray source and image receptor (film or electronic sensor) are placed outside the patient's mouth.

These include the lateral cephalometric projection of the sagittal or median plane, the submentovertex projection, Waters view, Reverse Towne's view, panoramic radiography and the oblique lateral projections of the mandibular body and ramus etc.

Q 1) Water's projection:

TNMGRU AUGUST 2013 (5 Marks)

Water's view also known as occipito-mental view is a postero-anterior view which is generally indicated to view the maxillary sinuses.

Indications:

(i) Evaluating maxillary sinuses.

(ii) Demonstrate the frontal and ethmoidal sinuses, orbit, the zygomatico frontal suture, and the nasal cavity.

(iii) Position of the coronoid of the mandible between the maxilla and the zygomatic arch.

(iv) Detecting the following middle third facial fractures:

- Le Fort 1
- Le Fort 2
- Le Fort 3
- Zygomatic complex
- Naso-ethmoidal complex
- Orbital blow out

Technique:

Image Receptor and Patient Placement:

The mid-sagittal plane of the patient should be positioned vertically and perpendicular to the film.

The head of the patient is extended such that the chin touches the cassette.

The centering of the cassette is around the acanthion.

The canthomeatal line forms a 37 degree angle with the plane of the ilm and the line joining the mental protuberance and the external auditory neatus should be perpendicular to the film.

The aim of this position is to extend the patient's head just enough so as to place the dense shadows of the petrous bone immediately below the antral floors.

When the head is extended too little the petrosal shadows are projected on to the lower part of the antrum.

When the head is extended too far back then the antral shadows are oreshortened and results in failure to show the antral floor.

In the year 1915, Water's suggested that the tip of the nose should be 0.5-1.5 cms away from the cassette. According to Mahoney in 1930, it was found that the shadow of the petrous bone can be correctly placed by adjusting the orbito-meatal line at 37 degrees to the horizontal.

If the patient's mouth is open, the sphenoid sinus will be seen superimposed over the palate.

Central x-ray beam position:

The central ray of the x-ray beam should be perpendicular to the image receptor and centered in the area of the maxillary. The x-ray cone is placed 2 cms above the occipital protuberance and x-rays travel through the middle of the maxillary sinus and on to the film. The x-rays thus enters from the vertex and exits through the acanthion. (anterior nasal spine)

Exposure Parameters:

KVp: 70-80
Ma: 10
Seconds: 1.6.

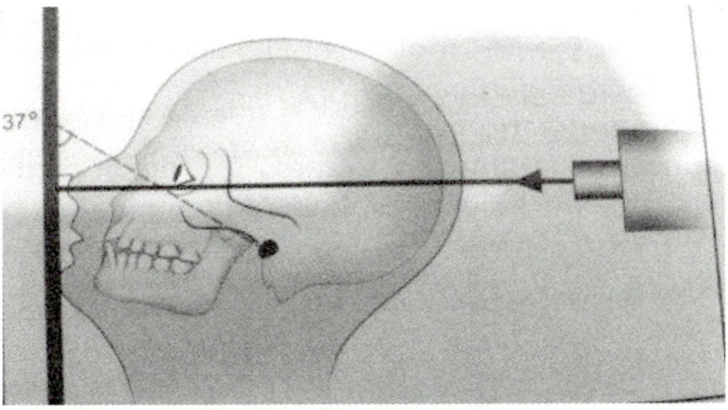

Fig. Canthomeatal line 37° above the horizontal plane, forming 37° angle with the film

Suggested reading:

1. Freny. R. Karjodkar, Essentials of Oral and Maxillofacial Radiology, 2nd edition, page 216.
2. Stuart C White, Michael J Pharoah, Oral Radiology, Principles and Interpretation 5th Edition, page 213.

Q 2) Lateral oblique view of mandible:

TNMGRU FEBRUARY 2007 (5 Marks

An open ended cylinder for aiming on a dental x-ray machine is mos suitable for this projection.

Film size is usually 5 × 7 inches and screen film is used.

Cassette should be hand held by the patient.

Consists of two projections:

1. Mandibular body projection.
2. Mandibular ramus projection.

Indications:

1. Lateral oblique view of the mandibular body:
   - Impacted teeth evaluation, fracture and lesions located in the body of the mandible.
   - Demonstrate the regions of the mandibular premolar anc molar regions and the inferior border of the mandible.
2. Lateral oblique view of ramus:
   - Impacted third molar evaluation, large lesions and fracture that extend into the ramus of the mandible.
   - Demonstrate the ramus view from the region of angle of the mandible to the condyle.

Technique:

1. **Body of mandible:**

   Head position:

   The head is tilted towards the side to be examined and the patient is asked to protrude the mandible.

   Film placement:

   Centered over the first molar, parallel and 2 cms below the inferior border of the mandible.

   Central ray projection:

   The central ray is directed towards the molar-premolar area at a point about 2cms below the angle of the mandible of the opposite side.

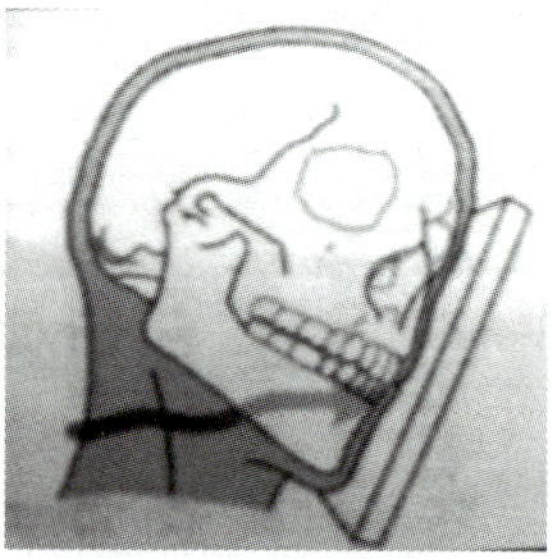

Fig. Head, cassette placement and central ray direction for lateral oblique view of body of mandible

A clear image of the teeth, alveolar ridges and the body of mandible can be obtained by the right technique.In case of distortion the reason could be excessive tilting of head and if there is superimposition of the other side of the mandible, it indicates inadequate tilting of head.

2. **Mandibular ramus:**

Position of the head:

The patient is asked to tilt the head towards the side to be examined such that the condyle of the area of interest and the contra lateral angle of the mandible form horizontal line.

To prevent superimposition of cervical spine on ramus protrude the mandible.

Film placement:

Placed over the ramus and far enough posteriorly to include the condyle .

Projection of the central ray:

Towards the center of the imaged ramus, from 2cm below the inferior border of the opposite side of the mandibular at the area of the first molar.

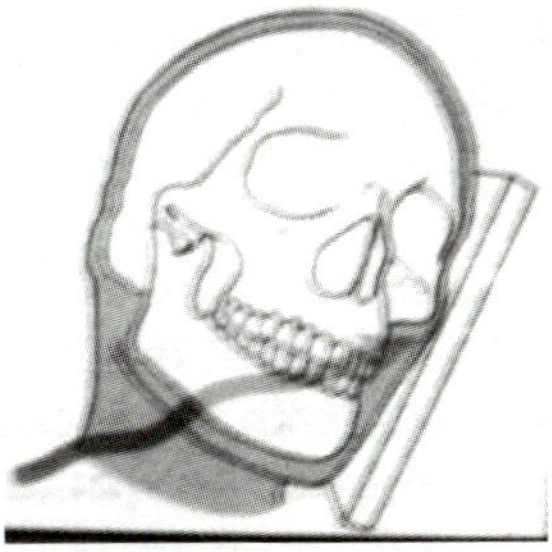

Fig. Head position, film placement and direction of central ray for ramus of mandible

If radiographs correctly taken then the third molar-retromolar area, angle of the mandible, ramus, and condyle head can be seen clearly. If head is excessively tilted there will be distortion, and if inadequately tilted, will show superimposition of the contralateral side of the mandible.

Exposure parameters:

Customary to use 65Kvp, 10 mA and about 1/4 second.

Suggested reading:

1. Stuart C White, Michael J Pharoah, Oral Radiology, Principles and Interpretation 5th Edition, 215-218.

Q 3) Transcranial projection:

BFU NOVEMBER 2013 (4 Marks)

A sagittal view of the lateral aspects of the condyle and the temporal component is obtained by the trans cranial view.

Indications:

(i) TMJ pain dysfunction syndrome.
(ii) Arthritic changes on the articular surface.
(iii) Study gross osseous changes on the lateral aspect of the joint.
(iv) Range and type of movements in open mouth position.
(v) Study spaces of the joint, condylar head postion, the condition and shape of the glenoid fossa and the articular eminence, especially in views with closed mouth position.
(vi) Comparison of both sides of TMJ.
(vii) Displaced condylar fractures.

Technique:

- The patient is positioned in a cephalostat.
- The film is placed flat against the ear.
- The film is positioned so that the TMJ is centered over the cassette and it is parallel to the sagittal plane.
- The head of the patient is adjusted in such a way that the sagittal plane is vertical and the ala-tragus line is parallel to the floor.
- The beam of x-ray is projected downward through the opposite side, through the cranium and above the petrous ridge of the temporal bone at an angle of +25 degree centered at the joint.
- The horizontal direction of the x-ray beam is corrected for individual long axis of the condyle and an average of 20 degree angle anteriorly is used.
- In routine transcranial projections, both the TMJs are examined in the closed and maximun mouth opening positions.

Three other types of approaches that are used

1. **Post auricular/Lindblom technique.**
   Tube head is positioned ½ an inch behind and about 2 inches above the external auditory meatus.
   The projection of the central ray of the x-ray is such that it passes along the long condylar axis.
2. **Grewcock method:**
   The central beam of the x-ray is passed from a point about 2 inches above the external auditory meatus.
3. **Gill's approach:**
   Central ray is directed 1/2 an inch anterior and about 2 inches above the external auditory meatus.

Disadvantages:

- As the angulation of the beam is positive, the central and the medial aspects of the joint are projected inferiorly and only the lateral part of the joint contours are seen in this view.
- The ipsilateral petrous ridge is often superimposed on the neck of the condyle, which can hide the bony changes occurring in the condyle or the temporal component.
- There is distortion of the image of the condyle, joint space and

the temporal component and the position of the condyle cannot be accurately assessed, especially if the horizontal beam is not individualised for each patient.

Suggested reading:

1. Freny R Karjodkar, Text Book Of Dental And Maxillofacial Radiography, 2nd edition, 225-226.
2. Stuart C White, Michael. J Pharaoh, Oral Radiology Principles and Interpretation, 5th edition, 543-544.

Q 4) Give uses of lateral skull projection:

MUHS DECEMBER 2005 (2 Marks)

Lateral skull projection can be of two types:

1. True lateral view.
2. Lateral cephalometric view.

Uses of true lateral skull view:

- Observe growth and development of facial bones.
- Used to assess developmental disorders of the facial bones.
- Fractures of the face of the middle third, to show the possible downward and backward displacement of the maxillary bone.
- Fractures of the cranium and cranial base.
- Investigations of the sinuses i.e frontal, sphenoidal and the maxillary sinuses.
- Diseases that affect the vault of the skull, especially:
  - Paget's disease.
  - Multiple myeloma.
  - Hyperparathyroidism.
  - Diseases that affect the sella turcica like the tumours of the pituitary gland in acromegaly.

Uses of Lateral cephalometric skull view:

(I) Orthodontics and
(ii) Orthognathic surgery

(i) Orthodontics:

- The initial diagnosis: to confirm the underlying skeletal and soft tissue abnormalities.
- Planning of treatment.
- Monitoring the progress of treatment eg. to assess the inclination of the incisors and anchorage requirements.
- Appraising the results of the treatment eg. To find out whether the treatment targets have been achieved by appraisal 1-2 months before the completion and to allow for the planning of retention.

(ii) Orthognathic surgery:

- Evaluation of the skeletal and the soft tissue patterns preoperatively.

- Assistance in planning the treatment.
- Appraisal of the post-operative results of the surgery and the long-term follow up studies.

Suggested reading:

1. Eric Whaites, Essentials of dental radiography and radiology, 3rd edition, chapter no.145
2. Stuart S White, Michael J Pharoah, Text book of Oral Radiology, principles and interpretation, 5th edition, pg no-211.

Q 5) Transorbital view:

MUHS JUNE 2004 (2 Marks)

Transorbital view is also called as transmaxillary or zimmer projection. Its a antero-posterior radiograph for TMJ examination.

This projection is successful in delineating the joint with minimum super imposition.

It is the frontal projection of the TMJ.

Indications:

- The entire mediolateral dimension of the articular eminence, condylar head, and condylar neck is visible, which makes this view particularly useful for visualizing condylar neck fractures.
- The morphology of the convex surface of the condylar head can be evaluated.
- Making this projection a useful adjunct to transcranial and transpharyngeal projections in the diagnosis of gross degenerative changes or other anomalies.

Technique:

1. The patient is seated in upright position.
2. The head is tilted downwards at 10 degree so that the cantho-meatal line is horizontal.
3. Position the x-ray cassette behind the patients head so that the central ray is projected to its center and perpendicular to it.
4. Place the tube head in front of the patient and direct the central ray through the ipsilateral orbit and through the joint of interest, exiting from the skull behind the mastoid process.

Open-mouth position:

1. Ask the patient to open the mouth as wide as possible or protrude the mandible so that the condyle is placed at the top of articular eminence preventing the superimposition of articular eminence and skull base on the condyle of interest.
2. In this profile the entire mediolateral dimension of the articular eminence, condylar head, and condylar neck is visible.
3. If the patient cannot open the mouth wide the condylar neck may still be well seen in the resultant view.

Limitations of transorbital technique:

If condylar motion is limited, only the condylar neck is visible because areas of the joint articulating surfaces are obscured by superimposition of the temporal component on the condylar head. A similar projection is the reverse open Towne's projection, which sometimes is used to image condylar neck fractures, particularly if medial displacement has occurred, because the condylar head and neck are visualized in the frontal plane.

Suggested reading:

1. Stuart C White, Michael J Pharoah, Oral Radiology, Principles and Interpretation 5th Edition, 544-54.

Q 6) Indications and technique of paranasal sinuses views:

TNMGRU AUGUST 2005 (5 Marks)

Paranasal sinuses are the air filled cavities of the craniofacial complex, comprising the maxillary, frontal, sphenoidal and the ethmoidal air cells.

Indications and various techniques for radiography are:

A) Posterioanterior projections:

I) Posteroanterior (granger) projection:

Indication: It is excellent to evaluate the inner and middle ear because the petrous pyramid can be viewed through the orbits.

- In this cassette is placed perpendicular to the floor and mid sagittal plane should be perpendicular to the plane of film, only forehead and nose should touch the cassette and central ray should pass through the canthomeatal plane perpendicular to the plane of film.

II) Modified method, inclined posteroanterior (Caldwell) projection:

Indication: This angulation will cause the petrous ridges to be superimposed on the maxillary sinuses, thus allowing more accurate examination of the orbits and ethmoidal air cells.

- In this cassette is placed perpendicular to the floor, only forehead and nose should touch to the cassette, so that the canthomeatal line is perpendicular to the cassette and the central ray is directed 23° to the canthomeatal line, entering the skull about 3 cm above the external occipital protuberance and exiting at the glabella.

III) Water's view:

Indications: This technique is used mainly to show the maxillary, frontal and the ethmoidal sinuses. If patient is asked to open his mouth then sphenoidal sinus can also be seen.

- In this technique cassette is placed perpendicular to the floor and mid sagittal plane needs to be vertical and also perpendicular to the film, and the head of the patient is extended so that only the chin touches the cassette. The cantho-meatal line is 37 degrees to the film and the line joining the external auditory meatus to the mental protruberance should be perpendicular to the film. Central ray should enter from vertex and acanthion.

IV) Standard Occipitomental projection (0° OM):

Indications:

- It exhibits the facial skeleton and the maxillary antra.
- Avoidance of the superimposition of the dense bones of the skull base.

Technique:

- **Film and patient position:** Long axis of cassette is positioned vertical, and it is placed perpendicular to the floor. Midsagittal plane should be vertical and perpendicular to the plane of the cassette. Only the chin and the nose should touch the cassette and radiographic base line should be 45 degree to the film.
- **Central x-ray beam:** It is directed horizontally through the occiput.

B) Lateral Paranasal sinuses view:

Indications:

It is used to detect the Pathologies like Inflammatory conditions and sinus polyps or cysts.

In this technique Place lateral aspect of head against table/upright Bucky surface, and central beam is perpendicular to the midsagittal plane of the patient and the plane of the image receptor and is centered over the external auditory meatus.

C) True lateral skull:

Indication:

- Used for the Investigation of Pathologies like Inflammatory conditions and sinus polyps or cysts associated with the frontal, sphenoidal and maxillary sinuses.

Technique:

- **Film and patient position:** In this technique Place lateral aspect of head against table/upright Bucky surface.
- **Central beam:** It is perpendicular to the midsagittal plane of the patient and the plane of the image receptor and is centered over the external auditory meatus.

D) Bregma Menton:

Indications:

Its especially used for showing the walls of the maxillary sinus, the orbits, zygomatic arches and the nasal septum.

Technique:

- Film and patient position: Cassette is placed parallel to the floor.

Mid sagittal plane is adjusted vertical and perpendicular to the plane of the film. The chin of the patient is extended as far as comfortable in such a way that the lower border of the mandible is parallel to the casette. Only the chin should be touching the cassette.The cantho-meatal line is perpendicular to the film.

- Projection of central ray:It enters through the bregma and exits through the menton.

E) Orthopantomogram:

- Orthopantomography can produce the image of the facial structures including the maxilla and mandible and their supporting structures.

Indication:

- It can be used to study the antrum, especially floor and posterior and anterior wall of maxillary antrum.

Technique:

- In panoramic radiography, the film and X- ray tube head move around the patient. The X-ray tube moves around the patient's head in one direction and film rotates in opposite direction and patient is in a stationary position.

F) Computed x-ray tomography (CT):

Indication:

Main antral cavity (floor, all walls, roof, allows comparison of both sides, hard and soft tissue structures) and all para nasal air sinuses can be seen.

- CT differs from conventional radiographic study in several ways. First, the x-ray tube is aligned with a detector crystal or banks of detectors rather than an x-ray film.

A highly collimated (very thin) x-ray beam is projected through the part being examined so that only a thin layer of the patient is exposed for each slice, in contrast to conventional tomography, in which the entire volume being studied is exposed even though only a small layer of the volume is in focus on each section.

Suggested reading:

1. Freny R. Karjodkar, Essentials of Oral and Maxillofacial Radiology, 2nd edition, 234.
2. Stuart C White, Michael J Pharoah, Oral Radiology, Principles and Interpretation 5th Edition, chapter 11, pg no.210-224.

CHAPTER **15**

Specialised Imaging Techniques

Introduction:

Apart from the conventional radiographic techniques some more advanced form of radiological methods are called specialised radiographic imaging which includes, panoramic radiography, computed tomography, MRI, CBCT etc.

Q 1) Indications and contraindications of sialography:

NOVEMBER 2011 MUHS (2 Marks)

Radiographic examination of the salivary glands is called sialography and usually involves injecting a small amount of the contrast medium into the duct of the salivary gland and then it is follwed by taking routine x-ray projections.

Indications:

(i) To demonstrate calculi or foreign bodies, residual stones or tumours.

(ii) **To evaluate the functional integrity of the glands:** To determine the extent of salivary gland destruction due to obstruction with calculi or foreign bodies. Sialography can help in determining whether a total excision or lithotomy should be performed.

(iii) Detection of fistulae, diverticuli or strictures.

(iv) Evaluation of chronic inflammatory diseases.

(v) To evaluate the ductal pattern.

(vi) In case there is swelling of the face, to rule out the any pathology involving the salivary gland.

(vii) **Intra-glandular neoplasms:** To demonstrate the tumour size, location, origin, and to find out whether it is benign or malignant.

(viii) **Selection of site for biopsy:** The facial nerve outline as a guide in the planning for biopsy or dissection.

(ix) Diagnosis of recurrent swellings and processes of inflammation.

(x) **As a therapeutic procedure:** Ductal dilatation achieved during sialography aids in drainage of debris if present. Therapeutic effect is achieved due the iodinated contrast medium which is injected into the ductal system.

Contraindications:

(i) Patients allergic to the contrast medium or the iodine content or experienced severe asthmatic attacks or anaphylaxis by use of iodine in prior sialographic procedure.

(ii) Cases where there is acute infection and inflammation:
   - (a) The contrast media can cause irritation.
   - (b) There is increased chance of rupture of duct.
   - (c) Potential for retrograde dissemination of pyogenic organisms through the gland.

(iii) Patients with thyroid function tests in the immediate future.

(iv) When the salivary calculus is located in the anterior part of the salivary gland duct.

(v) Congenital atresia or aplasia of the salivary glands.

Suggested reading:

1. Neville BW, Damm DD, Allen CA, Bouquot JE. Oral & maxillofacial pathology, 2nd ed. Philadelphia: W.B. Saunders. pp. 393–395.

Q 2) Advantages of radiovisiography

1. Reduced radiation of the patient compared to conventional X-ray, up to 80%. It can be told to the patients who will definitely feel better about this and increases the safety quotient.
2. Faster imaging and no need of processing.
3. Lack of any waste that can be of hazard in the form of processing chemicals and lead foils with the use of digital systems.
4. Digital intraoral sensor is used instead of X-ray film: In case flexible digital sensors are used, it becomes easier than the use of conventional x-ray films with less chance of gagging.
5. Immediate imaging on the computer screen: it is a real time procedure and the images come up instantly and can be enlarged.
5. High quality of the digital image that can be analyzed and processed.
6. Saving and storing images in files helps in better record maintenance.
7. Electronic transfer of images to other health providers without any changes in the quality of the original image is possible.
8. Children friendly for reduced radiation, if imaging is necessary.
9. With various softwares provided the measurement of periodontal bone height or other lesions can be done.After treatment progress can very well be quantified.
10. Digital Subtraction Imaging (DSR):
    When two images of the same object are taken and the intensity of the image of the corresponding pixels are subtracted, a uniform difference image is produced.
    It can thus be applied in following instances:

- Caries detection and progression:
- Periodontal bone loss: Using the DSR the changes in the alveolar bone of 1.5%/unit volume and differences that are significant in the crestal bone height of upto 0.78mm can be detected.
- The periapical lesions: Detection of morphological / structural changes in the tissue of periapical region.
- Implant: DSR can be used to assess the bone changes at each of the three phases of treatment of implants, evaluation and maintenance.

11. It is of great use in forensic odontology where in measurement of various tooth parameters can be effectively done and can help in age estimation and sex determination.
12. The technology is easier to sell to the patients as they can see the entire process and its advantages at real time.

Suggested reading:

1. Freny R Karjodkar, Essentials Of Oral And Maxillofacial radiology, edition 2nd, page 345.
2. Stuart C White, Michael J Pharoah, Oral Radiology, Principles and Interpretation 5th edi. pg.no.238.

Q 3) Advantages and limitations of MRI:

MUHS NOVEMBER 2010 (2 Marks)

Advantages of MRI:

- No usage of ionising radiation: RF pulses used in MRI do not cause ionization and hence are not harmful.
- It can thus be done on pregnant women and children.
- No biological effects due to absence of radiation exposure.
- Higher soft tissue contrast.
- It can differentiate between the acute and chronic phases of a disease.
- Superlative distinction between soft tissues is possible of normal and abnormal tissues.
- Blood vessels can be seen clearly.
- As the area of the body whose image is taken is electronically controlled, direct multiplanar imaging is possible, with out the need for re orientation of the patient.
- High resolution images can be constructed in all planes.
- Image manipulation can be done.
- There is no need of enhancement of images using intravenous contrast media with their associated risks.

Limitations of MRI:

- It is an expensive procedure as the equipment is expensive.
- Ferromagnetic metals present in the vicinity of the imaging magnet can prove to be potentially hazardous.

- Patients with cardiac pacemakers, insulin pumps, and ferromagnetic implants cannot be investigated with MRI.
- Metallic objects in the oral cavity such as appliances, crowns, etc. May cause artifacts.
- Endotracheal tubes need to be replaced by plastic.
- There is a possibility that the patient could develop an allergic reaction to the contrast agent.
- The procedure can cause claustrophobia.
- Patients who are overly obese cannot fit into the machine.
- Imaging times can be relatively long.
- Cortical bone is not imaged, as the signal obtainable is only for the bone marrow.
- False diagnosis: A MRI cannot always differentiate between a benign and malignant tumor, which can lead to a false positive result.
- The very powerful magnets prove difficulty in housing the equipment.
- The equipment is very expensive.
- Facilities are not widely and easily available.

Suggested reading:

1. Freny R Karjodkar, Essentials Of Oral And Maxillofacial radiology, edition 2nd, page 309-310.
2. Anil Govindrao Ghom, Basic Oral Radiology, 1st Edition, page 164-165.

Q 4) Digital Radiography:

TNMGRU FEBRUARY 2012 (5 Marks)

Its a method by which a radiographic image can be captured using a sensor, after which it is broken into electronic pieces and then presenting and storing the image with the use of a computer. In this type of radiography instead of receiving an analogue image on a film, a sensor is used to receive the analogue image and then using an analogue-to digital converter (ADC), it is converted to digital image which is mainly an array of picture elements called pixels, which has discrete gray values assigned to each. A special soft ware is used for storing and manipulation of the image in the computer. The image is thus directly displayed in seconds on the computer in front of the clinician and the patient.

Digital images are numeric and discrete in two ways:

1. in terms of the spatial distribution of the picture elements (pixels) and
2. in terms of the different shades of gray of each of the pixels.

A digital image consists of a large collection of individual pixels organized in a matrix of rows and columns.

Each pixel has a row and column coordinate that uniquely identifies its location in the matrix.

The formation of a digital image requires several steps, beginning with analog processes.

At each pixel of an electronic detector, the absorption of x rays generates a small voltage.

Production of a digital image requires a process called analog-to-digital conversion (ADC).

ADC consists of two steps:

Sampling and Quantization.

Sampling means that a small range of voltage values are grouped together as a single value.

Once sampled, the signal is quantized which means that every sampled signal is assigned a value.

These values are stored in the computer and represent the image.

In order for the clinician to see the image, the computer organizes the pixels in their proper locations and gives them a shade of gray that corresponds to the number that was assigned during the quantization step.

Equipment:

There are two essential components:

I) **Source of x-radiation:** Most commonly conventional dental units are used.

II) **Intra-oral sensor:** Its a small detector that can be placed intraorally and can capture the images and send to the computer for future processing.

Four types of sensors are being used:

1. **Charged couple device (CCD):**
   It is one of the most common image receptors used in digital radiography and is sensitive to x-rays or light, and is a solid state detector that consists of a silicon chip with an electronic circuit embedded in it.
2. **Complementary metal oxide semiconductor/active pixel sensor. (CMOS/APS):**
   In this type of sensor the silicon chip is less expensive to produce, and has greater durability and 25%more resolution than the CCD.
3. **Charged injection device (CID):**
   In this type of sensor, no computer is required for image processing. The CID uses the same docking platform with intra-oral camera, and within seconds it produces digital images directly that can be seen on the monitor.This image can also be saved on the computer or video disc recorder.
4. **Flat panel detectors:**
   Flat panel detectors are being used for medical imaging but have also been used in prototypes of extraoral imaging devices.
   The detectors can provide relatively large matrix areas with pixel sizes less than 100 microns.
   This allows direct digital imaging of larger areas of the body, including the head.

I) Direct digital imaging;

The x-ray photons that are emitted from the conventional radiographic unit come in contact with the intra-oral sensor and help the electrons to be released from the silicon chip, to produce a latent image. The electrons then travel to the computer unit where they are converted to pixels and can be seen on the monitor. The pixel is a digital equivalent of the silver halide crystal in conventional radiography. The CCD sensor has the ability to produce 640x480 individual pixels in size. The individual pixels are represented numerically by the levels of gray colour and varies from 0-255, which produces 266 shades of gray and are referred to as pixel's gray scale resolution. 0 indicates the maximum radiation measured and corresponds to the dark areas in the image and 255 represents no radiation at all and hence represents the radiopacity. The number of possible gray scale combinations/pixel is called the bit depth image. A digital image with 256 pixel resolution contains 8 bit-depth image.

II) Indirect digital imaging:

1. **Scanning of traditional radiographs:** In this method, a conventional radiograph is digitised using the CCD camera, that scans and converts image from analogue to a digital form and then displays the image on the computer.
2. **Photostimulable phosphor plate (PSP):** A reusable imaging plate is used which is coated with phosphors instead of sensors. After exposure to radiation, a high speed scanner is used to convert information into electronic image.

Advantages of digital radiography:

- The greatest advantage is the gray scale resolution of 266 colours of gray as compared to 16-25 shades of gray on a conventional film.
- This allows the manipulation of density and contrast so as to enhance the features or details of diagnostic importance, and that too with out additional exposure to the patient by taking another radiograph.
- Manipulation with contrast, sharpness, resolution, image orientation, colourisation and enlargement of the images are some unique features of the digital radiographic software.
- The use of subtraction radiography and reversing the gray scale with the use of the software, can be very useful for determination and analysis of patterns that may be typical of a particular disease or condition.
- Reduction in exposure is also a great advantage.
- It helps in reducing the processing time and hence can be of great help as a financial and professional value for a clinician.
- It takes only few seconds to a minute to take the radiograph and view it on the monitor.
- The storage of these images in small hard drives of the computer

also helps in saving space as compared to those of the conventional films.

- They can be easily relayed for referrals to other offices, lap tops removable CDs and discs and help in easy mobility of information
- Only the initial cost is higher, after which it is almost a money saver with no recurring expenditures like films and processing chemicals
- No need of extra space for darkroom.
- Use of digital radiography can make the dental office environment friendly as there is no hassle of disposing hazardous chemicals lead foil sheets etc.

Suggested reading:

1. Parks ET, Williamson GF. Digital radiography: an overview. J Contemp Dent Prac 2002; 3(4):23–39.
2. Stuart C White, Michael J Pharoah Oral Radiology, Principles And Interpretation 5th edition, page 225-231.

Q 5) Sialography:

TNMGRU FEBRUARY 2015 (5 Marks)

Sialography was first performed in 1902.

In 1913, Arcelin first presented a complete radiographic demonstration of the human salivary gland.

Barsony in 1925 utilized potassium iodide solution, Carlsten used lipiodol for the demonstration of stenson's duct dilatation.

It is a radiographic technique where in a radiopaque contrast medium is infused into the ductal system of the salivary gland after which imaging is done conventional films, fluoroscopy, panoramic radiography, tomography or CT.

Sialography remains the most detailed way to image the ductal system.

It can be performed on the parotid, submandibular and sometimes the sublingual salivary glands.

Indications:

- Detection of calculus or foreign body whether radiopaque or radiolucent.
- To determine the extent of destruction of the salivary gland due to obstruction.
- To detect and portray the fistulae, diverticuli and strictures.
- Demonstration of tumor, its location, size and origin.
- To help in outlining of the facial nerve as a guide for biopsy or dissection.

Contraindications:

- Sensitivity to Iodine compounds.
- During acute infection.
- May interfere with Thyroid function tests.

Method:

A radiograph is usually made before the infusion of the contrast solution into the ductal system so as to verify the optimal exposure factors and patient positioning parameters and for detecting radiopaque sialoliths or extraglandular pathosis.

With this technique, a lacrimal or periodontal probe is used to dilate the sphincter at the ductal orifice before the passage of a cannula (blunt needle or catheter) connected by extension tubing to a syringe containing contrast agent, fat-soluble (e.g., Ethiodol) or water-soluble (e.g., Sinografin) contrast solution is then slowly infused until the patient feels discomfort (usually between 0.2 and1.5ml, depending on the gland being studied).

These iodine containing agents render the ductal system radiopaque.

The filling phase can be monitored by fluoroscopy or with static films.

The intent is to opacify the ductal system all the way to the acini.

The ductal system opacification gives the appearance of branches of trees with no area of the gland devoid of ducts.

When the acinar filling phase occurs it appears as if the trees have blossomed.

The gland is allowed to evacuate for five minutes without stimulation. If the post evacuation radiographs show traces of contrast media then sialogogues such as lemon juice or 2% citric acid can be given to the patient to help evacuation of the contrast media by stimulating secretion.

Water soluble contrast agents are preferred as inflammatory reactions are observed due to inadvertent extravasation of the fat soluble agents.

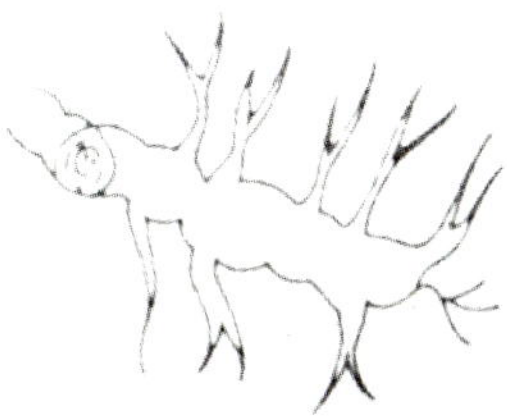

Figure a

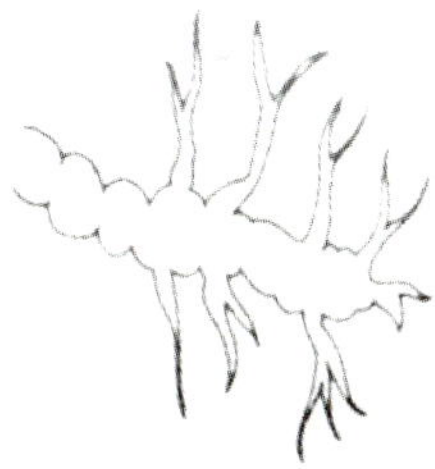

Figure b

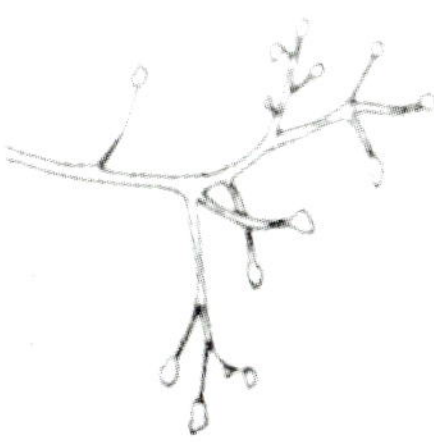

Figure c

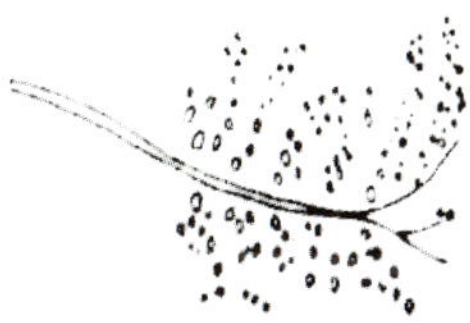

Figure d

Fig. (a) Calculus, (b) sialodochitis, (c) sialadenitis and (d) sjogren's syndrome respectively

Suggested reading:

1. Stuart C White, Michael J Pharoah, Oral Radiology, Principles and Interpretation 5th Edition, 660-663.

Q 6) Radiovisiography:

TNMGRU AUGUST 2013 (5 Marks)
BFU MAY 2007 (5 Marks)

Radiovisiography (RVG) was invented by Dr. Francis Mouyens and is the first direct digital system. It was first described in 1988 and then introduced commercially in the UK in 1989 and since then has undergone several changes.

Radiovisiography imaging systems produce a dynamic image that permits immediate display, image enhancement, storage, retrieval, and transmission.

It consists of four basic components:

- An X-ray set with electronic time.
- an intra-oral sensor.
- A display processing unit (DPU)
- Printer.
- Intra oral sensor comprises of a small detector which can be placed in the mouth and the radiographic image can be recorded. They are available as:
- Wired: The sensor is linked to the computer by a fiber-optic cable.
- Wireless: The sensor is not linked by a wire.

Radivisiography uses the digital sensors which are:

(i) Charged couple device (CCD): Uses a thin wafer of silicon as the basis for image recording. Most commonly used in RVG.

The silicon crystals are formed in a picture element (pixel) matrix.

When the sensor is exposed to radiation, the covalent bonds between the silicon atoms are broken, producing electron-hole pairs.

The amount of exposure is responsible for forming the number of electron hole pairs that an area receives.

The electrons are then attracted towards the most positive potential in the device, where charged packets are created.

One pixel corresponds to each packet.

The pattern of the charge formed from the individual pixels in the matrix represents the latent image.

The reading of the image is done by transferring each row of the pixel charges from one pixel to the next in the bucket brigade fashion.

When the charge reaches the end of the row, it gets transferred to a read out amplifier and is transmitted as a voltage to the analogue-digital converter which is located either within or connected to the computer.

Voltages from each pixel are sampled and assigned a numerical value representing a gray level.

The silicon matrix and its associated readout and amplifying electronics are enclosed within a plastic housing to protect them from the oral environment most detectors incorporate an electronic cable to transfer data to the analog to digital converter.

Because CCDs are more sensitive to the light rays than the x-rays, most manufacturers use a thin layer of scintillation material that is coated directly on the CCD surface or coupled to the surface by fiber optics.

This increases the x-ray absorption efficiency of the detector.

Gadolinium oxybromide compounds similar to those used in rare earth radiographic screens or cesium iodide are examples of scintillators that have been used for this purpose.

(ii) Complementary metal oxide semiconductor/active pixel sensor: (CMOS/APS): CMOS technology is the basis for typical consumer grade digital cameras. These detectors are also silicon based semiconductors but are fundamentally different from CCDs in the way that pixel charges are read.

(iii) Photo stimulable Phosphor: Its a wireless digital radiography system in which a reusable imaging plate coated with phosphor is used. The plates are flexible and can be used in the mouth. The storage phosphor imaging records diagnostic data on the plates following the exposure to the x-ray source and uses high speed scanners to convert the information to electronic files which can be displayed to electronic files & which can be displayed on the computer screen.

Advantages of RVG:

1. **Lower Dose Radiation:** Digital intraoral receptors require less radiation than film, thus lowering the patient absorbed dose. Dose reductions of up to 90 per cent compared to E speed film have been reported in the diagnosis.
2. **Image Manipulation:** This is perhaps the greatest advantage of digital imaging over conventional film. It involves selecting the information of greatest diagnostic value and suppressing the rest.
3. **Image Analysis:**
4. **No Film Processing:** Elimination of the difficulty of maintaining high-quality chemical processing solutions and conditions.
5. **Time Reduction:** The procedure is less time consuming.
6. **Storage:** There are no hassles of film storage.
7. **Easy and Quick Image Transfer:** Electronic transfer of images to other health providers without any alteration of the original image quality.
8. Digital Subtraction Imaging.

Disadvantages of RVG:

1. It cannot be sterilized. The bulk, lack of flexibility and the attachment to the handle leads to instability during exposure and correct positioning becomes difficult.
2. Greater thickness with relatively smaller sensor size than the conventional film.
3. The technique is simple, however the assessment of image may need some degree of familiarisation as the image is different from that of the conventional radiograph.
4. Relatively high initial expense of setting up a digital system.

Suggested reading:

1. Freny. R Karjodkar, Textbook Of Dental And Maxillofacial Radiology, 2nd edition, 227-228.

Q7) Advantages and limitations of Digital radiography.

MUHS MAY 2012- (3 Marks)

Latest advances in dental imaging is the digital radiography and is being used fruitfully by the dental professional. The digital radiography refers to the capturing of a radiographic image using a sensor, and then breaking it into electronic pieces and then presenting and storing of the image with the help of a computer.

Advantages of digital radiography:

- The gray scale resolution is superior.
- Can be easily reproducible.
- Reduced patient exposure to x-rays.
- The process is fast and image viewing is sped up.
- Lower recurrent cost.
- Increase in efficiency.
- The diagnostic quality of the image is enhanced.
- The quality of the image is excellent due to avoidance of conventional processing system.
- For specific diagnostic purpose it is possible to do image processing, enlargement and reconstruction.
- With the aid of the computer, detection of defects and three dimensional visualisation of the dental structures based on radiographic data is possible.
- Its an effective tool for patient education.

Limitations of Digital radiography:

- Initial set-up is costly.
- Image quality is still a debate.
- The thickness of the sensor is more than the intra-oral films.
- A disposable plastic wrapper has to be used every time for infection control.
- As the original image can be manipulated, legal issues could arise

and, it is debatable whether digital radiographs can be used as evidence in lawsuits.

Suggested reading:

1. Freny Karjodkar, Text Book Of Dental And Maxillofacial Radiology, Chapter 17, Pg No 343-344.

Q 8) Contrast media in sialography:

MUHS MAY 2015 (3 Marks)

Contrast sialography can be performed using either lipid soluble or water soluble agents.

Lipid or fat soluble contrast media:

Examples: Include ethiodol, lipiodol, todochioral, lipiodol U F.

Properties:

- Iodine content: They have iodine content ranging from 37-41% w/w.
- Specific gravity ranges from 1.28-1.36 at 150C.
- Their viscosity is high ranging from 80-100 centiposes.

Advantages:

- They produce satisfactory degree of radiographic opacification with sustained opacity, to study the post evacuation phase properly.
- Provides sharper visualisation with good resolution of the peripheral ducts.

Disadvantages:

- It is more discomforting for the patients.
- They may cause inflammatory reaction resulting in granuloma formation and subsequent fibrosis.
- Can cause clouding of glands.

Water soluble contrast media:

Examples: Hypaque 50, urograffin, Hypaque 73, Renograffin 60 and 73, Renograffin 60 and 75, Amipaque, Isopaque, Conray 80, Conray 420, Omnipaque.

Properties:

- They are easily mixed with saliva and body fluids.
- They have iodine content ranging from 28-30 w/w and viscosity ranging from 2-10 centiposes.
- They are hypotonic compared to saliva and plasma.

Advantages;

- As they are water soluble they help in filling the finer ductal system.
- There is less pain and discomfort to the patient.
- They are easily excreted from the tissues.

Disadvantages:

- Lesser degree of radiographic density and contrast.
- As they are evacuated faster, the radiographs have to be taken in shorter time.

Suggested reading:

1. Anil Govindrao Ghom, Textbook of oral medicine, 405-406.

Q 9) Scintigraphy in dentistry:

TNMGRU FEBRUARY 2008 (5 Marks)

It is a diagnostic technique in which a two-dimensional picture of internal body tissue is produced through the detection of radiation emitted by a radioactive substance administered into the body.

Scintigraphy uses radioactive compounds that have an affinity for particular tissues. These substances are injected into the patient, concentrated in the tissues of interest and their radiation emissions are detected and imaged using a gamma camera. This investigation allows to assess the function or the structure of the target tissue.

PET and SPECT are recent advances in radionuclide scanning where in three dimensional images can be obtained.

In dentistry commonly used scintigraphy are for salivary gland, bone and lymphoscintigraphy.

Salivary Gland Scintigraphy:

- It is a minimally invasive diagnostic test to assess salivary gland function and to determine abnormalities in gland uptake and excretion.
- It is the only salivary imaging technique that provides information on the functional capabilities of the glands.
- The estimation of severity of the involvement of the salivary gland and functional disorders can be done.
- Its simple and easy to perform, well tolerated by the patient and is reproducible.
- It is indicated for the evaluation of patient when sialography is contraindicated.

Procedure:

- Technetium is pure gamma ray emitting radionuclide that is given intravenously and is taken up by salivary gland.
- Then it is transported through the glands and secreted into oral cavity.
- Parotid, and submandibular glands are visualized distinctly as they bind and retain technetium.
- Both uptake and secretory phases can be recognized on the scan.
- Activity remaining in the salivary glands after the stimulation can suggest obstruction, tumours and inflammation.

Bone Scintigraphy:

Its a highly sensitive method that is used for demonstrating disease in the bone. It often permits earlier diagnosis or can demonstrate more lesions than can be done by conventional radiography.

This technique gives no information about the morphology of the lesion but can demonstrate areas of altered bone metabolism within and around the lesion, and hence allows good assessment of the growth of a lesion and extent of its borders:

This procedure procures the images of the distribution of the radioactive tracer in the skeletal system. It is done by following method:

Procedure:

Patient preparation:

1. The procedure should be explained to the patient. The patients should be well hydrated unless contraindicated and be asked to drink 2 or more glasses of water within the time of injecting and the time of delayed imaging.
2. The patient is asked to pass urine immediately before the delayed imaging and directed to drink plenty of water for a period of atleast hours after the administration of the radiopharmaceuticals.
3. For bone scintigraphy several 99m Tc -labelled radiopharmaceuticals are available.
4. In adults the usual dose of administration is 740-1, 110MBq injected by the intravenous route.
5. The dosages are different for obese and pediatric patients.
6. The radiopharmaceuticals for bone undergo oxidation. Extra care should be taken to prevent introducing air into the multidose vial. Quality control is essential before performing the procedure.

Lymphoscintigraphy:

It is turning out to be promising in the case of oral malignancies to assess metastasis to the nodes.

Uses of scintigraphy in dentistry:

- The bone scans are quite helpful in differentiating bony infections from the soft tissue ones.
- Increased uptake is seen in cases of inflammatory conditions of the TMJ. Scintigraphy helps in discovering early changes in the TMJ which could also lead to disc abnormalities. The radionucleide used is the 99mTc.
- SPECT images are used to detect pathologies of TMJ.
- Gallium scans are helpful in detection of abscesses, osteomyelitis and lymphomas.
- PET scans are especially helpful in the detection of oral squamous cell carcinomas and it is able to detect the pathology earlier than the CT or MRI. PET scan also is useful in determining the response to

treatment, diagnosis of recurrence, detection of residual pathology and distant metastasis and is quite helpful in locating the occult primary tumour.

- SPECT is especially helpful in implant dentistry where the effect of immediate prosthetic treatment on the peri-implant bone activity can be assessed. SPECT can also assess the osseo-integration process of the dental implant.
- To study metabolic disorders like Paget's disease and osteoporosis.
- Assess conditions like Fibrous dysplasia and other congenital conditions that are rare.
- Trauma and fractures of the dento-facial complex.
- Assessment of periodontal diseases.
- Salivary gland scintigraphy can help assess normal functioning as well as lesions of the salivary glands like aplasia, obstruction, trauma, acute inflammation etc.
- Lymphoscintigraphy is showing promising results in detection of oral malignancies. If the uptake is not noted in the first level of draining lymph nodes then the metastases to other nodes is considered negative.
- In forensic dentistry estimation of age at death for identification can be done with great precision upto the adolescent stage especially. The amount of radiocarbon present in the enamel as a result of nuclear testing can be an accurate indicator of the age of the person. Age estimation is done up to within 1.6 years.

Suggested reading:

1. Shazia Mushtaq, Role of nuclear medicine in dentistry, GJMEDPH 2012; Vol. 1 issue 6.
2. Vinita Boloor, Rajesh Hosadurga, Sruthy Pratap, Anupama Rao, Nuclear medicine in dentistry revisited: New avenues to explore, CCIJ, 2013, Volume, Issue : 3 189-194.

Q 10) Xeroradiography:

TNMGRU AUGUST 2004 (5 Marks)

The term xeroradiography is a greek word where 'xero' means dry. It is also called as edge enhancement radiography which means differentiating areas of different densities at the margins or edges. This technique simulates a Xerox machine. This process was developed by an engineer Dr. Robert. C, Mcmaster in the year 1950. In xeroradiography, the image acquisition is achieved by a photoelectrostatic process & not by photochemical process as in conventional radiography.

The image is recorded on a paper rather than on a film.

A selenium plate that rests on a thin layer of aluminum oxide, is given a uniform charge by passing it in front of a scorotron.

When the x-ray photons fall on this layer of selenium, charges diffuse out that are proportional to the energy of the x-rays. This effect occurs because of photoconduction. The resultant imprint, in the form of distribution of charges on the plate, attract the particles of the toner, which is then transferred to the reusable paper plates. This process doesnot require photographic developing.

Technique:

- Dental 110 xeroradiography unit system is used.
- The image is recorded on the aluminum plate coated with a layer of selenium. These selenium particles are given a uniform electrostatic charge and are stored in a unit called conditioner.
- The image receptor plates are the size no. 1 and no. 2 films and fit well in oral cavity.
- When x rays are passed on to the film, it causes selective discharge of the particles and this forms a latent image.
- Image is developed by passing cloud of oppositely charged powder particle called toner over the plate, which get attracted to variably charged areas depending on the intensity of the remaining charge.
- This formed image is fused to paper or laminated between a transparent & a translucent sheet of plastic & can be viewed by reflected or transmitted light.
- **Positive Image:** Darkest areas corresponds to most dense parts of anatomy.
- **Negative image:** Darkest areas corresponds to least dense parts of anatomy and dense objects appear white.

Uses:

1. Cephalometry
2. Evaluation of bone lesions in the mandible
3. Sialography
4. TMJ tomography.

Indications in head & neck region:

1. Assessment of Periodontal & periapical bone details.
2. Cephalometric radiography to show the required hard and soft tissue landmarks on one film.
3. Sialography to show fine duct structure.
4. Assessment of soft tissue shadows in larynx and pharynx.

Advantages:

1. Pronounced edge enhancement.
2. High contrast.
3. Easy to use.
4. Requires 1/3 rd exposure of conventional radiographs.
5. Image is easily reversible.
6. Visualisation of the alveolar crest height.
7. Caries seen more readily.
8. Useful in endodontics, cancer detection and imaging biomaterials.

Disadvantages:

1. High radiation exposure for extraoral technique. The main hazard is unavoidable larger skin radiation dose which is 2.4 to 16.2 times higher than conventional film techniques.
2. Edge enhancement causes artefacts.
3. Causes discomfort to the patient as humidity of oral cavity act as a medium for flow of current.
4. Expensive processors.

Suggested reading:

1. Freny R. Karjodkar; Essentials Of Oral &Maxillofacial Radiology edi: 1 st, pg no 144-145.

CHAPTER **16**

Dental Caries

Introduction:

Dental caries is a microbial disease of the calcified tissues of the teeth characterised by demineralisation of inorganic portion and destruction of the organic substance of the teeth.

It is defined by WHO as, a localised posteruptive, pathological process of external origin involving softening of the hard tooth tissues, and proceeding to the formation of a cavity.

Radiology can play an important role in diagnosis of dental caries because:

- It is non-invasive.
- Parts of teeth that cannot be visualized by the eye can be viewed.
- The depth of the lesion can be assessed.

Q 1) Diagnosis of dental caries:

BFU MAY 2006 (5 Marks)

In case of dental caries its better to initiate the therapy early so as to get the best resolution of the problem. For early therapy, its important to do early diagnosis.

The methods which are used for diagnosis of dental caries are as follows:

1. **Clinical methods:**
   - **(a) Visual inspection:** Sensitivity of test: it appears to have very low sensitivity and high specificity in diagnosing caries.
   - **(b) Tactile method by an explorer:** Sensitivity of test: the sensitivity of the explorer is reported to be low in occlusal lesion diagnosis. explorer should be used lightly or not at all on occusal surface.
   - **(c) Tooth separation:** Clinical manner proposed for the diagnosis of proximal surface decay is tooth separation. To improve the visibility and allow the application of blunt probe into the area.
2. **Radiographic and other methods:** Carious lesions are detectable radiographically when there is enough demineralization. They are valuable in detecting proximal caries which can go unnoticed in

clinical examination. 40% demineralistion is required to detect caries.

(a) Radiographic methods:

- Intraoral periapical radiography-Most commonly used conventional method.Easy to use and least expensive.
- **Bitewing radiography:** Gives very good diagnostic details of proximal caries.
- **Panoramic radiograph:** Can show various teeth involvement at a time but less sharp and accurate then IOPA and bitewing techniques.
- **Digital imaging (Radiovisiography):** Real time and accurate diagnostic method.
- Subtraction Radiography.
- **Cone beam computed tomography:** Gives accurate diagnosis and is recent advance.
- Xeroradiography.

(b) Optical coherence tomography: (OCT)

Its an imaging technology that can provide high resolution, 10-30micrometer morphologic depth images. It is similar to the ultrasound system, but uses light waves instead of sound waves.

(c) Polarized Raman Spectroscopy:

In order to aid in ruling out false-positive readings associated with OCT and increase the specificity of caries diagnosis, OCT is coupled with PRS to get a biochemical information so as to confirm the presence of caries.

(d) Terahertz pulse imaging (TPI):

Higher attenuation of terahertz radiation was observed in carious enamel as compared with healthy enamel.

(e) Fiberoptic transilluminator (FOTI):

(a) it is qualitative method for the diagnosis of dental caries.
(b) The surface of the tooth is examined using the transmitted light seen from the occusal view.
(c) Decayed tooth has decreased index and appears dark.
(d) the contrast between sound and carious tissue is then used for detection of lesions.
(e) diagnosis of interproximal surface is also done with FOTI.

(f) Digital imaging fiberoptic Transilluminator (DIFOTI): DIFOTI reduces the perceived shortcomings of FOTI by combining FOTI and a digital charge couple device camera. The resultant change in light distribution is captured by camera and sent to computer for analysis.

(g) Electrical conductance Measurement: Theory: sound surface should possess limited or no conductivity, whereas carious or demineralized enamel should have a measurable conductivity that will increase with increasing demineralization.

Results: Indicators for caries meter are:

- Green: no caries.
- Yellow: enamel caries.
- Orange: dentin caries.
- Red: pulpal involvement.

(h) **Visible luminescent spectroscopy:** The visible emission spectrum for decayed and nondecayed regions of teeth differs.

(i) **Quantitive light induced Fluorescence:** Acid dissolution of the structure results in a local decrease in fluorescence in area of acid exposure.

(j) **Infrared laser fluorescence:**

(k) **Use of caries detector dye:** various dyes such as silver nitrate, methyl red, procion, alizarin, calcein stain have been used to detect carious lesion by change in colour.

(l) **Ultrasound or ultrasonic imaging:** This method utilizes a sonar device in which beam of waves is directed against tooth surface and reflected wave is picked up by receiver.

(m) **Videoscope:** integration of a camera with the endoscope with resultant image that can be recorded and stored is called videoscope. It provides a magnified image for better visualization.

(n) **Newer methods for caries detection:** MINI D: It's a light weight pen sized device which is cordless and uses fibreoptic technology and light emitting diodes to accurately detect both occlusal and proximal caries.

DNA chip technology: It will be used to identify and rank genes associated with caries and periodontitis. Identified genes will serve as diagnostic markers.

Blue tooth technology for caries detection: It judges the pH levels of teeth and sends a warning or cautioning signal.

Dermatoglyphics is also a new method for caries diagnosis.

Suggested reading:

1. Anil Govindrao Ghom, textbook of oral medicine, 3rd edition, 485-487.
2. Crawley D.A. Longbottom C, Cole B.E, Ciesla C.M, Arnone D., Wallace V.P, Pepper M, Terahertz Pulse Imaging: A Pilot Study of Potential Applications in Dentistry, Caries Res 2003;37:352–359
3. Lin-P'ing Choo-Smith, Cecilia C.S. Dong, Blaine Cleghorn, Mark Hewko Shedding New Light on Early Caries Detection, J Can Dent Assoc. 2008 Dec; 74(10): 913–918.

Q 2) Radiation caries:

TNMGRU SEPTEMBER 2002 (5 Marks)

The patients with malignant lesion of the head and neck who have to undergo radiation therapy often presents with complex dental problems.

Radiation caries is a rampant form of caries that occurs in patients who receive a course of radio therapy that includes exposure of the salivary glands.

Etiology and Pathogenesis:

- The saliva often becomes thicker and more tenacious after irradiation. It loses its buffering capacity, flow is reduced and the pH is decreased.
- Because of reduced flow the cleansing action of saliva is interfered with and promotes caries formation.
- Xerostomia of varying degree favor the collection of debris on the teeth and thus initiates caries.
- This radiation induced xerostomia produces pronounced shifts in the oral microbial population resulting in cariogenic microorganisms such as streptococcus mutans and lactobacilli gaining prominence at the expense of non-cariogenic ones.
- There is no protection against demineralization since salivary electrolyte are lacking.

Clinical Manifestations:

- Radiation caries is a fast progressing severely destructive form of dental caries which is a common post irradiation complication in patients with head and neck malignant lesion.
- The common clinical manifestations of the injury is the destruction of tooth structure resembling dental caries, peculiar in that, it often begins in the cervical area of the teeth.
- The lesion resembles a demineralization process more than it does in true caries because of its pattern and the manner in which it sweeps across the teeth often causing amputation or snapping of tooth crown at its neck.
- The teeth seems brittle and pieces of enamel may fracture away from the tooth.

Clinically radiation caries can be seen in following patterns:

1. The most common is widespread superficial lesions attacking buccal, occlusal, incisal, and palatal surfaces.
2. Another type involves primarily the cementum and dentin in the cervical region. These lesions may progress around the teeth circumferentially and result in loss of the crown.
3. The superficial carious destruction of the neck of the teeth.
4. Change in tooth colour from brown to black.
5. An early gradual loss of the edges and occlusal plane of the teeth.
6. Generalized superficial defects.

Management:

- The patient should continue fluoride usage till xerostomia has subsided.

- If the teeth show evidence of demineralisation the fluoride gel should be used for 15 minutes, TID interspersed with the rinses of 1% fluoride.
- If a patient develops pulpitis, root canal treatment under antibiotic coverage is considered. Care should be taken not to put the necrotic debris beyond the tooth apex.
- Pulpotomy is not advisable because of the inherent risk of infection. Scaling root planing and curettage should be done as necessary with proper antibiotic coverage.
- Restorative treatment should be conservative and atraumatic. Careful use of rubber dam clamps and matrix band is advocated to prevent trauma.
- Xerostomia following radiation therapy is treated by indirect and palliative means. Salivary substitutes are available (salivart or xerolube). These are artificial substances which physically resemble natural saliva. However these substances do not contain lubricatory proteins antibacterial factors or other macromolecules that are normally found in saliva.
- Mild baking soda solution rinses and water can aid patients to keep their mouth moist. Sugar free chewing gums and mints appear to provide a degree of moisturizing relief.

Suggested reading:

1. Stuart C White, Michael J Pharoah, Oral Radiology, Principles and Interpretation 5th Edition, 34-36.
2. S Anil, Tara Philip, K Madhu, VT Beena, T Vijaykumar. Radiation caries – A rational approach towards its prevention and management. JIDA vol.64, No.1, January 1993.

Q 3) Radiological appearance of dental caries:

RGUHS OCTOBER 1997 (5 Marks)

Definition:

Dental Caries is an infectious disease caused by microorganisms which involves the calcified structures of teeth, and is characterised by demineralisation of the inorganic part and the destruction of the organic portion of tooth.

Since caries causes demineralization of the tooth, it can be diagnosed on radiograph (after approximate 40% demineralization is achieved), as the lesion allows greater passage of X-rays as compared to surrounding structures and hence appears more radiolucent.

Various radiographs for dental caries detection are:

- **Bitewing:** Aids in detecting caries in interproximal areas and distal ends of premolars and molars, and caries at CE junction.
- **Periapical:** Aids in detecting gross carious lesion, root caries and changes in apical and inter radicular bone due to caries.
- **OPG:** Useful to examine a case with multiple carious teeth or rampant caries.

Dental panoramic radiographs are not recommended for diagnosis of caries.

The limitation of radiograph is that it is a two dimensional representation of a three dimensional object, thus the exact site of caries cannot be located. Digital image receptors are now available for intraoral radiography.

Radiographic Appearance of Caries may be studied as:

According to the severity and extent of the lesion:

- Incipient
- Moderate
- Advanced
- Severe

According to the location

- Pit and fissure caries
  - Occlusal
  - Buccal/lingual pit
- Smooth surface caries
  - Proximal
  - Buccal or lingual surfaces
  - Root surface caries
- Recurrent caries

According to the etiology

- Recurrent caries
- Rampant caries
- Radiation caries

Proximal caries:

It is often difficult to detect because the surfaces of the posterior teeth are broad and the loss of small amount of mineral from incipient lesion and the advancing disease of the active lesion can be difficult to detect on a radiograph.

Lesions that only involve the enamel are generally not evident till about 30%-40% demineralization has occurred. This lesion can be differentiated from a cervical burn out because the lesion doesnot start below the gingival margin.

(i) **Incipient proximal lesion:** It appears as a classical triangle with its broad base at the tooth surface spreading along the enamel rods.

It may also appear as a notch, a dot, thin line or a band.

(ii) **Moderate proximal lesions:** More than the outer half of the enamel is involved but are not seen extending into the DE junction.

(iii) **Advanced proximal lesion:** When the demineralistion reaches the DE junction, it starts to spread along the junction and forms the base of a second triangle whose apex is towards the pulp chamber. This triangle has a wider base than that in the enamel, and progresses towards the pulp along the direction of the dentinal tubules.

(iv) **Severe proximal lesions:** Carious lesions are seen radiographically to have penetrated through more than half of dentine and are approaching pulp.

Occlusal caries:

- Occlusal lesions commonly start in the sides of a fissure wall rather than at the base and then tend to penetrate nearly perpendicularly toward the DEJ.
- Early lesions appear clinically as either chalky white, brown, yellowish or black discolorations of the occlusal fissures.
- When a lesion on the occlusal surface is confined to the enamel, it is obscured by the surrounding enamel. As the carious process progresses, a radiolucent line extends along the DEJ.
- The classic radiographic appearance of occlusal caries that extends into the dentin has a broad base, and is a radiolucent zone, usually below a fissure, with very little or almost no changes in the enamel.
- The deeper the occlusal lesion, the easier it is to detect on the radiograph.

Buccal/ facial/ lingual/ cervical caries:

- The caries on the buccal and lingual aspects of teeth usually involve the pit and fissures of the teeth.
- They appear round when small and as they enlarge they assume an elliptical or semilunar shape.
- They demonstrate sharp, well defined borders.

Caries of the root surface:

- The caries on the root surface involve both the cementum and dentine and is associated with gingival recession.
- It develops due to degradation by attrition, abrasion, and erosion.
- The caries process is best described as a "scooping", which results in radiographic appearance of an "ill-defined saucer like crater" or when the peripheral surface area is small it appears "notched".

Recurrent caries or secondary caries:

- When a caries develops at the margins of the existing restoration can be termed as recurrent or secondary caries.
- It should be noted, though, that a lesion developing in a restored surface is most frequently a new primary demineralization, either because of fault in the shaping or inadequate extension of the restoration that leads to accumulation of plaque.

Radiation caries:

- The lesion peculiarly starts at the cervical area and rapidly encircles the tooth, which results in the loss of entire crown and resulting in the root fragments remaining in the jaws.
- The appearance is characteristic with radiolucent shadows occurring at the necks of the teeth and most commonly involving

the mesial and the distal aspects.

- Variations in the depth of destruction may be present, but generally there is uniformity within a given region of the mouth.

Radiographic Differential Diagnosis

- Erosion cavity
- Nonopaque filling
- Cervical burn out
- Internal resorption
- External resorption
- Hypoplasia of enamel

Suggested reading:

1. Freny Karjodkar, Textbook of dental and maxillofacial radiology, 2nd edition, pg no. 406-418.
2. Syriopoulos K, Sanderink GC, Velders XL, Van Der Stelt PF. Radiographic detection of approximal caries: a comparison of dental films and digital imaging systems. Dentomaxillofacial Radiology. 2000 Sep 1; 29(5):312-8.
3. White & Pharoah, Textbook of oral radiology, 5th edition, pg no. 297-312

CHAPTER 17

Infections and Inflammatory Lesions of the Jaws

Introduction:

Inflammatory lesions are by far the most common pathologic conditions of the jaws.

The jaws are unique from other bones of the body in that the presence of teeth creates a direct pathway for infectious and inflammatory agents to invade bone by means of caries and periodontal disease.

The body responds to chemical, physical, or microbiologic injury with inflammation.

The inflammatory response destroys or walls off the injurious stimulus and sets up an environment for repair of the damaged tissue.

It is important for the dental clinician to be able to diagnose these conditions and give proper treatment.

Q 1) Osteoradionecrosis:

TNMGRU AUGUST 2009 6 Marks

Definition:

(a) Necrosis of bone caused by excessive exposure to ionizing radiation.

(b) Osteoradionecrosis is defined as an area of exposed necrotic bone in one or more locations of the maxillary or mandibular alveolar process, with failure to heal during at least three months.

The sequence leading to osteoradionecrosis is as follows:

1. Treatment of oral cancers involves radiation of the jaws as therapy following which an area of bone may not heal.
2. Irradiation leads to damage to the osteocytes and causes impairment of the blood supply and the obliteration of the inferior alveolar artery is thought to be the main cause leading to ischemic necrosis of the mandible.
3. Radiation treatment leads to osteitis which occurs due to radiation, trauma and infection, which was old theory and now can be

replaced by theory of sequence of metabolic and cellular changes resulting in chronic non-healing wounds.

4. Marx redefined the pathophysiology of osteoradionecrosis by stating that endarteritis is induced by radiation therapy which results in hypoxia of the tissues, hypocellularity and hypovascularity and this results in breakdown of tissues and non-healing wounds that are chronic.

Risk factors in osteoradionecrosis:

(i) Primary site of cancer.
(ii) Proximity of tumor to bone.
(iii) Extent of mandible included in the primary radiation field.
(iv) Poor oral hygiene including odontogenic and periodontal disease.
(v) State of dentition.
(vi) Radiation dose (above 60 gray).
(vii) Chronic trauma from ill fitting dentures.
(viii) Acute trauma from surgical procedures of jaws.
(viii) Nutritional status.

Staging as given by Marx:

Stage:

I) The alveolar bone is exposed but there is no pathologic fracture and hyperbaric oxygen therapy gives good results.
II) Disease does not respond to hyperbaric oxygen therapy, and requires sequestrectomy and saucerisation.
III) There is damage to the entire thickness of the bone and pathologic fracture could be present, and complete resection is required with reconstruction with free tissue.

Clinical Signs And Symptoms:

1. More common in mandible than maxilla due to rich vascular supply of the maxilla.
2. Posterior mandible is more affected than the anterior.
3. Ulceration or necrosis of the mucous membrane with exposure of necrotic bone.
4. Symptoms of pain, dysesthesia or anesthesia, may be present along the inferior alveolar nerve in the mandible.
5. Foul smell from mouth, abnormal taste sensation, and food impaction may also be found.
6. Exposure of rough, irregular denuded bone may result in physical irritation to the adjoining tissues, and later on may lead to pathologic fracture and intra- or extraoral fistula formations.
7. Disturbances with limitations in mouth opening and difficulty in mastication, swallowing and speech may also occur.
8. Radiographically areas of increased density interspaced with osteolytic regions and late forming sequestra are seen. It resembles osteomyelitis, but is more widespread.

Prevention:

(i) The jaws, teeth and oral mucosa should be shielded before radiation therapy in the area.
(ii) Removal of unhealthy teeth before radiation therapy.
(iii) As a general rule, teeth that are in direct line of radiation should be rendered healthy enough to require little or no treatment for 5 years after radiation.

Treatment:

Osteoradionecrosis is best managed by topical antibiotic or antiseptic mouth rinses. Hyperbaric oxygen therapy promotes the oxygenation of tissues, increases angiogenesis and promotes osteoblastic fibroblastic function. It is carried out for about Dives at 100% oxygen and 2-2.5 atmospheric pressure.

Sequestrated bone may be managed with limited resection or may require mandibulectomy. If surgery is required, post surgical hyperbaric oxygen therapy of 10 dives is recommended.

Stage wise treatment regimen:

A) Early stage:

There is no discomfort present due to the lesion, which has been present only for a short time.

1. The irradiated patient should be followed up periodically that is every 3 months during the first year and then every 6 months.
2. Avoiding oral mucosal irritants like smoking, alcohol, removable dentures.
3. Introduction of good oral hygiene.
4. Irrigation of the lesions with 0.2% chlorhexidine TDS.
5. Pentoxyphylline 800mgs/day+vitamin A and D 1000IU/day.

B) Intermediate stage:

In this stage pain can occur which may or may not improve with antibiotics.

1. The observation of good oral hygiene should be continued.
2. Irrigation with 0.2% chlorhexidine of the lesions should be continued.
3. Antibiotic treatment: Amoxycillin/clavulanic acid is given 875 mgs TDS+ciprofloxacin 500mgs BD daily until disappearance of the pain.
4. If the pain and discomfort persist, minorly invasive surgery can be carried out, provided the lesion is small 0.5-1cm and is not causing invasion of the neighboring structures.

C) Advanced stage:

Complications like fractures of the mandible, trismus and cutaneous fistula can occur.

1. The above measures mentioned apply.Apart from those,

2. Elimination of the osteolytic areas with ablation surgery.
3. Reconstruction surgery of the posterior region with bone grafts, vascularized flaps or free grafts.

Suggested reading:

1. Bouquot, Brad W. Neville, Douglas D. Damm, Carl M. Allen, Jerry E. (2002). Oral & maxillofacial pathology (2.ed.). Philadelphia: W.B. Saunders. p.263.
2. Epstein JB, Wong FL, Stevenson-Moore P J, Osteoradionecrosis: clinical experience and a proposal for classification. Oral Maxillofac Surg. 1987 Feb; 45(2):104-10.
3. Javier Silvestre-Rangil, Francisco-Javier Silvestre Clinico-therapeutic management of osteoradionecrosis: A literature review and update, Med Oral Patol Oral Cir Bucal. 2011 Nov 1;16 (7):e900-4.
4. Lyons A, Ghazali N. Osteoradionecrosis of the jaws: current understanding of its pathophysiology and treatment. Br J Oral Maxillofac Surg. 2008;46:653–660.

Q 2) Describe the radiographic appearance of chronic osteomyelitis:

MUHS OCTOBER 2004 (2 Marks)
TNMGRU OCTOBER 2003 (5 Marks)

Osteomyelitis is an infection of bone and bone marrow. Can affect long bones pelvic bones and may also affect the jaws. Mandible is more commonly affected especially the posterior part.

Definition:

Osteomyelitis is inflammation of bone where in the inflammatory process may spread through the bone to involve the marrow, cortex, cancellous portion, and periosteum.

Radiographic appearance:

The earliest changes in bone in chronic osteomyelitis is blurring and unsharpness, fuzziness of trabeculae.

Gradually solitary or multiple radiolucent areas may be seen on the radiograph, representing enlarged trabecular spaces due to foci of necrosis and frank bone destruction.

There is loss of lamina dura around involved teeth.

Multiple areas of radiolucency with ill defined borders are seen resembling, moth eaten appearance.

As the lesions progress segments of necrotic bone detach and get calcified, and appears as more dense bone, called sequestra.

Chronic osteomyelitis has a tendency to stimulate the formation of new periosteal bone appearing as single or multiple layers of bone giving, onion peel appearance.

There is gradually formation of involucrum. An involucrum denotes a layer of living bone that has formed about dead bone. Later an opening in the involucrum termed cloaca is formed which is typical of chronic osteomyelitis.

Types of Chronic osteomyelitis:

- Chronic suppurative osteomyelitis:
- Chronic Non Suppurative Osteomyelitis.
  - (a) Focal Sclerosing Osteomyelitis
  - (b) Diffuse Sclerosing Osteomyelitis.
- Chronic Subperiosteal Osteomyelitis.
- Garre's Osteomyelitis (proliferative periostitis).
- Actinomycotic Osteomyelitis.

1. **Chronic suppurative osteomyelitis:**
   - Multiple radiolucencies of variable size with outlines that are irregular and poor in definition of borders are present.
   - Moth eaten appearance: The bone gradually develops a moth eaten appearance as radiolucent areas enlarge and are separated by islands of normal bone. (This is due to enlargement of medullary spaces and widening of volksman's canals secondary to lysis of bone and replacement with granulation tissue.)
   - Sequestrum formation: Segments of necrotic bone detach from normal bone and form sequestra. There is formation of involucrum which is deposition of shell of new bone by the periosteum surrounding the sequestra and has holes called the cloaca in the regions where there is rupture of the subperiosteal abscess that opens on the skin with the help of multiple sinuses which discharge pus.
   - Periosteal new bone formation: Often stimulates periosteal bone formation as a single layer or multiple layers of radiopaque lines parallel to cortical bone.
   - Roots of the involved teeth may undergo resorption and loss of lamina dura.
2. **Chronic non-suppurative osteomyelitis:**
   - (a) Focal sclerosing osteomyelitis: Well circumscribed radiopaque apical mass looking like a benign cementoblastoma can be seen. Root outline is clearly visible on the radiographs.
   - (b) Diffuse sclerosing osteomyelitis: Ill defined osteoclastic and osteosclerotic areas can be seen.
3. **Chronic subperiosteal osteomyelitis:**
   May show moth eaten appearance, multiple small radiopaque flakes in occlusal projection, and mottling of adjacent trabeculae.
4. **Garre's osteomyelitis:**
   - Its a peculiar type of osteomyelitis that is chronic and affects the children and young adults. It typically involves the mandible and is often associated with an odontogenic infection due to caries.
   - It presents as localised overgrowth of bone on the outer aspect of the cortex. This bony mass is supracortical but subperiosteal and is smooth, fairly calcified, and can be described as a duplication of the cortical layer of the mandible.
   - There is a thin convex shell of bone overlying the cortex with

radiolucent space between the bone and cortex.

- Onion peel appearance-thickening and lamination of the cortex may show alternating radiopaque and radiolucent lines.

5. **Actinomycotic osteomyelitis:**
   Produces dense bone and scarring of soft tissues which has been described as lumpy jaw.

Suggested reading:

1. Collert S, Isacson J. Chronic sclerosing osteomyelitis (Garré). Clin. Orthop. Relat. Res. 1982; (164): 136-40.
2. Freny R Karjodkar, Essentials of Oral And Maxillofacial Radiology, chapter 20, page no 283-290.
3. H.M Worth, Principles and practice of Oral Radiologic Interpretation, page 215-230.

Q 3) Differential diagnosis between periapical abscess and periodontal abscess:

MUHS MAY 2008 (2 Marks)

Sr. no	Periapical Abscess	Periodontal Abscess
1.	Periapical abscess can be due to trauma or chemicals or mechanical irritation of the pulp.The bacterial invasion leads to pulpitis and later periapical abscess.	It is culmination of a long period of chronic periodontitis.
2.	**Pathogenesis:** • Microorganism: Streptococci viridians and staphylococci are frequently associated with abscess formation. • They produce the enzyme called coagulase which causes fibrin deposition and thus helps in walling off the lesion. Coagulase promotes virulence by inhibition of phagocytosis. • Bacterial invasion: bacterial invasion of pulp which spreads to periapical tissues, causing acute periodontitis, tender tooth and alveolar swelling. • Necrosis of periapical tissue. • Abscess formation: necrosed tissue coalesces and enlarge causing pus.	**Pathogenesis:** • Pre-existing periodontal pocket. • Multiplication of bacteria: bacteria multiply in the depth of pocket and cause sufficient irritation to form as acute abscess, with exudation of pus into this area. It results in sufficient swelling to destroy the cortical plates of bone.

Sr. no	Periapical Abscess	Periodontal Abscess
	✪ progress of abscess: purulent material travels through path of least resistance.	
3.	**Clinical features:** ✪ It develops in the periapical region of the tooth as sequelae to necrosis of pulp. ✪ Route of infection – through pulp	**Clinical features:** ✪ It starts at the gingival crevice and extends down on one or more surface of the root, frequently as far as apical region.
	✪ Pulp is non vital. ✪ Tenderness is positive on vertical percussion. ✪ Destruction of bone around the apex of root. ✪ Patients experience sensitivity or pressure in the affected area. Ice relives the pain and heat intensifies it. ✪ Associated teeth or tooth are firm. Pain is severe and throbbing type.	✪ Route of infection – periodontium. ✪ Pulp is vital. ✪ Tenderness is positive on lateral percussion. ✪ Destruction of alveolar bone at lateral to the root or interdental region. ✪ Associated teeth are tender and mobile. ✪ Acute episodes usually has sudden onset with extreme pain. There is also distension and discomfort.
4.	**Radiographic appearance** ✪ Widening of the radiolucent line of the periodontal ligament space or no apparent changes evident. ✪ Loss of the radiopaque line of the lamina dura at the apex. ✪ Area of bone loss at the tooth apex No apparent bone destruction but dense sclerotic bone evident around the tooth apex (sclerosing osteitis). ✪ Circumscribed, well-defined radiolucent area of bone loss at the apex, surrounded by dense sclerotic bone.	**Radiographic appearance** ✪ Loss of the corticated interdental crestal margin, the bone edge becomes irregular or blunted. ✪ Widening of the periodontal ligament space at the crestal margin. ✪ Loss of the normally sharp angle between the crestal bone and the lamina dura — the bone angle becomes rounded and irregular. ✪ Localized or generalized loss of the alveolar supporting bone.

Sr. no	Periapical Abscess	Periodontal Abscess
		✪ Patterns of bone loss — horizontal and/or vertical — resulting in an even loss of bone or the formation of complex intra-bony defects. ✪ Loss of bone in the furcation areas of multirooted teeth — this can vary from widening of the furcation periodontal ligament to large zones of bone destruction.
5.	**Diagnosis** ✪ Clinical diagnosis : carious tooth, tenderness positive with involved tooth, sinus formation, non-vital teeth will give clue to the diagnosis. ✪ Laboratory diagnosis: central region of necrosis contain dense accumulation of polymorphonuclear leukocytes, surrounded by inflamed connective tissue wall of varying thickness.	**Diagnosis** ✪ Clinical diagnosis : severe pain with swelling in the apical region will give clue to the diagnosis. ✪ Laboratory diagnosis : There is central cavity filled with pus walled off on one side by the root and on the other side by connective tissue.

Suggested reading:

1. Eric whaites, textbook of essential of dental radiography and radiology, third edition, chapter 21, page no. 246.

Q 4) How will you distinguish between reversible and irreversible pulpitis?

MUHS MAY 2011 (2 Marks)

Sr. No	Reversible pulpitis	Irreversible pulpitis
1.	It is a mild to moderate inflammatory condition of pulp caused by noxious stimuli in which pulp is capable of returning to the uninflammed state after removal of stimuli.	It is a persistent inflammatory condition of pulp caused by noxious stimuli in which pulp is not capable of returning to the uninflammed state after removal of stimuli.

Sr. No	Reversible pulpitis	Irreversible pulpitis
2.	It is caused by injury to the pulp by trauma, disturbed occlusal relationship, thermal shock, excessive dehydration, chemical stimulus.	It is caused by bacterial involvement of pulp through caries.
3.	Pain is less severe, sharp and of short duration.	Pain is more severe, piercing or shooting, radiating and of longer duration.
4.	Pain subsides after removal of stimulus.	Pain does not subside after removal of stimulus.
5.	Patient does not give history of night pain.	Patient gives history of night pain.
6.	Pain is increased by cold beverages or cold air.	Pain is increased by heat and sometimes relieved by cold.

Suggested reading:

1. Louis I grossman, Endodontic Practice: Endodontic Emergencies, 11th ed, 83-87.

Q 5) Garre's osteomyelitis:

RGUHS APRIL 2001 (5 Marks)

Carl Gaffe in 1893 first described Garre's osteomyelitis as a focal gross thickening of the periosteum with peripheral reactive bone formation due to infection. It was at one time reported only in the long bones especially the tibia, but in 1948 Berger reported a case involving the mandible. It specifically affects the children and young adults and is often associated with an odontogenic infection caused mainly due to dental caries.

It is also known as 'proliferative periostitis'.

This is non-suppurating sclerosing osteomyelitis characterized by formation of hard, bony swelling at periphery of jaw.

It is induced by a mild infection below the periosteum from cancellous portion of jaw that penetrates the cortex.

For lesion to develop following conditions should be satisfied:

1. The periosteum should possess a high degree of osteoblastic activity.
2. Mild infection should be present to serve as a stimulus.
3. A fine balance has to be maintained between the resistance of the involved host and the virulence and the number of organism.

Etiology:

The organisms that cause this are mainly staphylococcus pyogenes of the aureus and albus variety and streptococci and some mixed organisms can also be the cause.

Typical evolution of this lesion can be because of the osteogenetic potential that is high in young patients that allows the osteoblastic process to be superior to the osteoclastic one and this pattern resembles that of the condensing osteitis that is seen in the periapical area of the carious teeth, however the bone proliferation is periosteal rather than endosteal.

Clinical features:

(a) Males affected more than females and generally below 30 years of age.
In the young patients due to the considerable activity of the osteoblastic cells in the periosteum, there is condensation of the cortical bone and it usually affects the mandible which results in a swelling that is hard over the jaws causing facial asymmetry and there is little or no pain.
(b) Mandible more commonly involved than maxilla especially inferior border of mandible and 1st molar region.
(c) Presents as hard non tender swelling with medial and lateral expansion of jaw.
(d) Size vary from 1-2 cm to involvement of the entire length of affected side. Cortex may become 2-3 cm thick.
(e) If secondarily infected it causes considerable discomfort.
(f) Generally the skin over the swelling is normal, but in some cases if there is pain it could be inflammed.
(g) Other associated symptoms: lymphadenopathy, hyperpyrexia, leukocytosis. However these findings are milder than the other types of osteomyelitis, in which cases there is high fever. increased WBC count, sedimentation rate or alkaline phosphatase values.

Radiologic features:

(a) An intra oral periapical radiograph will show a carious tooth opposite the hard bony mass.
(b) Shadow of the thin convex shell of the bone overlying the cortex, with radiolucent space between the two is seen.
(c) Panoramic and occlusal views will reveal a typical localised bony overgrowth on the outer cortical surface. This bony mass is supracortical but subperiosteal and is smooth, fairly calcified, and can be described as the duplication of the cortical layer of the mandible.
(d) A lateral oblique view of the mandible will show the expansion of the lesion which can be both inferior and lateral to the lower border of the mandible, where as the panoramic and the occlusal views will show a vertical and lateral apposition of the bone respectively.
(e) As infection persists cortex becomes thick and becomes laminated having alternate radiolucent/radiopaque layers giving an onion peel like appearance.
(f) Adjacent cancellous bone may remain normal.
(g) Following removal of irritation cortical bone may remodel to a normal appearance.

Histopathologic findings:

The chief characteristic is the new bone formation or osteoid tissue, bordered with osteoblasts and some areas of bone resorption. In the marrow spaces, lymphocytes can be seen commonly.

Differential diagnosis:

1. Ewing's sarcoma
2. Caffey's disease (infantile cortical huperostosis)
3. Osteosarcoma.
4. Peripheral osteomas, tori, exostoses should be clinically distinguished.
5. Ossifying subperiosteal hematoma.

Treatment:

The usual treatment options are observation, analgesics and NSAIDs, and bone curettage.

Removal of the offending teeth or source of infection along with antibiotic therapy will help in resolution of the condition.

Resection and bone transport using a circular external fixator for the treatment of sclerosing osteomyelitis of Garré might be an effective and safe method.

Suggested reading:

1. McWalter GM, Schaberg Garre's osteomyelitis of the mandible resolved by endodontic treatment. SJJ Am Dent Assoc. 1984 Feb;108(2):193-5.
2. Nikomarov D, Zaidman M, Katzman A, Keren Y, Eidelman M., New treatment option for sclerosing osteomyelitis of Garré, J Pediatr Orthop B. 2013 Nov;22(6):577-82.
3. Stephane Schwartz, Huan Pham, Garre's osteomyelitis: a case report, The American Academy of Pedodontics/Vol. 3, No. 3, 283-285.

CHAPTER 18

Cysts of the Jaws

Introduction

Cyst is pathological cavity containing fluid, semifluid or gaseous contents, and which is not created by accumulation of pus.It is frequently but not always lined by an epithelium.

They appear mostly as radiolucencies on a radiograph and many cysts have distinctive radiological characteristics of their own.

Many cysts are asymptomatic in their initial stages and are observed by chance on routine radiography. Radiography plays an important role in the study of cysts and helps in assessing their extent and nature and helps to decide a strategy on their surgical management.

Q 1) Radiographic appearance of dentigerous cyst:

MUHS MAY 2012 (2 Marks)

Dentigerous cyst which is also known as the follicular cyst is a cyst of odontogenic origin and is a developmental cyst which is associated with the crown of an unerupted tooth. The cavity of the cyst is lined with epithelial cells derived from the reduced enamel epithelium and occurs because of the accumulation of fluid between the reduced enamel epithelium and the crown of the tooth.

Radiographically the difference between a normal dental follicle and the dentigerous cyst is just about the size. When a follicular space is more than 3mm, its considered to be a dentigerous cyst.

Location:

- More than 75% of the cases of dentigerous cyst occur in the mandible and the teeth commonly involved are:
- Most commonly mandibular third molar.
- Second most common is the maxillary third molar.
- Maxillary canine.
- Mandibular second premolar.
- An important diagnostic point is that this cyst attaches at the cemento-enamel junction.

Radiographic features:

Periphery and shape:

The common appearance is a well demarcated radiolucency attached at an acute angle to the cervical area of the unerupted tooth. The border of this lesion is usually sclerotic.

Dentigerous cysts typically have a well-defined cortex with a curved or circular outline. If infection is present, the cortex may be missing.

It's a commonly unilocular lesion with well defined margins and radiopaque borders but rarely could be multilocular. If the cyst gets infected, the margins can get ill-defined.

Radiographically three types of dentigerous cysts occur:

1. Circumferential
2. Lateral
3. Radicular

The internal aspect is completely radiolucent except for the crown of the involved tooth.

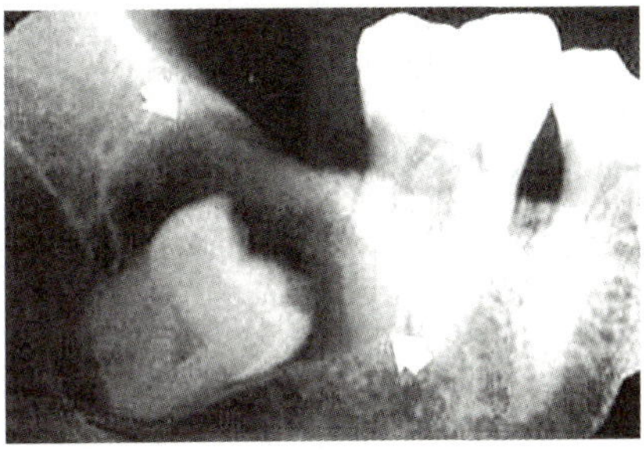

Fig. Dentigerous cyst with cystic lining surrounding the crown of tooth

Effect on surrounding structure:

The size of the cyst can vary greatly from being just about slightly bigger than a dental follicle to involving large areas of the jaws causing hollowing out of the majority of the bone. There can be erosion, resorption of roots and displacement of the teeth as well.

Suggested reading:

1. Stuart C White, Michael J Pharoah, Oral Radiology, Principles and Interpretation 6th edition, 347 .

Q 2) Radiographic appearance of periapical cyst:

BFU MAY 2006 (5 Marks)

Periapical cyst also called as a radicular cyst and can be termed as the most common cyst of the jaws.

Dental caries and trauma leading to pulpitis and then necrosis is the most common cause.

Periapical or radicular cyst occurs when rests of epithelial cells of the periodontal ligament proliferate due to stimulation and undergo cystic change degeneration by inflammatory products which are common sequelae in the progressive changes associated with bacterial invasion of the pulp and its death.

Radiographic features:

- Appears as a pear shaped or round radiolucency at the apex of a tooth mainly due to caries or trauma, resulting in death of the pulp, rendering the tooth non-vital.

- The epicenter of the periapical cyst lies at the apex of the non-vital tooth. However some times they may occur at the mesial or distal surface of the root apex coinciding with the opening of an accessory canal.
- Most periapical cysts occur in the maxilla involving the incisors or canines.
- When they involve the lateral incisor, there is chance of invagination into the antrum.
- They may also form in relation to roots of deciduous molars.
- The size of the radiolucency is more than 1.5cm but less than 3cms.
- It has well defined sclerotic borders and is usually curved or circular unless it is hindered by the neighboring structures like the cortical plates.
- The borders are smooth, well corticated and well defined unless it is secondarily infected.
- The radiopaque border is continuous with the lamina dura of the associated tooth. Infection may cause the borders to become blurred or indistinct.
- Long standing cysts may displace the adjacent teeth.
- The cyst may push the floor of the maxillary antrum and may appear as if it has involved it. However the presence of cortex between the cystic border and contents of the antrum can help to determine otherwise. It may also penetrate maxillary antrum.
- There can be expansion in a curved or circular shape of the outer cortices of the maxilla or mandible.

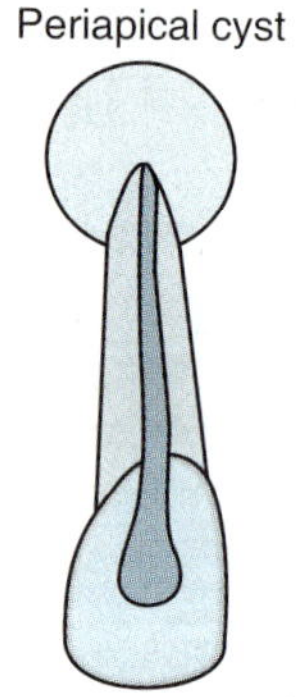

Fig. Periapical cyst associated with maxillary incisior

- These cysts may displace the mandibular alveolar canal in the inferior direction.
- Radicular cysts of long duration may cause resorption of roots.
- Dystrophic calcifications may occur in some long standing cysts and may appear as sparsely distributed small particulate opacities.

Suggested reading:

1. Freny R Karjodkar, Text Book Of Dental And Maxillofacial Radiology, 2nd Edition, 513.
2. Stuart C White, Michael J Pharaoh, Oral Radiology Principles And Interpretation, 5th Edition, 385-386.

CHAPTER 19

Benign Tumours of Jaws

Introduction:

Benign tumours represent a new uncoordinated growth that generally has the following characteristics.

Benign tumours are slow-growing and spread by direct extension and not by metastases.

They tend to resemble the tissue of origin histologically.

For example, an ameloblastoma, a tumor thought to be derived from odontogenic epithelium is often composed of cells that resemble ameloblasts.

It is thought that benign tumors have unlimited growth potential.

Q 1) Radiographic appearance of Pindborg's tumour (CEOT):

MUHS NOVEMBER 2010 2 Marks

The Pindborg's tumours account for about 1% of all odontogenic tumours. These are located in the bone and produce a mineralised substance within amyloid like material.

Though it is seen in the same age group as that of ameloblastoma, it is less aggressive than it.

This neoplasm is more common in men and the average age of occurrence is about 42 years though the range is from 8-92 years.

Expansion of the jaws is the usual feature and probably the only symptom.

Radiographic features:

Site: As with ameloblastoma the calcifying epithelial odontogenic tumours (CEOT) have the predilection for the mandible and develop most commonly in the premolar-molar region. About 52% are associated with an unerupted or impacted tooth.

These tumors show a area of radiolucency surrounding the crown of a mature, unerupted tooth.

The borders are well defined and have a cyst like cortex. In some cases the boundaries could be irregular or ill-defined.

The tumour can be unilocular or multilocular and generally have radiopaque foci scattered within of varying size and density.

This gives a driven snow like appearance.

The most characteristic and diagnostic finding is the appearance of varying radiopaque foci around the crown of the embedded tooth. The lumen of the tumour may have a crisscrossing of small, thin radiopaque trabeclae in several directions.

Effects on the surrounding structures:

The CEOT has the capability of displacing or preventing the eruption of a developing tooth. It can cause expansion of the jaws and has a maintained boundary of cortical bone.

Suggested reading:

1. Stuart C White, Michael J Pharoah, Oral Radiology, Principles and Interpretation, 5th Edition, page 422-424.

Q 2) Radiographic appearance of adenomatoid odontogenic tumor

MUHS MAY 2008 (2 Marks)

These tumours are non-aggressive, uncommon tumours originating from the odontogenic epithelium.

The lesion was first reported by Stafne, and has distinctive clinical-and microscopic features and behavior patterns that sharply differ from ameloblastomas.

The origin of adenomatoid odontogenic tumors may be from enamel organ epithelium, and it is classified as a mixed tumor because dentinoid material and occasionally enamel matrix is manufactured.

Adenomatoid odontogenic tumors comprise 3% of all oral tumors.

The central and peripheral type of tumours have been reported.

The central tumours are further divided into two types, that is the follicular type which are associated with the crown of the embedded tooth and the extrafollicular type which are not associated with any embedded tooth.

About 73% of the central lesions are the follicular type.

Location:

- At least 75% of adenomatoid odontogenic tumors occur in the maxillary bone.
- The most common region is the incisor-canine-premolar area and especially the canine region, is the usual area involved in both jaws.

Borders:

- The borders are generally well defined and are sclerotic.

Internal structure:

- Within the lumen, radiographically, radiopacities develop in about 2/3rds of the cases.
- One tumor may be completely radiolucent, another may show faint radiopacities while some may contain clusters of dense radiopaque foci which could be ill-defined.
- Quite often the calcifications are small in size and have well defined borders and may resemble cluster of pebbles.
- Intra-oral radiographs may be required to demonstrate the calcifications within the lesion, which may not be seen on panoramic radiographs.
- Effects on the surrounding structures:
- The enlargement of the tumour can be accompanied by the displacement of the adjacent teeth.
- Resorption of the roots is rare.
- This lesion can hinder the eruption of the tooth that its involved with. It can cause expansion of the jaws but the cortex is preserved.

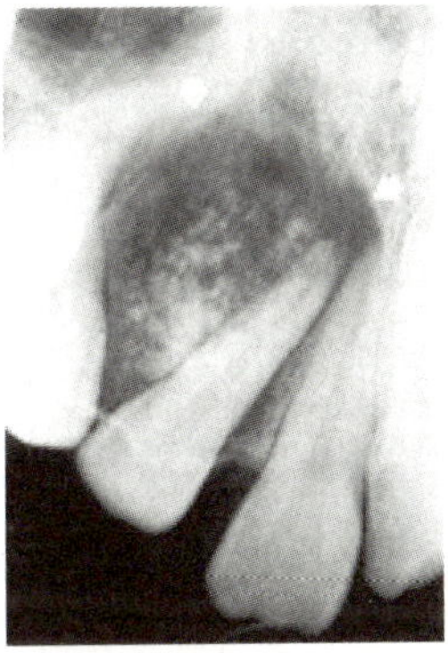

Fig. Adenomatoid odontogenic tumour in the maxillary anterior region

Suggested reading:

1. Stuart C White, Michael J Pharoah, Oral Radiology, Principles and Interpretation fifth edition, chapter 21, page no. 431-432.

Q 3) Ameloblastoma:

RGUHS OCTOBER 2002 (4 Marks)

A true neoplasm of the odontogenic epithelium, ameloblastoma is a persistent, locally invasive tumour and is aggressive but has benign growth traits.Cusack in 1827 recognised this condition first and was designated as adamantinoma by a french physician, in 1885, Louis-Charles Malassez.It was renamed as ameloblastoma in 1930 by Ivey and Churchill.

It arises from remnants of the dental lamina or enamel organ.

Etiology:

(i) Irritation.

(ii) Infection: Robinson observed that 1/3rd of the cases have a history of oral infection.
(iii) Trauma.
(iv) Dietary deficiency.
(v) Viruses: Polyoma viruses.

Classification:

(i) Unicystic.
(ii) Peripheral.
(iii) Multicystic.
(iv) Conventional.
(v) Pituitary ameloblastoma.
(vi) Adamantinoma of long bones.
(vii) Malignant ameloblastoma.

Clinical features:

It has a slight predilection for men and can occur in the age range of 20-50 years.These tumours are quite often associated with unerupted teeth. These generally occur as painless swellings, causing facial deformity to quite a severe extent, and pain can occur if the swelling impinges on other structures and can lead to loose teeth, ulcers and periodontal disease.

It can be associated with paresthesia.

Lesions can occur in the mandible and maxilla, but the mandibular molar-ramus region is most commonly involved.

It can cause severe expansion of the maxilla and mandible and can lead to grotesque deformities.

When the maxilla is involved it can encroach upon the maxillary sinus and the floor of the nose.

As the lesion is slow growing, it can cause expansion of the bony cortices, because the periosteum gets enough time to develop thin bony shell ahead of the expanding lesion.

This thin bony shell crackles when pressed and the phenomenon is called the typical egg-shell cracking or crepitus which is an important diagnostic feature.

Radiographic features:

They occur commonly in the molar-ramus region of mandible but symphysis may be involved.

When in maxilla it can involve the maxillary antrum and the nasal cavity.

The lesions appear as well defined radiolucencies with smooth, scalloped, corticated borders.

The lesion consists of septa which are arranged in different forms and can vary from honey comb, soap bubble, spider nevus like appearances.

They can mimic a typical dental cyst like appearance.

Multilocular appearance is a common type of radiological presentation.

It can cause expansion and thinning of cortex and some times a window formation also can be seen where the periosteum is unable to cope up with the expansion of the lesion.

There is a tendency to cause extensive root resorption and some times displacement of teeth.

The expansion can lead to egg shell crackling of the bone.

Differential diagnosis:

When associated with unerupted teeth it can look like dentigerous cyst.

It should be differentiated from odontogenic keratocyst, ossifying fibroma, giant cell granuloma and odontogenic myxoma.

Management:

Surgical resection or enucleation is the most effective and definitive treatment for this condition, though chemotherapy, radiation therapy, curettage and liquid nitrogen have been used with some efficacy. During surgery, due to its invasive nature, excision of the normal tissue around the margins of the tumour needs to be done.

Smaller lesions can be removed by intraoral approach and for large lesions jaw resection may be required.

Maxillary lesions are treated more aggressively due to tendency to involve the maxillary sinus and nasal cavity and other adjacent vital structures.

Suggested reading:

1. Stuart C White, Michael J Pharoah, Oral Radiology, Principles and Interpretation 5th Edition, 419-422.

Q 4) Radiographic appearance of giant cell reparative granuloma:

TNMGRU APRIL 1996 (4 Marks)

Reparative giant cell granulomas (RGCG) are classified according to the site of occurrence as central (bone) and peripheral(gingival tissues).

RGCG is a reactive process rather than a true neoplasm.It can begin due to trauma or inflammation and accounts for about 1-7% of the benign tumours of the jaws.

The lesion is generally slow growing and the fast growing lesions are rare, and though it has a benign histological appearance, it behaves in an aggressive manner like a malignant lesion.

In 1953 Jaffe first called this lesion as giant cell reparative granuloma, in which he described this lesion as a local reparative reaction to hemorrhage, intraosseously which was induced by trauma.Before this the lesion was termed as a giant cell tumour.

Most of the cases of these lesions are reported in the maxilla or mandible and there few cases involving the other cranio-facial bones and small tubular bones of the hands and feet.

Radiological features:

Central giant cell granuloma:

Begins as a small radiolucent lesion and grows slowly and enlarges, and thin bony trabeculae become noticeable and gives the lesion a honeycomb like multilocular appearance. It can cause expansion, resorption of root and erosion through the overlying cortex.

Location:

- Found in mandible twice as often as in maxilla.
- In younger patients it is more likely to occur anterior to the 1st molar in mandible and anterior to the cuspid in maxilla.
- In older patient, greater frequency in the posterior aspect of jaw.

Periphery:

- The lesion grows slowly and is likely to have well defined margins especially in the mandible.
- The periphery seldom shows cortication.
- Lesions that affect the maxilla can have ill-defined margins which may mimic the borders of a malignant lesion.

Internal structures:

- Generally small lesions show very little evidence of trabeculation.
- Some cases may have fine granular pattern of calcification which can be visible against bright light.
- This granular bone can get organised in to an ill defined fine wispy septa which is typical trait of this lesion.
- When they emanate at right angles from the periphery it is very much suggestive of this lesion.
- Presence of a small indentation in the region of the origination of the septa strongly indicates this lesion.
- In some cases the septa could be well defined and may divide the internal aspect into separate compartments creating a multilocular appearance.

Effects on surrounding structures:

- Paresthesia is not usually observed with this lesion because though it can grow and expand and be invasive, it doesnot affect the perineural sheets.
- Displacement and resorption of teeth.
- Resorption may be profound and irregular in outline.
- Loss of lamina dura involving the teeth within the lesion can be seen.
- There could be displacement of the inferior alveolar nerve in the inferior direction.
- This lesion could have a potential to expand the cortical boundaries of maxilla and mandible.
- Expansion is usually uneven or undulating and when viewed in an occlusal film it could demonstrate a double boundary.
- The bone which forms the border of the expanded mandible can often have a granular texture when compared to the cortical bone.
- Sometimes there is destruction of the outer cortical bone instead

of expansion, and this effect is seen more often in the maxilla which can make the lesion look like a malignant one.

- There are chances that these lesions might transform into osteosarcoma or fibrosarcoma.

Peripheral giant cell granuloma:

Radiographic appearance:

The lesions of peripheral giant cell granuloma develops in the soft tissue and may show superficial resorption sometimes of the underlying crest of the alveolar bone which is called cupping.

Suggested reading:

1. Freny R Karjodkar, Text Book Of Dental And Maxillofacial Radiology, chapter 26, pg no 595.
2. K. A. Jeevan Kumar, S. Humayun, B. Pavan Kumar, and J. Brahmaji Rao, Reparative giant cell granuloma of the maxilla, Ann Maxillofac Surgv.1(2); Jul-Dec 2011.
3. Padam Narayan Tandon, S. K. Gupta, Durga Shanker Gupta, Sunit Kumar Jurel, and Abhishek Saraswat Peripheral giant cell granuloma Contemp Clin Dent. 2012 Apr; 3(Suppl1): S118–S121.

CHAPTER 20

Malignant Tumours of Orofacial Region

Introduction:

Malignant tumours are aggressive fast growing lesion that can affect the oro-facial region. They are generally ill defined and cause destruction of the tissues as they grow. Soft tissue tumours may show changes in radiography only when the bone is involved where as those arising from bone will show radiographic changes from the beginning and various tumours may have typical radiographic features and their knowledge is important for diagnosis as well as treatment.

Q 1) Radiographic Appearance of Osteosarcoma

BFU MAY 2006 (5 Marks)

Osteosarcoma is a malignant neoplasm of bone in which osteoid is produced directly by malignant stroma as opposed to adjacent reactive bone formation.

Radiographic Features:

- Mandible is more commonly affected then the maxilla.However any part of the jaw can be involved. Posterior part of the mandible along with the tooth bearing areas, angle and the vertical part of the ramus is most commonly involved.

  In the maxilla, the alveolar ridges, antrum and the palate are most commonly involved.
- The borders of the lesion are ill defined, and the lesion is radiolucent with no sclerotic border or encapsulation.
- When the periosteum is invaded directly by the lesion the periosteum may show a typical sun-ray or sun-burst appearance. This occurs when the periosteum is partly destroyed, displaced or disorganised.
- Another type of periosteal reaction is called the Codman's triangle which occurs when the periosteum is elevated and maintains its osteogenic potential but is breached in the centre.

- When sometimes, laminar periosteal new bone is formed it may give onion peel appearance of periosteum.
- Osteosarcomas could be completely radiolucent, mixed radiopaque/ radiolucent or totally opaque.
  - (i) **Osteolytic or radiolucent type:** They have ill defined borders, are unicentric and may have moth eaten appearance. There could be perforation and expansion of the cortical bone.
  - (ii) **Mixed type:** The lesion will have small amount of new bone formation. This bone formation is in the form of strand and the trabecular pattern may resemble the honeycomb pattern.
  - (iii) **The osteoblastic type:** The lesion has a ragged, ill defined borders, and there is combination of excessive bone deposition along with areas of radiolucent bone destruction. This type gives a dense granular appearance.
- Thus there is loss of normal trabecular pattern in this disease.
- It is a destructive lesion and may result in widening of the periodontal membrane. Mandibular lesions can destroy the cortex of the inferior alveolar canal, and the adjacent lamina dura.
- In the lesions involving the maxilla, the walls of maxillary antrum and nasal cavity may be lost.
- Due to severe destruction of bone pathological fractures of bone is common in cases of osteosarcoma.

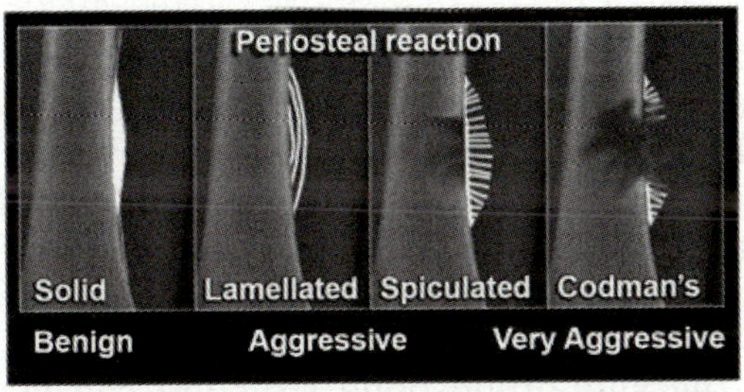

Fig. Periosteal reactions of bone in osteosarcoma.

Suggested reading:

1. Freny R Karjodkar, Text Book Of Dental and Maxillofacial Radiology, 2nd Edition, 620-621.
2. Stuart C White, Michael.J Pharaoh, Oral Radiology, Principles and Interpretation, 469.

Q 2) Discuss clinical and radiographic features of squamous cell carcinoma originating in bone.

5 Marks (Not specific to any university)

Synonyms:

Squamous cell carcinoma originating in the bone is also known as,

Primary intraosseous carcinoma, intra-alveolar carcinoma, central squamous cell carcinoma, and primary epithelial tumour of the jaw etc.

Definition:

According to the World Health Organization's International Histologic Classification of Tumors, its a squamous cell carcinoma originating within the jaw, which has no initial connection with the oral mucosa, and presumed to develop from the residues of the odontogenic epithelium.

Classification:

The proposed classification is as follows:

Type 1. Arising ex odontogenic cyst.

Type 2. Arising ex ameloblastoma.

- A. Well-differentiated (malignant ameloblastoma)
- B. Poorly differentiated (ameloblastic carcinoma)

Type 3. Arising de novo.

- A. Nonkeratinizing.
- B. Keratinizing:

Clinical Manifestations:

- They are rare in occurrence and may remain unobserved till it reaches large size.
- It is more common in men (male:female ratio is 3:1 approximately) and occurs in the 4th -8th decade.
- It occurs more commonly in the mandible than the maxilla and the first molar region is more involved.
- It can be associated with pain, pathologic fractures, and involvement of the sensory nerves leading to paresthesia of the lip, and lymphadenopathy also occurs commonly.
- The epithelium above the lesion appears normal. These lesions can cause destruction of the antral or the nasal floors, loss of outline of cortication of the inferior alveolar canal and loss of lamina dura. Resorption of roots is not usual and the teeth that loose the lamina dura and the supporting bone structure can lead to the floating tooth appearance.

Radiographic Features:

- The lesions are most commonly seen in the mandible than the maxilla and the molar region is more commonly involved, the anterior region being rarely affected.
- The lesions appear in the tooth bearing areas as they originate from the remnants of the dental lamina.
- The lesions are radiolucent with no reduction of bone and very little residue of bone remaining in the center of the lesion. In case of small lesions the buccal and lingual plates can cast shadows which might look like the lesions having a trabecular pattern.
- It presents as a diffuse radiolucency, with ill-defined to well-defined periphery. The peripheral shape shows destruction of the bony

structures and varying degrees of extension into the periphery. The degree of ill definition or raggedness can show the aggressiveness of the lesion.

- If the lesion is large in size, it can lead to pathologic fractures, step deformities, thinning of the cortical borders and consequently the soft tissue mass.
- Radiographs may show the destruction of the antral and nasal floors and loss of cortical outline of the inferior alveolar canal.
- There can be loss of lamina dura and the teeth may give, floating tooth appearance.

Differential Diagnosis:

- **Periapical cysts or granulomas:** These are non-aggressive and have smooth borders.
- **Odontogenic tumors:** the margins are usually well-defined.
- **Metastatic carcinoma, multiple myeloma, fibrosarcoma, and carcinoma arising in the dental cyst:** the margins are not infiltrative and there is no extensive bone destruction.
- **Peripheral squamous cell carcinoma:** the surface epithelium is involved.

Diagnostic Criteria:

As proposed by a few authors:

1. In order to differentiate it from the squamous cell carcinomas arising from the mucosa, there should be no ulceration on the overlying mucosa except in case of trauma or tooth extractions.
2. To differentiate from other odontogenic carcinoma, the serial sections of the histologic specimens must demonstrate the squamous cell carcinoma without other odontogenic cells or cystic components.
3. The distant primary tumour can be ruled out by taking chest radiographs, which should be clear at the time of diagnosis and also through out the follow up period of six months and more.

Treatment:

- The tumours are excised with the surrounding bony structures in an en bloc resection.
- Radiotherapy and chemotherapy maybe used as adjunctive therapies.

Suggested reading:

1. Elzay RP. Primary intraosseous carcinoma of the jaws: review and update of odontogenic carcinomas. Oral Surgery, Oral Medicine, Oral Pathology. 1982 Sep 1;54(3):299-303.
2. Freny Karjodkar. Textbook of dental and maxillofacial radiology, 2nd edition, pg no. 605, 606.
3. Suei Y, Tanimoto K, Taguchi A, Wada T. Primary intraosseous carcinoma: review of the literature and diagnostic criteria. Journal of oral and maxillofacial surgery. 1994 Jun 1; 52(6):580-3
4. White & Pharoah, Textbook of oral radiology, 5th edition, pg no. 463, 464.

CHAPTER 21

Fibro-Osseous Lesions

Introduction:

Fibro osseous lesions constitute a group of lesions in which normal bone is replaced by fibrous tissue containing abnormal bone or cementum. These lesions should be differentiated from tumours as the treatment approach is very different.

Q 1) Radiographic features of periapical cemental dysplasia

MUHS MAY 2012 (2 Marks)

Its a condition associated with localised alteration in the metabolism of bone which results in the replacement of the components of the normal cancellous bone with tissues that are fibrous and cementum like material, abnormal bone, which is similar to that seen in fibrous dysplasia or can be a mixture of both.

Radiographic appearance:

- The epicenter of the lesion is usually present at the apex of a tooth.
- It is mostly seen in the anterior teeth of the mandible, though any tooth can be involved and in some cases even the maxillary teeth can be involved.

The periphery and shape:

- In most of the cases the periapical cemental dysplasias have a well defined border and most often a radiolucent border with different widths is present and may be surrounded by a sclerotic band that also can vary in width.
- The lesion is usually round or oval in shape and is centered at the apex of the tooth but can also have an irregular outline some times.

Internal structure:

In the early stage:

- There is loss of lamina dura.

- Can appear as a radiolucency at the apex of the tooth involved.

The mixed stage:

The radiolucent structure develops presence of radiopaque tissue. These structures sometimes are called cementicles.

The mature stage:

The internal part of the lesion can become completely radiopaque and can be devoid of any particular pattern and is usually surrounded by a thin radiolucent margin as the lesion matures from the center to outward.

Suggested reading:

1. Stuart C White, Michael J Pharoah, Oral Radiology, Principles and Interpretation, 6th edition, 432-437.

Q 2) Differentiate periapical cemental dysplasia from benign cementoblastoma radiographically.

MUHS MAY 2011 (2 Marks)

Definition:

(i) **Periapical cemental dysplasia:** Periapical cemental dysplasia (PCD) is a localized change in normal bone metabolism that results in the replacement of the components of normal cancellous bone with fibrous tissue and cementum-like material, abnormal bone (similar to that seen in fibrous dysplasia), or a mixture of the two.

(ii) **Benign cementoblastoma:** Benign cementoblastomas are slow-growing, mesenchymal neoplasms composed principally of cementum.

	Benign cementoblastoma	Periapical cemental dysplasia (PCD)
1.	The mandible is the most common location; the mandibular permanent second premolar and first molar.	It is most common in mandibular anterior teeth, and in rare cases the maxillary teeth may be involved.
2.	It appears as a well-defined radiopacity.	It is well defined with total radiolucent, mixed or radiopaque appearance.
3.	Well defined radiolucent band just inside the cortical border.	It may or may not have a well defined radiolucent band.
4.	It is a mixed radiolucent-radiopaque lesion which is majorly radiopaque.	It shows radiolucent, mixed or radiopaque appearance depending upon the stage.
5.	It has a more uniform circular shape	It has more irregular undulating outline.

6.	Cemental mass obscures the outline of the enveloped root.	It dose not obscure the outline of the root .
7.	Does not cause loss of the lamina dura.	It generally causes loss of the lamina dura.
8.	In most of cases it shows root resorption.	It shows root resorption rarely.
9.	It causes expansion of the mandible with intact cortex.	Smaller lesions do not cause expansion of the involved jaw. However, larger lesions may rarely cause expansion of the jaw.

Suggested reading

1. Stuart C White, Michael J Pharoah, Oral Radiology, Principles and Interpretion, fifth edition, chapter 23, page no457, 492.

Q 3) Radiographic appearance of fibrous dysplasia:

RGUHS APRIL 2003 (5 Marks)

Localised change in the normal bone metabolism leading to replacement of all the components of the cancellous bone with fibrous tissue which contains differing amounts of abnormal bone is called fibrous dysplasia.

Radiographic appearance:

Site:

The maxilla is involved twice as commonly as the mandible and affects the posterior region most commonly.The lesions are usually unilateral except in very extensive cases involving the maxillo-facial area where it can be bilateral.

Borders:

The borders of this lesion are usually irregular or ill defined and there is a gradual blending of the normal trabecular bone with the abnormal trabecular pattern.

In the early lesions there could be a distinction in the boundary between normal and abnormal bone which could be sharp and also corticated.

The internal structure:

The lesions of fibrous dysplasia could vary greatly in the density and pattern of the trabeculae. The variations being more significant in the mandible and quite homogenous in the maxilla.

The internal structure of the lesion can be very radiolucent or radiopaque or a mixture of the two as compared to the normal bone. The density of the lesion is more radiopaque in the maxilla and the base of the skull. The lesions in their early phase can appear more radiolucent than the mature ones or in some cases even may have granular septa giving a multilocular appearance.The trabeculae that are abnormal are more in number, shorter, thinner and irregular in shape than those that are normal. This leads to creation of a radiographic pattern that is radiopaque and can vary.

It can have a granular, typical ground glass appearance similar to that of a shattered windshield.

It can also have the pattern of the surface of the orange peel which is called as peau de orange, a wispy cotton wool appearance or amorphous, dense pattern.

A typical feature of this condition is the orientation of the abnormal trabeculae giving the impression of a thumb print.

In some cases cyst like radiolucent areas may be seen in the mature lesions which are bony cavities almost like those of the simple bone cyst.

Effects on the surrounding structures:

If the lesions are small, they may have no effect on the peripheral structures. When the lesions grow they can cause expansion of the bone, while maintaining the thinned outer cortex.It can encroach the maxillary antrum displacing its cortical boundary, and may end up involving the whole of the antral cavity.The involvement of the antrum starts from the lateral wall. The cortices of the structures involved like the floor of the antrum can be changed to an abnormal pattern of bone. Though the dentition is not affected, the bone surrounding the teeth can be altered and there is disappearance of the lamina dura due to a change into an abnormal bone pattern. In case the density of the bone is increased in the cases of fibrous dysplasia, there can be narrowing of the periodontal ligament space.

There can be displacement of teeth, interference with the normal eruption of teeth and it may pose complications for the normal orthodontic treatment.

In some cases there may be resorption of roots.

Fibrous dysplasia has an unique tendency to cause displacement of the inferior alveolar nerve canal in a direction that is upwards.

Suggested reading:

1. Stuart.C White And Michael.J.Pharaoh, oral radiology, principles and interpretation, 5th edition, 485-489.

Q 4) Radiographic appearance of Paget's disease:

BFU NOVEMBER 2013 (4 Marks)

Paget's disease is fibro osseous lesion where there is resorption and apposition of osseous tissue in one or more than one bone simultaneously. It is not a generalised skeletal disease. It may involve pelvis, femur, skull and vertebrae. Jaws are involved infrequently.

The maxilla is more commonly involved than the mandible.

Radiographic appearance: It has three stages.

I) Early radiolucent resorptive stage:

- When the mandible is involved the inferior cortex appears osteoporotic.

- The trabeculae change shape, decrease in number, and long linear trabeculae may be seen aligned in a horizontal manner.These linear, coarse and sparse, trabecule which converge towards the midline of mandible is quite typical of paget's disease.
- Root resorption might occur.
- In the skull discrete lytic lesions called osteoporosis circumscripta can be seen with somewhat irregular margins, and appearance of denser bone surrounding them.

II) Granular or ground glass stage:

- With the progress of the disease the trabeculae become short and orient randomly giving a granular pattern similar to that in fibrous dysplasia.
- Rounded patches of abnormal bone of greater density within radiolucent areas of bone is seen more commonly in the mandible than the maxilla.

III) Dense, radiopaque, appositional stage:

- In the later stages the trabeculae may become organised into rounded radiopaque patches of abnormal bone creating the cotton wool appearance.
- The opaque areas coalesce to form larger opacified areas causing increased density of bone.
- There is enlargement of bone and thinning of cortex which however remains intact. The outer cortex may appear laminated in occlusal radiographs.
- Mandible may appear prognathic due to increased thickness.
- Pagets disease when affects the maxilla may encroach the maxillary antrum and its cortical boundaries may appear more granular than sharp.
- Hypercementosis may develop in few or most of the teeth, with obliteration of periodontal membrane and loss of lamina dura. There may thus be generalised loss of lamina dura. The roots of the teeth may get ankylosed.
- Sarcomas might develop in these lesions which might result in destruction of bone.

Suggested reading:

1. Freny R. Karjodkar, Text book of dental and maxillofacial radiology, 2nd edition, 646-650.
2. Stuart C White, Michael .J Pharaoh, oral radiology, principles and interpretation, 5th edition, 507-508.

CHAPTER 22

Radiopaque Lesions of the Jaws

Q1) Differential diagnosis of periapical radiopacities:

TNMGRU FEBRUARY 2012 (5 Marks)

1. True periapical radiopacities are produced by lesions that surround the apex or are located in the periapex.
2. False (projected) periapical radiopacities are produced by entities that are situated buccally or lingually to the apex and whose radiopaque images are superimposed over the apical region.

I) True periapical radiopacities:

1. **Condensing or sclerosing osteitis:** Induced by an inflammation or infection that most often occurs as a pulpo-periapical lesion.
   The highly concentrated products of infection are thought to act as irritants and produce bone resorption, whereas the diluted irritants may induce bone proliferation.
   No pain, swelling, drainage, or associated lymphadenitis.
   - The radiographic image varies greatly in size, shape, contour, Small lesions are often cupped around the apex.
   - majority are found in the mandible, principally at the apices of the first molars and premolar.
2. **Periapical idiopathic osteosclerosis:** Periapical sclerosis that is idiopathic (enostosis, dense bone island, bone whorls, bone eburnation) is a relatively common finding on full-mouth radiographs of dentulous patients over 12 years of age.
   The term idiopathic emphasizes that the cause of the lesion is not readily apparent or understood are located in the periapex of the mandibular first premolar and canine.
   The radiopacity of periapical idiopathic osteosclerosis may vary from a few millimeters to 2 cm in diameter. Its shape may range from generally round to very irregular, and sometimes triangular configuration is observed.
3. **Periapical cemental dysplasia:** This condition can affect the apex of a vital tooth and is totally asymptomatic. (PCOD) 90% occur in the mandible and 80% occur in women.

The shape is mostly round or oval and the borders have smooth contour.The size may vary from 0.5-2 cms.

This mature lesion is uniformly dense, and may have a thin radiolucent border.

The condition to be ruled out will be condensing osteitis which involves usually a non-vital tooth at the apex, where as the PCOD and FCOD doesnot.

4. **Hypercementosis:** Excessive formation of cementum on the surface of the tooth. The early stages are only microscopically detectable, but as additional layers of cementum are added, the accumulation becomes apparent on the radiograph.

   The premolars are more often affected than the remaining teeth, and the first molars are next in order of involvement.

   An isolated nodule or the characteristic club shaped root may be seen. In either case the root is surrounded by a normal space of periodontal ligament and the lamina dura.

   Hypercementosis may be differentiated from the false radiopaque images that are projected over the apex by feature of the projected images:The projected radiopacities are not delineated by the space of periodontal ligament and the lamina dura like Hypercementosis.
5. **Unerupted succedaneous teeth:** When the permanent crowns of succedaneous teeth are completely formed and the resorption of the root ends of the corresponding deciduous teeth is initiated, the images of the permanent tooth crowns represent periapical radiopacities
6. **Foreign Bodies:** Radiopaque foreign bodies in the periapex are usually root canal-filling materials.

   The images produced by extruded gutta percha, silver points, sealer, or retrograde amalgam restoration and the filled root canal, coupled with the history of a related procedure, contribute to the easy recognition of these periapical radiopacities.

II) False radiopacities:

1. **Anatomic Structures:** Soft tissue or bony anatomic structures may be projected as radiopaque shadows over tooth apices. Examples of such configurations include the anterior nasal spine, ala of the nose, malar process of the maxilla, external oblique ridge, mylohyoid ridge, mental protuberance. and hyoid bone.

   Identification of these structures depends on the knowledge of regional anatomy.
2. **Impacted Teeth, Supernumerary Teeth, And Compound Odontomas:** Since it is unusual for impacted or supernumerary teeth or those in a compound odontoma to be situated directly at the apices of the unerupted teeth these can be categorised as false radiopacities.

   The radiopaque images at the periapex of the impacted, supernumerary teeth or an odontoma can be easily identified by the density and their shape.

3. **Osteoma:** Osteomas can form from membranous bones of the skull and face. Osteomas originate from the periosteum.
   The mandible is more commonly involved than the maxilla.
   Osteomas are found most frequently on the posterior aspect of the mandible commonly on the lingual side of the ramus or on the inferior mandibular border below the molars.
   Osteomas have well-defined borders.
   Radiograph taken with a different angulation may change the position of the lesion and clinical examination will help in diagnosis.
4. **Tori:** Maxillary tori: It may be superimposed over the apical areas of the maxillary teeth, especially if the torus has developed in the middle or anterior region of the palate.
   Mandibular tori: On mandibular periapical radiographs, a torus mandibularis appears as a Radiopaque shadow, usually superimposed on the roots of premolars and molars and occasionally over a canine or incisor.
5. **Tips of retained roots:** Tips of retained roots which are especially in the molar area can be so situated so that their radiopaque shadows are seen over the apices of the adjacent teeth.
6. **Foreign bodies:** Various foreign bodies in the jaw bone or their surrounding soft tissues can be projected at the apices of teeth and be seen as periapical radiopacities which include fragments of metal, buttons, hooks, zippers, other metal dress acccessories, jewellery and dental materials and instrument fragments.
7. **Mucosal Cyst of the Maxillary Sinus:** The mucosal cyst of the maxillary sinus occurs in approximately 2% of the population. This entity represents a retention cyst in the lining mucosa of the maxillary sinus.
   On radiographs the cyst usually appears as a relatively dense, dome-shaped mass with its base on the floor of the maxillary sinus; the apices of the maxillary first and second molars may appear to be within the opaque image of the cyst.
8. **Ectopic Calcifications:** Ectopic calcifications in the soft tissues surrounding the jaw may be mistaken on radiographs for calcified odontogenic structures. Such deposits of abnormal calcific salts may be readily distinguished from calcified odontogenic structures and lesions by considering that the latter radiopacities are usually surrounded by a periodontal ligament type of space and a lamina dura, whereas the former do not have such characteristic borders.
9. **Sialoliths:** Although sialoliths in the submandibular gland and duct may be seen on periapical films, they are best visualized on occlusal, lateral oblique, and panoramic radiographs.
   When present in the parotid duct, on periapical films, they may be superimposed over the maxillary molars or the posterior maxillary alveoli.

10. **Rhinoliths and Antroliths:** Rhinoliths and antroliths are calcified masses occurring in the nasal cavity and maxillary sinus, respectively.
    Their images may be cast over the apices of adjacent maxillary teeth on periapical radiographs.
11. **Lymph nodes that are calcified:** Lymph nodes that are calcified occur in the cervical and submaxillary regions . The majority are calcified tuberculous nodes. On certain radiographic views, their images are projected over the mandibular bone and occasionally over the apex of a mandibular tooth.
12. **Phleboliths:** Phleboliths (angioliths) are thrombi that are calcified in veins, venules, or the sinusoidal vessels of the hemangiomas. They are always coincidental with vascular stasis.
    When these phleboliths are projected at the apex of the mandibular teeth or the bone, they can be confused with sialoliths.
13. **Arterial Calcifications:** When just a small segment of the artery is involved, however, and the radiopaque image of this segment is cast over the body of the mandible near the inferior border, the artery may simulate a sialolith within the submaxillary gland or duct or a small, calcified lymph node.

Suggested reading:

1. Norman K Wood, Paul W Goaz, Differential Diagnosis Of Oral And Maxillofacial Lesions, 5th Edition 457.

CHAPTER 23

Radiolucent Lesions of the Jaws

There are various normal radiolucencies of the oral and paraoral structures and they can also be produced by pathological conditions like abscess, cysts, tumours. It is important to understand the difference between the two.A thorough knowledge of various pathological radiolucencies is important for the dental clinician to diagnose them and render a proper treatment plan.

Q 1) Multilocular Radiolucencies:

TNMGRU FEBRUARY 2015 (5 Marks)

Multilocular radiolucencies can be enumerated as follows:

(i) Anatomic Patterns
(ii) Multilocular Cyst
(iii) Ameloblastoma
(iv) Central Giant Cell Granuloma
(v) Giant Cell Lesion Of
(vi) Hyperparathyroidism
(vii) Cherubism
(viii) Odontogenic Myxoma
(ix) Odontogenic Keratocyst
(x) Aneurysmal Bone Cyst
(xi) Metastatic Tumors To The Jaws
(xii) Vascular Malformations And
(xiii) Central Hemangioma Of Bone

Rarities:

Ameloblastic variants, Arteriovenous malformations, Burkitt's lymphoma, Calcifying epithelial odontogenic tumor, Cementoossifying fibroma, Central calcifying odontogenic cyst, central giant cell tumours, Central salivary gland tumors, Central odontogenic and nonodontogenic fibromas, Chondroma, Chondrosarcoma, Fibromatosis, Langerhans' cell disease (eosinophilic granuloma), Fibroodontogenic dysplasia, Fibrous dysplasia,

Hemangiopericytoma, Immature odontoma, Leiomyoma, Lingual mandibular bone defect,

Neurillemoma, Neuroectodermal tumor of infancy, Osteomyelitis,

Pseudo tumor of hemophilia, Squamous odontogenic tumour

1. **Anatomic variations:** Bone marrow spaces and the maxillary sinuses may show multilocular appearance.
2. **Multilocular cysts:** Primordial cyst occurs in patients between 10-30 years. Well defined radiolucency, oval or round, with border that is sclerotic and it can be uni or multilocular. It can be generally seen below and between the roots or can be near the alveolar ridge.
   Odontogenic keratocyst is a non inflammatory cyst of odontogenic origin arising from the dental lamina and is common in 2nd or 3rd decades. It is generally well demarcated and grows mesiodistally than buccolingually and may have multilocular appearance.
   Cysts like primordial cyst and odontogenic keratocyst can show multilocular appearance.
3. **Ameloblastoma:** Common benign odontogenic tumor of the jaws mostly involving the mandibular posterior region, which is more common in males. It can have multilocular appearances ranging from soap bubble, honey comb, spider nevus like that is from centre radiating trabeculae to the periphery.
4. **Giant cell lesions of hyperparathyroidism:** May appear as multilocular lesions.
5. **Cherubism:** This condition occurs in the age group of 2-20 years and generally starts in the rami of the mandible bilaterally. It become noticeable as swellings that are painless of the face in these areas. In some cses the entire mandible may be involved.
6. **Central giant cell granuloma:** It may occur initially as a solitary, cyst like radiolucent lesion, but with gradual increase in size it develops architecture that leads to a soap bubble type of multilocular radiolucency.
7. **Odontogenic myxoma:** May produce multilocular appearance and the appearance can be soap bubble, tennis racket or honey comb pattern.
8. **Aneurysmal bone cyst:** Can produce multilocular radiolucencies and when large can balloon out the cortex.
9. **Malignant tumors' metastaic lesions:** In women are those from the breast, adrenal gland, colorectal area, genital organs, and thyroid gland.
   In men the most common examples are from prostrate, kidneys, bone, lungs and adrenal glands. These can produce multilocular radiolucencies.
10. **Vascular malformation (VM) in bone:** In about 50% of cases a multilocular appearance can be detected.
    Another form these lesions can take reveals trabeculae that are coarse and linear which happen to radiate from an approximate center of the lesion.

Suggested reading:

1. Norman K. Wood, Paul W. Goaz, Differential Diagnosis of Oral and Maxillofacial Lesions, 5th Edition, Chapter 20, Page no 333-355.

Q 2) Multiple punched out radiolucencies in the jaws:

RGUHS APRIL 1997 (4 Marks)

The lesions that are usually bilateral, radiolucent, well defined but not corticated, with an oval or a cystic shape are described as punched out radiolucent lesions. At times it may appear ragged and even infiltrative.

1. **Anatomic variations:**
   - Osteoporotic bone marrow defects which are focal:common in mandible posterior region, female predilection, seen at the apices of the teeth.
   - Radiographic features: Vary from lesions that are cyst like to multilocular or irregular with well defined borders and shows cortical expansion.
   - Multiple separate cyst like marrow spaces: trabecular pattern of mandible shows large marrow spaces and sparse trabeculations.
   - Multiple post extraction sockets :patients history and by telltale depressions on the alveolar ridge.
2. **Multiple cysts or granuloma:** It may be either radicular, dentigerous or primordial cyst or keratocyst in a non syndromic patients.
3. **Basal cell nevus syndrome:** Its an autosomal dominant trait with female predilection occurring in the age group of 5-30 years, shows cutaneous & skeletal abnormalities such as multiple cystic lesions of the jaws, bifid ribs, fusion of vertebrae, polydactyly, mild prognathism ectopic calcification, basal cell nevoid carcinoma, palmar and plantar dyskeratosis, jaw cysts-dentigerous cysts, primordial or radicular.
4. **Multiple myeloma:** Synonyms: plasma cell myeloma, plasma-cytoma, myeloma.

   Can be defined as neoplastic proliferation of the plasma cells that produce immunoglobulins, which is chronic, progressive, and occurs mainly in the bone marrow but may appear in other organ systems.

   Radiographic manifestations:
   - Multiple rounded, with margins that are well defined, but with lack of cortication(punched out) and others may be irregular.
   - The lesions adjacent to each other coalesce and enlarge and remnant of bone is left between lesions.
   - In advanced cases there are thousands of rounded radiolucency scattered giving a rippled appearance.
5. **Metastatic carcinoma:** There is formation of new foci of the malignant tumour from a malignant disease that occurs by way of the blood vessels. Usually occurs in the age group of 50-70 years of life, with female predilection, and affects mostly posterior mandibular region, and causes erosion of cortical plates.

   Radiographic features: Multiple, rounded, well defined radiolucencies.

6. **Langerhan's cells disease:** Synonyms: Idiopathic histocytosis, histocytosis X.

Classification:

(a) Acute disseminated type form–Letterer-Siwe Disease.
(b) Chronic disseminated form–Hand Schuller-Christian Disease.
(c) Chronic localized form–Eosinophillic Granuloma.

(a) Acute disseminated type form–letterer-siwe disease: Usually affects infants under I year of age, associated with enlargement of organs and other swellings, petechiae, necrotic ulcers, severe pancytopenia, mobility of teeth and gingival bleeding.

Radiologic features:

(a) Multiple small, round radiolucencies with well defined borders.
(b) Chronic disseminated form-Hand Schuller-Christian disease :affects children and young adults with 3 principal manifestations-bony lesions, exophthalmos, and diabetes insipidus. Oral lesions like loosened teeth, ulcerations, edema of the gingiva are sometimes seen.

Radiographic features: Bony lesions appear ragged and patchy and coalesce giving a geographic appearance, multiple punched out lesions are seen on the radiographs of jaw.

(a) Chronic localized form- eosinophillic granuloma :It affects both adults and juvenile, (1.5-15 yrs) marked male predilection in adults, proliferative periostitis, destruction of dental follicles and missing teeth are seen in juvenile not in adult type.

Radiographic features: Proliferative periostitis with radiolucent ragged borders in juveniles, where as definitive radiolucencies with sclerosing borders in adults.

Rareties :

1. Ameloblastoma
2. Cherubism
3. Craniofacial dysostosis
4. Florid cementoosseous dysplasia
5. Giant cell granuloma
6. Hyperparathyroidism
7. Lymphomas
8. Neurofibromatosis
9. Noonan's syndrome
10. Oxalosis
11. Papillon – lefevre syndrome
12. Scleroderma
13. Traumatic bone cyst
14. Systemic sclerosis

Suggested reading:

1. Norman K.Wood, Paul W. Goaz.; Differential Diagnosis of Oral and Maxillofacial lesions; Ch-22, Pg no: 380-390.

CHAPTER 24

Miscellaneous

Q 1) Sunray Appearance:

RGUHS APRIL 2006 (4 Marks)

Introduction:

A reaction of a peculiar type which gives the appearance of sunray or sunburst kind of appearance secondary to an aggressive periostitis.

The sunburst appearance is basically calcified streaks that appear on the radiographs, radiate from a primary lesion from the surface of the bone.

It is a description for the appearance of a layered periosteal reaction which occurs as a result of the extension of the tumour, sclerosis and formation of dense, filliform spicules of the periosteum, in the surrounding tissue perpendicular to the periosteum.

It occurs when the lesion grows too fast and the periosteum has very short time to lay down new layer of bone and instead the sharpy's fibers are stretched out perpendicular to bone.

This phenomenon occurs when the periosteum is very rapidly stripped from the coretx. Several types of substances that can come in contact with the inner surface of the periosteum that is exposed can lead to new bone formation. The substances responsible are inflammatory products from infection, blood from trauma, granulomatous reactions or neoplasms. The sun-ray appearance is very typical feature of osteosarcoma and chondrosarcoma, but some other lesions can also lead to this feature, like hemangioma, benign cementoblastoma, odontogenic myxoma, multiple myeloma, complex odontoma. In rare cases fibrous dysplasia may show this appearance.

It is seen in following conditions:

- Osteosarcoma.
- Ewing's Sarcoma.
- Fibrous Dysplasia.
- Multiple Myeloma.
- Central Hemangioma.
- Odontogenic myxoma.
- Benign cementoblastoma.
- Complex odontoma.

1. **Osteosarcoma:** It is a malignant tumour, characterized by the formation of bone or osteoid by tumor cells.

Radiographic features:
3 types, Frankly Osteolytic, Mixed, Frankly Osteoblastic are seen.

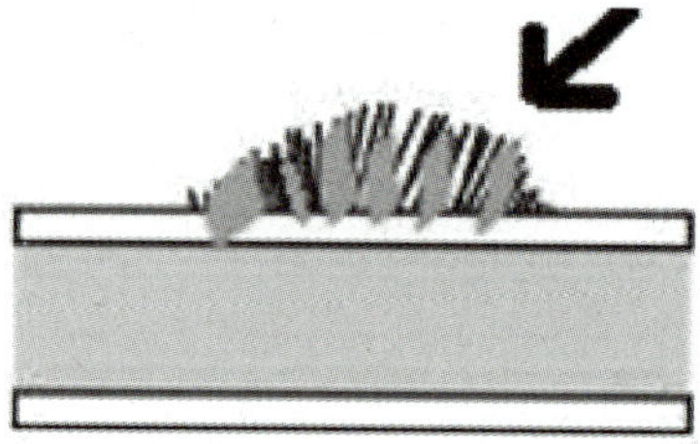

Fig. Diagramatic representation of sun-ray appearance

(a) The mandible is more commonly affected than the maxilla.
(b) The lesion has an ill-defined border.
(c) It can be either radiolucent or radiopaque with no peripheral sclerosis or encapsulation.
(d) If the tumor has invaded the periosteum several thin spicules that are irregular and of new bone which are directed outward and perpendicular to the surface of lesion are seen producing a sunray appearance.

2. **Ewing's Sarcoma:** It is also called as 'round cell sarcoma' or 'endothelial myeloma'. It is derived from mesenchymal connective tissue of bone marrow.

   Radiographic features:
   - It is ill-defined destructive radiolucent lesion which may be unilocular or multilocular.
   - It has ill-defined margins and is never corticated.
   - If it penetrates the cortex, it may stimulate the periosteum to produce thin layer of bone which are laid down in layer more or less parallel to shaft, resulting in laminated or onion skin effect along the bone surface.
   - In advanced cases, where osteophytes formation is present, it may present as sunray appearance.

3. **Multiple Myeloma:** It is also called as myeloma, plasma cell myeloma, and plasmacytoma.
   It is a malignant neoplasm of plasma cell.

   Radiographic features:
   - It is commonly seen in mandible.
   - In mandible the lesion is more common in posterior body, ramus and condyle.
   - The periphery of the lesion is well defined, without corticated radiolucencies, with an oval or cystic shape called as punched out lesion.
   - The lesion affects any cortical boundary it encounters.
   - Periosteal reaction is less common, if present then it appears as a single radiopaque line or rarely sunray appearance.

4. **Fibrous dysplasia:** Fibrous dysplasia is a fibro-osseous lesion in which the normal bone is replaced with fibrous tissue.
   It can affect a single or several bones and is monostotic and polyostotic types.

   Radiographic features:
   - It shows extremely variable pattern which can range from a

cystic type radiolucency to dense osteoblastic lesions, with the orange peel and ground glass or print of a finger kind of appearance.

- The margins of the lesions usually blend with the surrounding normal bone and the cortex could sometimes be perforated.
- The sunray kind of periosteal reaction generally can be seen when the bone is formed along the Sharpey's fibres that are perpendicular and attach between the cortex and the periosteum.
- It could be a true periosteal reaction or the pattern of calcification of the lesion itself.

5. **Central hemangioma:** Hemangioma is a type of hamartoma in which there is proliferation of the blood vessels which create a mass, to resemble a neoplasm, central hemangioma is often found in the vertebrae and skull. It may be developmental or traumatic.

   Radiographic features:
   - It mainly affects mandible in the posterior region of the body and the ramus region and also within the inferior alveolar canal.
   - Periphery is well defined and corticated in some cases, but sometimes it may be ill defined.
   - The hemangioma can break through the outer part of the cortex and can cause displacement of the periosteum and can lead to formation of fine linear spicules of bone that emerge from the surface of the bone causing a sun-ray appearance.

6. **Complex odontome:**
   - Appear as a dense radiopaque object, sometimes lying in a clear space. Density is greater than bone and to more than or equal to the teeth.
   - Internal structure shows a well defined radiolucency containing irregular masses of calcified tissue which is associated with unerupted teeth.
   - Rarely shows sun-ray appearance.

7. **Benign cementoblastoma:**
   - Radiographically it can be seen as a well defined radiopaque lesion with a cortical border, surrounded by well-defined radiolucent band just inside the cortical border.
   - Appear as mixed radiolucent radiopaque lesion may have amorphous or a wheel spoke pattern and may show sun ray appearance.

8. **Odontogenic myxoma:**
   - The lesion is usually well defined with a corticated margins. Most of the time it appears multilocular having a mixed radiolucent- radiopaque internal pattern.
   - There is presence of septa which give it multilocular appearance – tennis racket like or step ladder like when septa are straight and thin etched.

- Sometimes septa are curved or coarse with two or three straight septa.
- Rarely may give a sunray appearance.

Suggested reading:

1. Freny R Karjodkar Essentials of Oral and Maxillofacial Radiology, ch no23, pg no393.
2. S Prapayasatok, A Iamaroon, DA Miles and T Kumchai, A rare, radiographic 'sunray' appearance in Fibrous dysplasia, Dentomaxillofacial Radiology (2000) 29, 245 – 248.
3. Stuart C White, Michael J Pharoah, Oral Radiology, Principles and Interpretation 5th Edition, 24 pg no 427.

Q 2) Mixed radiolucent and radiopacities of the jaws

TNMGRU AUGUST 2015 (5 Marks)

1. **Calcification of crown of developing tooth:** Depending upon stage of tooth development the crypt along with tooth can give mixed appearance.
2. **Root of a tooth with rarefying osteitis:** Retention of tooth roots with accompanying rarefying osteitis will appear as mixed radiolucent-radiopaque areas in the jaws.
3. **Rarefying And Condensing Osteitis:** Quite often rarefying and condensing osteitis will occur in a non-vital tooth at its apex or root that is retained giving a mixed appearance.
4. **Periapical Cementosseous Dysplasia (PCOD):** The mixed stage of PCOD will appear as a radiolucent-radiopaque lesion usually at the apices of mandibular anteriors or in the molar premolar teeth region. They have well defined outer borders.
5. **Healing Surgical Site:** After treatment of benign conditions, primary healing takes place through ossification of the surgically produced hematoma, which is then slowly transformed to normal bone under favourable conditions.
   If the radiograph is made after some calcification of the hematoma has taken place, the radiolucency contains foci of patterns that progress from ground glass to spiculed to trabecular. Thus during healing of a treated lesion mixed radiolucent and radiopaque appearance can be seen.
6. **Chronic Osteomyelitis:** The radiographic appearance of chronic osteomyelitis is most often a mixed radiolucent-radiopaque image. In many cases the borders are ragged and poorly defined but in others they are well defined.
   The radiolucent areas usually consist of infected granulation tissue containing areas of necrosis, fibrosis or both.
   The radiopacities represent sclerosed, quite often non-vital bone, sequestra, or both.
7. **Osteoradionecrosis:** Osteoradionecrosis (ORN) is generally regarded as a disease of the hard and soft tissues after radiation therapy of the area.

The lesion shows areas of osteolysis and radiopaque areas of sequestration and thus a mixed radiopaque radiolucent lesion over significant region of the jaw bones can be seen.

8. **Focal Cementosseous Dysplasia:** These lesions fit into the category of benign reactive fibrocemento osseous lesions that range from the local periapical cementosseous dysplasia to florid cementoosseous dysplasia.
   Occur mostly at the apical region of molar-premolar teeth.
   It passes through three stages that is radiolucent, mixed and radiopaque. In the mixed stage it gives the radiolucent-radiopaque appearance.
   The distinctness of the margins varies, as do the radiopaque patterns scattered throughout the lesion. Usually, there is a radiolucent periphery, but bone peripheral to this may show a thin radiopaque border or in other cases a smudged, often ground-glass, thick radiopaque pattern.
9. **Fibrous Dysplasia:** It is a fibro-osseous lesion which again has three stages, ie radiolucent, mixed and radiopaque.
   The intermediate stage is recognized by its smoky, hazy, or mottled radiolucent-radiopaque pattern which is produced by poorly defined aggregates of spicules of bone distributed throughout the radiolucent area. This gives a typical ground glass appearance to the lesions.
10. **Paget's Disease:** The maxilla is involved more often than the mandible. The intermediate stage gives a mixed appearance.
    There is the first indication of a developing radiopacity in the osteolytic stage to the dense opaque appearance of calcification in areas intermixed with areas of radiolucency showing the distinctive cottonwool appearance.
11. **Cemento-ossifying Fibroma:** The cementifying and ossifying fibromas usually occur as periapical lesions that are basically round and well marginated.
    More commonly occur in the mandible in the molar-premolar region. They are usually solitary entities and in the cementifying stage will show mixed radiolucent-radiopaque appearance.
12. **Osteogenic Sarcoma:** The radiolucent-radiopaque lesion usually has ragged, ill-defined borders, and its opaqueness results from areas of excessive bone production intermingled with radiolucent foci of bone destruction.
    In some lesions, sequestra are formed, and these usually appear as well-defined, dense radiopacities. Another mixed appearance is the cumulus –cloud appearance due to formation of lot of neoplastic bone.
13. **Osteoblastic Metastatic Carcinoma:** Usually the osteolytic metastatic tumours can induce osteoblastic activity in the tumour or the bone that is neighboring.These kind of lesions will appear as a combination of radiopaque-radiolucent with usually vague, irregular borders.

The dissemination may be so wide that the resultant picture may mimic Paget's disease.

14. **Chondroma And Chondrosarcoma:** Both may appear as radiolucent lesions of the jaws. The radiopacities that develop in chondromas are more orderly than the chondrosarcomas and both may show mixed radiolucent-radiopaque appearances.
15. **Ossifying Subperiosteal Hematoma:** They occur when a subperiosteal hematoma of the jawbone is induced by trauma.
    The hematoma ossifies rapidly. The new bone is often formed in perpendicular columns from the cortical plate outward.
    Such an osseous arrangement gives a sunburst pattern or at times the appearance of an irregularly thickened cortex.
16. **Desmoplastic Ameloblastoma:** It occurs more commonly in the maxilla and in the anterior region of both the jaws.It has been reported to take on a mixed radiographic pattern in a significant number of cases.
17. **Odontoma:** The odontoma is a benign tumor that contains various components of tissues of teeth.
    Initially there is bone resorption and radiolucent stage and then intermediate stage because of the partial calcification of the odontogenic tissues, this stage is characterized by a radiolucent-radiopaque image.
18. **Adenomatoid odontogenic tumour:** The AOT is an uncommon tumor that may undergo different stages of development.
    It is a pericoronal cyst like radiolucency that mimics the radiographic appearance of a dentigerous cyst.
    In the maturing stage clearly defined foci of radiopacity can be seen within the radiolucency.
19. **Calcifying odontogenic cyst:** The radiographic appearance a cyst type radiolucency that contains distinct foci of radiopacity although a considerable number do not show radiopaque foci because the calcifications are still too small to show on radiographs.
20. **Ameloblastic fibro-odontoma:** It is frequently located in a position that is pericoronal to a tooth that is embedded and in the beginning is totally radiolucent, but gradually it acquires an increasingly prominent radiopaque foci as the hard dental tissues within it become mineralized.
21. **Calcifying epithelial odontogenic tumour:** The CEOT (Pindborg tumor) is considered rare, representing approximately 1% of odontogenic tumors. The most common appearance are of a pericoronal radiolucency and of diffuse radiopacities within radiolucent areas.

Suggested reading:

1. Norman K wood, Paul.W.Goaz, Differential Diagnosis of Oral and Maxillofacial Lesions, 5th edition. 433-446, 415-430.

ORAL MEDICINE

LONG ANSWERS QUESTIONS

CHAPTER 1

Ulcerative, Vesicular and Bullous Lesions

Q 1) Classify vesiculo-bullous lesions of oral cavity. Describe ANUG in detail.

MUHS DECEMBER 2005 10 Marks

Definition:

Vesicle: A fluid filled blister less than 1 cms in diameter.
Bulla: A fluid filled blister more than 1 cms in diameter.

I) Primarily Vesicular Lesions:

1. Primary Herpetic gingivostomatitis:
2. Herpangina.
3. Hand-foot and mouth disease.
4. Primary varicella zoster (chicken-pox).
5. Secondary varicella zoster (Shingles)
6. Recurrent Herpes Stomatitis.
7. Recurrent Herpes Labialis.
8. Contact Vesicular stomatitis.
9. Impetigo.

II) Primarily Bullous Lesions:

1. Pemphigus vulgaris.
2. Bullous pemphigoid.
3. Benign mucous membrane pemphigoid.
4. Bullous lichen planus.
5. Erythema multiforme.
6. Steven's johnson's syndrome.
7. Epidermolysis bullosa.
8. Dermatitis herpetiformis.

Acute Necrotising Ulcerative Gingivostomatitis: (ANUG)

Definition:

ANUG is a painful, progressive infection associated with ulceration, swelling and sloughing off of necrosed tissue mainly affecting the gingiva especially the interdental papilla caused by fusiform bacilli, spirochetes and bacteriointermedius.

ANUG came to be known as Trench Mouth at the time of World war I because it was commonly seen in the individuals in the combat trenches.

The destruction of the tissues is thought to be caused by the endotoxins which act directly on the tissues or act indirectly by the triggering of the immunologic and inflammatory reactions.

Etiology And Predisposing Factors:

1. Most common causative organism is fusiform bacillus and spirochetes.
2. Maintenance of continuous anerobic flora of the organism, Treponema spp and selenomonas spp.
3. The occurrence of ANUG in patients in the absence of a medical disorder is seen mostly in ages between 16-30 years and is associated with three factors that are major:
   (a) Maintenance of poor oral hygiene and association of pre-existing marginal gingivitis or presence of dental restorations that are faulty.
   (b) Smoking.
   (c) Emotional stress.
4. **Predisposing Factors:**

   Local:

   (a) Poor oral hygiene and associated marginal gingivitis and restorations that are faulty.

   Systemic:

   (a) Nutritional deficiency causing malnutrition.
   (b) Debilitating diseases/Immunosuppression.
   (c) Psychosomatic factors like stress.
   (d) Leukemia, Aplastic anemia, AIDS and Malignancies.
   (e) Lack of sleep.
   (f) Smoking or chewing tobacco.

   Clinical Features:

   (i) Sudden onset of localised or diffuse gingival pain, acute gingival bleeding, bad taste and fetor oris and some times metallic taste in mouth, profuse salivation.
   (ii) there is ulceration of the interdental papillae and presence of necrotic slough. The necrosis associated with the dental papillae has been described as "punched out".
   (iii) Teeth seems slightly extruded and have a woody sensation, mobile teeth, blunting of interdental papillae.
   (iv) The presence of malaise, fever, enlargement of the cervical lymph nodes occurs rarely.
   (v) The systemic presentations can be more often seen in children.
   (vi) The features similar to ANUG, but with greater intensity of

pain can be seen in necrotising periodontitis in the HIV/AIDS cases.

(vii) Typical lesions of necrotic, punched out ulcerations which become covered by gray, yellow slough and pseudomembrane with pronounced linear erythema.

(viii) Develops most often on the marginal gingiva and the interdental papilla.

(ix) If left untreated may cause destruction of periodontium.

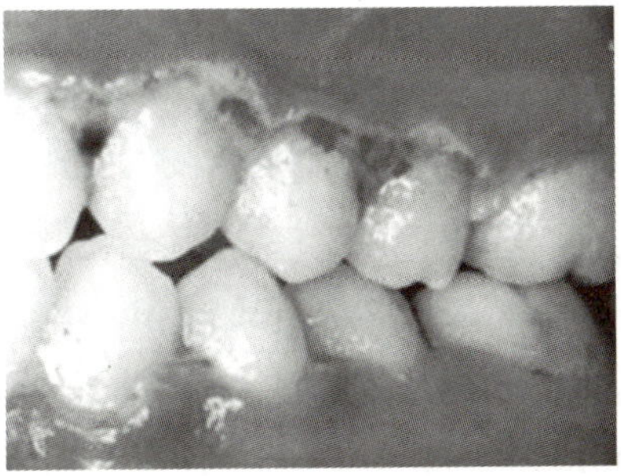

Fig. Necrotising ulceration in interdental papillary region

Differential Diagnosis:

(i) **Benign mucous membrane pemphigoid:** Its a bullous disease and sub epithelial bulla are present. Necrosis and punched out ulcers are absent.

(ii) **Pemphigus:** It is also a bullous lesion and has muco-cutaneous lesions. Nikolskys' sign is positive and follows a chronic course with classical histological picture. Skin changes are also seen and hence can be differentiated from ANUG.

(iii) **Syphilitic gingivitis:** Primary lesions present only on gingiva and do not spread to neighboring structures.

(iv) **Tubercular ulcer:** These are chronic ulcers and have typical undermined margins and donot have grey pseudomembrane like ANUG.

Treatment:

1. Manage the underlying factors.
2. Well balanced diet and regular meals.
3. Gently removing the necrotic material with swab.
4. 3% hydrogen peroxide diluted with equal amounts of water which is used to rinse the mouth every 2 hours on first day and 3-4 times/ day for the next 4 days.
5. Penicillin V(oral): 400, 000 units/day for 5 days/ OR Penicillin V 250-500mgs 6 hourly OR amoxicillin 250-500mg TID for 5-7 days OR Erythromycin 250-500 mgs 6 hourly with Metronidazole 400mgs TID for 5 -7days.
6. Oral prophylaxis with gingival curettage and root planing can be undertaken after acute symptoms subside.

Suggested reading:

1. Anil Govindrao Ghom, Text book of oral medicine, 3rd edi. pg no. 549-550
2. Burket's Text book of oral medicine, 10 thedi. pg no. 61-63
3. Karring, edited by Jan Lindhe, Niklaus P. Lang, Thorkild (2008). Clinical periodontology and implant dentistry (5th ed.). Oxford: Blackwell Munksgaard. pp. 413, 459.
4. Scully, Crispian (2008). Oral and maxillofacial medicine: the basis of diagnosis and treatment (2nd ed.). Edinburgh: Churchill Livingstone. pp. 101, 347.

Q 2) Classify ulcerative and vesiculobullous lesions. Describe the etiology clinical features and treatment plan for recurrent aphthous stomatitis:

MUHS OCTOBER 2004 10 Marks

Classification of Ulcerative And Vesiculobullous Lesions:

Classification of ulcerative lesions:

1. **Single ulcers:**
   - (a) Traumatic
   - (b) Tuberculous
   - (c) Syphilitic
   - (d) Histoplasmosis
   - (e) Blastomycosis
   - (f) Mucormycosis
   - (g) Neoplastic ulcers
2. **Multiple ulcers:**
   - (i) **Acute Ulcers:**
     - (a) Primary herpetic gingivostomatitis.
     - (b) Herpangina.
     - (c) Hand-foot-mouth disease.
     - (d) Varicella–zoster virus infections: chicken pox and herpes zoster.
     - (e) Erythema multiforme.
     - (f) Contact allergic stomatitis.
     - (g) Oral ulcers occurring secondary to cancer chemotherapy and /or radiotherapy.
     - (h) Acute necrotising ulcerative gingivitis.
   - (ii) **Chronic Ulcers:**
     - (a) Pemphigus.
     - (b) Subepithelial bullous dermatoses.
     - (c) Herpes simplex virus infection in immunosuppressed patients.
3. **Recurring oral ulcers:**
   - (a) Recurrent aphthous stomatitis.
   - (b) Behcets syndrome.
   - (c) Recurrent herpes simplex virus infection.
   - (d) Cyclic neutropenia.

(e) Chronic idiopathic neutropenia.

Classification of vesicular lesions:

1. Primary Herpetic gingivostomatitis.
2. Herpangina.
3. Hand-foot and mouth Disease.
4. Primary Varicella-zoster (Chickenpox).
5. Secondary Varicella-zoster (Shingles).
6. Recurrent Herpes Stomatitis.
7. Recurrent Herpes Labialis.
8. Contact Vesicular stomatitis.
9. Impetigo.

Classification of bullous lesions:

1. Pemphigus Vulgaris.
2. Bullous Pemphigoid.
3. Benign Mucous Membrane Pemphigoid.
4. Bullous Lichen Planus.
5. Erythema Multiforme.
6. Stevens-Johnson Syndrome.
7. Epidermolysis Bullosa.
8. Dermatitis Herpetiformis.

Recurrent Aphthous stomatitis:

Definition:

Its derived from the greek word aphtha, "mouth ulcer" which is quite a commonly occurring lesion and is characterised by the formation of repeated benign and non-contagious oral ulcers in persons who are otherwise healthy.

Thought to be associated with an immune response that is T-cell mediated which is triggered by a variety of factors.

The factors that can trigger these lesions could be deficiency in nutrition, local trauma, stress, imbalances of the hormones, allergies, genetic predisposition or other factors.

There is a tendency for the ulcers to occur periodically and there is complete healing between the attacks. The ulcerations usually last for 7-10 days and the episodes can occur about 3-6 times in a year.

The ulcers most commonly involve the non-keratinised areas of the oral cavity, however in severe forms, though less common, they may also involve keratinized epithelial surfaces.

Precipitating Factors:

I) **Trauma** – Self inflicted bites.
- Oral Surgical procedures.
- Overzealous use of tooth brushes.
- ill fitting dentures.
- Fish bone, biscuit crumbs or fruit Skin.

- Sharp and broken carious tooth.

II) **Endocrine Factors:** relation between RAS & menstruation (Increased incidence during premenstruation week).

III) **Psychological factors:** chronic anxiety states, hysteria, hypochondriasis, epilepsy etc.
Stress amplifies perception of pain rather than truly acting as a precipitating factor.

IV) **Allergy:** asthma, hay fever or food allergies.
Exact mechanism not known but may occur due to conjugation of foods with epithelial proteins & precipitating Type IV hypersensitivity reaction.

V) Cessation of smoking: cause aphthae.
Exact mechanism not clear but smoking keratinizes the mucosa and hence stopping of smoking predisposes to aphthae.

Etiology:

I) **Heredity:** Probability of 90 % in offspring when both parents have the disease.
: 60 % when only one parent has the disease.
: 20 % when both parents show negative history.

II) **Immunological Factors:** A local immunological response against antigenically altered mucosa produced by bacteria or viruses or may represent a central immunologic fault where aberrant clone of lymphocytes damage the oral mucosa.

III) **Microorganisms & RAS:** Streptococcus sanguis, Adenovirus type I, L form of streptococci, herpes simplex virus, varicella-zoster virus, adeno virus and the cytomegalo virus.
However their isolation is not sufficient to implicate them in pathogenesis.

IV) **Deficiencies in nutrition:** Iron, folic acid & vit.B12, deficiency allows expression of unrelated underlying tendency to ulceration, without itself playing a primary role

V) **Zinc deficiency:** Role not fully established.

Classification:

(i) Minor ulcers < 1 cm in diameter and heal without scar.

(ii) Major ulcers > 1cm in diameter, take longer time to heal and often scar on healing.

(iii) Herpetiform ulcers manifest as recurrent crops of dozens of small sized ulcers involving the entire oral mucosa.

Clinical Manifestations:

1. The initial episodes of this condition begin frequently in the 2nd decade of life and could be precipitated by incidents like minor trauma, menstruation, upper respiratory tract infections, or the contact with certain food substances.
2. There is a prodromal phase of burning from 2-48 hours prior to the

appearance of the lesions and the ulcers are confined to the oral mucosa.

3. At the beginning of the lesions, an area of erythema develops. After several hours there is development of a white papule which ulcerates and gradually increases in size over the next 48-72 hours.
4. The ulcers are round and shallow, symmetrical and no tissue tags are present at the edges of the ulcers.
5. Though the ulcers are often multiple, their number, size and frequency of occurrence varies considerably.
6. The buccal and labial mucosa are most commonly involved.
7. The heavily keratinised palate and the gingiva are rarely involved.In mild cases of RAS, the lesions attain a size of about 0.3-1 cm and the healing starts within a week and occurs without scarring and is complete in about 10-14 days.
8. The major form of the ulcers are deeper and larger than 1cms and can reach a size of about 5 cms. Large areas of the oral mucosa are involved in such cases and these deep ulcers can conjoin to form even larger lesions. They are round or ovoid with well defined margin, erythematous edge, and floor of yellowish slough. These major aphthae can be extremely painful and can interfere with speech and eating.

   They heal slowly and leave scars especially in major ulcers which can cause reduction in the mobility of the uvula and the tongue and can lead to destruction of portions of the oral mucosa. The lesions in major aphthae may persist for upto 6 week and leave a scar upon healing.

   Some major ulcers may involve the deeper mucosal tissue with inflammatory cellular infiltration of periglandular submucosa (periadenitis) also known as Sutton's disease.

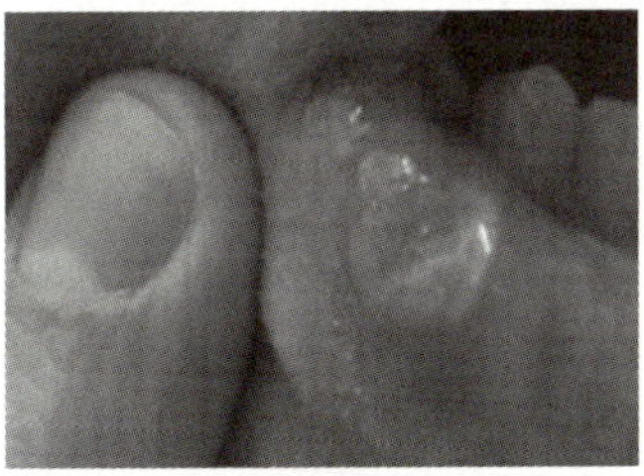

Fig. Major aphthous ulcer

9. The least common variety of the RAS is the herpetiform ulcers and generally affect the adults.

   Crops of multiple, small, shallow ulcers, often upto 100, may occur at any site of oral cavity, the ventral surface of tongue being the most common.

   Lesions begin as small pinched sized erosions that gradually enlarge & coalesce to produce ragged margins and are more painful.

   Heal in 7-30 days, occasionally with scarring.

Diagnosis:

Detailed history and clinical examination will generally help in diagnosis.

Laboratory investigations should be done if ulcers take long time to heal and also when they first develop after 25 years of age.

Biopsy should be done when in doubt and to exclude other diseases.

Smears taken of aphthous ulcers quite often show typical Anitshkow cells in abundance and though not pathognomonic of the disease could help in diagnosis.

Differential Diagnosis:

1. **Herpetic stomatitis:** These lesions usually are vesicular lesions and involve the more keratinised areas of oral mucosa commonly. There is generalised malaise, fever and sense of ill being and typical is generalised marginal gingivitis which is absent in aphthous stomatitis. Laoratory investigations may show giant cells and ballooning degeneration of the keratinocytes with ground glass nuclei which is absent in aphthous stomatitis.
2. **Erythema Multiforme:** It is a vesiculobullous disease and typical iris or bulls eye lesions may be present, hence can be differentiated from aphthous. Eye, skin and genital lesions are commonly present which is not so in aphthous stomatitis.
3. **Erosive lichen planus:** There are skin lesions also that could be present and intraoral lesions are present bilaterally and presence of wickham's striae at the periphery could be present. Histopathologically epithelium has typical saw tooth like reteridges. All these are absent in aphthous.
4. **Pemphigus and pemphigoid:** These are bullous lesions and in pemhigus nikolskys sign will rule out aphthous. In case of pemhigoid, sub epithelial bulla can be seen histopathologically and can be differentiated from aphthous.

Treatment:

I) Immune enhancement:
   (a) Levamisole
   (b) vaccines

II) Immune & inflammatory suppression:
   (i) **Local steroids:** Orabase often combined with 0.1% triamcinolone gives relief and helps in healing and reducing pain and inflammation.

   Hydrocortisone sodium succinate, beclomethasone dipropionate, fluocinonide, clobetasol, dexamethasone, betamethasone sodium phosphate.

   Hydrocortisone hemisuccinate pellets, of 2.5 mgs can be given QID.

   Carboxy methyl cellulose paste with triamcinolone acetonide, can be administered 4 times/day.

   0.5mg tablet of betamethasone phosphate which is

dissolved in 15 ml of water, which can be used as a mouth rinse 4 times/day for 4 minutes each time.

(ii) **Systemic steroids:** In severe cases 30-60 mg/day prednisone can be given orally in divided doses and can be tapered off in about 21 days regimen.

III) **Antibiotics/ antiplaque agents/ antiseptics:** Tetracycline, doxycycline, minocycline, chlorhexidine gluconate, triclosan. Tetracycline mouth wash using 250 mg capsule powder in water as mouth wash can be used to rinse the mouth.This can prevent secondary infection.
A 100 mg doxycycline capsule in 10 ml of water can used as a mouth rinse for 3 minute each time, or 500mg of tetracycline plus 500mg of nicotinamide can be administered 4 times/ day to provide relief and reduce the duration of the ulcer.
Mouth rinses of chlorhexidine gluconate can reduce the pain and severity of the ulcers but not the frequency.

IV) **Antihistamines:**
 (a) Diphenhydramine Hydrochloride.
 (b) Cromoglycic acid.

V) **Local anaesthetics /analgesics:** Amlexanox paste, benzydamine hydrochloride spray or mouth wash, viscous lidocaine, and diclofenac in hyaluronan can be effective.

VI) **Thalidomide:** About 50-100mg/day can be effective in cases of severe RAS, but the ulcers do tend to recur in about 3 weeks.But has serious side effects.

VII) **Homeopathy:**

VIII) **Enhancement of Salivary peroxidase system:**
 (a) dentifrice with aminoglucosidase & glucose oxidase.

IX) **Longovital:**

X) **Diet supplementation:** It is reported that supplementation with vitamin B12 can prevent recurrences in some cases.

XI) There can be avoidance of trauma by avoiding the usage of rough or hard food stuff and also important to brush teeth gently. In case sodium lauryl sulfate is suspected to be the reason, the products containing this chemical should be avoided and can prevent recurrence in some patients.

XII) If patch testing give results to the effect that there is allergy to food, then the diet can be modified.

XIII) Other treatment modalities, though not proven are used and research is being carried out includes myrtus communis, aloevera, rosa damascena, zinc sulphate, nicotine, polio virus vaccine and prostaglandins.

Suggested reading:

1. Brocklehurst P, Tickle M, Glenny AM, Lewis MA, Pemberton MN, Taylor J, Walsh T, Riley P, Yates JM (September 12, 2012). “Systemic interventions for recurrent aphthous stomatitis (mouth ulcers)”.

2. Neville BW, Damm DD, Allen CM, Bouquot JE (2008). Oral & maxillofacial pathology (3rd ed.). Philadelphia: W.B. Saunders.
3. Odell W (2010). Clinical problem solving in dentistry (3rd ed.). Edinburgh: Churchill Livingstone. pp. 87–90.
2. Scully C (2013). Oral and maxillofacial medicine: the basis of diagnosis and treatment (3rd ed.). Edinburgh: Churchill Livingstone. pp. 226–234.

Q 3) Classify vesiculo bullous lesions of oral cavity. Describe erythema multiforme in detail:

RGUHS OCTOBER 1998 (10 Marks)

Classification of vesiculobullous lesions:

I) Lesions that are primarily vesicular:

1. Primary Herpetic Gingivostomatitis
2. Herpangina
3. Hand-foot-mouth disease
4. Primary varicella-zoster (chicken pox)
5. Secondary varicella zoster (Shingles)
6. Recurrent Herpes Stomatitis.
7. Recurrent Herpes Labialis.
8. Contact Vesicular stomatitis.
9. Impetigo.

II) Lesions that are primarily bullous:

1. Pemphigus vulgaris
2. Bullous pemphigoid
3. Benign mucous membrane pemphigoid
4. Bullous lichen planus
5. Erythema multiforme
6. Steven's johnson's syndrome
7. Epidermolysis bullosa
8. Dermatitis herpetiformis

Erythema multiforme:

This condition is an acute and self limiting disorder, that is, inflammatory, hypersensitivity reaction affecting skin and mucous membrane which leads to different types of skin lesions and that is why called as "Multiforme".

Etiopathogenesis:

It is hypersensitivity reaction which may be due to:

- Immune mediated diseases.
- Immune complex formation and subsequent deposition in microvasculature may play a role in the pathogenesis of erythema multiforme.
- Drug like sulfonamides, NSAIDS, anticonvulsants barbiturates oral contraceptives, etc.
- Infections mainly by bacterial, viral fungal and protozoal infections.
- Other infections, such as mycoplasma.

- Vaccination, radiation, occasionally disease like crohn's disease, ulcerative colitis.
- Precipitating factors are herpes simplex virus, epstein barr virus, and histoplasmosis.
- The majority of cases follow outbreaks of HSV infection. HSV-1 is the most common strain implicated.

Classification:

Types of Erythema Multiforme (EM):

1. **EM Minor:** typical target or raised edematous papules involving skin of the extremeties, with minimal mucosa involvement.
2. **EM Major:** The lesions are peculiar target or bull's eye lesions, or raised papules that are edematous involving the extremeties along with the involvement of one or more mucous membranes and detachment of the epidermis with involvement of less than 10% of the total area of the surface of the body (TBSA).
3. **Steven's johnson's syndrome and toxic epidermal necrolysis:** There is presence of blisters that are widespread and prominently on the trunk and the face. There are pruritic macules and erosions of one or more mucous membranes.

The detachment of the epidermis is less than 10% of TBSA in case of Steven's -johnson's syndrome and 30% or more in case toxic epidermal necrolysis.

Clinical features:

- Erythema multiforme is seen commonly in young adults and children and rarely affects adults after 50 years.
- Males are affected more than females.
- The onset can be acute and even explosive and sudden and there are systemic symptoms such as fever, malaise in cases that are severe.
- The skin areas of the hands and feet and the extensor surfaces of the elbows and knees are commonly involved.
- In most cases the neck and the face are involved and in more severe case the trunk is affected.
- The peculiar lesions of this condition on the skin can be non-specific macules, papules and vesicles and in severe case bullae.
- The typical lesions on the skin consist of petechiae in the center of the lesions.
- The very typical diagnostic feature of this lesion is the target or iris or the bull's eye lesions that consist of a bulla in the center or a pale area which is surrounded by bands of erythema and edema.
- Stevens–Johnson Syndrome: The condition always has the presence of oral lesions which consist of extensive vesiculations and are followed by erosive lesions that are painful and covered with a grayish-white or hemorrhagic pseudomembrane. The lesions can also involve the larynx, pharynx and the esophagus. The lesions

in the eye comprise of uveitis, conjuctivitis, symblepheron and in some cases pan-ophthalmitis.The genital lesions consist of scrotal erosions, vulvo-vaginitis and balanitis. The lesions on the skin can be very minor to severe.

TEN: It is characterised by conjunctivitis, pharyngitis, and pruritis.There is epidermal detachment of more than 30%of the TBSA. The mucosal involvement is in the order of oropharynx, eyes, genitalia and anus.

Oral manifestations:

- The lesions in this condition begin as bullous lesions on an erythematous base and they break down soon and form irregular ulcers. They can be rarely witnessed as intact bullae.
- The erythema multiforme lesions are large, irregular and there is often bleeding from the lesions, but the viral lesions are small, round and shallow and symmetric.
- In the oral mucosa the lesions of EM can occur any where but more commonly the lips are involved and the gingivae are rarely involved. This is an important difference between EM and primary herpes simplex infections where the gingival involvement is common.
- In severe and full blown cases the lips show extensive erosion, and large areas of the mucosa are denuded of the epithelium.
- The patient has great difficulty in eating and swallowing and there is drooling of blood tinged saliva.
- The lesions of the lip begin to crust within 2-3 days.
- In most of the cases the healing starts in 2 weeks, but in some severe cases it can go on for several weeks.

Diagnosis:

- Bulls eye lesion with hemorrhagic crusting of lips is typical of EM.
- Positive serology – for HSV antibodies or mycoplasma pneumonia when its hypersensitive response to HSV or mycoplasma pneumoniae.
- Biopsy of perilesional tissue: intracellular edema of spinous layer of epithelium and edema of superficial connective tissue which may produce subepidermal vesicles.
- Immune deposits: fibrin and C3 at the basement membrane zone.

Differential diagnosis:

1. **Viral lesions like primary herpetic gingivostomatitis:** Less severe form and gingival involvement is more common and typically generalised marginal gingivitis present.
2. **Pemphigus vulgaris:** Antibodies are directed against intercellular substance. Nikolsky's sign is positive.
3. **Mucous membrane pemphigoid:** More chronic course and eye involvement is typical.
4. **Allergic reaction:** Target lesions are absent.
5. **Erosive lichen planus:** It is more commonly seen in elderly women and bilaterally present on the buccal mucosa.Wickham's striae may

be present at the periphery.

6. **Recurrent aphthous ulcers:** They are recurrent and less severe. Iris lesions are absent.
7. Paraneoplastic pemphigus.
8. **Systemic lupus erythematous:** Multisystem involvement and typical butterfly erythematous patches on skin.

Management:

- The mild cases of EM can be treated by supportive measures that include local anesthetic and mouth washes and inclusion of soft and liquid diet.
- Supportive care, electrolytes, a liquid diet and nutritional support should be started as early as possible. If patient is dehydrated due to pain then intravenous rehydration should be carried out.
- Removal of cause: If it is possible to identify causative drug, its use should be discontinued.
- Early ophthalmologic and dermatological consultation are recommended.
- Topical anesthetic agent (lidocaine gel) antiseptic mouth washes with hydrogen peroxide or chlorhexidine and topical corticosteroids. May help to remove discomfort.
- A short course of systemic corticosteroids in patients of EM without contraindications to it can be used for the treatment of moderate or severe cases.
- It has been proved that corticosteroids are very effective on EM and SJS, if treated in high doses for a short time with proper tapering of dosages.
- Minor EM: 20-40 mg per day prednisolone is administered for 4-6 days and then taper the dose. Major erythema multiforme usually required 40-80 mg / day with gradual tapering over 2-3 weeks.
- Treatment protocols such as early therapy by giving systemic prednisone (0.5 to 1.0 mg/kg/day or pulse methyl prednisolone (1mg/kg/day for 3 days), intravenous pulsed dose methyl prednisolone (3 consecutive daily infusions of 20-30 mg/kg to a maximum of 500 mg given over 2 to 3 hours), and dexamethasone pulse therapy (1.5mg/kg over 30-60 minutes on 3 consecutive days), all have been shown to be effective.
- The use of systemic corticosteroids should be done by expert clinicians, who know the side effects as well the benefits of this drug and should be used with care.
- In patients with severe recurrent form of this condition, dapsone, levamisole, azathioprine or thalidomide can be administered.

Suggested reading:

1. Bastuji-Garin S, Rzany B, Stern RS, Shear NH, Naldi L, Roujeau JC. Clinical classification of cases of toxic epidermal necrolysis, Stevens-Johnson syndrome, and erythema multiforme. Arch Dermatol. 1993 Jan. 129(1): 92-6.
2. Scully, Crispian (2008). Oral and maxillofacial medicine: the basis of diagnosis and treatment (2nd ed.). Edinburgh: Churchill Livingstone. pp. 196–198.

Q 4) Classify vesiculobullous lesions of oral cavity and write in detail clinical features, diagnosis, investigations, differential diagnosis and treatment of

Recurrent herpetic gingivostomatitis

BFU MAY 2010 (15 Marks)

Acute Herpetic Gingvostomatitis

TNMGRU AUGUST 2010 20 Marks

Also known as primary herpetic gingivostomatitis or labial herpes, is a combination of gingivitis and stomatitis which results in inflammation of the oral mucosa and the gingiva. It is often the the initial manifestation in case of primary herpes simplex infections.

In 90% of cases the PHGS is caused by HSV-1 but in rare instances HSV-2 might also cause herpetic gingivostomatitis.

It can be acute or chronic and recurrent.

Classification of Vesiculobullous Lesions:

a. Non febrile associated lesions:
   - Recurrent herpes labialis
   - Recurrent herpes stomatitis
   - Reiter's syndrome
   - Dyskeratosis congenital

b. Febrile associated lesions:
   - Herpetic gingivostomatitis
   - Herpangina
   - Hand-foot-mouth disease
   - Chickenpox
   - Herpes zoster
   - Smallpox
   - Bullous lesions:
   - Phemphigus
   - Familial benign chronic pemphigus
   - Bullous pemphigoid
   - Epidermolysis bullosa
   - Dermatitis herpetiformis
   - Erythema multiforme
   - Steven's johnsons' syndrome

(i) **Primary herpetic gingivostomatitis:** Also called as acute herpetic gingivostomatitis and develops in both children and young adults with incubation period 5 to 7 days.

Prodromal symptoms – fever, headache, malaise, nausea, vomiting, mouth becomes painful, irritability, pain upon swallowing and cervical lymphadenopathy.

Location:

The lesion mainly occurs on hard palate, attached gingiva, dorsum of tongue, buccal mucosa, lips and may be on skin and there is appearance of multiple small vesicles having thin walls and an inflammatory base surrounding it. They are quickly rupturing vesicles, small, shallow, oval shape, discrete ulcer, and grayish white or yellow plaque covers the base of the ulcer.

- Ulcers are 1 to 5 mm and coalesce to form large irregular ulcers.
- In severe cases, lips become hemorrhagic and matted with fibrin like exudates.
- It becomes painful during mastication and speech.
- Gingiva becomes swollen and ulcerated, also causes pharyngitis.
- The typical feature is the generalised marginal gingivitis.
- There may be fetid breath, drooling of saliva and difficulty in maintaining oral hygiene.
- Difficulty in chewing and swallowing may lead to improper nutrition and electrolyte imbalance.
- The disease is self-limiting and starts healing in a week to 14 days without leaving any scars.

Diagnosis:

1. History: History of close contact with patient having disease.
2. Clinical findings of typical features.
3. HSV isolation from exfoliative cytology.
4. Antibody titre: antibodies to HSV appear in a week and reach peak in 3 weeks, direct fluorescent antigen detection testing is more accurate than routine cytology.

Investigation:

1. **Direct smear:** material obtained from base of smear and stained- the finding of multinucleated cells with swelling, ballooning and degeneration is adequate for diagnosis, isolation of virus from suspected site, to tissue culture.
2. **Serological studies:** Serological assays include (anti-HSV IgM and IgG), the Tzanck test and immunofluorescence. The gold standard is considered to be the culture of viral isolates. Testing the HSV antibody can help in detecting both the types of virus, HSV-1 and HSV-2. Primary HSV infection is associated with an increase in IgM titer followed several weeks later by permanent IgG titers.

Individuals with recent infections are more likely to test positive for herpes IgG and IgM or herpes IgM alone.

Differential diagnosis:

- **Hand, foot and mouth disease:** Vesicular lesions are present in mouth as well as hands and feet, where as primary herpetic gingivostomatitis is present only in the mouth.
- **Herpangina:** These lesions are more commonly seen on the posterior part of oral cavity, especially the hard palate, tonsillar areas and sometimes pharynx. It is caused by Coxackie virus.

- **Recurrent apthous ulcer:** History of recurrence and family history is present in most of the cases. Marginal gingivitis is absent.
- **Herpes zoster infection:** Occurs unilaterally and more common in adults.
- **Erythema multiforme:** Apart from oral mucosa, skin, genitals and eyes are involved.
- **Bullous lichen planus:** These are more commonly seen in adults and frequently in women. Presence of Wickham's striae is characteristic and histology will reveal liquefaction degeneration of basal cell layer.
- **Benign mucosal phemphigoid:** These are bullous lesions and involve other parts of the body apart from mouth which is not the case in PHGS. The bulla are typically sub epithelial.
- **Pemhigus:** The lesions are bullous and involve the skin of other parts of the body as well. Nikosky's sign will be positive.
- **Allergic stomatitis:** History of allergy to a particular agent can be elicited.The general symptoms like prodrome and high fever and malaise will be absent. Treatment with antiallergic will resolve the lesions.

Treatment:

1. **Symptomatic treatment:**
   - **Pain control measures:** topical anesthesia 2% lidocaine, 0.5% benzocaine hydrochloride, solution of diphenhydramine hydrochloride 5 mg mixed with equal amount of milk of magnesia can also reduce pain.
   - **Topical anti-infective agents:** given to prevent secondary infections, agents used are 0.2% chlorohexidine gluconate, tetracycline mouth wash.
2. **Supportive care:**
   - Fluid is given to maintain proper hydration and electrolyte balance.
   - **Good oral hygiene:** good oral hygiene is maintained to prevent infection, avoidance of hard and spicy food.
3. **Specific treatment:**
   - Acyclovir suspensions 15 mg /kg or acyclovir tablets 200mg five times daily for 5 days initiated in first 3 days of onset can decrease duration of lesions.
   - Acyclovir 800mg/day may be used as prophylactic regimen.
   - Val acyclovir tablets 500mg or famciclovir 250mg twice/day for 5 days may be used as alternative. Tosca met is drug of choice against acyclovir resistant HSV.

(ii) **Recurrent herpetic gingivostomatitis:** It is often seen in adults and the manifestation clinically is as an attenuated form of the primary herpetic stomatitis. It is mostly associated with Trauma, fatigue, menstruation, pregnancy, upper respiratory tract infection, emotional upset, allergy, exposure to sunlight or ultraviolet light and gastrointestinal disturbances.

Clinical features and oral manifestations:

- The occurrence of this lesion is varied and may occur nearly every month in some cases and could appear only once a year or less in others.
- **Site:** It appears in the area of primary inoculation or the adjacent areas which are supplied by the ganglion involved. It occurs on keratinised mucosa that is closely bound to like palate, attached gingiva or alveolar ridge. It could also occur on the lips. (Recurrent herpes labialis).

Signs and symptoms

- Burning or tingling sensation.
- Feeling of tautness.
- There can be swelling or pain and soreness in the area in which the vesicles subsequently develops.
- Vesicles are small (1mm or less in diameter) tend to occur in localized cluster and may coalesce to form larger lesion.
- These gray or white vesicle rupture quickly, leaving a small red ulceration, sometimes with red erythematous halo.
- On lips ruptured vesicles covered with the brownish crust.
- Lesions heals within 7-10 days and leave no scar.

Histopathologic features:

- Fresh scraping from the base of vesicle shows 'ballooning degeneration', 'chromatin margination' and typical 'Lipschutz bodies' and multinucleated giant cells.

Treatment:

- Specific antiviral drugs are used like topical 5% Acyclovir cream topically 3-6 times/day.
- Systemic therapy with valacyclovir or famicyclovir 500-1000 mg three times a day.

Suggested reading:

1. Annie Kitty George, and Sukumaran Anil, Acute Herpetic Gingivostomatitis Associated with Herpes Simplex Virus 2: Report of a Case, J Int Oral Health. 2014 Jun; 6(3): 99–102.
2. Burket's, Oral Medicine Diagnosis and Treatment, 10th edition, chapter 3, pg no 44-46.
3. Shafer's, text book of oral pathology, sixth edi. chapter 6, pg no.337-338.

Q 5) Classify ulcers of the oral mucosa. Discuss the differential diagnosis of recurrent multiple ulcers:

RGUHS 1999 (10 Marks)

Classification of ulcerative lesions:

1. **Single ulcers:**

(a) Traumatic
(b) Tuberculous
(c) Syphilitic
(d) Histoplasmosis
(e) Blastomycosis
(f) Mucormycosis
(g) Neoplastic ulcers

2. Multiple ulcers:

(i) Acute Ulcers:

(a) Primary herpetic gingivostomatitis.
(b) Herpangina.
(c) Hand-foot-mouth disease.
(d) Varicella-zoster virus infections: chicken pox and herpes zoster.
(e) Erythema multiforme.
(f) Contact allergic stomatitis.
(g) Oral ulcers secondary to cancer chemotherapy and / or radiotherapy.
(h) Acute necrotising ulcerative gingivitis.

(ii) **Chronic Ulcers:**

(a) Pemphigus.
(b) Subepithelial bullous dermatoses.
(c) Herpes simplex virus infection in immunosuppressed patients.

3. Recurring oral ulcers:

(a) Recurrent aphthous stomatitis.
(b) Behcets syndrome.
(c) Recurrent herpes simplex infection
(d) Cyclic neutropenia.
(e) Chronic idiopathic neutropenia.

Differential diagnosis of recurrent multiple ulcers:

1. Recurrent aphthous stomatitis:

Aphthous word is derived from Latin word 'aphthae' meaning thrush.

A chronic inflammatory disease characterised by painful, recurring, ulcerations of the oral mucosa.

There are three forms:

Minor ulcers: Generally less than 1 cms in size. There may be a prodrome of burning sensation in the area of future ulcer, generalized edema of oral cavity, especially tongue, paraesthesia, malaise, low grade fever, localized lymphadenopathy. There is no vesicle formation. There is involvement of the buccal and lip mucosa, buccal and lingual sulcus, tongue, soft palate, pharynx, gingiva, all areas not attached to periosteum (non-keratinised surfaces)

The ulcers persist for 7 – 14 days & heal without scarring.

Major ulcers also called as Sutton's disease, or periadenitis mucosa necrotica recurrence or Mickulicz's scarring aphthae): Usually more than 1 cms in size.They take longer time to heal and often may heal with scarring. Large painful ulcers.

1 -10 in no. on lips, cheeks, tongue, soft palate and fauces.

The lesions may persist for upto 6 week and leave a scar upon healing.

Round or ovoid with well defined margin, erythematous edge floor of yellowish slough.

Herpetiform ulcers: Appear as crops of small ulcers and look like herpetic ulcers and hence the name. Crops of multiple, small, shallow ulcers, often upto 100, may occur at any site of oral cavity, the ventrum of tongue being the most common. Heal in 7-30 days, occasionally with scarring.

These ulcers can be differentiated from other ulcers especially by taking history. Heredity is the most common etiological factor. There will be history of similar ulcers in the family and many a times one or both the parents may suffer from these.

History of allergy to pineapples, strawberries, chocolates will be present. These ulcers can be precipitated by minor trauma like eating biscuits, brushing or fish bone, self inflicted bites, sharp, broken carious teeth and minor oral surgical procedures, or ill fitting dentures.

They occur especially in students during exams, that is stress and anxiety can cause these lesions to erupt. Their occurrence increases in women especially during the premenstrual and menstrual time. Thus proper history will help in diagnosis of aphthous ulcers.

These are common in people with zinc deficiency and also occur in smokers after their cessation of smoking.

The typical shallow ulcer with erythematous margins which almost always heal on their own in 7-10 days will help in diagnosis.

Biopsy or cytology of the ulcer will reveal the typical Anitschkow cells characteristic of aphthous ulcers.

2. Behcet's disease (BD):

Its a chronic condition with multisystem involvement and characterised by a triad of:

(i) Recurrent aphthous stomatitis. 2) Ulcers of the genitals. 3) Lesions of the eyes.
This condition affects individuals more commonly of the mediterranean origin from places like the middle east, china and korea.

(ii) For a patient to be diagnosed with Behçet's disease the patient should be affected with oral aphthous ulcers, which can vary in shape and size and number and occurs at least 3 times/year along with 2 of the 4 hallmark symptoms:

(iii) Inflammation of the eyes(uveitis, iritis, and retinal vasculitis).

(iv) pathergy reaction that is a papule more than 2 mms in diameter, that appears about 24-48 hours after the needle -prick.The pathergy test show a specificity of about 95-100.

- The most common area of involvement in the BD is the oral mucosa.
- In above 90% of the cases recurring oral ulcers occur.

- These lesions cannot be distinguished from recurrent aphthous stomatitis.
- The second common site is the genital area in which there occurs ulcers of the scrotum and the penis in males and ulcers of the labia in females.
- The lesions involving the eyes are uveitis, optic atrophy, retinal infiltrates, edema, vascular occlusion, conjunctivitis and keratitis.
- The other symptoms include Arthritis. central nervous system involvement venous thrombosis, thrombophlebitis, ulcerations of the intestine, and renal and pulmonary disease.
- The oral ulcers are difficult to distinguish from aphthous ulcers. But the concurrent presence of genital and eye lesions will help distinguish and establish the diagnosis.The pathergy test also is very typical for diagnosing these lesions and the multisystem involvement will help in differentiating it from other recurrent ulcers like recurrent herpes labialis or recurrent herpes simplex infection.

3. Recurrent herpes labialis: Its a recurrent herpes simplex infection which can occur every month or once or twice in a year. As the name suggests these lesions occur on the lips and there is prodrome of burning or tingling sensation in the area of occurrence and there may be swelling or edema followed by outbreak of clusters of vesicles which might rupture to form ulcers which are small and may have an erythematous halo. Females are more commonly affected and the typical site of the lesions that is vermilion border of the lips and surrounding skin and formation of brownish crust can help in distinguishing from other recurrent ulcers.

4. Recurrent intraoral herpes: These lesions occur typically on the keratinised mucosa involving the gingiva, hard palate, tongue dorsum. These are also small short lived vesicles which rupture to form ulcers with erythematous halo and they may coalesce to form larger irregular ulcers.

In aphthous ulcers and Behcets ulcers vesicles donot appear and this can be used to differentiate recurrent herpes labialis and recurrent intraoaral herpes lesions from them.

5. Cyclic neutropenia: Cyclic (periodic) neutropenia is a rare benign, hematologic disorder characterized by cyclical depression of the peripheral blood polymorphonuclear leukocyte (PMNL) count at 21-day intervals that occurs secondary to a periodic failure of the stem cells in the bone marrow.

This condition is characterised by fever, malaise, ulcerations of the oral mucosa with scarring, periodontitis, gingivitis and disappearance of the neutrophils from the blood and bone marrow at approximate intervals of 21 days.

Oral lesions are common in cyclic neutropenia and may be the major clinical manifestation of the disease.

The two most common oral manifestations are oral mucosal ulcers and periodontal disease.

The oral ulcers recur with each new bout of neutropenia and resemble the large deep scarring ulcers seen in major aphthous stomatitis.

The periodontal manifestations range from marginal gingivitis to rapidly advancing periodontal bone loss caused by bacterial infection of the dental supporting structures.

The typical 21 day cyclical appearance of ulcers especially in children associated with fever and malaise and severe periodontal involvement can help in distinguishing from other recurrent ulcers. Also the cyclical drop in neutrophil counts during the episodes to below 500/mm3 can help to confirm the diagnosis.

6. Recurrent erythema multiforme: Erythema multiforme is a self limiting but acute condition and sometimes there are recurrent skin lesions that are considered to be hypersensitivity reaction type IV which is associated with certain medications or infections, and various other triggers.

It is called multiforme because it manifests variety of skin lesions.

Most frequently in children and young adults and is rare after age 50 years.

It has an acute or even an explosive onset.

Vesiculobullous lesions involve the skin, eyes and genitals.

The lesions on skin are typical target or iris or bulls eye type of lesions. Intra oral vesicles also form but breakdown to form ulcers. There is peculiar bloody crusting of the lips and drooling of saliva.

When they occur in recurrent episodes they need to be differentiated from other recurring ulcers like aphthous ulcers and behcets syndrome.

The tetrad of oral, skin, eyes and genital lesions with typical bull's eye lesions on the skin and out break especially after taking certain drugs can help differentiate from other recurring ulcers.

More over it is vesiculo bullous lesion which aphthous ulcers and Behcet's disease are not.

Recurrent herpes labialis occurs on the lips and recurrent intraoral herpes lesions occur on the keratinised oral mucosa and donot have concurrent lesions any where else in the body and hence can be differentiated from recurrent episodes of erythema multiforme.

7. Chronic Idiopathic Neutropenia: This term is usually used when chronic neutropenia occurs due to unknown reasons.

This rare blood condition is typically characterised by abnormally low white blood cells in the body.

The features associated with this disorder includes recurring fever, ulcerations in the oral cavity, and/or periodontitis.

As the WBCs are low in count, the patients are more prone to develop recurrent infections that can result in life threatening consequences in some cases. This condition may persist for months or years and can affect adults as well as children.

However most of the cases are less severe than the congenital form of neutropenia and may not require specific treatment. But in some cases of idiopathic neutropenia, the infections can lead to life threatening consequences.

The persistent low levels of neutrophils and recurrent infections and also occurring in adults can help in diagnosis. In cyclic neutropenia the fall in neutrophils and the other symptoms occur in 21 day intervals and thus can be differentiated from it.

Suggested reading:

1. Allen CM, Bouquot JE. (2008). Oral & maxillofacial pathology (3rd ed.). Philadelphia: W.B. Saunders. p. 336.
2. Criteria for diagnosis of Behçet's disease". Lancet 335 (8697): 1078–80.
3. Burket's, Oral Medicine Diagnosis and Treatment 10th edi. 63-68.

Q 6) Classify vesiculobullous lesions. Discuss the etiology, clinical features, diagnosis, differential diagnosis and management of pemphigus vulgaris:

TNMGRU FEBRUARY 2006 (15 Marks)

I) Primarily Vesicular Lesions:

1. Primary Herpetic gingivostomatitis.
2. Herpangina.
3. Hand-foot and mouth Disease.
4. Primary Varicella-zoster (Chickenpox).
5. Secondary Varicella-zoster (Shingles).
6. Recurrent Herpes Stomatitis.
7. Recurrent Herpes Labialis.
8. Contact Vesicular stomatitis.
9. Impetigo.

II) Primarily Bullous Lesions:

1. Pemphigus vulgaris
2. Bullous pemphigoid
3. Benign mucous membrane pemphigoid
4. Bullous lichen planus
5. Erythema multiforme
6. Steven's johnson's syndrome
7. Epidermolysis bullosa
8. Dermatitis herpetiformis

Etiology:

- It is an autoimmune disorder characterized by intraepithelial bulla formation due to breakdown in intercellular adhesion.
  - Antigen antibody reaction leads to epithelial cell separation (IGg antibody+pemphigus antigen) and separation of cells takes place in lower layers of stratum spinosum.
  - Autoantibodies against desmosomal components results in epithelial cell separation called acantholysis.
  - The main antigen is Dsg3, but 50% of patients also have autoantibodies to Dsg1.
  - The autoantibodies are mainly IgG4 and IgG1.

- Complement mainly C3 can act as antibody causing acantholysis.
- Activation of proteases.
- Acantholysis and spongiosis occur due to the loss of syndecan 1 expression.

Clinical features:

Typical features are:

- Intra Epithelial Bulla.
- Supra Basilar Split.
- Acantholysis.
- Nikolskys Sign.
- Tzanck Cells.
- Seen in 5th-6th decades, male /female 1: 1
- A total of 80-90% of patients develop oral mucosal lesions and in about 60% cases oral lesions may appear before the skin lesions.
- Vesicles or bullae which are thin walled may vary from few mms to several cms, on skin or mucosa.
- Lesions are thin walled and contain watery fluid, which may become purulent or sanguinous and break down easily and may extend peripherally to involve large areas.
- Buccal mucosa most commonly involved followed by gingiva, palate and the ventral tongue surface and the lips.
- There may be severe desquamative gingivitis and lips may be covered with thick hemorrhagic crusts.
- Lesions begin as bulla and break down easily to form ulcers.The lesions bleed easily have ragged borders, are covered with white or blood tinged exudate, are very tender causing difficulty in eating.
- Nikolskys sign could be present.It is formation of fresh bulla when pressure is applied to normal appearing skin.
- If the surface of the blister is applied with vertical pressure, the blister extends laterally, known as the Asboe-Hansen signs.

Diagnosis:

Histopathological features:

Bulllae are intra epithelial/acantholysis in stratum spinosum/loss of intra cellular bridges/nuclei are large & hyperchromatic/connective tissue may be inflammed with chronic inflammatory cells/as the bullae rupture they are infiltrated with polymorphonuclear leucocytes and surface may show suppuration.

- There is attachment of the basal cell layer to the lamina propria and they project into the bulla in a tombstone pattern.
- Though there is scanty inflammatory cells, eosinophils can be spotted.
- Acantholytic stratum spinosum cells occur singly or are in the form of clumps that can be seen lying free in the fluid of the blisters.The cells tend to get rid of their polyhedral shape and are small and

rounded and consist of hyper chromatic nuclei called the Tzanck Cells.

Clinical examination:

Patients will show active blistering and positive Nikolsky's sign.

Biopsy: Biopsy of intact bulla will show acantholysis.

Tzanck smear: Scraping of the base of bulla will show floating and free, rounded or ovoid, acantholytic cells, with hyperchromatic, enlarged nuclei.

Compressed air test: A stream of compressed air directed on the gingival tissue will cause a bleb to form.

Direct immunofluorescence: Circulating antibodies of IgG type which is bound to the intercellular cement area of the oral mucosa.

Indirect immunofluorescence: patients will show antikeratinocyte antibodies against the intercellular substance which show up under a fluorescent microscope.

ELISA test: It can help in the detection of DSG1 and DSG3 in the samples of the serum.

Upper gastrointestinal endoscopy: Can reveal in identifying esophageal involvement.

Differential diagnosis:

- **Bullous pemphigoid:** Lesions are subepithelial and usually present on skin rather than intraoral. Autoantibodies are directed against BP 230 and BP 180 antigen.
- **Mucous membrane pemhigoid:** Unlike the blisters in pemhigus, they donot get cloudy or change into erosions. Nikolsky's sign is absent. Skin involvement is less frequent. Eyes are involved in 80% of cases which is not so in pemphigus vulgaris.Blisters are not painful which in pemphigus are.
- **Recurrent aphthous stomatitis and Behcet's disease:** These are recurrent ulcerative lesions and heal on their own and recur. The lesions of pemphigus continue for weeks or months and the lesions are not round or symmetrical as in aphthous but shallow and irregular and extend laterally and have detached epithelium at the periphery.
- **Erythema multiforme:** It has an acute onset and protean manifestations and eyes and genitals are involved commonly unlike pemphigus. The skin lesions have typical iris or bull's eye lesions on the skin in erythema multiforme but not in pemphigus.
- **Herpetic gingivostomatitis:** Have an acute onset and there is fever, malaise, lymphadenopathy and the oral lesions affect the attached gingiva and the lesions are smaller and typical feature is the generalized marginal gingivitis.
- **Erosive and bullous lichen plnus:** Histopathology will show saw tooth appearance of epithelium and liquefaction degeneration of basal cells which is not present in pemphigus. Direct immunofluorescence will also help in diagnosis.

- **Linear IgA disease:** Immunofluorescence will show linear homogenous deposition of IgA antibodies along the basement membrane.
- **Dermatitis herpetiformis:** Mucosal involvement is rare. Tzanck test and Nikolsky's sign are negative.
- **Drug induced stomatitis:** History of drug intake before eruptions will be present and Nikolsky's sign and Tzanck test will be negative.

Treatment:

There is no single treatment for treatment of pemphigus vulgaris. Each individual case needs to be dealt with separately.

The initial aim of treatment to help disease remission.

Mild cases: Topical analgesics and anesthetics. Benzydamine hydrochloride mouth rinses can be given. Antiseptic mouth washes like chlorhexidine gluconate 0.2% or hydrogen peroxide.

Topical steroids: Mouth rinse consisting of betamethasone sodium phosphate tablet of 0.5 mgs dissolved in 10ml of water QID/TDS. Triamcinolone 0.1 application in adhesive base, 2.5 mg hydrocortisone lozenges can be given. Topical cyclosporine 100 mg/ml can be beneficial.

Severe cases:

Systemic steroids:

If extensive lesions involving the oral cavity are present systemic prednisone may be indicated. It is prescribed as 40mg tablets per day for 7 days with no tapering. Patients are treated with initial prednisolone 40-60 mg/day and in severe cases 60-100mg/day. If doses above 100 mg are required pulsed intravenous corticosteroid therapy can be considered. Topical steroids in the form of ointment or solutions either alone or in combination with systemic steroids can be given to control the disease.

Pulsed intravenous corticosteroids: Intermittent high doses of intravenous steroids usually methyl prednisolone 250-1000 mgs or equivalent doses of dexamethasone given on 1-5 consecutive days to achieve a rapid control of the disease.

Adjuvant drugs: Include Azathioprine, oral cyclophosphamide, pulsed intravenous cyclophosphamide with dexamethasone or methyl prednisolone, mycophenolate mofetil, intravenous immunoglobulins, tetracycline and nicotinamide, 8-methoxy-psoralen which is followed by peripheral blood exposure to Uv radiation, extracorporeal photopheresis and plasma exchange need to be considered.

Suggested reading:

1. Anil Govindrao Ghom, Text Book Of Oral Medicine, 3rd edition, 371-376.

CHAPTER 2

Red and White Lesions of the Oral Mucosa

Q 1) Classify red and white lesions of the oral cavity. Describe etiopathogenesis, clinical features, differential diagnosis and treatment for oral leukoplakia:

MUHS MAY 2009 (10 Marks)

1. **White lesion:** Any abnormal area of the oral mucosa that appears whiter than the surrounding tissues on clinical examination and is usually slightly raised, roughened or otherwise of different texture.
2. **Red lesions:** These are areas of mucosa that have reddened appearance and is generally smooth and atrophic or could reveal a granular or velvety texture and may occur alone or with area of hyperkeratosis.

Classification of Red and White Lesions (Burket's):

I) Hereditary White Lesions:

- (a) Leukoedema
- (b) White Sponge Nevus
- (c) Hereditary benign intraepithelial dyskeratosis.
- (d) Dyskeratosis Congenita

II) Reactive/Inflammatory white lesions.

- (a) Linea alba
- (b) Frictional (Traumatic) Keratosis
- (c) Cheek biting
- (d) Chemical, Thermal and Physical Injuries of the Oral Mucosa
- (e) Actinic Keratosis (Cheilitis)
- (f) Smokeless Tobacco–Induced Keratosis
- (g) Stomatitis nicotina
- (h) Sanguinaria-induced leukoplakia

III) Infectious white lesions and red and white lesions:

- (a) Oral hairy leukoplakia.

(b) Candidiasis.
(c) Mucous Patches (Syphilitic)
(d) Parulis

IV) Idiopathic or true leukoplakia
V) Bowen's disease
VI) Erythroplakia
VII) Oral Lichen Planus
VIII) Lichenoid reaction:
(a) Drug induced lichenoid reaction
(b) Graft-versus-Host Disease

IX) Lupus Erythematosus (Systemic And Discoid)
X) Developmental white lesions: Ectopic lymphoid tissue
XI) Fordyce's Granules.
XII) Gingival and palatal cysts of the new born and adults
XIII) Miscellaneous Lesions:
(a) Geographic Tongue.
(b) Hairy tongue
(c) Oral Submucous Fibrosis.

Definition of Leukoplakia:

Leukoplakia is a white patch that cannot be scraped or rubbed off and cannot be classified clinically or histopathologically as any other lesion.

A white patch or plaque that cannot be clinically or histopathologically characterised as any other disease and is not associated with any physical or chemical agent except the use of tobacco. This definition was put forth in 1984 in an international symposium but there were confusions and problems to accept this definition.

Etiopathogenesis:

A. Local factors.
B. Systemic factors.

A. Local factors:

1. **Tobacco:**
   - **Smokeless tobacco:** When the tobacco is chewed variety of materials leach out which contains various chemical content, such as nitrosonornicotine, nicotine, pyridine etc along with alkaline ph of snuff act as local irritant and causes alteration in mucosa. They produces sublethal injury of the cell, within the deeper layers of oral epithelium which leads to epithelial hyperplasia.
   - **Smoking tobacco:** It is more harmful as it contains polycyclic hydrocarbon, carbon mono-oxide, nicotine along with production of heat.
2. **Alcohol:** The prevalence of leukoplakia is higher among alcoholics as alcohol facilitates the entry of carcinogen into exposed cells and thus alter the oral epithelium and its metabolism.

3. **Sanguinaria:** Herbal extract used in toothpaste and mouth rinse causes true leukoplakia.
4. **Chronic irritation:** Continuous trauma or local irritation eg, sharp broken teeth, ill-fitting dentures, malocclusion etc. Leukoplakia is a protection of the traumatised mucosa against chronic irritation but now a days maximum lesions seen due to mechanical irritation are frictional keratosis with very low precancerous potential.
5. **Candidiasis:** The presence of candida albicans is seen in association with nodular type of leukoplakia.
6. **Electromagnetic reaction or galvanism:** Galvanism caused due to the generation of current between dissimilar, opposing or adjacent restoration.

It causes metallic taste, persistent pain and inflammatory changes in oral mucosa. These mucosal changes may promote, malignant transformation of leukoplakia.

B. Regional or systemic factors:

1. **Syphilis:** Predisposing factor for the development of leukoplakia. Leads to diffuse vasculitis resulting in the atrophy of filliform and fungiform papillae and results in bald smooth lingual surface and this makes it susceptible to oral irritation and leukoplakia frequently develops on it.
2. **Vitamin deficiency:** Deficiency of vitamin A causes metaplasia and keratinisation of certain epithelial structures and thus can lead to leukoplakia, vitamin B complex deficiency has also been suggested as predisposing factor.
3. **Nutritional deficiency:** Sideropenic anemia and other nutritional deficiency can be predisposing factors for the occurrence of leukoplakia.
4. **Xerostomia:** Some factors such as salivary gland diseases, anticholinergic drugs and radiation that causes xerostomia can lead to leukoplakia.
5. **Drugs:** Anticholinergic, antimetabolic drugs may predispose to the occurrence of leukoplakia.
6. **Virus:** Herpes simplex virus and human papilloma virus have been associated with etiopathogenesis of leukoplakia.
7. **Idiopathic cryptogenic leukoplakia:** Leukoplakia without any underlying cause is termed as idiopathic leukoplakia and it has a higher potential for malignant transformation.

Clinical Features:

Classification:

1. **Homogeneous leukoplakia:** It is generally a well defined patch which is white, and can be localised or extensive and which is slightly elevated, and has a fissured and wrinkled surface resembling cracked mud appearance and could be leathery in feel to touch.

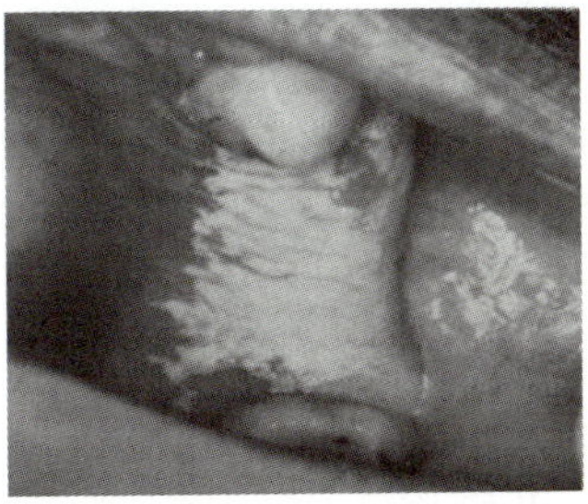

Fig. Homogenous leukoplakia

2. **Nodular (speckled) leukoplakia:** Is granular or non-homogeneous. Its a combination of mixed red and white areas in which white nodules or patches are spread over an atrophic or erythematous background.This variety of leukoplakia is more prone to change in to a malignancy and upto 2/3rds of the cases may some times may show epithelial dysplasia or carcinoma.

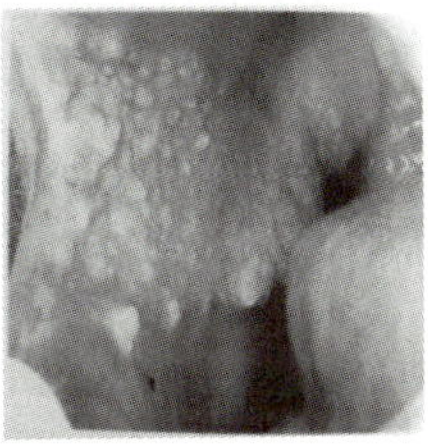

Fig. Nodular or speckled leukoplakia

3. **Verrucous leukoplakia:** It is a term that is used for describing the lesions that are thick white and have papillary surfaces in the oral mucosa. These lesions are seen in older adults in the 6th and 8th decades and are heavily keratinised.Some lesions exhibit a exophytic pattern of growth.
4. **Proliferative verrucous leukoplakia:** In this type the leukoplakia is extensively papillary or has a verrucoid white plaque like appearance and can gradually involve multiple sites in the oral mucosa and is highly prone to change into dysplasia, squamous cell carcinoma or verrucous carcinoma.

Sharp's staging of leukoplakia:

1. **Stage I:** It is a very early lesion and is non-palpable, its translucent faintly and is a white discolouration.
2. **Stage II:** localized or diffused has slight elevation of plaque, and its outline is irregular, is opaque white in colour and has fine granular texture
3. **Stage III:** The lesion is thick and white and is indurated and shows fissuring.

Higher risk of malignant transformation is seen in non-homogenous type of leukoplakia, however, any type of leukoplakia can undergo malignant change.

1. The geographic location of an individual and habits of patients dictate the incidence of leukoplakia. eg, in countries where there is frequent usage of smokeless tobacco, there are greater chances of affectation with leukoplakia.
2. The adults above 50 years of age are affected and is more frequently found in men.
3. Prevalence increases with age and about 8% men who are older than 70 years are affected.
4. Most commonly affected regions are the buccal mucosa, vermilion border of the lower lip and the gingiva.
5. In bidi smokers bilateral leukoplakia at the corners of the mouth is commonly seen.
6. These lesions are less frequently seen in the maxillary areas, retromolar region, palate, floor of the mouth and the tongue.
7. However contradictory to this, 90% of the lesions of the tongue and floor of the mouth show dysplasia or carcinoma.
8. The range of prevalence is about 0.2-5% and India has a whopping prevalence of 0.2-4.9%.
9. Leukoplakia can be either solitary or multiple.
10. Sublingual keratosis: When it involves the floor and ventral surface of the tongue. Ebbing tide type: Variant of leukoplakia occurring in the floor of the mouth, appears similar to the undulations left on the sand by ebbing tide.
11. Extent varies from small, well localized, irregular patches to diffuse lesions involving considerable portion of oral mucosa.
12. Color: White or yellowish white.
13. Surface: Rough on palpation, wrinkled or shriveled in appearance.
14. Symptoms: There is feeling of thickness of the mucosa in the affected area and the ulcerated and the nodular type may be associated with burning sensation.

Differential diagnosis:

- **Lichen planus:** Distinguished by presence of wickham's striae and multiple skin and oral lesion. In the oral cavity these lesions are usually bilateral and more common in middle aged women, where as leukoplakia is more common in men.
- **Lupus erythematosus:** There is an area of atrophy in the center and there is a border of slightly elevated zone and white dots, or radiating white striae. Systemic symptoms of this conditions might be present and will help in differentiating from leukoplakia.
- **Leukoedema:** Occurs on buccal mucosa milky appearance that is faint and has wrinkled and folded pattern when compared to whiteness of leukoplakia and will disappear on stretching, which leukoplakia will not.
- **White spongy nevus:** It tends to occur soon after birth or at puberty and has folded appearance and is seen in younger individuals and

is distributed widely through out the oral mucosa which is not so in leukoplakia. Proper history will help in differentiating.

- **Psoriasis:** Auspitz's sign is positive and skin lesion are also present.
- **Habitual cheek biting:** These lesions are more extensive and may have tissue tags at periphery which leukoplakia doesn't. More commonly seen in younger age group and more so in those with parafunctional habits, or presence of nervous disorders which can help in differentiating from leukoplakia.
- **Tobacco pouch keratosis:** These are keratotic lesions that occur in areas where smokeless tobacco is generally kept as a habit. These lesions may lack the whiteness of leukoplakia and on stretching may disappear which leukoplakia will not.
- **Burns:** Chemical, physical or thermal burns can cause white patches. Proper history, easy scrapability, pain and associated inflammation of the lesions will help to differentiate from leukoplakia.
- **Syphilitic mucous patches:** Systemic symptoms and presence of split papule or condyloma latum may be present as differentiating factors.
- **Hairy leukoplakia:** These lesions are folded grayish white lesions along the lateral border of the tongue and will have associated other features of AIDS in the individual.
- **Verruca vulgaris:** These are elevated white lesions about 0.5 cms or more in diameter but well defined, where as leukoplakia will be more wide spread.
- **Electrogalvanic white lesion:** These lesions will disappear when the dissimilar metals are removed or when teeth are extracted having metal restorations.

Treatment of Leukoplakia:

I) Removal of Etiological Factors:

1. **Prohibition of Smoking:** patient should be asked to cease smoking immediately and advise Nicotine substitutes.
2. **Removal of any chronic irritant:** Enameloplasty in case of any broken or sharp teeth.
3. Eliminating other factors like syphilis, alcohol, tobacco chewing, dissimilar metal restorations, vitamin and iron deficiencies.

II) Medical Management:

1. **Antioxidant therapy:**
   - Beta-carotene alone in dose of 30mg daily for 3-6 months.
   - Lycopene capsules 4mg bid or 8 mg OD for 3months.
2. **Vitamin therapy:**
   - Vitamin B complex is given as supplements in cases of commissural and lingual leukoplakia.
   - L-Ascorbic Acid (Vitamin C): Protective effect on epithelium.
   - therapeutic dose-75000-300000IU for 3 months.

- 13-Cis-Retinoic acid: A vitamin A analogue, 1.5 mg-2 mg/body wt for 3 months.

3. **Bleomycin:** A cytotoxic antibiotic, topical bleomycin in dosages of 0.5% -1% per day for 12 to 15 days.
4. **Nystatin therapy:**
   - It is given in candidal leukoplakia, twice/day of 500000 IU along with application locally of 20% borax glycerol or 1% gentian violet or mouth washes with clorogen solution.
   - 100000 units/ml of nystatin oral suspension; 300ml: rinse with one teaspoonful (5ml) for 2 minutes, use QID and spit out.

   Photodynamic Therapy:
   - Photodynamic therapy (PDT) is a non invasive method for the treatment of oral premalignant lesions and head and neck cancers.
   - The principle of PDT is a non-thermal photochemical reaction, which needs the simultaneous presence of a photosensitising agent (photo sensitizer), oxygen, and visible light.

6. **Green tea:** Tea inhibits formation of mutagens and reduces lipid peroxidation.
7. **Gene therapy:** Gene therapy is a new treatment procedure in which an existing gene is manipulated, or a new gene is introduced, in order to slow the growth of the lesion or cause the death of the dysplastic cells.

III) Surgical Treatment:

1. **Conventional surgery:** The lesions are removed surgically by wide excision, including safe margins.
2. **Cryosurgery:** In this process the tissues are exposed to very cold stimuli to produce irreversible cell damage. The death of cell occurs at -20 degrees centigrade.A cryoprobe which is refrigerated by liquid nitrogen can be used.
3. **Electrocautery:** Tissue destruction by current of high voltage. The reduction of bleeding is of great advantage. Foul odour is a disadvantage, hazards of explosion, under local or general anesthesia, slow healing, pain and scar.
4. **Laser:** Its commonly used in leukoplakic cases for biopsy or peeling of the lesions when large areas are involved and ablation which is used to paint away a lesion which is removed by laser. Ablation is non contact surgical application in which the tissue is simply vapourised.

Generally CO_2 lasers are used which contains CO2, nitrogen and helium gases. Neodymium-doped yttrium aluminum garnet: ((NDYAG)lasers also used.

Suggested reading:

1. Blaggana A, Blaggana V, Vohra P. Oral leukoplakia: A Therapeutic Challenge-An

Update. Journal of Innovative Dentistry, vol 1, Issue 2 May-August 2011.
2. Burket's Textbook of oral medicine chapter 5, page 85.
3. Lodi, G; Sardella, A; Bez, C; Demarosi, F; Carrassi, A (Oct 18, 2006). "Interventions for treating oral leukoplakia." Cochrane database of systematic reviews (Online) (4): CD001829.doi: 10.1002/14651858
4. Ravi Kiran Ongole Text book of oral medicine &radiology, Chapter 6 pg, 144.
5. Soames, JV; Southam, J.C. (1999). Oral pathology. page no 139–140, 144–151.

Q 2) Classify oral candidiasis, describe the etiology, clinical features, differential diagnosis and management of oral thrush.

MUHS NOVEMBER 2006 (10 Marks)

"Candidiasis" is an opportunistic infection the cause of which is a fungus that is yeast like, candida, and is a very common fungal infection of the oral cavity in humans.

Classification of Oral Candidiasis:

(i) Acute:
- Acute Pseudomembranous.
- Acute atrophic (antibiotic sore mouth).

(ii) Chronic: Atrophic
  (a) Denture stomatitis.
  (b) Angular chelitis.
  (c) Median rhomboid glossitis.

Hyperplastic:
  (a) Candidal leukoplakia.

(iii) Chronic Mucocutaneous Candidiasis:
  (a) Familial.
  (b) Endocrine candidiasis syndrome.
  (c) Localized.
  (d) Generalized (diffuse).

(iv) Immunocompromise (HIV) associated.

Acute Pseudo membranous Candidiasis (Thrush):

Thrush or acute pseudomembranous candidiasis is caused by fungus that is yeast like, candida albicans. Also caused by Candida tropicalis, C parasilopsis, C guilliermondii, C krusei, Cpsedotropicalis, candida rugosa, stelltoidea, candida famata and candida rugosa.

It is a superficial infection of the upper tiers of the epithelium and the result is formation of white plaques that are patchy and flecks with curdy white appearance on the mucosal surface.

Gentle rubbing or scraping of the lesions leaves a region of shallow ulcers or erythema.

As a reason of the characteristic plaque or curdy white appearance, and ease of scrapability, lesions of thrush are easily recognized, and diagnosed.
Etiology and predisposing factors:

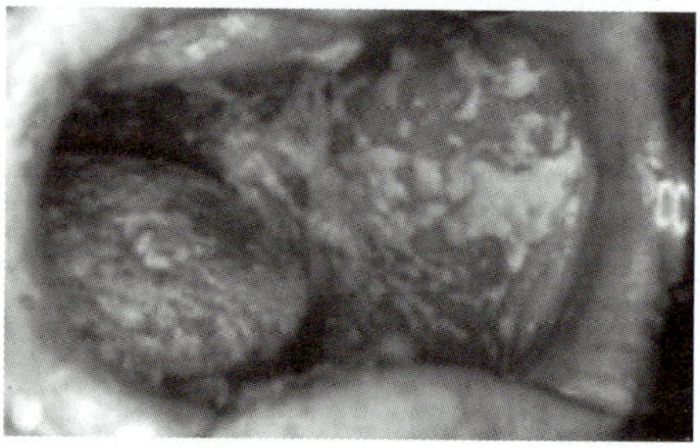

Fig. Curdy white Lesions of Thrush

1. Excessive use of antibiotics, antibacterial mouth rinses.
2. Xerostomia due to anticholinergics and salivary gland diseases.
3. Local irritation due to heavy smoking and orthodontic appliances & dentures.
4. Drugs like corticosteroids, cytotoxic drugs and immunosuppresives, and radiation t/t.
5. The corticosteroids in aerosol form or topical application can lead more often to candidiasis than its administration systemically.
6. Diseases like leukemia, diabetes, lymphoma, tuberculosis.
7. Malnutrition and malabsorption.
8. Infancy, old age and pregnancy.
9. Hypoparathyroidism, hypothyroidism, addisons disease.
10. Poor oral hygiene.
11. Immunodeficiency states: Primary and acquired immunodeficiency states like hypogammaglobulinaemia.

Clinical features:

- In infants:
- Starts between 6th or 10th day.
- Contracted through mother.
- Any part of the oral mucosa and the circumoral region also can be involved.
- Can be noticed on careful examination.
- They are often painless and can be removed easily or with some difficulty.
- The lesions look typically soft white, bluish or curdy white.
- In adults:
- Can occur on any mucosal surface but most common on roof of mouth, mucobuccal fold and retromolar area.
- More common in females than males.
- Prodrome like rapid onset of bad taste.
- There may be burning sensation or dryness of mouth.
- There may presence of inflammation, painful areas of erosion or erythema.
- The lesions are typical curdy, bluish, pearly white lesions. Lesions may simulate the appearance of cottage cheese or curdled milk.

- Adjacent mucosa may be erythematous.
- Can be easily wiped out but might leave eroded areas.
- Some lesions may be inconspicuous.
- May occasionally be associated or coexist with dysplastic or carcinomatic changes.
- Deeper lesions may cause ulcers.
- Erythematous areas or white patches may develop under dentures.
- Histopathologically, diagnosis can be made and confirmed by presence of tangled mass of Yeast cells and mycelia or hyphae of candida species, and debris.
- Submucosa could be free from infection.

Differential diagnosis of thrush:

(a) **Food debris:** This can be scraped off and will not leave behind painful erosive areas. The prodrome and fever and other systemic symptoms.

(b) **Habitual cheek biting:** These are keratotic lesions and cannot be scraped off easily. Tissue tags are present at the periphery and history will elicit habit of cheek biting or other causes like nervous disorder.

Lichen planus (plaque type): It is a keratotic lesion and cannot be scrapped off, and are usually bilateral. Histopathologically saw tooth appearance of reteridges and degeneration of the basal cell layer of the liquefaction type is present, and absence of candida hyphae, will help in differentiating from thrush.

(c) **Leukoplakia:** This is also a keratotic lesion and cannot be scrapped off easily. It lacks the curdy white appearance. The lesions have cracked mud, speckled or papillary keratotic lesions. Histopathologically, the drop shaped retepegs and varying degrees of epithelial dysplasia and lack of candidal hyphae will help to differentiate from thrush.

(d) **Gangrenous stomatitis:** Pseudomembrane is usually dirty in color.

(e) **Burns:** History of consuming hot beverages or pizza, keeping of aspirin in mucobuccal fold to reduce tooth ache, or any chemical like creosote, guiacol or phenol derivatives in toothache drops, or clove oil application, will be present. They are superficial white material of burns and are thin, delicate and more friable than of thrush.

(f) **White sponge nevus:** This has typical thickened white corrugated, folded appearance and could be present since birth. Cytological smear with absence of candida hyphae will help to differentiate from thrush.

Management:

- Removal of the cause and predisposing factors.
- Stopping or changing the antibiotic.

- In denture wearers replacing the denture or relining with addition of mycostatin suspension.
- Washing the denture at night with hypochlorite solution.
- **Topical Treatment:**
  1. **Clotrimazole:** Tablets of 10mg to be dissolved in the mouth 5 times daily.
  2. 1% gentian violet locally.
  3. **Nystatin:** One tablet, 100000 units to be dissolved in mouth 3 times a day.
- Nystatin oral pastilles 200000 units /oral pastille to be dissolved slowly in the mouth 5 times /day.
- Nystatin oral suspension 100000 units/cc, 1 tsp with 1/4 cup of water as oral rinse.
- Topical creams and ointment containing nystatin, ketoconazole, or clotrimazole.
- AmphotericinB (0.1 mg/ml) as oral rinse.
- Addition of corticosteroids and antibiotics added for faster action.
- Amphotericin B 0.08mg/kg 2-3 hourly in cream or ointment.
- Rinses:
- Mycostatin rinses for 7-10 days 3-4 times/day.
- 0.2 -1% chlorhexidine solution for rinsing.

Systemic management:

- 250 mgs of nystatin TDS for 2 weeks followed by 1 troche /day for 3rd week.
- Ketoconazole in a 200 mg tablet with food once /day. It can cause hepatotoxicity. Careful monitoring of liver function in case of long term use is important.
- Fluconazole, a triazole is given as 100mg tab once a day for 2 weeks.
- Itraconazole 100mg capsule in a dose of 200mg /day orally for 14 days.
- AmphotericinB (0.1 mg/ml) as oral rinse.

Suggested reading:

1. Anil Govindrao Ghom, Textbook of oral medicine 3rd edi. Pg no.154
2. Burket's, Oral Medicine Diagnosis and Treatment 10th edi. Pg no.94-101.

Q 3) Classify red & white lesion of the oral cavity. Describe in detail, clinical features, differential diagnosis and management of lichen planus.

MUHS SUMMER 2015 10Marks

Classification Of Red And White Lesions (Burket's):

I) Hereditary White Lesions:
- (a) Leukoedema
- (b) White Sponge Nevus

(c) Hereditary benign intraepithelial dyskeratosis.
(d) Dyskeratosis Congenita

II) Reactive/Inflammatory white lesions.

(a) Linea alba
(b) Frictional (Traumatic) Keratosis
(c) Cheek biting
(d) Chemical, Thermal and Physical Injuries of the Oral Mucosa
(e) Actinic Keratosis (Cheilitis)
(f) Smokeless Tobacco–Induced Keratosis
(g) Stomatitis nicotina
(h) Sanguinaria-induced leukoplakia

III) Infectious white lesions and red and white lesions:

(a) Oral hairy leukoplakia.
(b) Candidiasis.
(c) Mucous Patches(Syphilitic)
(d) Parulis

IV) Idiopathic or true leukoplakia

V) Bowen's disease

VI) Erythroplakia

VII) Oral Lichen Planus

VIII) Lichenoid reaction:

(a) Drug induced lichenoid reaction
(b) Graft-versus-Host Disease

IX) Lupus Erythematosus (Systemic And Discoid)

X) Developmental white lesions: Ectopic lymphoid tissue

XI) Fordyce's Granules.

XII) Gingival and palatal cysts of the new born and adults

XIII) Miscellaneous Lesions:

(a) Geographic Tongue
(b) Hairy tongue
(c) Oral Submucous Fibrosis.

Lichen Planus:

Erasmus Wilson described it in 1869. The term 'lichen planus' is derived from the algae, lichens on the rocks which it resembles and 'planus' stands for flake. It is a common dermatological disorder occurring on skin and mucous membrane and has a form of lace like pattern resembling lichens.

Clinical Features:

- Occurs in adulthood and the age range for males is 35-44 years and for females 45-54 years. It has more predilection for females.
- It may involve skin, oral and other mucous membranes.
- Other mucosal surfaces including larynx, esophagus, stomach, nasal and vulva and glans penis may get involved.
- There is usually intense pruritus. The itching associated with LP usually provokes rubbing of the lesion rather that scratching.
- They are characterised by violaceous or purple hued pruritic

papules or plaques.

- It is dry with thin adherent scales.
- On skin they occur on flexor surfaces of wrist and fore arm, inner surfaces of knees, and on thighs and trunk.
- Koebner Phenomenon: Fresh lesions may appear on scratch marks or at sites of other non-specific trauma.

Oral Lichen Planus:

- Occurs on buccal mucosa in 84% of cases and involves the tongue, lips, floor of the mouth and palate also.
- Patient may report with burning sensation of oral mucosa.
- Oral lesions are characterised by white and gray striae that are velvety thread like papules that radiate in a linear, reticular, or angular pattern forming a lacy pattern of reticular or rings and streaks over the buccal mucosa. Tiny white elevated dots are present at the intersection of these grayish white lines are called Wickham's striae.

Classification:

- Reticular
- Papular
- Annular
- Plaque
- Atrophic
- Erosive
- Bullous
- Hypertrophic

a. Reticular Type:

1. Most common form and is mostly bilateral.
2. It consists of fine whitish lines that produce lace like pattern.

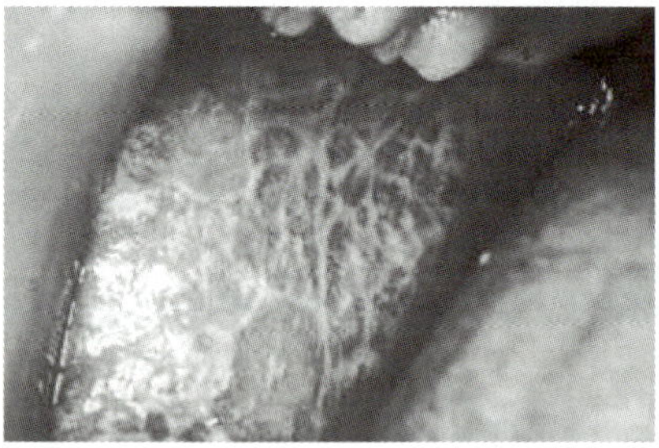

Fig. Reticular lichen planus with interlacing white striae

b. Papular:

- Whitish elevated lesions of 0.5 to 1mm in size and seen on keratinised areas of oral mucosa.
- Papules are spaced apart yet close enough to give pebbled white or gray color.

- Most often papules are seen at the periphery of reticular pattern.

c. Plaque:

- Seen on dorsum of tongue and buccal mucosa.
- Plaques are either pearly white or grayish white.
- These plaques range from slightly elevated and smooth to slightly irregular form.

d. Atrophic Type:

- Appears as smooth, red, poorly defined area, with peripheral striae evident.
- Attached gingiva is frequently involved.
- At the margins of atrophic areas whitish keratotic striae are evident radiating peripherally.
- It is always symptomatic with complaints of pain and burning.

e. Bullous Form:

- Consists of vesicles and bullae which are short lived. When ruptured leave ulcerated areas.
- Buccal mucosa is most commonly involved and posterior and lateral surface of tongue.

f. Hypertrophic Form:

It appears as elevated white lesion that has resemblance to leukoplakia and is well circumscribed.

g. Annular Type:

- Appears as round or ovoid, white outline with either pink or reddish center.
- In about 11% of cases Lichen Planus may be associated with pigmentation.

Histopathological Features:

- Hyperortho or hyper parakeratosis.
- Acanthosis with inter cellular edema of spinous cell layer in some cases.
- Civatte bodies which appear as round or ovoid. Well defined eosinophilic globule can be seen in spinous and basal cell layer and lamina propria.
- Saw tooth reteridges are typical of Lichen Planus.
- Thickening of granular cell layer.
- Band like dense inflammatory cell infiltrate containing lymphocytes and plasma cells in upper lamina propria.
- Positive for direct immunofluorescense reaction with IgA, IgM, and IgG antisera.

Malignant Potential:

- The incidence of malignant potential ranges from 0.4% to 12.3%.
- Carcinoma development is more in women than in men.

- Atrophic, erosive, and ulcerative lesions are more prone to develop into malignancy.

Differential diagnosis of lichen planus:

1. **Leukoplakia:** Men are more commonly affected. Lichen planus is more common in women. The lesions are generally unilateral, more white and leathery as compared to those of lichen planus and wickham's striae are absent.
2. **Candidiasis:** These are curdy white in appearance and more wide spread generally and the pseudomembranous lesions can be easily rubbed off in case of candidiasis.
3. **Pemphigus:** Pemphigus is a bullous lesion and lacks the white appearance of lichen planus and the wickham's striae. Nikolsky's sign is positive and histopathology examination will reveal suprabasilar split and show acantholysis.
4. **Lupus erythematosus:** These lesions are flaky and feathery in appearance.
5. **Drug induced lesion:** History of drug administration will be present.
6. **White sponge nevus:** Seen at birth and puberty where as lichen planus is seen over the age of 30 years.
7. **Geographic tongue:** The lesions are circinate with slightly raised white margins and red centre. The lesions are seen on tongue and they change location, which is not seen in lichen planus.
8. **Cheek bite:** History of trauma is usually present.The lesions are extensive and tissue tags at margins are present. Wickham's striae are absent.
9. **Lichenoid drug reaction:** A course of systemic steroids will show improvement in cases of lichen planus within 2 weeks, whereas no improvement in lichenoid drug reaction.

Management of oral lichen planus:

- The lesions of lichen planus are more often asymptomatic, but the atrophic form can result in symptoms like burning sensation or severe pain, interfering with speaking, eating, and swallowing.
- The oral lichen planus lesions that cause symptoms generally require therapy and should be treated if symptoms are significant.

I) Elimination of Risk Factors:

(a) Plaque and calculus deposits are associated with a significantly higher incidence and should be removed.

(b) Mechanical trauma of dental procedures, trauma from sharp cusps, dental restorations that are rough and sharp, ill fitting prosthetic appliances, can cause the exacerbation of the symptoms of oral lichen planus and should receive attention.

(c) Stress is one of the most frequent causes of acute exacerbations in these patients and should be dealt with.

II) Pharmacological Treatment:

A) Immunosuppressive Agents:

I) **Corticosteroids:**

The most predictable and successful drugs in the treatment of oral lichen planus are the corticosteroids.

Their use can be topical, intra-lesionally or systemically. These medications are successful in the treatment because of their anti-inflammatory and immunosuppressive properties.

(i) **Topical Corticosteroids:**

(a) To reduce the pain and inflammation of these lesions the topical corticosteroids are widely used as a treatment module. The use of triamcinolone either as a orabase or in lozenges form is used most frequently.

(b) Corticosteroids like betamethasone, clobetasol, flucinolone acetonide, fluocinonide and triamcinolone acetonide are used in adhesive paste giving very good result.

(c) 0.1% Triamcinolone acetonide a more potent steroid-2 to 3 times a day showed - improvement in patients' symptoms.

(d) A very potent anti-inflammatory agent, betamethasone valerate has shown improvement in one month.

(e) fluocinonide 0.5% in an adhesive base: fluorinated and so-called "superpotent" corticosteroid and given five to six times daily shows improvement in signs or symptoms in 2 weeks.

(f) Clobetasol propionate 0.025% in an Orabase paste three times daily showed improvement in 1 month in erosive lichen planus.

Intralesional Injections:

This mode of treatment is used in erosive lichen planus as three to four weekly or biweekly treatments with intralesional triamcinolone acetonide and topical corticosteroids. Doses of 5 to 10 mg/ml-appear to be a safe choice .

Inj. Triamcinolone 0.5 ml (Amcort), OD per week for 4 weeks.

Or

Inj. Methylprednisolone 40 mg / ml, OD per week for 4 weeks.

(ii) **Systemic:**

I) Prednisone: 10mg (Wysolone, Emsolone) TID for 2 weeks, then taper the dose of 30mg/day for the first of 3 weeks, 15mg/day for second week, then 5mg/day for 3rd and final week.

II) Dexamethasone(decadron) in elixir form in 0.5 mg/ml for 3 days to be used as a rinse with 15 ml QID and then to be swallowed.

- For 3 days, rinse with teaspoonful (5 ml) QID and

swallow.

- Another 3 days, rinsing to be done with 5 ml QID and to be swallowed every other time.
- After this rinsing with 5 ml QID and expectorate.

B) Calcineurin inhibitors:

1. **Cyclosporine:** Its an immunosuppressive drug that is very commonly used. Used as 0.025% cyclosporin in an adhesive base to apply four times daily.
2. **Tacrolimus:** 0.03% QID for 4-8 weeks.
3. **Pimecrolimus:**

C) Antifungals:

1. Amphotericin B
2. Griseofulvin
3. Nystatin
4. Azole derivatives.

Clotrimazole 1% (Candid cream) T.I.D. / day for a week.

D) Immunomodulatory Agents:

I) **Retinoids**

1. **Topical:** Fenretinide, Isotretinoin, Tazarotene, Tretinoin.
2. **Systemic:** Acitretin, Etretinate, Isotretinoin, Temarotene, Tretinoin.

   Topical retinoid vitamin A: concentration of 0.1% for the treatment of oral lichen planus, showed improvement in atrophic and erosive lesions when used four times for 2 months.

   0.1 % isotretinoin gel applied twice daily for 2 months. Reticular and plaque like lesions improved or resolved with therapy, whereas erosions diminished in size.

II) **Levamisole:**

It is used as an antihelminthic drug but also has immunoregulatory properties.

It is available as Ergamisol and Vermisol in doses of 50-150 mg tablets.

Can be given as 50mg TID for three consecutive days/week for 4-6 weeks.

E) Miscellaneous Drugs:

(i) **Antibiotics:** Tyldesley successfully treated severe and painful erosive oral lichen planus with 2% aureomycin mouthwash.

(ii) Tetracycline (doxycycline) was also found to be useful in the treatment of gingival lesion.

(iii) **Azathioprine:** The efficacy of azathioprine in the treatment of erosive and generalized oral LP has been reported.

Azathioprine (Imuran®, Azoprin®) is available as 50 mg / 100 mg tab. 1mg/kg/day for one month: Dosages can be increased up to

2mg/kg/day and should not be given for more than 3months.

(iv) Dapsone: Is used as an antibacterial agent.
It is available as 5% gel and in the form of 25mg, 50mg and 100mg tablets.

(v) **Interferon:** A topically applied gel preparation containing human fibroblast interferon (HuIFN-beta)and interferon-alpha (IFN-alpha) cream may improve erosive oral LP.

III) Non-Pharmacological Treatment:

(a) **Ultraviolet Irradiation(Puva):** In the treatment of lichen planus, 8-methoxypsoralen and long wave UV light (PUVA) therapy is being used with some success.

(b) **Photodynamic therapy:** Photosensitising compounds like methylene blue, which is activated at a specific wave length of the laser beam is used so as to destroy the targeted cells via oxidisers that are strong, and can cause cellular damage, lysis of the membranes, and inactivation of the proteins.

(c) **Surgery:** Plaques that are isolated and the erosive lesions resistant to healing can be surgically excised because it provides excellent tissue specimens for histopathological confirmation of diagnosis and may cure localized disease.

(d) **Laser Therapy:** In cases of painful erosive oral lichen planus that show unresponsiveness to the topical applications with super potent corticosteroids, management by surgery like cryosurgery and other treatment modalities like lasers have been tried.

(e) **Pulse Therapy:** 'THE BIG SHOT' – was first described by Pasricha and Ramji in 1984.

It has been defined as discontinuous and intermittent intravenous infusion of very high doses (mega doses) of drugs over short time.

Generally Dexamethasone Cyclophosphamide Pulse (DCP) combination therapy is used and there are 4 phases of treatment.

Suggested reading:

1. Burket's Oral Medicine, Diagnosis & Treatment, 10th ed. 2008, BC Decker, Inc.
2. Drore Eisen et al. The Therapy of Oral Lichen Planus. Critical Reviews in Oral Biology and Medicine, 4(2): 141-158 (1993).
3. J S Pasricha et al. Pulse therapy as a cure for auto immune disease.Ind J Dermatol, Venereol, Leprol 2003 ; 69(5): 323–28.

Q 4) Classify Red and White lesions. Describe oral submucous fibrosis in detail.

MUHS MAY 2003 (10 Marks)

Classification of Red and White Lesions (Burket's):

I) Hereditary White Lesions:

(a) Leukoedema
(b) White Sponge Nevus
(c) Hereditary benign intraepithelial dyskeratosis.

(d) Dyskeratosis Congenita

II) Reactive/Inflammatory white lesions.

(a) Linea alba
(b) Frictional (Traumatic) Keratosis
(c) Cheek biting
(d) Chemical, Thermal and Physical Injuries of the Oral Mucosa
(e) Actinic Keratosis (Cheilitis)
(f) Smokeless Tobacco–Induced Keratosis
(g) Stomatitis nicotina
(h) Sanguinaria -induced leukoplakia

III) Infectious white lesions and red and white lesions:

(a) Oral hairy leukoplakia.
(b) Candidiasis.
(c) Mucous Patches(Syphilitic)
(d) Parulis

IV) Idiopathic or true leukoplakia

V) Bowen's disease

VI) Erythroplakia

VII) Oral Lichen Planus

VIII) Lichenoid reaction:

(a) Drug induced lichenoid reaction
(b) Graft-versus-Host Disease

IX) Lupus Erythematosus (Systemic and Discoid)

X) Developmental white lesions: Ectopic lymphoid tissue

XI) Fordyce's Granules.

XII) Gingival and palatal cysts of the new born and adults

XIII) Miscellaneous Lesions:

(a) Geographic Tongue.
(b) Hairy tongue
(c) Oral Submucous Fibrosis.

Definition (OSMF):

Oral submucous fibrosis is a complex, chronic, and potent precancerous condition which is characterised by juxta-epithelial inflammatory reaction and progressive fibrosis of the submucosal tissues that is the lamina propria and the deeper connective tissues.

Classification of Osmf: Khanna and Andrade in 1995:

- **Group I:** Its the earliest stage and there are no limitations of mouth opening and the interincisal distance is greater than 35 mm.
- **Group II:** The interincisal distance is 26-35 mm.
- **Group III:** These are moderately advanced cases and the interincisal distance is 15-26mm. There are visible fibrotic bands in the soft palate, pterygomandibular raphe and the anterior faucial pillars.
- **Group IV A:** The trismus is severe and the interincisal distance is less than 15 mm and there is presence of extensive fibrosis involving the entire oral mucosa.

- **Group IV B:** The disease is in advanced stage and there are premalignant and malignant changes all over the oral mucosa.

Staging:

Stage 1-Early Osmf:

- Mild blanching
- No restriction in mouth opening, tongue protrusion
- Burning sensation

Stage 2-Moderate Osmf:

- Moderate blanching.
- There is reduced mouth opening by 33%, tongue protrusion reduced.
- Burning sensation even in absense of stimuli.
- Presence of palpable bands.
- Lymphadenopathy.

Stage 3-Severe Osmf:

- Burning sensation very severe
- More than 60% reduction in mouth opening
- Ulcers over buccal mucosa
- Thick palpable band
- Bilateral lymphadenopathy

Etiology:

1. **Chillies:** capsaicin is the active ingredient of chillies. It is vanillyamide of 8-methyl-6-nonenic acid, which is the active irritant of the chillies.
2. **Tobacco:** Its the most common irritant known and the causative factor in malignancy of the oral cavity.
3. **Lime:** lime is used with betel nut for chewing it acts as local irritant.
4. **Betelnut:** The presence of areca alkaloids, predominantly arecoline.
5. **Nutritional Deficiency:** the subclinical vit.B complex deficiency suspected in such cases.
6. **Defective Iron Metabolism:** microcytic hypochromic anemia with high serum iron have been reported in submucous fibrosis.
7. **Bacterial Infection:** streptococcal toxicity and klebsiella rhinoscleromatis may be a factor in cause of submucous fibrosis.
8. **Collagen Disorders:** it is thought to be localized collagen disease of oral cavity.
9. **Immunological Disorders:** raised ESR and globulin levels are indicative of immunodeficiency disorder.
10. **Altered Salivary Composition:** increased pH, increase in salivary amylase, low level of calcium increases in phosphatase and potassium and normal level of salivary immunoglobulin.
11. **Genetic Susceptibility:** The occurrence of OSMF in a familial pattern has also been reported.

Pathogenesis:

1. Tannins, flavanoids and catechin from areca nut reduces the susceptibility of collagen to degradation by collagenase that leads to fibrosis.
2. Tobacco along with nicotine and other carcinogens, causes mechanical trauma.
3. Lime that is mixed with tobacco causes chemical burns to the mucosa.
4. Alcohol and other spirits cause hypersensitivity and the three factors cause altered immunity and along with genetic susceptibility causes fibroblastic proliferation leading to OSMF.

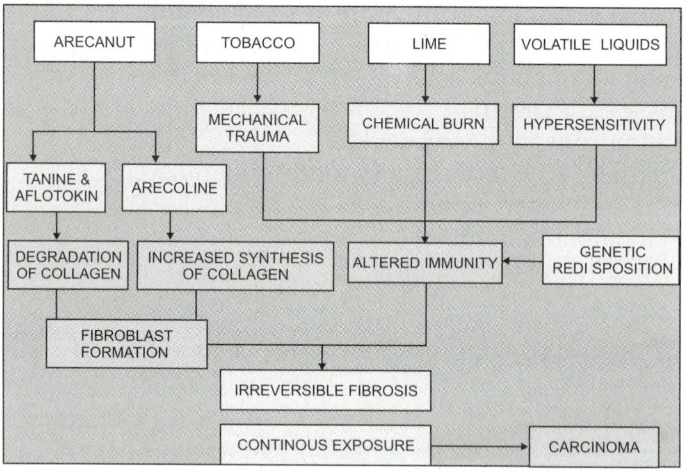

Fig. Flow chart of pathogenesis of OSMF

Clinical Features:

1. **Age and Sex Distribution:** Patients in the age group of 20-40 years are commonly affected.
2. **Site Distribution:** The most frequent location is buccal mucosa and retromolar areas, soft palate, uvula, tongue and labial mucosa. sometimes involves floor of mouth and gingiva.
3. **Prodromal Symptoms:** There is a sensation of burning in the oral mucosa, aggravated by spicy food, followed by either hypersalivation or dryness of mouth.
   Vesiculation, ulceration, pigmentation, and gustatory sensation.
4. **Late Symptoms:** Trismus, difficulty in tongue protrusion, difficulty in swallowing, reffered pain.
5. **Blanching of the oral mucosa:** The impairment of the vascularity of the local area is responsible for the blanching and the blanched mucosa becomes slightly opaque and white.
6. **Betel Chewer Mucosa:** It is brownish red discoloration of mucosa with irregular surface that tend to desquamate.
7. **Fibrous Band:** As disease progresses the mucosa becomes stiff

and vertical bands appear. These bands can be palpated easily and feel rough on palpation.

8. **Lip Features:** Mucosa is blanched, becomes rubbery, and is characterized by presence of circular bands around the rima oris like a thin band.
9. **Buccal Mucosa:** It becomes coarse, blanched and inelastic in advanced cases, the mucosa becomes tough and leathery with numerous vertical fibrous bands.
10. **Soft Palate and Uvula:** It is marked by fibrotic changes and clear delineation of the soft palate from hard palate. Uvula is shrunken and in extreme cases it becomes bud like or hockey stick appearance.
11. **Palatal Fauces:** The pillars of the fauces become short and thick and tonsils may get pressed in between fibrosed pillars.
12. **Tongue:** Depapillation in the lateral margin. It becomes smooth. Patient can not protrude beyond the incisal edges.
13. **Floor Of Mouth:** It becomes inelastic.
14. **Gingiva:** It becomes fibrotic, blanched, and inelastic.
15. **Associated Features:** Pigmentation, vesicles, ulceration, petechiae. Screening by biopsy is essential before starting the treatment.

Histopathology:

Shows severely atrophic epithelium with loss of reteridges and inflammatory cell infiltration.

Epithelial atypia of varying degrees is present.

Connective tissue shows severe hyalinisation and homogenisation of collagen with inflammatory cell infiltration.

Treatment:

- Giving up habits of chewing as betel nut and tobacco.
- Reducing consumption of spicy foods, including chillies.
- Maintaining proper oral hygiene.
- Consumption of diet that are rich in vitamins, A, B complex and C and iron.
- Giving up drinking fluids which are taken hot like tea and coffee.
- Alcohol abstention.
- Cuspal grinding of sharp teeth and extraction of third molars.

Medical Treatment:

- The prescription of chewable tablets of hydrocortisone (Efcorlin); one tablet that has to be chewed at intervals of 3-4 hours for 3-4 weeks.
- Hyaluronidase injection given intralesionally as 0, 5ml, 1500 IU mixed with 1 ml of lignocaine to be injected into each buccal mucosa/week for 3 weeks or more depending on the severity of the condition.
- Hyaluronidase as intralesional injections, 0.5 ml, 1500 IU and 0.5 ml of hydrocortisone acetate 25mg/ml, to be injected in each

buccal mucosa once a week alternatively for 4 weeks or more according to the condition.

- Hydrocortisone 100mg once or twice daily as submucosal injections can be given according to the severity of the disease for a period of 2-3 weeks.
- Placentrax 2-3 ml can be given as submucosal injections /sitting twice or thrice in a week for 3-4 weeks.
- A methylxanthine derivative, Pentoxyphyllin has vasodilating properties which helps to increase the vascularity of the oral mucosa and is recommended as an adjunct therapy in the management of OSMF.
- Interferon-gamma, which is an antifibrotic cytokine, alters the synthesis of collagen and helps in reducing the symptoms of OSMF.
- 0.5mg tablet of colchicine to be given twice/day.
- 16 mg of lycopene /day has shown improvement in the condition of OSMF.
- Lately it has been proven by scientists that the intra-lesional injections of autologous bone marrow stem cells is supposed to be a safe and effective treatment in cases of OSMF.Angiogenesis is induced by the injections of autologous bone marrow stem cells injections in the region where the lesion is present and helps reduce the extent of fibrosis and helps in increasing mouth opening to a significant extent.

Surgical treatment:

- When the interincisal distance becomes less than 20 mm in cases of progressive fibrosis, treatment with surgery is recommended.
- Multiple incisions deep into the mucosa, submucosa and the fibrotic tissue are given to release the bands and then this gap is filled with mucosal graft obtained from tongue and this gap is sutured.
- Z -plasty: Z-shaped incisions that are multiple and deep are made in the fibrotic tissue and suturing is done in a straight pattern.

Physiotherapy:

Physical therapy using muscle-stretching exercises for the mouth may be helpful in preventing further limitation of mouth movements. This is often combined with medical and surgical therapy.

Active and passive stretching:

- The patient is instructed to actively open the mouth as wide as possible. The opening position should be held for 5 seconds followed by relaxation in the rest position for 5 seconds.
- In passive stretch patient is instructed to actively open the mouth. Then finger pressure is applied by therapist to the maxillary and mandibular dentitions with use of thumb and index finger.
- Stretching exercises is performed by using ice cream sticks for about 5-10 minutes with 3-4 repetitions 4 times in a day. Stretching

exercises is performed at home using ice cream sticks for 5-10 minutes and 3-4 repetitions 4 times in a day.

Suggested reading:

1. Aziz, SR (1997). "Oral submucous fibrosis: an unusual disease". Journal of the New Jersey Dental Association 68 (2): 17–9.
2. Cox, S. C.; Walker, D. M. (1996). "Oral submucous fibrosis. A review". Australian Dental Journal41 (5): 294–9.
3. Ravikiran Ongle text book of oral medicine chapter no 6, pg no 169.

Q 5) Describe the differential diagnosis of oral precancerous lesions and conditions:

TNMGRU, APRIL 2004, (15 Marks)

Definitions:

The world health organistion (WHO) defined the potentially malignant disorders as, the risk of malignancy being present in a lesion or condition either during the time of initial diagnosis or at a future date.

They are classified as:

Precancerous lesions: It is defined as a morphologically altered tissue in which cancer is most likely to occur than its normal counterparts.

Precancerous conditions: They are defined as generalised state or condition that is associated with significantly increased risk for cancer development.

According to Hamed Mortazavi et.al following are the precancerous lesions and conditions.

Precancerous lesions	Precancerous conditions
Leukoplakia	Oral lichen planus
Erythroplakia	Discoid Lupus erythematosus
Proliferative verrucous leukoplakia (PVL)	Epidermolysis bullosa
Viadent leukoplakia	Verruciform xanthoma
Candida leukoplakia	Graft- versus- host- disease
Reverse smokers' palate	Cheilitis glandularis
Verrucous hyperplasia	Xeroderma pigmentosum
Oral verrucous carcinoma	Syphilis (third stage)
Actinic keratosis, cheilitis	Plummer-Vinson syndrome
Dyskeratosis congenita	Malnutrition
Keratoacanthoma	Vitamin A, B, C deficiency
Oral submucous fibrosis –Latest hypothesis is, it being considered as a premalignant lesion.	Immunosuppressive diseases

A) Precancerous lesions:

Leukoplakia:

- Its a white patch or plaque that cannot be scraped or rubbed off and cannot be clinically or histologically diagnosed as any other lesion. (by WHO 1980)
- More commonly seen in males at 35-45 years of age and can appear on any site of the oral cavity but mostly seen on buccal mucosa, alveolar mucosa, floor of mouth, lateral border of tongue, lips, palate etc. It occurs coincident with the area in which irritants are kept.
- Clinically seen as elevated grayish white plaque with leathery appearance, irregular surface or wrinkled surface usually nonscrapable.
- More common in males of 35-50 years.
- The typical cracked mud like or speckled or sometimes verrucous appearance with the history of tobacco abuse or the presence of sharp teeth and broken restorations causing irritation can help in differentiating from other premalignant disorders.
- Histopathologically it shows typical drop shaped reteridges which is peculiar for leukoplakia.

Proliferative verrucous leukoplakia:

- Its an aggressive and distinct form of leukoplakia and Hansen etal in 1985 first described it.
- The male-female ratio is 1: 4 without the usage of tobacco.
- It can be differentiated clinically from other lesions because the PVL appears on the oral mucosa as white plaque or patch that is multifocal and has rough surface projections and exophytic growth. The lesions of PVL spread gradually to involve the other areas of the oral mucosal region. The gingiva is most commonly involved but there could be involvement of other sites also.

Sanguinaria associated keratosis(Viadent leukoplakia):

- This type of leukoplakia appears as a white patch or plaque and is commonly associated with the use of mouth rinse containing sanguinaria or tooth paste.
- Most commonly seen in the maxillary mucosa of the alveolus in the persons using the mouth wash containing sanguinaria.
- Studies show that the extracts of sanguinaria have a carcinogenic effect. Hence the viadent leukoplakia can be considered as a premalignant lesion. The history of use of such a mouth wash or tooth paste with typical clinical appearance especially involving the maxillary area can help in differentiating.

Candida leukoplakia(CL)(chronic hyperplastic candidiasis):

Its a chronic form of candidiasis and the typical characteristics are the presence of firm, white, leathery plaques on the cheeks, lips, palate and the tongue.The rate of epithelial dysplasia is about 4-5 times more in CL than in leukoplakia.

Presence of candida hyphae and the firm leathery plaques will help in diagnosis and differentiation.

Erythroplakia:

- A fiery red patch which cannot be clinically or histopathologically diagnosed as any other condition.
- Occurs on all mucosal surface of head and neck region but in men mostly floor of mouth is involved and in women mostly mandibular alveolar mucosa, sulcus and mandibular gingiva is involved.
- It is asymptomatic. Clinically, non elevated macule that is red or a patch on the epithelial surface which is soft, velvety, straight or scalloped, well demarcated margins. Homogenous & smooth erythroplakia has smooth velvety surface while granular or speckled erythroplakia has granular rough surface.
- Clinical diagnosis is made on the basis of red demarcated patch with no signs of inflammation and infection and biopsy shows atrophic epithelium and dysplastic features.

Snuff dippers lesion: (Tobacco pouch keratosis):

- This lesion has a typical appearance of a white plaque in the buccal or the labial vestibule where the patient is used to keeping the tobacco quid. Its thin grayish white or gray lesions whose margins blend with surrounding mucosa.
- There is loss of periodontal and gingival tissue, which is painless in that region and teeth shows extrinsic staining.
- The degree to which there is alteration of the mucosa depends on the quantity, frequency, type of tobacco, and host susceptibility.

Keratosis of the palate associated with reverse smoking:

- It refers to specific white lesions which appears in heavy pipe or cigarette and bidi smokers on the hard and soft palate.
- In early cases mucosa is reddened and subsequently becomes grayish white, thickened, fissured, irregular and having dried mud appearance with erythematous spots of orifice of salivary glands.
- It can be differentiated from other lesions by the history of cigar or pipe smoking with generalized lesion on palate and biopsy shows acanthosis and hyperkeratosis of epithelium.

Verrucous hyperplasia (VH):

- It was described first as a thick, extensive, white plaque by Shear and Pindborg in the year 1980.
- Verrucous carcinoma and VH are histopathologically different, in that the VH has thickened epithelium which is superficial to the underlying normal epithelium, while the verrucous carcinoma has a hyperplastic epithelium characterised by invaded pushing border

into the underlying connective tissue, but with an intact basement membrane.

Oral verrucous carcinoma (Ackerman's tumour):

- They appear as white lesions which are papillary in nature with pebbly surface which is sometimes covered with white leukoplakic film. They have rugae like folds with deep clefts.
- Biopsy shows marked epithelium proliferation, parakeratin plugging and pushing margins.

Dyskeratosis congenita (DC):

- Its an inherited disease that is rare and is characterised by a triad of nail dystrophy, skin pigmentation that is reticular and oral leukoplakia. And mostly seen in males during first 10 years of life.
- Nail changes are the first manifestation. Nails become dystrophic and show shedding. Later shows grayish pigmentation on trunk, neck, thigh. Skin becomes atrophic, telangiectatic.
- Intraorally the most common sites are the tongue and the buccal mucosa which shows diffusely distributed vesicles and ulcerations, followed by accumulation of white patches of necrotic epithelium. Recurrent ulcerations and erosive leukoplakia also seen.
- The typical triad of signs will help in differentiating from other precancerous disorders.

Actinic cheilitis (AC):

Its a premalignant condition and most commonly involves the lower lip.Diffuse poorly defined areas of atrophic, ulcerative, erosive or keratotic plaques are the typical features of this condition. Scaly patches, dryness, swelling, fissures that are transverse, crusting and blotching are the other features. Typical lesions especially involving lips can help in differentiating from other oral premalignant disorders.

Keratoacanthoma:

- This lesion appears as a firm, sessile, painless nodule, with a central plug of keratin. It commonly occurs on sun exposed hair-bearing skin.
- Some cases have been reported on lips and some have arisen from intraoral mucosa and hence can be considered in differential diagnosis of oral premalignant disorders.
- Elevated lesion with central keratin plug on sun exposed area will help to differentiate it from other lesions.
- Biopsy will show thickened layer of parakeratin or orthokeratin with central plugging.

Actinic keratosis:

- Cutaneous premalignant lesion caused due to ultraviolet radiation.
- More commonly seen on face, neck, dorsum of hand, scalp, forearm.

- Appears as whitish grey irregular plaques usually less than 7 mm in diameter, rough surface feel like sandpaper.

Precancerous conditions:

Oral submucous fibrosis:

- Earlier the oral submucous fibrosis was considered as premalignant condition but now a days it is considered as premalignant lesion.
- Its a chronic, insidous disease that can affect any part of the oral mucosa and some times the pharynx. Most frequent location of oral submucous fibrosis is the buccal mucosa and retromolar areas. It also commonly involves soft palate, palatal fauces, uvula, tongue and labial mucosa.
- In the early stages:
    - Blanching and mottled, marble-like appearance.
    - Burning sensation.
    - Hyper or hyposalivation.
    - Vesicles, erythematous mucosa, ulcers on the mucosa, mucosal pigmentation that is blotchy and melanotic, and petechiae of the mucosa
    - Defective taste sensation.
- Late symptoms:
    - There is difficulty in opening the mouth.
    - the sunken cheeks are present out of proportion to age.
    - Depapillation and rigidity of the tongue.
    - There is blanching of the floor of the mouth and the gingival tissues are fibrotic.
    - The soft palate becomes stiff and there is reduced mobility and the uvula is shrunken, bud like with hockey stick appearance, and blanched and atrophic tonsils.
- A clinical diagnosis of OSF is quite easily made because of the typical signs and symptoms described above and can be differentiated from other oral premalignant disorders clinically on that basis. The leathery bands and marble like appearance with limited mouth opening makes diagnosis very obvious.
- Biopsy further helps in differentiation as it shows typical atrophic epithelium and hyalanisation of the collagen bundles in the connective tissue which is pathognomonic of this condition. It also exhibits dilated and congested blood vessels with infiltration of inflammatory cells.

Oral lichen planus:

- It is a common chronic immunological and inflammatory disorder that has an appearance that varies from keratotic to erythematous and ulcerative.
- Buccal mucosa is most commonly involved, but can be seen on tongue, gingiva, palate, lips, floor of mouth and appears as radiating white and gray velvety thread like papules in a linear, angular or

reticular pattern which forms a typical lacy reticular pattern.

- The buccal mucosa is bilaterally involved which helps in differentiating from other oral premalignant disorders.
- Wickham's striae are the tiny white elevated dots present at the intersection of white lines. Patient may report with the burning sensation of oral mucosa.
- Clinical diagnosis is made on the basis of white nonscrapable lesion with lacy pattern and presence of wickham's striae. Koebner phenomenon also helps in diagnosing.

Histopathologic features shows typical saw toothed appearance of rete ridges, liquefaction degeneration of basal layer, eosinophilic band just beneath the basement membrane. Presence of civatte bodies is unique to this condition.

Discoid lupus erythematosus (DLE):

- This condition is chronic and is a typical scarring immunologic disease, muco-cutaneous disorder that has characteristic white plaques that are keratinised and have elevated borders and white striae that are radiating and telangiectasia.
- Most common intraoral sites are buccal mucosa, palate, lip.
- Patient may complain of burning sensation, xerostomia, soreness of mouth.
- It begins as erythematous area, sometimes slightly elevated, but more often depressed, with white spot and Fine white striae radiate out from the margins.
- Central healing may result in depression.
- Clinical diagnosis is made on the basis of skin lesion with lesions present on oral mucosa which is atrophic and erythematous.

Epidermolysis bullosa (EB):

- Its a bullous lesion of the skin and the mucosa.
- There are three varieties of this condition.EB simplex, junctional and dystrophic. Involvement of the oral cavity is reported in the junctional and the dystrophic form of the disease and is characterised by formation of vesicles and bulla which form after mild trauma. Dental defects like, congenitally missing, hypoplastic teeth may be seen.

Verruciform Xanthoma:

- Verruciform xanthoma (VX) is a rare benign lesion first described by Shafer in 1971.
- It mainly occurs in the oral mucosa. The gingiva is the most commonly affected site, followed by tongue, buccal mucosa, vestibular mucosa, floor of the mouth, soft palate and lower lip.
- The lesions appear as a well-defined, asymptomatic, slightly elevated mass with a yellow-white or red color and a papillary or verruciform surface.

Graft-versus host disease:

- Its a common complication in patients treated with allogenic peripheral stem cell transplantation.
- Oral involvement has been observed in 80% of patients, characterized by atrophy, erythema, erosion, ulcers, lichenoid lesions, xerostomia, and oral pain.
- It can be differentiated with other lesions as clinically there is lichenoid lesions with the history of transplantation.

Cheilitis Glandularis:

- Cheilitis glandularis (CG) is characterized by hyperplasia of minor salivary glands, first described by von Volkman in 1870.
- Frequently the lower lip is involved but lesions on the upper lip have also been reported.
- It can be differentiated from any other condition because there is presence of chronic inflammation of suppurative type of the lower lip and typical swelling of the mucous glands which is associated with the purulent discharge from the dilated openings of the ducts.

Xeroderma Pigmentosum:

- It is an autosomal recessive rare disease, which is associated with cutaneous malignant transformation.
- Occurs in early age and shows Increased frequency to sun burn.
- Patient shows freckled pigmentation and patchy depigmentation.
- Oral involvement is usually observed in patients under 20.
- Squamous cell carcinoma of the lower lip and tongue has been reported in patients with XP.

Syphilis (Third Stage) Iron deficiency anemia, Malnutrition, Vitamin A, B, and C Deficiency and Immunosuppressive Diseases (HIV). Although the above conditions have been mentioned with malignant potential, data regarding their malignant transformation is controversial. However, they should be considered as predisposing factors of oral malignancy.

Suggested reading:

1. Burket's, Text book of Oral Medicine, Diagnosis and Treatment, 10th edition, chapter 5. Pg no 85-125.
2. Eversole LR, Leider AS, Alexander G. Intraoral and labial keratoacanthoma. Oral Surg Oral Med Oral Pathol. 1982 Dec; 54(6): 663-7.
3. Hamed Mortazavi et.al, Oral Potentially Malignant Disorders: An Overview of More than 20 Entities from the journal of Dental Research, Dental Clinics, Dental Prospects. Vol. 8, No. 1 Winter 2014.

Q 6) Essay on oral candidiasis:

TNMGRU AUGUST 2006 (20 Marks)

'Candidiasis' is a disease caused by infection with a fungus that is yeast like, candida albicans and is probably the most common manifestation of human candidial infection.

Classification

(i) Primary oral candidiasis

- **Acute form**
- Pseudomembranous.
- Erythematous.
- **Chronic form**
- Hyperplastic
- Erythematous
- Pseudomembranous
- **Candida associated lesion**
- Denture Sore Mouth
- Angular cheilitis
- Median rhomboid glossitis
- **Keratinized primary lesion super infected with candida**
- Leukoplakia
- Lichen planus
- Lupus erythematosus

(ii) Secondary candidiasis

Systemic mucocutaneous candidiasis and its oral manifestation.

Predisposing factors for oral candidiasis:

- Excessive use of antibiotics, antibacterial mouth rinses, dry mouth due to various drugs like anticholinergics, and diseases of salivary glands can change the oral microbial flora and fauna.
  Defense against candida is dependent on the quantity as well as the quality of the saliva. Any changes in saliva like decreased flow of saliva or a change in its constituents is called as salivary hypofunction or hyposalivation and could be an important predisposing factor for development of candidiasis.Xerostomia is most often quoted as the causative reason for this lesion.
- Chronic irritation like broken dentures, other restorations, orthodontic appliances, heavy smoking.
- Diseases like leukemia, tuberculosis, diabetes, lymphomas, and tuberculosis can compromise the immune system and lead to oral candidiasis.
- Excessive use of corticosteroids, cytotoxic drugs and radiotherapy for head and neck area can precipitate candidiasis.
- Old age, pregnancy, infancy, hospitalisations, oral epithelial dysplasias can cause this condition.
- Hyperparathyroidism, Addison's disease, hypothyroidism.
- Immunodeficiency states like hypogammaglobulinemia, AIDS.
- Diet: Malnutrition whether by poor diet or due to malabsorption, especially of iron, folic acid and vitamin B12, can lead to oral candidiasis. According to some studies vitaminA or pyridoxine can also be the cause.

Causative organisms:

This lesion is caused by yeast like fungus, candida albicans and the other species which can cause candidiasis are candida stellatoidea, candida tropicalis, candida pseudotropicalis, candida famata, candida rugosa, Candida geotrichium, Candida guilliermondii, Candida dubliniensis,

It is present in two forms i.e. yeast form and hyphal form.

I) Primary oral candidiasis:

1. **Thrush or pseudomembranous candidiasis:**

   It is the superficial infection of upper layer of oral mucous membrane, which leads to the formation of white plaques which can be patchy or flecks on the surface of the mucosa.

   Pathogenesis:

   There is excessive proliferation of the candidal hyphae leading to desquamation of the oral epithelial cells. There is also accumulation of bacteria, keratin and necrotic tissue entangled in the hyphae. This debris helps to form the pseudomembrane that adheres firmly to the oral mucosal surface.

   Clinical features:

   - In infants starts on the 6th to 10th day of birth due to infection contracted from the mother.
   - The lesions appear as soft curdy bluish white, and can be easily scraped off.
   - In adults any part of the oral mucosa such as floor of mouth retro molar area, muccobuccal fold, palate, tongue can be involved. Extensive areas can be involved.
   - More common in women as compared to men.
   - Prodrome of bad taste may occur.
   - Patient may complain of burning sensation and difficulty in eating spicy foods.
   - The lesions appear bluish white and curd like in nature and areas of erythema may surround the lesion.
   - The lesions can be scraped off and will leave erythematous erosive areas.
   - Deeper invasion of the hyphae can occur and may be difficult to scrape off the lesions.

   Diagnosis:

   Clinical diagnosis can be done by the presence of Pseudomembranous lesions that can be easily scraped off.

   Differential diagnosis:

   - Plaque type of lichen planus
   - Leukoplakia
   - Gangrenous stomatitis
   - Chemical burns

2. **Acute atrophic candidiasis:**

   Also called as 'antibiotics sore mouth'.On scraping the white patch, raw erosive areas are left and the atrophic or erosive red component is more prominent in this type.

Clinical features:

- Commonly involves the tongue and tissue underlying the prosthesis.The tongue appears atrophic and red.
- lesion appears red or erythematous rather than white.
- Vague pain or burning sensation exists.
- A few white thickened foci that rub off leaving a painful surface lesion closely resembling erosive lichen planus and erythroplakia.

Diagnosis:

History of excessive use of antibiotics along with erythematous areas and especially red atrophic tongue can help in diagnosis.

Differential diagnosis:

- Chemical burn
- Drug reaction
- Syphilitic mucus patches
- Necrotic ulcer
- Traumatic ulcer

3. **Chronic hyperplastic candidiasis:**

It is also called as 'candidial leukoplakia' because of firm adherent white patches occurring in oral mucosa.

Clinical features:

- Occurs most commonly in men of middle age or above, who are heavy smokers.
- Can occur on lips, cheeks and tongue.
- firm and white leathery plaques are present.
- lesions may persist without any symptoms for years.
- Does not rub off by lateral pressure. Lesions range from slightly white to dense white with cracks and fissures, occasionally present.

Diagnosis:

A firm white leathery appearance seen which cannot be rubbed off.

Differential diagnosis:

- Leukoplakia
- Hairy leukoplakia

4. **Candida associated lesion:**

(a) Denture stomatitis:

Also called as Denture Sore Mouth.

Clinical features:

- As the name suggests, usually found under complete denture or partial denture and found mostly in women and most commonly occurring under upper complete denture and hence palatal involvement.
- Patchy distribution often associated with specked curd like white lesion.
- Maxillary denture bearing area can be extensively involved and may appear atrophic or show white lesions distributed all over.
- Typical feature is palatal papillary hyperplasia giving it raspberry

look.

- Petechiae can be seen distributed over the denture bearing area.
- The atrophy and redness caused by the lesion can be very sharply demarcated restricted to the tissue in contact with the denture.
- Soreness and dryness are common complaints.

(b) Median rhomboid glossitis (MRG):

- It is also known as central papillary atrophy and is a condition in which there is a typical area of loss of papillae of the tongue and redness, and the location is the dorsum of the tongue in the midline just in front of the circumvallate papillae.
- It occurs due to failure of the tuberculum impar to retract before the fusion of the two lateral halves of the tongue and can said to be developmental condition.
- How ever the reason quoted is also that it is caused by a fungal infection.It is thought to be a type of oral candidiasis.
- More common in males.
- Location is anterior to the foramen caecum on the dorsal surface of the tongue anterior to circumvallate papillae.
- It is rhomboid or diamond shaped and appears reddish and may be flat or raised. Texture may vary from granular, lobulated or indurated.
- Usually asymptomatic but burning and pain have been reported.

Diagnosis:

The typical diamond shape of the lesion and site, anterior to foramen ceacum helps in diagnosis.

Biopsy will show loss of papillae and varying degrees of hyperparakeratosis.

(c) Angular cheilitis:

Its a condition that is inflammatory and can affect one or both the corners of the mouth. There is typical presence of erythema, scaling, painful cracks or fissures, bleeding and ulceration at the angles of the mouth.

Etiology:

(i) Candida albicans mainly but also there can be role of staphylococci and streptococci.
(ii) over closure of jaws as in edentulous patients or patients with artificial dentures, with reduced vertical dimensions.
(iii) General protein deficiency can also cause this condition.
(iv) Atopic dermatitis involving the face is frequently associated with angular cheilitis.
(v) Hypersalivation, Down's syndrome, large tongue where in constant dribbling of saliva could be a causative factor.

Clinical Features:

(i) Can occur in children as well as in adults.

(ii) There is feeling of dryness and burning sensation at the corner of the mouth.
(iii) There is triangular area of erythema and edema at one or commonly both the corners of the mouth.
(iv) Wrinkling, fissuring and ulceration with mild bloody crust in some cases may be seen.
(v) From the corners of the mouth can be seen linear fissures or furrows that radiate which are seen in severe cases especially in denture wearers.
(vi) Spontaneous remissions may occur.

Diagnosis:

Erythematous, furrowed, wrinkled, maserated appearing lesions at the corner of the mouth are highly suggestive of angular cheilitis.
There is need to take a complete history which includes the status of dentition, oral hygiene practices and the occupation of the patient.
The patient has to be asked about the presence of any medical illness like anemia and other disorders that can lead to immunodeficiency, habits of smoking, chewing tobacco, alcohol consumption, certain skin diseases like lichen planus and psoriasis, allergic conditions and the use of medications. The swabbing of the corners of the mouth and microbiological examination can also be done.

II) Secondary candidiasis:

Systemic/ chronic muco-cutaneous candidiasis:

This disorder is rare and shows persistent or recurrent candidal infections of the skin, nails and the mucous membranes and there can be a combination of occurrence of failure of the endocrines and immunodeficiency.

The typical characteristic oral manifestations are that they are of long duration and the lesions are hyperplastic, whitish and nodular and present with deep fissures and seen in most of the patients. The area affected commonly is the tongue. There was no difference in the histologic findings between chronic mucocutaneous candidiasis and other forms of candidal infection.

Diagnosis of oral candidiasis:

The typical clinical appearance can easily help in the diagnosis but some times can be a challenge. As the lesions of candidiasis are white, red or a combination of both, several lesions can be considered in differential diagnosis.

Oral swabs, oral rinses and oral smears are the special investigations that can help in detecting the presence of candida.

The lesions can be gently scraped with a tongue blade or spatula and the debris can be applied to the glass slide directly. When cultures are necessary, oral swabs can be taken. According to some, it is better to take the swabs from 3 different oral regions.

In case of using the oral rinse for detection, the mouth is rinsed with phosphate buffered saline for one minute and then the patient is asked to spit in a vessel and then sent for laboratory analysis.

Biopsy is considered important in case of candidal leukoplakia.

Periodic acid-Schiff stain is used for biopsies and smears which stain the carbohydrates in the cell walls of the fungus into magenta. As the candida also stains vividly gram+ve, Gram's staining is also used.

Sometimes to rule out some underlying medical conditions blood tests for full blood counts, and complete hemogram may be done.

Treatment of oral candididiasis:

Oral candidiasis can be treated either topically or systemically.

It is generally treated with anti-fungals like nystatin, miconazole, amphotericin B and gentian violet, as topical application.

Very important aspect of treatment is the removal of cause.

Removal of cause:

In patients who are immunocompromised and suffer from HIV/AIDS or due to chemotherapy will need systemic treatment with antifungals given orally or intra-venously.

If the antibiotics or corticosteroid use has lead to this condition, then their usage should be stopped although many a times this is not a desirable option depending on the reason the drug was prescribed. Underlying immunosuppression may be medically managed after it is identified and it can help in preventing the recurrence of these infections.

The candida hyphae in the oral cavity can be controlled by improvement in the oral hygiene methods like regular brushing of teeth, and the use of anti-microbial mouth washes.

Cessation of smoking can be beneficial as it can lead to many forms of oral candidiasis.

In case the infection is due to the use of inhaled steroids then rinsing the mouth with water after the use of steroids may be beneficial.

Replacement of broken dentures and restorations are essential.

Maintenance of good denture hygiene is important and it can be achieved by regular cleansing of the same and taking out the dentures at night before sleeping. This helps the mucosa to recover from the infection. In cases of oral candidiasis the dentures can act as a constant source of these candida species and may continually keep infecting the mucosa after the antifungals are stopped.Disinfection of the dentures is hence important for the treatment of this lesion.Commercial denture cleaners are available but the dentures can be readily kept clean with the help of soaking them overnight in a 1: 10 sodium hypochlorite solution. If the denture has metal parts it can be soaked in chlorhexidine solution.

Before the dentures are replaced in the mouth, they can be coated with antifungal medication.In case of presence of angular cheilitis, inadequate occlusal vertical dimension may need to be corrected to cure the lesion.

Topical treatment:

They are preferred because they limit systemic absorption, but effectiveness totally depends on patient compliance, following are most commonly used topical treatment.

- Nystatin in the dosages of 100000IU/ml, at 5ml QID and Amphotericin B at 50mg as 5ml TDS has been the choice for local treatment for years.
- The suspension of fluconazole is given at a dosage of 10mg/ml aqueous suspension and given as 5ml/day for 7-14 days.
- Miconazole in dosages of 200-500mg/day 4 times daily as a gel form applied directly over the lesion can give good results.
- 50mg of miconazole mucoadhesive buccal tablet 1/day is a new form that is developed.
- Clotrimazole: 1 oral troche (10mg tablet) when dissolved in mouth 5 times daily, the drug has got antibacterial and antifungal properties.
- Gentian violet as 1% can be used but may lead to superficial mucosal necrosis.
- Nystatin preparation: it includes a suspension and oral pastille, vaginal tablets. Nystatin oral pastille (available as 200,000 units oral pastille, 1 or 2 pastille dissolved slowly in mouth 5 times/day)
- Amphotericin B: 5 to 10 ml oral solution can be used as a rinse and then expectorated, 3-4 times/day.
- Elixir containing both tetra cycline and amphotericin B may also provide beneficial effect in acute atrophic candidiasis.
- Mycostatin cream: 1 lac. unit or lactose containing vaginal tablet can be kept under the tongue.
- The addition of absorbable corticosteroids and antibiotic agents to symptomatic effect mycostatin can be used as rinse for 7 to 10 days 3 to 4 times a day.
- Idoquinol: it has antifungal and antibacterial property, when this is combined with corticosteroids, it is very helpful in management or angular cheilitis.

Systemic treatment:

- **Nystatin:** it is polyene agent given 250mg TDS for a period of 2 weeks followed by 1 troche / day for 3rd week, Nystatin has better taste, so to avoid patient discomfort, sucrose, or flavoring agent should be added.
- **Ketoconazole:** it is an imidazole derivative and taken as 200 mg tablet with food once daily. Careful liver monitoring is must, because excessive use leads to hepatotoxicity.
- **Fluconazole:** It is triazol antifungal agent effective in treating candidiasis (100 mg tablet taken once daily for 2 weeks) and is well tolerated.
- A potent drug which is a new triazole antifungal called variconazole has been found to be effective.

- **Itraconazole:** it (100mg capsules) may be used for the treatment of oral candidiasis (200 mg daily orally for 14 days) Itraconazole oral suspension is now available (200mg daily 2 weeks) salivary levels of itraconazole are maintained for several hours after administration. Itraconazole is contraindicated in patients taking astemizole, triazolam, midazolam and cisapride.

Suggested reading:

1. Carla Garcia-Cuesta Maria-Gracia Sarrion-Pérez, and Jose V. Bagán Current treatment of oral candidiasis: A literature review, J Clin Exp Dent. 2014 Dec; 6(5): e576–e582.
2. Liu X, Hua H, Oral manifestation of chronic mucocutaneous candidiasis: seven case reports. J Oral Pathol Med. 2007 Oct;36(9): 528-32.
3. Lynch, DP, "Oral candidiasis. History, classification, and clinical presentation." Oral surgery, oral medicine, and oral pathology 78 (2): 189–93.
4. Scully, Crispian (2008). Oral and maxillofacial medicine: the basis of diagnosis and treatment (2nd ed.). Edinburgh: Churchill Livingstone. pp. 191–199.

Q 7) Enumerate the red lesions of oral cavity and describe in detail etiopathogenesis, clinical features and management of erythroplakia:

BFU NOVEMBER 2013 (12 Marks)

Red lesions:

1. **inflammatory conditions:**
   A. Inflammation associated with traumatic injury:
   Mechanical: cheek biting ill fitting denture, sharp edge, over hanging restoration, and ecchymoses due to trauma.
   Chemical: aspirin, formocresol.
   Thermal: hot food, hot beverage, hot instrumentation.
   Radiation: mucositis, cheilitis.
   B. Inflammations associated with Infection:
   Bacterial:
   - Scarlet fever, red fever
   - Gonococcal stomatitis
   - Vincent infection on gingivostomatitis
   - Acute pharyngitis, tonsillitis

   Fungal:
   - Atrophic candididasis
   - Angular cheilitis
   - Acute pseudomembranous candidiasis

   Viral:
   - Measles kopliks
   - Herpes simples infection
   - Herpes zoster
   - Herpangina
   - Chicken pox
   - Hand foot mouth disease

C) Allergic/immunological
- pyogenic granuloma
- giant cell epulis
- pregnancy tumours
- inflammatory fibrous hyperplasisa
- desquamative gingivitis

2. Congenital and developmental condition:
- hemangioma
- sturge- weber syndrome
- median rhomboidal glossitis
- geographic tongue
- melkerrson – Rosenthal syndrome
- crohns disease

3. vascular disease and blood disorder:
- purpura
- polycythemia
- agranulocytosis
- polyarteritis nodosa
- leukemia

4. Dermatological disorder:
- erythema multiforme
- Stevens Johnson syndrome
- lichen planus
- lichenoid reaction
- psoriasis
- lupus erythematosus

5. Other systemic disorders:
- diabetic stomatitis
- beriberi
- pernicious anemia
- ulcerative stomatitis

6. Premalignant and malignant lesions:
- Speckled leukoplakia
- Erythroplakia
- Squamous cell carcinoma
- Carcinoma -in -situ
- kaposis sarcoma.

Erythroplakia:

The term erythroplakia is applied to any area of reddened, velvety textured mucosa that cannot be diagnosed clinically or histopathologically as being caused by inflammation or any other disease process.

Etiopathogenesis:

- In most of the cases the cause is uncertain and it is idiopathic.
- Consumption of alcohol and smoking are important contributing factors.

- A specific type of oral erythroplakia occurs in chutta smokers in India. The etiology shows a strong relationship with the consumption of tobacco and the usage of alcohol.
- Candida albicans has been isolated in many erythroplakic conditions.

Clinical features:

Shear described following clinical variants of erythroplakia:

1. **Homogenous erythroplakia:** Appears as bright red velvety lesions which are about 1-1.5 cms in diameter and many are less than 1 cms in diameter. The borders can be straight or scalloped but well demarcated from surrounding structures.
2. **Erythroplakia interspersed with patches of leukoplakia (erythroleukoplakia):** Quite a few times there is co-existence of erythroplakia and leukoplakia and appears interspersed. The red part of the lesion appears less prominent and has more whitish colour.
3. **Granular or speckled erythroplakia:** These are also red slightly elevated patches with irregular outlines and granular or nodular surface and may be interspersed with small white plaques.
4. **Smooth erythroplakia:** It is soft to palpation and velvety in texture.
   - Common in 6-7th decades of life and shows male predilection.
   - Can occur on any mucosal surface of the oral cavity and may involve the larynx and pharynx.Common on the vermilion border of lip, lateral and ventral surfaces of tongue, buccal mucosa, mouth floor, and the soft palate.
   - The most frequently involved site of occurrence of the lesion in males in some studies was the floor of mouth, but in females the combined mandibular alveolar mucosa-mandibular gingiva-mandibular sulcus was most common.
   - The retromolar area in both males and females and the floor of the mouth in females was the next most common site of occurrence.
   - Non elevated red macule which is rarely multiple and may not be as extensive as leukoplakia can get.
   - Almost always symptomatic.
   - The colour is red and the texture is velvety mainly due to lack of keratin or extreme thinness of the epithelium.

Management:

- The treatment given for leukoplakia can also be applied to erythroplakia.
- Elimination of suspected irritants is mandatory, but prompt biopsy for lesions that persists is important.
- Vital staining with toulidine blue can be repeated after the period of getting rid of the suspected irritants.Extensive dysplasia or

early carcinoma may be shown by lesions that stain on second application. When the epithelial dysplasia is severe or carcinoma in-situ has intervened complete removal of the lesion is mandatory.

- Incisional biopsy is preferred so as to establish microscopic diagnosis and also because it is often associated with a epithelial dysplasia that is severe, carcinoma in situ and invasive carcinoma.
- Surgical stripping is often performed with minimal damage to the underlying connective tissue.
- Laser ablation, electrocoagulation and cryotherapy are also effective.
- Long term follow up is mandatory and prime key to therapy for this lesion as recurrence and multifocal involvement is common.
- When there is actual invasive carcinoma it should be treated promptly according to the guidelines for the treatment of cancer.

Suggested reading:

1. Reichart PA, Philipsen HP, Oral erythroplakia--a review. Oral Oncol. 2005 Jul;41(6): 551-61.
2. William G. Shafer, And Charles A. Waldron, Erythroplakia Of The Oral Cavity, Cancer36, 1021-1028, 1975.

CHAPTER 3

Pigmented Lesions of Oral Mucosa

Q 1) Write The Causes Of Endogenous And Exogenous Pigmentation Of Oral Mucosa And Write In Details About Peutz-Jegher's Syndrome And Bismuthism:

MUHS NOVEMBER 2011 10 Marks

The endogenous pigments are either normal constituents of cells or accumulate under special circumstances.

Endogenous Pigments are colored substances which originate within the body:

1. **Hemoglobin- derived:**
   - (a) Hemosiderin
   - (b) Bilirubin
   - (c) Porphyrin
2. **Non-hemoglobin-derived:**
   - (a) Lipofuscin
   - (b) Melanin
   - (c) Homogentisic acid

- Hemoglobin gives a red or bluish appearance to the mucous membrane and it is a representation of the pigmentations associated with lesions that are vascular. The colour is imparted due to the erythrocytes that are circulating and flowing through the patent vessels.
- Hemosiderin gives a brownish appearance and it is deposited as a result of extravasation of blood which could be due to trauma or a problem with the hemostatic mechanism. Generalised deposition of hemosiderin in the tissues, known as hemochromatosis can occur as a result of various pathological conditions.
- The pigment derivative of tyrosine is melanin which is synthesised in the melanocytes and they then transfer the melanin granules to the adjacent basal cells so as to protect from the damage caused by the effects of actinic radiation.Over

synthesising by the melanocytes or over population results in increased melanin pigmentation. Over production can result due to various mechanisms that can include exposure to sun, certain drugs, genetic factors, pituitary ACTH. In benign nevi and malignant melanomas melanocyte over population occurs.

Endogenous Pigmentation in Oral Mucosal Disease:

Pigment	Color	Disease Process
Hemoglobin	Blue, red, purple	Varix, hemangioma, Kaposi's sarcoma, angiosarcoma, hereditary hemorrhagic Telangiectasia
Hemosiderin	Brown	Ecchymosis, petechiae, thrombosed varix, hemorrhagic mucocele, hemochromatosis
Melanin	Brown, black or gray	Melanotic macule, nevus, melanoma, basilar melanosis with incontinence

Pigments that are exogenous usually are deposited traumatically directly in the submucosa. But in some cases they may be ingested, absorbed and distributed through the hematogenous route and get precipitated in the connective tissues and most commonly in areas that are prone for chronic inflammation like the gingiva.

Lesions that occur due to heavy metal therapy are no longer seen frequently as these metal containing medications are prescribed rarely now-a days. The exception to this is the lesions caused by gold because it is still used regularly to treat cases of arthritis. Certain chromogenic bacteria may also generate exogenous pigmentation that are commonly present on the keratinised surface of the tongue.

Exogenous Pigmentation of Oral Mucosa:

Source	**Color**	**Disease Process**
Silver amalgam	Gray, black	Tattoo, iatrogenic trauma
Graphite	Gray, black	Tattoo, trauma
Lead, mercury, bismuth	Gray	Ingestion of paint or medicines.
Chromogenic bacteria	Black, brown, green	Superficial colonization

Causes of Endogenous Pigmentation:

- Developmental Disorders:
  - Pigmented cellular nevus
  - Labial and Oral melanotic macule
  - Forbes-Albright syndrome
  - Polyostotic fibrous dysplasia
  - Neurofibromatosis

- Peutz-Jeghers syndrome
- Hyperfunction of the pituitary gland
- Hemangioma
- Hereditary hemorrhagic Telangiectasia

- Post inflammatory pigmentation:
- Functional/Physiologic Variants:
  - Racial pigmentation
  - Chloasma
  - Pregnancy
- Drugs:
  - Tetracycline
  - Busulfan
  - Chlorpromazine
  - Minocycline
  - Quinacrine
- Deficiency Disorders
  - Vitamin B 12 deficiency
- Endocrine disorders:
  - Addison's disease
  - Cushing's syndrome
  - Acromegaly
  - Hyperthyroidism
- Neoplastic Disorders:
  - Compound Nevus
  - Melanoacanthoma
  - Kaposi's sarcoma
  - Malignant melanoma/melanoma

Causes of Exogenous Pigmentation:

- Iatrogenic pigmentation due to Specific Agents:
  - Dental Amalgam
  - Chewing/Smoking of Tobacco
  - Betel nut chewing
- Pigmentation due to Drugs and metals:
  - Bismuthism – Bismuth poisoning
  - Plumbism – Lead poisoning
  - Argyria – Silver poisoning
  - Arsenism
  - Auric Stomatitis or Gold poisoning
  - Pigmentation due to Copper, Chromium and Zinc
- Brown Heme associated lesions:
  - Ecchymoses and Petechiae
  - Hemochromatosis / Bronze Diabetes
  - Carotenemia
  - Jaundice
  - Hematoma
  - Cyanosis

Peutz-Jeghers Syndrome:

In 1921 Jan Peutz, a Dutch physician described this syndrome who noticed that there was a relationship between the occurrence of intestinal polyps and muco-cutaneous macules. This syndrome is an inherited disorder that is autosomal dominant and has typical presence of intestinal polyps in association with the presence of skin and the mucosal macular melanin deposition.

There is an increased chance of developing cancer of the intestines in patients with this syndrome.

Etiology:

Germ line mutations have been detected on the LKB1 (STKI11) gene on chromosome 19pl3.3. Inactivation of this gene by germline mutations or loss of normal allele can result in hamartomatous polyps.

Clinical Features:

- It is usually of childhood onset with no sex predilection.
- The major manifestation is the intestinal polyps that are found anywhere in the gastrointestinal tract, but most frequently in the small intestine. The number and rate of growth of this polyps are variable.
- The polyps become symptomatic between the ages of 10-30 years and may cause ulceration with bleeding, obstruction, diarrhoea and intussusceptions. Patients can get anemic due to chronic blood loss.The polyps are usually benign but malignant transformation can occur.
- Tuberous sclerosis is a frequent neurological problem encountered in this syndrome.
- There are characteristic multifocal macular melanin pigmentation in perioral location. Freckle like macules can be seen on hands, perioral skin, and intraorally involve the gingival, buccal and labial mucosa.
- The macules appear as freckles or ephelides, usually they measure less than 0.5 cm in diameter and bluish black color.The anterior part of the tongue, buccal mucosa, mucosa of the lips, can also show similar lesions. Ephelides can also be seen on the fingers and hands.
- Intraorally the pigmented macules are seen most commonly on the lower lip and buccal mucosa.
- The freckles are bluish black on the skin and brownish intraorally.
- The perioral freckling often fades as the affected individual matures, leaving oral mucosal pigmentation that may be indistinguishable from racial pigmentation or pigmentation associated with Addison's disease.
- Children with unexplained recurrent abdominal pain should be examined for cutaneous and mucosal pigmentation and this syndrome. Patients with this syndrome should be evaluated for

cancer and family screening should be considered.

- Basilar melanogenesis without the proliferation of the melanocytes are the histologic features of this lesion.
- This condition should be treated by gastroenterologist and the oral lesions require no treatment.

Bismuthism:

It is systemic metallic intoxication due to bismuth compound.

Medicinal use- nowadays it is rare, in past it was used in the treatment of venereal disease.

Occupational exposure: Working in bismuth factory can cause intoxication.

Pigmentation is produced by the action of hydrogen sulphide on the bismuth compound, which is formed through bacterial degradation.

Clinical features: Gastrointestinal disturbances, nausea, bloody diarrhea, bismuth grippe, jaundice. Bismuth line- sometimes in long bone, white bands of increased density seen at the diaphyses is called bismuth line.

Oral features:

Metallic taste, increase salivation with burning sensation in oral cavity.

Ulcerative gingivostomatitis.

Tongue frequently enlarges and can become sore.

Bismuth line: blue black line appears to be well demarcated to eye on gingival papillae

Management:

Removal of cause, oral hygiene maintenance, topical anesthetics.

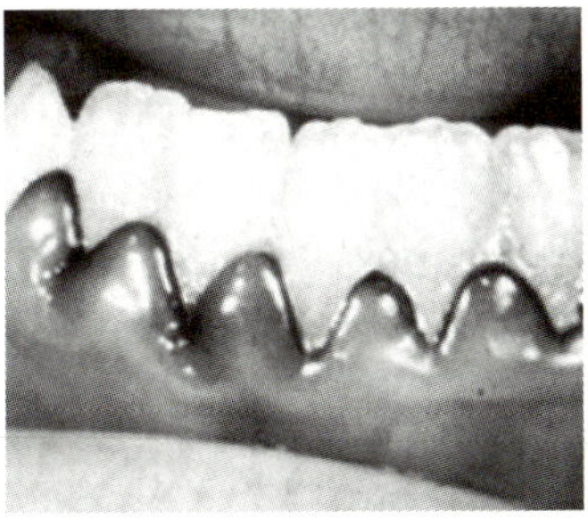

Fig. Bluish black line of bismuth poisoning on marginal gingiva

Suggested reading:

1. Harsh Mohan, Essential Pathology For Dental Students, 4th edition, 50-55.
2. Burket's Oral Medicine, Diagnosis & Treatment, 10th ed, 107-108.

CHAPTER 4

Oral Cancer

Q 1) What is oral cancer? describe in detail etiology, clinical features, investigation, treatment modalities of oral cancer.

TNMGRU AUGUST 2015, 10 Marks

Definition:

Oral cancer is a growth of malignant cells in any part of the oral cavity, which includes the lips, tongue, hard and soft palates, salivary glands, buccal mucosa, ventral tongue surface, mouth floor and gingiva.

90% of oral cancers are squamous cell carcinomas.

Etiology:

1. **Tobacco and alcohol:**
   - Tobacco contains potent carcinogens which includes nitrosamines, polycyclic hydrocarbons, nitrosodiethanolamine, polonium and nitrosoproline.
   - There are about 28 known carcinogens in smokeless tobacco. They include the non-volatile alkaloid derived tobacco specific, N-nitrosamine, and N-nitrosamino acids as a major group and the volatile tobacco specific nitrosamines, volatile aldehydes. Smokeless tobacco also is known to contain some poly nuclear agents.
   - Tobacco used as smoke in cigars, pipe and bidi more so than cigarettes can also lead to oral cancer.
   - Nicotine is powerful and addicting drug, so it is considered as major etiological factor.
   - Alcohol, acting both independently as well as synergistically with smoking, has been implicated in oral carcinogenesis. More importantly, alcohol may act as a solvent and enhance the penetration of carcinogens into target tissues. Acetaldehyde, which is the alcohol metabolite, has been identified recently as a tumor promoter.

2. **Betelnut:**
   - People with betel quid chewing habit, with or without added tobacco are at a higher risk of developing oral cancer.
   - The use of betel quid, containing both areca nut and tobacco, is associated with a much higher relative risk of oral cancer, between 8-15 times as compared to that of 1-4 times, associated with using the quid, without tobacco.
3. **Viruses:**
   - HPV and Herpes simplex virus in recent years have been implicated as causative agents of oral cancers.
   - HPV-16, HPV-18, HPV-31, HPV-33 are considered high-risk subtypes due to their association with malignant tumor.
   - The other organisms considered as causative agents and risk factors for oral squamous cell carcinoma are the epstein barr virus, cytomegalo virus and the human herpes virus 8.

4) Oral carcinoma initiation has been suggested to be due to candida also. It has been observed by clinical studies that the nodular type of leukoplakia that is infected with candida has a higher rate of dysplasia and tendency to undergo malignant transformation.

5) **Dental Hygiene and Related Factors:** Persistent irritation with sharp teeth and poor oral hygiene have also been implicated as factors for development of oral carcinoma. Dental sepsis and bad oral hygiene are suggested to increase the carcinogenic potential of tobacco.

6. **Genetic susceptibility:** It has now been proved that about 10% of all types of cancer have a strong component, that is heredity. Role of the same is now being suggested even in oral cancers.
7. **Nutritional factors:** Diet deficient of vegetables and fruits can increase the risk of developing cancer because fruits and vegetables contains vitamin A and C and antioxidants which are associated with reduced risk of oral cancer.
8. A defective immune response, as seen in a human immunodeficiency virus (HIV)-infected individual, may predispose to cancer.
9. **Molecular changes:** The genetic alterations observed in head and neck cancer are mainly due to oncogene activation and tumor suppressor gene inactivation, leading to de-regulation of cell proliferation and death.
10. Growth regulators and TSGs (tumour suppressor genes) act as transducers of negative growth signals. Genetic alterations involving the tumor suppressor genes p16 and p53, are frequently observed in head and neck tumours.

Clinical features:

- Oral cancer is commonly seen on lower lip, anterior floor of mouth, and lateral border of tongue, hard and soft palate, buccal mucosa.
- "coffin corner" at the posterior tongue/floor of the mouth is a common site for cancer but may be missed often on preliminary

inspection, These lesions need special care and very close and minute examination to be noticed.

- Oral cancer can have various clinical appearances like ulcers, red or white lesions, lumps, fissures etc. After the initial inspection, palpation of lesions is must to detect the presence of induration and their fixation to the deeper tissues.

Oral squamous cell carcinoma can manifest as any of the following:

- As a red lesion that is erythroplakia.
- An ulcer with a granular appearance associated with fissuring or exophytic margins that are raised.
- A mixture of red and white lesion.
- As a lump with abnormal supplying blood vessels.
- A lump or ulcer that is indurated.
- An extraction socket that shows non-healing.
- A lesion that is fixed to the overlying skin or mucosa or to the deeper tissues.
- Involvement of the cervical lymphnodes showing enlargement or hardness and fixation. Node enlargement is a typical feature of oro-pharyngeal cancers.

Signs and symptoms:

- Discomfort is the most common symptom.
- Patient may also present with awareness of mass in the mouth or neck.
- Dysphagia, odynophagia, otalgia, limited movement, oral bleeding, neck masses, and weight loss.
- Loss of sensory function, when it is unilateral.
- Loss of function involving the tongue affect speech, swallowing and diet.
- Tissue changes seen are red, white, or mixed red and white lesion.
- Smooth, granular, rough or crusted lesion or the presence of mass or ulceration.
- It may take different shape such as papillary, verruciform, fungating, or cauliflower like.
- Lymphatic spread commonly involves sub mandibular and digastrics nodes and the upper cervical nodes.
- Involved lymph nodes becomes enlarged and firm to hard in texture, fixed and immobile.
- The lesion may be flat or elevated and minimally palpable or indurated.

Investigation:

(a) **Biopsy and histopathological examination:** The biopsy should be sufficiently large to include the suspected lesion and apparently normal tissue to make a diagnosis without further need of another specimen. Since red rather than white areas are most likely to show any dysplasia present in the lesion, a biopsy should include the former.

(b) **Vital staining:**
 1. Toluidine blue:
 2. Methylene blue:
 3. Lugol's iodine:

(c) **Brush biopsy:** The brush biopsy uses a small nylon brush to gather cytology samples then sent for computer scanning and analysis (Oral CDx) to identify and display individual cells.

(d) **Velscope:** It is useful for evaluation of surgical borders and post surgical evaluation.

(e) **Orascoptic dk:** It enhances the ability of detection of potential cancer at early stage.

(f) Chemiluminescent devices generates light based on chemical reactions. The suspected area appears brighter.

(g) **Exfoliative Cytology:** It is used to asses cellular morphology.

(h) **Molecular analysis:** Molecular markers obtained from tissue are used for detection and evaluation of cancerous lesion.

(i) **DNA ploidy:** DNA ploidy is the measurement of nuclear DNA content. Can provide a measure for gross genetic damage.

(j) **Saliva-based oral cancer diagnostics:** The concept of a saliva test to diagnose OSCC is gaining importance.

(k) **Optical coherence tomography (OCT):** Has the potential to be applied in OSCC diagnosis.

(l) **Imaging:** Imaging can decide whether the lesions could be resected, and help in planning the precise extent of resection, and indicate whether the therapy should be minimally invasive.

Routine radiology like intraoral periapical technique, Lateral oblique for the body and ramus of mandible, Conventional and digital panoramic radiography, Computed tomography provides a better assessment of cortical bone involvement. Nuclear scintiscanning, magnetic resonance imaging, positron emission tomography, and Ultra sonography.

Treatment:

I) Surgery:

- Surgery is the preferred first line treatment of small, accessible oral SCCs.
- The treatment involves the local excision of the malignancy and should include clear oncologic margin, which is generally 2 cms and in addition selective dissection of the cervical lymph nodes in the neck.
- At the time of primary surgery, care has to be taken to do immediate reconstruction to replace the excised tissue.
- Advanced-stage oral SCC is treated by a combined treatment program of surgery, chemotherapy, and radiotherapy.

II) Radiotherapy:

- Destruction of the cancer cells and their stoppage of multiplication is brought about by high energy radiation.
- This is generally done either by giving an external beam therapy or implantation of radio-isotopes within the cancerous lesion.
- The dose of radiation is dependent on the size of the tumour, but for early stage of the disease, dosages of 66-74 gray is given as 2.0Gy/fraction, everyday from monday-friday in 7 weeks, which gives quite good results.

III) Chemotherapy:

- The use of drugs that are cytotoxic and are delivered orally or intravenously to destroy the cancer cells selectively.
- Cisplatin 100 mg/m2 IV on days 1.22 and 43 or 40-50 mg/m2 IV weekly for 6-7wk or
- Cetuximab 400 mg/m2 IV loading dose 1 week prior to the start of radiotherapy and then 250 mg/m2 weekly.
- Chemotherapy is usually used as an adjunct to surgery or radiotherapy or both and very rarely alone.

Suggested reading:

1. Crispian Scully, José V. Bagan & Joel B. Epstein, Oral cancer: Current and future diagnostic Techniques.
2. Mehrotra R, Yadav S.Oral Squamous cell carcinoma: Etiology, pathogenesis and prognostic value of genomic alterations.Indian J Cancer 2006;43: 60-6.
3. R V Chandra, J K Hoang, MBBS, and P M Phal, Imaging the oral cavity: key concepts for the radiologist. Br J Radiol. 2011 Oct; 84(1006): 944–957.

Q 2) Enumerate malignant tumors of the oral cavity. Describe the clinical and radiological features of squamous cell carcinoma involving the mandibular alveolus. Briefly mention the treatment modalities and complications of the treatment modalities.

MUHS OCTOBER 2003 (10 Marks)

A. Odontogenic:

(i) Odontogenic carcinoma:
- Malignant ameloblastoma
- Primary intraosseous carcinoma
- Other odontogenic epithelial tumours and their malignant variants
- Malignant changes in odontogenic cyst

(ii) Odontogenic sarcoma:
- Ameloblastic fibrosarcoma
- Ameloblastic fibrodentinosarcoma
- Odontogenic fibrosarcoma

B. Nonodontogenic:

(i) Epithelial:

- Squamous cell carcinoma
- Metastatic carcinoma
- Basal cell carcinoma
- Transitional cell carcinoma
- Malignant melanoma
- Verrucous carcinoma
- Spindle cell carcinoma
- Primary intra-alveolar carcinoma
- Intra-epidermoid carcinoma
- Adenoid squamous cell carcinoma

(ii) Fibrous connective tissue:
- Fibrosarcoma
- Malignant fibrous histocytomas
- Miscellaneous locally aggressive fibrous lesions

(iii) Adipose tissue:
- Liposarcoma

IV. Cartilage:
- Chondrosarcoma

V. Bone:
- Osteosarcoma
- Osteochondrosarcoma
- Ewing sarcoma

VI. Vascular tissue:
- Hemagioendothelioma
- Hemangiopericytoma
- Angiosarcoma

VII. Neural tissue:
- Neurosarcoma
- Neurofibrosarcoma
- Neuroblastoma
- Ganglioneuroma

VIII. Muscle:
- Leiomyosarcoma
- Rhabdomyosarcoma
- Malignant granular cell myoblastoma

IX. Lymphoid tissue, R-E system:
- Hodgkins lymphoma
- Non-Hodgkins lymphoma
- Primary reticular cell sarcoma
- Burkitts lymphoma
- Leukemia
- Lymphosarcoma
- Giant cell follicle lymphoma
- Multiple ediopathic hemorrhagic sarcoma of Kaposi

X. Myeloma:
- Multiple myeloma
- Plasmacytoma

XI. Tumors of salivary gland:

- Mucoepidermoid carcinoma
- Adenoidcystic carcinoma
- Adenocarcinoma
- Acinic cell adenocarcinoma
- Malignant pleomorphic adenoma
- Central mucoepidermoid carcinoma of the jaws
- Adenocarcinoma of miscellaneous form
- Epidermoid carcinoma
- Stromal salivary gland tumor

Clinical features:

- This lesion affects the males more commonly than the females. Mostly in older age group of more than 50 years.
- Squamous cell carcinoma of mandibular alveolus begins as a red or white or mixed lesion that is irregular and patchy of the epithelium that is affected.
- The premolar-molar areas are more commonly affected.
- Initially the lesion may begin as an erosion, ulceration or an exophytic, granular, serpiginous, verrucous tumour which may or may not be painful.
- With progress of time the lesions develop an area of ulceration in the center, and the borders are rolled out and indurated which is representation of invasion by the malignant cells of the peripheral tissues and there is infiltration into the adjacent muscles and bone that can be palpated.
- The ulcerative lesions are very often painful.
- Extension along the periodontal membrane with destruction of alveolar bone and loosening of teeth may be present.
- There is also superficial pressure erosion of the alveolar process from an alveolar ridge lesion which proliferates as a flat elongated ulceration, that characteristically bleeds easily.
- Extension on to the cheek, floor of the mouth and the mandible and later pathologic fractures of the mandible may occur.
- The occurrence of pain can vary from case to case and there is regional lymphadenopathy characterized by rubbery-hard lymph nodes that can be attached to the underlying structures.
- The submandibular and jugulodigastric nodes are most frequently involved.
- Other clinical features include symptoms of paresthesia, dysesthesia, anesthesia, pain, bad odour, inability to open the mouth, severe mobility of teeth or hemorrhage.
- Extensive lesions of mandibular alveolus can lead to airway obstruction, and also of the eustachian tube and the naso-pharynx.

- There is a general complaint of feeling of illness and significant weight loss.
- The condition is often fatal if untreated.

Radiographic Features:

- The lesions of squamous cell carcinoma of the jaws appears totally radiolucent, with occasional residual normal bone as small islands.
- The periodontal ligament space is widened, with loss of lamina dura, which is evidence of invasion of bone around the involved teeth.
- The teeth have a floating appearance that are within the soft tissues that are without any bony support and is described as floating or hanging teeth.
- The tumor may grow along the inferior alveolar canal and through the mental foramen that can result in increased width and loss of cortical boundary of the canal.
- It may invade the adjacent structure such as, buccal and lingual mandibular plates by destruction of cortical boundary.
- There is thinning and destruction of the inferior border of the mandible, with occurrence of a pathological fracture.

Treatment modalities for the squamous cell carcinoma involving the mandibular alveolus:

- A variety of modalities of treatment that include excision, resection, radio-therapy, chemotherapy and blocking of the epithelial growth factor, or a combination of them, either in concurrence or in a orderly sequence.
- The locoregional control of the primary tumor is the primary step towards the successful treatment outcome.The lesions of the early stage (I/II) of mandibular alveolus can be successfuly treated with a single treatment modality like surgery or Radiation Therapy.
- The treatment of choice usually is surgery because transoral resection is possible, achieving complete tumour removal and also adequate control of the margins. Surgically, tumors excision is done including a normal margin of 1 cm in all the dimensions from the primary tumour and margins less than 5 mm are considered inadequate.
- In carcinoma of alveolus chemotherapy alone cannot be a definitive way of treatment.
- in patients who have the lesions that cannot be resected, it is reported that a combination of chemo and radiotherapy can lead to improvement in overall survival of 10%-20%.
- For the lesions of the early stage radiotherapy may be suitable for the superficial lesions that measure less than 3cms and which are away from the bony structures and can be accessible for brachytherapy.
- The treatment for the stage III and IV tumours a combination

treatment modality is essential.

- In cases of the tumours that are locally advanced and are operable, surgery is done and is followed by radiotherapy.
- Radiotherapy as a adjuvant treatment is suggested in cases where there are multiple pathologically positive lymph node involvement in the neck region, perineural invasion, invasion of the lymphatics and blood vessels high grade histopathology and advanced T (III and IV) stage.
- Adjuvant combination of chemo-radiation is suggested when the surgical pathology exhibits extracapsular spread in the cervical lymph nodes and positive and close margins of less than 5mm at the primary site.
- In cases where the tumour is in close proximity to the mandible marginal versus segmental mandibulectomy has to be taken into consideration.
- Along with the treatment of the primary tumour, the cervical lymph nodes that are at risk of metastases need to be managed.

Management of the mandible:

- As mentioned above in case of close proximity of the tumour to the mandible, marginal versus segmental resection will have to be considered.
- In cases which are treated prior by radiotherapy, the marginal mandibulectomy is contraindicated because there is multifocal involvement of bone and the vascularity is compromised.
- Horizontal or vertical marginal mandibulectomy can be done.In certain cases the posterior part of the ramus can be spared in appropriate cases of segmental madibulectomy.
- In order to achieve a good surgical access for the larger and more posteriorly located lesions a paramedian step-type of mandibulectomy is considered.

Complications of treatment modalities used in squamous cell carcinoma:

Radiation therapy complication:

- Acute complication such as Mucositis.
- Alterations in salivary glands leading to xerostomia.
- In bone, hypovascularity and hypocellularity lead to the risk of osteoradionecrosis.
- Dysgeusia or impaired sense of taste.

Chemotherapy complication:

- Mucositis.
- Xerostomia.
- Loss of taste.

Surgical Complications:

- Surgical resection of cancer affects speech, swallowing and chewing.

- Oral cancer that is managed surgically adversely affects the function of mastication.
- Neurologic complications also occur because the nerves can either be directly involved or may be in close proximity.

Suggested reading:

1. Freny R. karjodkar, Essentials Of Oral And Maxillofacial Radiology. Chapter 23, Page No. 393-402
2. Liviu Feller, Johan Lemmer Oral Squamous Cell Carcinoma: Epidemiology, Clinical Presentation and Treatment. Journal of Cancer Therapy, 2012, 3, 263-268.
3. Stuart C White, Michael J Pharoah, Oral Radiology, Principles and Interpretation Chapter 22, 5th edition, page no.459-46
4. Yogesh More, Anil K. D'cruz Oral Cancer: Review Of Current Management Strategies The National Medical Journal Of India Vol. 26, No. 3, 2013.

CHAPTER 5

Salivary Gland Diseases

Q 1) What are function of Saliva? Enumerate the causes of xerostomia and note on its management:

RGUHS OCTOBER 2004 9 Marks

Saliva is a liquid secreted in the mouth by the salivary glands and is clear and slightly alkaline.

Functions of saliva:

- The fluidity of saliva helps in solubility of food and taste substances and helps in bolus formation with help of the enzymes lipase and amylase.
- Keeps the oral cavity moist and lubricated and aids in speech, swallowing and helps in preventing the oral mucosa from thermal and chemical insults.
- Salivary flow and its flushing effect clears the tooth surfaces.
- Saliva with its wide variety of substances acts as the host's main defense against dental caries.
- It dilutes hot and irritating substances and prevents injury to the oral mucosa.
- The salivary mucin which has low solubility, high viscosity and elasticity and adhesiveness helps to prevent the mucosa from environmental damages.
- The defense factor and antibacterial properties of saliva are due to lysosome, lactoperoxidase, lactoferrin and agglutinins and passive factor include immunoglobulin's, bicarbonate and carbonate system.
- The physical flow of the saliva helps in removing the bacteria and debris and helps maintain a hygienic oral environment.
- Saliva helps in wound healing due to nerve growth factor and epidermal growth factor.
- After eruption of teeth, the presence of calcium, phosphorous, magnesium, fluoride, as well as other trace elements in the saliva, through diffusion and interaction with the enamel of teeth helps

in maintaining the integrity, hardness, decreased permeability and resistance to caries.

- Helps to maintain the pH balance in oral cavity and neutralises the acids produced by the bacterial plaque.The salivary bicarbonate help to maintain the pH balance.
- Many drugs and alcohol is excreted into the saliva and may serve as route of elimination.
- Helps in maintaining the hydration of the oral cavity.Dry mouth creates the need of thirst and fluid intake.
- Also has hormonal function in the form of polypeptide hormone known as epidermal growth factor. Found in submandibular and parotid gland.
- Anticarcinogenic activity is the function of mucins present in saliva that limit the penetration of various potential toxins and irritants in foods, beverages, as well as from hazardous agents like tobacco smoke and smokeless tobacco, snuff etc.

Xerostomia:

Xerostomia refers to a subjective sensation of dry mouth; it is frequently, but not always, associated with salivary gland hypo function.

The dry mouth is common during periods of anxiety, mouth breathing and with advancing age.

Among older adults xerostomia is a common complaint and affects about 20% of elderly.

Causes of xerostomia:

(i) Temporary conditions that can cause xerostomia are dehydration, use of certain drugs, viral infections, and psychogenic cause like fear.

Dry mouth can occur due to various types of drugs such as those used to treat motionsickness, anti-depressants, anthistaminics, anxiolytics, anti-parkinsonisn drugs, decongestants, anti-psychotics.

Duct calculi: Commonly involving the submandibular salivary gland can produce dryness on affected site. Once removed may revert the condition.

(ii) Chronic inflammatory disease, such as Sojgren's syndrome, sarcoidosis, and amyloidosis can cause dry mouth due to changes in the salivary glands.

(iii) In some patients with HIV, there is enlargement of the salivary glands and xerostomia.

(iv) Diabetes that is uncontrolled, cystic fibrosis, primary biliary cirrhosis, Hepatitis C virus infection are some of the systemic diseases that can lead to xerostomia.

(v) Radiation therapy to head and neck region almost always causes the patients to develop xerostomia.Secretory cells, especially the serous cells show changes due to radiation and there is a reduction in the salivary flow causing dry mouth.It also changes the viscosity of saliva.

(vi) Patients who undergo chemotherapy treatment, show dryness of the mouth but the change is temporary.

(vii) Local factors like decreased mastication, chronic smoking, and mouth breathing can cause xerostomia.

(viii) Developmental abnormalities like aplasia, tumours, autoimmune diseases, certain disorders affecting the afferent or efferent portions of neural transmission can cause xerostomia.

(ix) Nutritional deficiencies like pernicious anemia, iron deficiency anemia, deficiency of vitamin A and hormonal imbalances can cause xerostomia.

(x) Systemic conditions associated with high temperature and dehydration may lead to reduced salivary flow.

(xi) Fluid loss associated with vomiting, diarrhoea, hemorrhage can cause reduced salivary flow.

(xii) Rare causes include, Amyloidosis, Hemochromatosis, Wegener's disease.

Management of xerostomia:

Treatment that is available for dry mouth may be divided into five categories

1. Preventive therapy
2. Symptomatic treatment
3. Local or topical salivary stimulation
4. Systemic salivary stimulation
5. Therapy that is directed to an underlying systemic disorder.

Based on current literature and clinical practice the overall management strategy for xerostomia and salivary gland hypo function should include a combination of supplemental fluoride topical palliative agent, and a secretogogue.

I) Preventive therapy:

- Topical use of fluoride in a patient with salivary gland hypofunction is absolutely critical to control dental caries. Oral health care practioners may also use fluorides varnishes.
- Gels or rinses of topical fluoride can be used once or twice/ day and sodium fluoride mouth rinse should be retained in the oral cavity for at least a minute before its expectoration. The prevention of demineralisation of the enamel in patients following radiotherapy has been shown to be effective by the use of 0.05% sodium fluoride rinse which is used twice daily.
- A tooth brush can be used to apply fluoride gels which can be left in the mouth for 2-3 minutes before rinsing.
- It is essential that patients maintain meticulous oral hygiene, they require more frequent dental visit, patients should be counseled as to diet, avoiding cariogenic food and beverages and brushing immediately after meal, use of alcohol and caffeine should be minimized.
- Appropriate antifungal therapies should be instituted in case

of oral candidiasis which is common in xerostomic patients. Topical medications that are prescribed for oral applications include, clotrimazole as 10mg tablets where 1 tablet is to be dissolved slowly in the mouth about 5 times/day. Nystatin oral pastilles.200000 units, 1-2 tablets to be dissolved slowly in the mouth 5 times/day.

- Denture wearers are instructed to remove them before the use of topical antifungal applications.In the treatment of angular cheilitis, nystatin and triamcinolone acetonide cream, or the cream containing ketoconazole have been found to be useful adjuncts.

II) Symptomatic treatment:

Several symptomatic treatments are available. Water is most important and patient should be encouraged to sip it through out the day; this will help to moisten the oral cavity, hydrate the mucosa and clear debris from the mouth.

Salivary substitutes which contain generally, hydroxyethylcellulose or carboxymethylcellulose and come in various flavors can give very good symptomatic relief.

There are number of rinses, mouthwashes and gels available to provide symptomatic relief.

Patients should be cautioned to avoid products containing alcohol, sugar or strong flavouring that may irritate sensitive dry mucosa.

Frequent use of product containing Aloe Vera and vit E should be encouraged.

III) Local/topical salivary stimulation:

Chewing will stimulate salivary flow as well as sour and sweet taste. The chewing of gum, paraffin, mint, and use of lozenges containing citric acid, can be very effective in relieving symptoms.

Electrical stimulation has also been examined as a therapy for salivary hypofunction.

Acupuncture with application of needles in the parotid and other region for therapy of salivary gland hypofunction and xerostomia has been suggested.

IV) Systemic stimulation:

Use of several sialogogues for salivary stimulation have long been examined and include anethole-trithione, bromhexine, pilocarpine hydrochloride and anecdotally, bethanecol hydrochloride.

- Bromhexine is given as 8 mgs TID in adults, and 4mgs BD or TID in children.
- Anethole Trithion is given as 25 mgs tablets one or two tablets TID.
- Pilocarpine should be administered 30 minutes before meals, in 5 mg tablets, 3 to 4 times a day, with the usual dose range being approximately 3 to 6 tablets a day, not to exceed two tablets per dose. It is contraindicated in patients with

pulmonary disease, asthma, cardiovascular disease or narrow angle glaucoma.

V) **Treatment of underlying systemic disorder:**
Most clinical work has been done in sjogren's syndrome and various therapeutic modalities have been established to reduce the symptoms. Lot of latest therapies using various compositions are being used to reduce or minimise salivary gland dysfunction during head and neck radiotherapy.

Suggested reading:

1. Nishat Sultana, M. Ehtaih Sham, Xerostomia: An overview, International Journal Of Dental Clinics 2011: 3(2): 58-61.

Q 2) Classify Salivary gland disorder. Write in detail about etiology, clinical feature, Investigation & treatment of Sjogren's syndrome.

TNMGRU FEBRUARY 2013 (10 Marks)

Classification of salivary Gland Disorder:

(i) **Developmental Disorder:**
- Aberrancy
- Aplasia
- Hypoplasia
- Hyperplasia
- Atresia
- Accessory ducts
- Diverticuli
- Congenital Fislula

(ii) **Functional Disorder:**
- Sialorrhea
- Xerostomia

(iii) **Obstructive Disorders:**
- Sialolithiasis
- Mucus Plug
- Stricture & Stenosis
- Extraductal Causes

(iv) **Cysts:**
- Mucocele
- Ranula

(v) **Enlargement:**
- Sialosis
- Allergic
- Sarcoidosis
- Obstructive
- Infections

(vi) Infection:

- Viral Infection
- Bacterial Infection
- Mycotic infection

(vii) Autoimmune Disorder:

- Sjogren's syndrome
- Mickulicz's Disease
- Uveoparotid fever
- Recurrent non-specific parotitis

(viii) Tumours:

Benign:

Pleomorphic adenoma.
Warthins tumour
Basal cell adenoma
Myoepithelioma
Canalicular adenoma

Malignant:

Muco epidermoid carcinoma
Adenocystic carcinoma
Malignant pleomorphic adenoma

Sjogren's Syndrome:

A. Definition:

Sjogren's syndrome is an autoimmune disorder that is chronic and has typical characteristic symptoms of oral and ocular dryness and the exocrine glands show lymphocytic infiltration and destruction.

B. Types:

(i) Primary Sjogren's Syndrome:
It is also called as sicca syndrome & it consists of dry eyes (xerophthalania) & dry mouth (Xerostomia).

(ii) Secondary Sjogren's syndrome:
It consist of dry eyes, dry mouth & collagen disorders usually rheumatoid arthritis or systemic lupus erythematous.

C. Etiology, risk factors & Pathogenesis:

Etiology:

Though not very well understood and multifactorial there are four events:

(i) Initiation by an exogenous factor.
(ii) Disruption of salivary gland epithelial cells.
(iii) T lymphocyte migration and lymphocytic infiltration of exogenous glands.
(iv) B-lymphocyte hyperactivity and production of rheumatoid factor and antibodies to RO(SS-A) and La(SS-B)

Risk factors:

(i) Genetic predisposition.

(ii) Viruses that have been implicated are Epstein barr virus, Hepatitis C virus and human T-cell leukemia virus -1.

(iii) Sex hormones: As females are more affected than males, it suggests that the immune regulatory properties of sex hormones are involved in its development.

Pathogenesis:

(i) Autoantibodies Ro/SSA and La/SSB, are found commonly in the serum of 60-70% of patients with primary Sjogren's syndrome.

(ii) There is chronic lymphocytic infiltration and subsequent damage of salivary gland acini.

(iii) Up regulated expression of human leukocytic antigen molecules leads to destruction of exocrine glands.

(iv) Autoantibodies to Muscarinic M3 receptors: Autoantibodies to salivary and lacrimal glands muscarinic M3 acetylcholine receptors are produced in Sjogren's syndrome.

(v) B cell hyperactivity.

D. Clinical Features:

- Generalised dryness, which typically includes xerostomia and kerato conjunctivitis sicca, which are components of the sicca syndrome are the major symptoms of Sjogren's syndrome.
- The sicca syndrome also includes dryness of the vagina and chronic bronchitis. Apart from causing skin, nose and vaginal dryness, Sjogren's syndrome may also affect other organs of the body like the kidneys, blood vessels, lungs, liver, the biliary system, brain, pancreas and the peripheral nervous system.
- Xerostomia is major complaint in most of the patients resulting in unpleasant taste and difficulty in eating dry food.
- The mouth may develop soreness and burning sensation.
- Angular stomatitis & denture stomatitis, cracking of lips also occurs mainly due to lack of saliva.
- Increased incidence of caries is seen.
- Lateral or bilateral enlargement of parotid gland may occur due to dryness of mouth.
- Clinically the mouth may appear moist in early stages of sjogren's syndrome but in later there may be lack of usual pooling of saliva in floor of mouth.
- In advanced cases the mucosa is glazed, dry and tends to result in candidal infection.
- In some patient there may be clicking quality of speech.
- Tongue typically develops characteristic lobulated usually red surface with partial or complete depapillation.
- The patient usually complains of dry eyes & continuous irritations in the eyes.
- In the patient with secondary Sjogren's syndrome, rheumatoid arthritis is typically long standing & clinically obvious.

Investigations:

(i) Eye test:

(a) Dryness on the surface of the eyes can be revealed by the slit-lamp examination.

(b) Shirmer's test: In this test the production of tears can be measured by the use of paper strips that are inserted in the eyes for several minutes. At the same time both eyes are tested. In this test a small strip of filter paper is placed in the lower eyelid and the patient is asked to close the eyes for 5 minutes.When the paper is removed and the moisture is measured, and in cases of Sjogren's syndrome less than 5mm is moistened in 5 minutes.

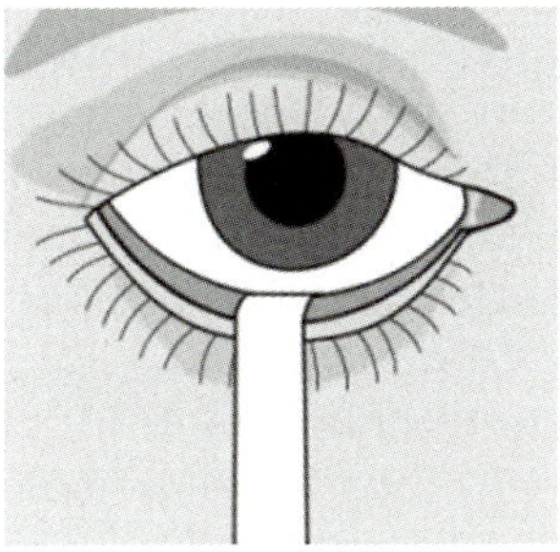

Fig. Schirmer's test

(c) **Rose Bengal dye test:**

In this test the physician instills a red vegetable dye on the surface of the eyes that stain cells that have lost mucin coating.

The distinctive colour of the dye helps to detect the state and the functioning of tear film and the rate of evaporation of the tears.In case of distinctive change of colour will indicate presence of Sjogren's syndrome.

Method:

A. 1% rose bengal dye is instilled in both the eyes.

B. Conjunctival staining is scored quantitatively.

The rose bengal stain is taken up by the devitalised cornea and the conjunctiva.

Interpretation:

A. The conjunctiva that gets stained is suggestive of Sjogren's syndrome.

B. The staining test is capable of identifying Sjogren's syndrome even before the development of symptoms.

(ii) Salivary flow test:

(a) Salivary flow test is conducted to check the status of the salivary glands and the production of saliva. The patient is asked to spit as much saliva as possible which is collected in a cup and weighed. This test helps to determine the functioning of the salivary glands and if the sample collected is not optimum then this condition can be considered to be present. Other test is collection of whole unstimulated saliva which is collected in a test tube every minute for 15 minutes. If the collection is less than 1.5 ml it is positive for Sjogren's syndrome.

(b) **Lip/ minor salivary gland biopsy:** In the biopsy specimen the histopathologic findings of presence of autoantibodies against the extractable nuclear antigens SS-A/Ro or SS-B/La and the objective finding of lacrimal dysfunction can be diagnostic of this condition.

The minor salivary gland biopsy specimen along with the grading system for quantifying the salivary histologic changes can be the best diagnostic tool for the salivary component of the Sjogren's syndrome. The grading system is as follows:

1. The infiltrating mononuclear cells are counted and an aggregate of 50 or more cells is called a focus.
2. The surface area of the specimen and the total number of foci are measured.
3. The number of foci/4mm^2 is calculated.

Thus the focal score is calculated and the range can be 0-12 that denotes the confluent infiltrates. The focal score of 1 is considered to be positive for Sjogren's syndrome, however some criteria require the score to be more than 1.

(c) **Sialography:** It may show characteristic changes and can be useful for evaluation of this syndrome. It may show a cherry blossom appearance of salivary gland and duct. Parotid gland involvement may show honey comb or salt and pepper appearance.

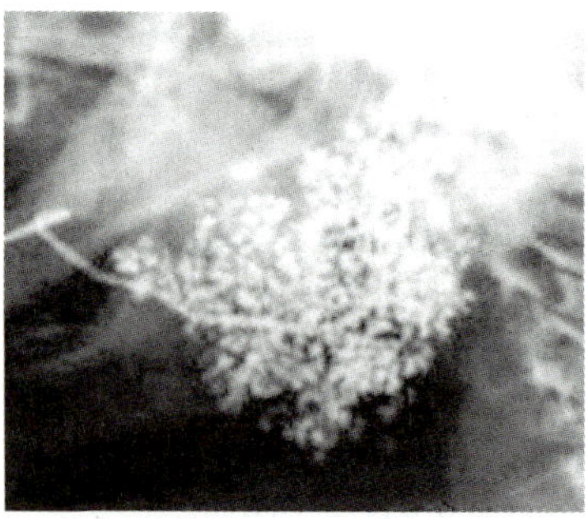

Fig. Cherry blossom appearance of the ductal acini in Sjogren's syndrome (SS)

(d) **MRI or CT:** These tests can help in the assessment of enlarged glands and the potential lymphadenopathies.

MRI is preferable to CT as it gives a better resolution of the soft tissues.

(e) **Ultra sound scans:** The salivary glands show a uniform grey appearance but in SS round black areas will be seen in the scan.

(iii) **Blood tests:** Patient's with SS quite often have antibodies in their blood which are at high levels. These can be measured with blood tests. The ESR test is performed as it can show the high levels of antibody that makes the blood thicker. The ESR can show and measure the rate at which the cells in a tube of blood settle. Thicker the blood higher is the ESR.

Treatment:

1. **Eye care:** Eye drops containing artificial tears can be used to successfully treat mild to moderate cases of dry eyes. In case of irritation of the eyes. A short term dose of eye-drops containing corticosteroids can be effective but due to side effects long term use has to be avoided.

2. **Oral care:**
   - (i) Prevention of caries can be achieved by maintaining good oral hygiene.
   - (ii) Increasing your fluid intake.
   - (iii) Stimulation of saliva can be achieved by use of sugar-free chewing gums.
   - (iv) In order to lubricate the mouth and reduce the dryness ice cubes can be asked to suck regularly.
   - (v) regularly using mouth rinses for soothing effects and protect it against infection.
   - (vi) Use of Saliva substitutes can be prescribed that are available as spray, lozenges, gels or gum.

3. **Medical treatment:**

   Pilocarpine: It is used often to treat the symptoms of dry eyes and mouth. It has the ability of stimulating the glands to produce more saliva and tears. Cevimeline can also be used. Both these drugs can help increase production of saliva and sometimes tears.

   Hydroxychloroquine: It has the ability to slow down the attack by the immune system on the salivary and lacrimal glands.It also helps to reduce the other symptoms like the joint and muscle pain and stiffness.

Treatment of other symptoms:

Dry skin:

There are several types of soaps and cream to be used for dryness of the skin.

Dryness in the vagina:

A lubricant can be used to treat this condition. Estrogen creams or hormone replacement therapy can be considered.

Pain in the muscle and joints:

These can be treated with NSAIDs like ibuprofen.

Suggested reading:

1. Borchers, A. T., Naguwa, S. M., Keen, C. L. & Gershwin, M. E. Immunopathogenesis of Sjögren's syndrome. Clin. Rev. Allergy Immunol. 25, 89-104 (2003)
2. Delaleu, N., Jonsson, R. & Koller, M. M. Sjögren's syndrome. Eur. J. Oral Sci. 113, 101-113 (2005)
3. Voulgarelis, M. & Tzioufas, A. G. Pathogenetic mechanisms in the initiation and perpetuation of Sjögren's syndrome. Nature reviews.Rheumatology 6, 529-537 (2010)Sjogren's syndrome. Nature Reviews Rheumatology 9, 544-556 (2013)

Q 3) Write the differential diagnosis of dryness of mouth:

RGUHS OCTOBER 2002 (10 Marks)

Dry mouth also known as xerostomia is a subjective feeling of dryness which is often but not always associated with hypofunction of salivary glands. It is usually associated with changes in the salivary composition, or reduction in the rate of salivary flow, and may have no identifiable cause.

Differential diagnosis:

1. **Physiologic:**
   (i) During sleep, there is a decrease in flow rate of saliva. This results in a temporary feeling of dry mouth on waking. It goes away after eating and drinking or with proper oral hygiene.
   (ii) Anxiousness and stress can lead to dry mouth and proper history will help in diagnosis.
   (iii) Dehydration can lead to dry mouth which is because the body tries to conserve the fluid. History of diarrhea, vomiting or blood loss may help in diagnosis.
   (iv) Some older people may have symptoms of dry mouth which is due to changes in the salivary glands related to age that can cause moderate decrease in salivary flow.
2. **Drugs:** There are about 500 drugs that can cause dryness in the oral cavity. The drugs that can do so are, ones which are used to control motion sickness, anti-depressants, anti-psychotics, anxiolytics, anti-histamines, anti-parkinsonism drugs, anti-hypertensives, diuretics and narcotics, decongestants, anticonvulsants, antiemetics, anti-histaminics, and antispasmodics. The symptoms of dryness starts shortly after intake of offending drug or by increase in the dosages. Many of the above mentioned drugs lead to dryness due to their anti-cholinergic effects. The history of taking these medicines will help in diagnosis.
3. **Mouth breathing:** Is often a cause of dryness of the mouth and often occurs in patients with malocclusion or just as a habit. If the patient is aware the dry mouth can be correlated.

4. **Duct calculi:** Commonly involving the submandibular salivary gland can produce dryness on affected site. Once removed may revert the condition.The symptoms of pain and swelling of the involved salivary gland especially while eating and the radiographic evidence of calculus will help in diagnosis.
5. Chronic inflammatory disease, such as Sojgren's syndrome, amyloidosis, sarcoidosis, can lead to xerostomia because of changes in the salivary glands.
   - The typical clinical triad of dry eyes, dry mouth and the presence of other conditions like rheumatoid arthritis and other connective tissue disorders will help to locate the cause of dry mouth as due to Sjogren's syndrome.
   - In amyloidosis the dry mouth occurs due to direct involvement of salivary glands. Macroglossia with amyloid deposits can be seen on the face. Congo red is used to diagnose amyloid which shows birefringence and dichroism.
   - Sarcoidosis is a multisystem granulomatous disease and when the salivary gland is involved can lead to dry mouth. Salivary gland involvement with lymph nodes involvement and non-specific ulcer in the oral cavity can help in clinical diagnosis. Laboratory investigation includes Kveim-Siltzbach test which is positive in some cases.
6. Patients in some cases who are infected with HIV can have enlargement of salivary glands and dry mouth. The typical clinical features of AIDS and laboratory diagnosis can help establish the cause.
7. Some systemic conditions like uncontrolled diabetes, cystic fibrosis, primary biliary cirrhosis, Hepatitis C virus infection can lead to xerostomia.
   - Patients with diabetes are generally aware of their condition and the cause of dry mouth can be easily correlated.

     Clinical features include polydipsia, polyphagia and polyuria. There is acetone breath and patients feels fatigue and tiredness. Diabetic neuropathy is also present.

     Patients may have weight loss or obesity, difficulty in sleeping and hypertension.

     Plasma glucose concentration will be elevated above 140mg/dl.

     Glucose tolerance test will reveal plasma glucose concentration of about 200 mg/dl.
   - Hepatitis C is caused by Hepatitis C virus and is seen in intravenous drug users and patients with renal dialysis.

     Systemic complaints may be malaise, high fever, morbiliform skin rash, anorexia, vomiting. There will be tenderness and enlargement of liver. There will be yellowing of skin and dark urine. Intraorally yellowing will be seen on the palate and sublingual areas.

Laboratory diagnosis will reveal billirubin levels in excess of 3mg/dl. SGOT and SGPT levels rise 10 times.

- Primary biliary cirrhosis is an autoimmune disorder affecting the liver. It is a rare disorder and the symptoms are sleepiness during the day, severe fatigue and itching in about 20-70% patients. Patients with severe disease may have jaundice.

  Laboratory test will show abnormalities in liver enzyme tests are usually present and elevated gamma-glutamyl transferase and alkaline phosphatase are found in early disease.

  Elevations in bilirubin occur in advanced disease.

8. Most of the patients who undergo radio-therapy to the head and neck region can develop xerostomia. Radiation affects the secretory cells especially the serous cells and causes reduction in the saliva out put and also changes the viscosity of saliva. The history of malignancy and radiation therapy can be easily established from patient history.
9. Decreased mastication due to painful teeth or any systemic disorder or due to fever or any other cause can lead to dryness of mouth. Patient history can point out to the cause of dry mouth.
10. Developmental abnormalities like aplasia, tumours, autoimmune diseases, certain disorders affecting the afferent or efferent portions of neural transmission can cause xerostomia.

    Proper patient history and physical examination can help in determining the exact cause of dry mouth.
11. Nutritional deficiencies like pernicious anemia, iron deficiency anemia, deficiency of vitamin A and hormonal imbalances can cause xerostomia.
    - Clinical diagnosis of iron deficiency anemia can be done due to presence of koilonychias, angular cheilitis, depapillation of tongue and neuropathy. Laboratory diagnosis will show abnormal RBCs in the peripheral smear and there will be microcytic, hypochromic anemia.
    - In pernicious anemia the clinical features like generalised weakness, painful and sore tongue and tingling and numbness of the extremities will be present. Laboratory diagnosis will reveal the oral epithelial cells having enlarged hyperchromatic nuclei and prominent neucleoli and serrated nuclear membranes. Cells exhibit poikilocytosis and macrocytosis. Schilling's test will help in confirming the diagnosis.
    - Vitamin A deficiency will reveal night blindness, dry conjunctiva, corneal ulceration. Skin may have boils, acne, pimples and premature wrinkling. Histopathology will reveal squamous metaplasia.
12. Rare causes include Hemochromatosis, Wegener's disease.

- Hemochromatosis is a disorder where there is excess iron deposition which results in sclerosis and dysfunction of the organs and tissues involved. There is a tetrad of bronzed skin, liver cirrhosis, diabetes and cardiac failure.
  More common in men and intraorally diffuse brown pigmentation will be seen at the junction of hard and soft palate.
- Wegners granulomatosis occurs especially in the 4th and 5th decades, and the typical clinical features are nasal stuffiness and chronic discharge which can sometimes be bloody.
  Intraorally there is tumour like vegetations in the mouth and nose. There is oral ulceration which is perforating in nature.
  Clinical diagnosis consists of typical strawberry gingivitis with necrotic ulcerations in the mouth.
  Laboratory diagnosis includes cytoplasmic localisation and histopathologically chronic inflammatory cells and multinucleated giant cells are seen.

13. In ectodermal dysplasia salivary glands including the accessory salivary glands may be hypoplastic leading to dryness of mouth and cracked and fissured lips.
14. **Oral submucous fibrosis:** This premalignant condition has marked symptom of dry mouth due to fibrotic bands that form in the oral mucosa. This could be due to occlusion of the ductal openings of the major and minor salivary glands.
15. **Renal failure:** Patients may complain of dry mouth due to direct involvement of salivary glands, dehydration, chemical inflammation and mouth breathing.
16. **Kidney transplantation:** These patients develop enlarged salivary glands and reduced salivary flow leading to dry mouth.

CHAPTER **6**

Temporomandibular Joint Disorders

Q 1) Classify TMJ disorder and discuss in detail about clinical manifestations radiographic appearance and management of osteoarthritis of TMJ.

BFU NOVEMBER 2013 (11 Marks)

Temporomandibular joint disorders (TMDs) affect the temporomandibular joint (TMJ) or / and the muscles of mastication. The most common symptom is pain, localized predominantly in the preauricular area. To a lesser extent, the ear, temple, and muscles of the neck are involved.

Classification by WALDEN BELL:

- Masticatory Muscle Disorders
  - Protective muscle splinting
  - Masticatory muscle spasm (MPD)
  - Masticatory muscle inflammation (myositis)
- Derangement of TMJ
  - Incoordination
  - Anterior disk displacement with reduction (clicking)
  - Anterior disk displacement without reduction (close lock)
- Extrinsic Trauma
  - Traumatic arthritis
  - Dislocation
  - Fracture
  - Internal disk derangement
  - Myositis
  - Myospasm
  - Tendonitis
- Degenerative Joint Disease
  - Non-inflammatory phase (Arthosis)
  - Inflammatory phase (osteoarthritis)
- Inflammatory Joint Disease
  - Rheumatoid arthritis
  - Infective arthritis

  - Metabolic arthritis
- Chronic Hypomobility
  - Ankylosis
  - Fibrosis of articular capsule
  - Contracture of elevator muscles
  - Internal disk derangement
- Growth Disorders Of The Joint
  - Developmental
  - Acquired
  - Neoplastic

Osteoarthritis (Degenerative Joint Disease):

- Osteoarthritis / Degenerative joint disease (DJD) is primarily a disorder of articular cartilage and sub-chondral bone associated with synovial membrane inflammation which is secondary.
- It is a localized joint disease without systemic manifestations.
- It is a non-inflammatory disorder of the joint with typical characteristics of:
  - Deterioration of the joint, loss of articular cartilage and bone erosion.
  - Proliferation, which is characterized by new bone formation at the articular surface and in the sub-chondral region.
- It occurs when the ability of the joint to adapt to excessive forces is exceeded.
- Excessive loading on the articular cartilage leads to thinning of the cartilage and during joint activity can break away.
- This leads to subcondylar cysts, sclerosis of the underlying bone, and osteophyte formation.
- The fibrous tissue covering in patients with degenerative disease is preserved.
- Degenerative joint disease (DJD) may be categorized as:
  - Primary degenerative joint disease is often due to wear and tear. It is often asymptomatic and is most commonly seen in patients above the age of 50 years.
  - Secondary degenerative joint disease results from a known underlying cause such as, congenital dysplasia, trauma or presence of metabolic disease. This is more common in younger individuals.

Etiology:

Its etiological factors are:

- Chronic para-functional activity such as tooth clenching, bruxism that leads to dental attrition and degenerative diseases of TMJs.
- Ageing
- Acute trauma
- hypermobility

Risk factors include gender, diet, genetics and psychological stress:

- Gender: female are more predisposed to the osteoarthritis. Role of estrogen in the disease is unknown, but estrogen receptors have been identified on TMJ articular tissues.
- Diet: of excessively hard or chewy foods increase the load on TMJ leading to degenerative diseases.
- Psychological stress: leading to para-functional habits such as tooth clenching, bruxism. Stress also leads to biological, biochemical, and hormonal changes that might contribute to the changes in joints.

Clinical manifestations:

Very common symptoms and signs include:

- Many patients with mild to moderate DJD of the TMJ are asymptomtomatic.
- Pain, which is generally of the dull aching type and there could be sharp pain on moving the joint.
- In the initial phases due to synovitis, pain is prevalent.
- The pain is often associated with stiffness in the joints, mouth opening limitations, and increased sensitivity to cold and dampness, and relief is brought about by use of NSAIDs.
- There is presence of stiffness in the mornings, crepitus of the joints, clicking and popping sounds.
- In advanced stages there can be deviation of the joint to the affected side.
- There can be unstable or fluctuating malocclusion, and discrepancies in the occlusion like skeletal anterior open bite, reduced overbite and an increase in the over jet with the osteoarthritic TMJ.
- Internal derangements may coexist in the same joint in about 1/3rd of the cases.

Depending upon the clinical features TMJ osteoarthritis is divided in to three stages / phases:

1. The initial stage/ early phase where there is evolution of the condition which takes an average of 2.5-4 years. There are clinical signs like clicking sounds and intermittent locking.
2. TMJ destruction occurs in the intermediate phase and lasts for about 6 months to a year, and the patient may have symptoms like sudden pain in the joints during rest or function, opening limitations, and grating sounds.
3. In the late phase the degenerative activity stops and the joints become stable and the phase is called as burn out, which lasts for about 6 months and the the joints become stable. There is usually absence of pain in the joints, presence or absence of mouth opening limitations and grating sounds. The complete process from initiation to the burnout phase takes about 5-6 years.

Radiographic findings:

- Narrowing of the joint space, irregular joint space, flattening of the articular surfaces, subchondral sclerosis, osteophytic formation, anterior lipping of the condyle may be evident depending on the stage of the disease.
- Sometimes small, round, radiolucent areas with irregular margins surrounded by varying area of increased density are seen on articular surface of the joint, these are called as Ely's cysts.
- In the latter stage of the disease there is bony proliferation at the periphery of articulating surface, increasing the surface area. This new bone is called an osteophyte.
- Osteophytes typically appears on the anterosuperior surface of condyle and lateral aspect of the temporal component.
- The osteophytes may break off and lie free within the joint space (joint mice).
- In severe DJD the glenoid fossa may appear grossly enlarged due to erosion.
- The enlargement of fossa and reduced size of the condylar head allow the condyle to move forward and superiorly in to an abnormal anterior position that may lead to anterior open bite.

Treatment:

Management is largely symptomatic. Treatment includes educating the patient and training them in self-management, regular communication by phone, pharmacological treatments, use of topical ointments, injections of steroids and hyaluronic acid, referring to a physiotherapist, muscle strengthening, physical therapy and TENS therapy.Acupuncture and low level laser therapy can also be used.

Patient Education and self-management:

- Patient counseling and educating the patient in the disease's natural course.
- Elimination of oral habits e.g. tooth clenching, chewing gum.
- Provide information about jaw care associated with daily activities.
- Modification of activity includes instruction to the patient to take soft diet, avoid foods that require wide mouth opening and eating food that is cut into small pieces.
- Modification of habits, avoiding mouth opening excessively and chewing gums.
- Avoiding jaw clenching consciously.

Physiotherapy:

- The use of jaw movements, active and passive, techniques of manual therapy, body posture correction, and techniques of relaxation.
- Physical therapy: TENS, acupuncture, low-level laser therapy and ultrasound are often used to reduce pain.

Oral Appliance Therapy:

Joint stabilization appliances:

- This is most commonly used intraoral appliance in TMD.
- It provides stabilisation of joints, teeth protection, redistribution of forces, elevator muscles relaxation, reduce bruxism, decrease in loading of joints, and can also stabilise the occlusion secondarily and help in relaxation of masticatory muscles.
- The splint therapy may be used in combination with pharmacotherapy.

Pharmacological modalities:

- **Acetaminophen:** given in the dosages of up to 4gms/day.It has to be used carefully in patients with history of alcoholism and liver disorders.
- COX-2 non-selective and selective oral non-steroidal anti-inflammatory drugs (NSAIDs).
- **Topical NSAIDs:** Diclofenac sodium 1% gel, apply onto the area affected 3-4 times/day.
- **Capsaicin:** capsaicin applied topically 0.025% / 0.075% concentration for 4 times a day for several weeks.
- Intra-articular injections of corticosteroids and hyaluronates, glucosamine and/or chondroitin sulphate.
- **Opioid analgesics:** Tramadol: 50- 100mg tablets every 4-6 hr.
- Tricyclic antidepressants:
- **Amitriptyline:** at doses of 10–25 mg HS, may increase upto 75-100 mg daily if needed. (Amline, Sarotena, Tryptomer 25mg, 75mg tablets SR tablets.)
- **Nortriptyline:** at usual doses of 10–30 mg HS the total daily dose can be given once a day. (Nortriptyline HCL 10 mg capsule, pamelor 10/25 mg capsule).

Suggested reading:

1. Burket's Textbook of oral medicine, 11th Edition, Chapter 9, Temporomandibular disorder. Page no. 223-250.

CHAPTER 7

Orofacial Pain

Q 1) Classify facial pain. Describe the etiopathogenesis, clinical features, and management of atypical facial pain.

TNMGRU APRIL 1995 1(5 Marks)

The International Association for the study of pain's widely used definition which states: "Pain as an unpleasant emotional and sensory experience which is usually initiated by a noxious stimulus and transmitted over a specialised neural network to central nervous system where it is interpreted as such."

Orofacial pain (OFP) is the presenting symptom of a broad spectrum of diseases. As a symptom, it may be due to disease of the orofacial structures, generalized musculoskeletal or rheumatic disease, peripheral or central nervous system disease, or psychological abnormality; or the pain may be referred from other sources (eg; cervical muscles or intracranial pathology).

Classification of facial pain (Bells Classification)

1. **Somatic pain:**
   - A. Superficial somatic pain:
     1. Cutaneous pain
     2. Mucogingival pain
   - B. Deep somatic pain
     1. Musculoskeletal pain
        - (a) Muscle pain
          1. Protective splintic pain
          2. Myofascial trigger point pain
          3. Muscle Spasm pain
          4. Muscle inflammation pain
        - (b) Temporomandibular joint pain
          1. Disc attachment pain
          2. Retrodiscal pain
          3. Capsular pain
          4. Arthritic pain
        - (c) Osseous and periosteal pain

(d) Soft connective tissue pain
(e) Periodontal dental pain

2. Visceral pain
- (a) Pulpal dental pain
- (b) Vascular pain
  1. Migrainous neuralgia
  2. Atypical odontalgia
  3. Common migraine
  4. Classic migraine
  5. Vascular inflammation pain
- (c) Visceral mucosa pain
- (d) Glandular, ocular, and auricular pain

(ii) Neuropathic pain:

A. Neuropathic pain
1. Traumatic neuroma pain
2. Paroxysmal neuralgia
   - (a) Idiopathic neuralgia
   - (b) Symptomatic neuralgia
3. Neuritic neuralgia
   - (a) Peripheral neuritis
   - (b) Herpes zoster
   - (c) Postherpetic neuralgia

B. Deafferentation pain
1. Reflex sympathetic dystrophy (causalgia)
2. Anesthesia dolorosa
3. Atypical odontalgia / Phantom pain

(iii) Psychogenic pain:

A. Chronic Face pain

B. Psychoneurotic pain
1. Conversion hysteria pain
2. Delusional pain

Atypical facial pain:

- The use of this term as a diagnostic classification has been discouraged recently. It was used originally to describe the condition in cases where the response to the neurosurgical procedures was not typical. It has been considered to represent a psychological disorder but no diagnostic criteria that is specific has been established.
- Atypical facial pain has been defined as condition where there is pain which is continuous, nagging, variable intensity, deep, migrating and diffuse and is typically in the absence of any other diagnoses.
- By virtue of revision of the Classification of the International Headache Society, ATFP has been recently defined as persistent idiopathic facial pain, and is a condition that is not properly

understood and there is lack of proper diagnostic criteria and lacks proper treatment plan. The pain is typically a persistent pain which lacks the characteristics of cranial neuralgias and cannot be attributed to any other disorder.

- According to the IHS, ATFP can be diagnosed when there is facial pain daily and persists all day long. At the onset the pain is limited to one side of the face especially in the region of the naso-labial fold or one side of the chin, but can spread to involve areas of the upper and lower jaw, or wider areas of the face and neck and is generally poorly localised and deep in nature.

Aetiopathogenesis:

- It is usually psychogenic and occurs in patients who suffer from depressive reaction, hysteria or schizophrenia.
- The initiation of pain can occur due to surgery or trauma of the face, teeth or gingiva and may persist without any local cause that can be demonstrated.
- Nasopharyngeal carcinoma, vascular disease and thalamic infarcts can all produce pain around the face, but are frequently not identified by a standard physical examination.
- Dental and oral diseases including temporo-mandibular joint (TMJ) dysfunction are the commonest causes, and atypical facial pain should be regarded as dental in origin until proven otherwise.
- Dental caries in a lower molar tooth or ulceration of the pharynx, tongue or buccal mucosa may be referred to the ear via the auriculo-temporal branch of the trigeminal nerve, tympanic branch of the glossopharyngeal nerve, or the auricular branch of the vagus nerve.
- Paranasal sinus disease, and cerebrovascular disease, pain may be experienced in the face or forehead.

Clinical manifestations:

- The most common manifestation of ATFP is a pain that is dull and constant and not the brief and severe attacks of pain that are characteristic of trigeminal neuralgia. Examination and laboratory studies can help in diagnosis.
- There is absence of trigger zones, and rarely there is lancinating pain. There is no associated sensory loss or other physical signs.
- It affects women most commonly in the 4th-5th decades. There are often reports of the pain starting soon after a dental procedure such as surgery or restoration.
- Past dental history: The patients give history of taking help of several dental procedure for alleviating the pain and these procedures, give temporary relief and the pain returns in days or weeks.
- In some cases the patients could give a history of procedures of the sinus or of receiving trials of several medications like antibiotics,

corticosteroids, anticonvulsants or decongestants.

- After a surgical procedure spontaneous pain may be localised to an area or migrate. The pain could be unilateral, cross the midline or involve both the maxillary and mandibular regions.

Treatment:

- After the establishment of diagnosis and after exclusion of other conditions, the symptoms should be taken seriously and not ignored.
- The patients need counseling regarding the nature of atypical odontalgia and they should be assured that they donot suffer from undetected and life-threatening disease and they can be helped with non-invasive procedures.
- Sometimes consultation with otolaryngologist, neurologist or psychiatrist can be helpful.
- Amitryptiline, nortryptiline and doxepine, tricyclic antidepressants that are given in low to moderate doses can be effective in reducing or eliminating pain.
- The drugs that may be recommended are gabapentin and clonazepam. Topical desensitisation with capsaicin, anesthetics or doxepin can be effective.

1. Tricyclic Antidepressants:
   (a) **Amitriptyline:** Is the antidepressant that has been found to be effective in chronic OFP treatment. Analgesic trials with TCAs reveal that drugs with mixed serotonin/nor-adrenaline (e.g., imipramine and amitriptyline) or selective serotonin reuptake inhibitors (SSRI), such as fluoxetine or paroxetine. Venlafaxine (75 mg) was found to be modestly effective (B, IIb) in the treatment of atypical facial pain TCAs are given initially at low dosages and are increased gradually to help reduce the adverse effects.

   Dose: 10–25 mg HS, may increase upto 75mg daily if needed.(Amline, Sarotena, Tryptomer 25mg, 75mg tablets SR tablets.)

   (b) **Nortriptyline:** 10–30 mg HS, total daily dosage may be given once a day. (NortriptylineHcl 10 mg capsule, pamelor 10 / 25 mg capsule)

   Drug should be gradually tapered up until the desired therapeutic effect is achieved or side effects develop, such as drowsiness, dry mouth, or weight gain, nausea, vomiting, loss of appetite, anxiety, decreased sex drive.

2. **Gabapentin:** Gabapentin is widely used for neuropathic pain. It is an antiepileptic drug has shown promise in relieving neuropathic pain. It is considered as first line of drug for post herpetic neuralgia, prophylactic effect in migraine, diabetic neuropathy.

   Dose: Treatment should be started at a dose of 100 mg TDS. The dose can also be increased to a maximum of 1200 mg/d for greater efficacy. (Neurontin 300 mg, 400 mg capsule, Gabantin, Gabapin100, 300, 400 mg capsule)

Adverse effect: Hyperlipidemia is one of the important side effects known to occur while other side effects such as dizziness, coordination problems, infections, nausea, vomiting are usually self limiting within ten days of initiation of therapy.

3. **Clonazepam:** It is in a group of drugs called benzodiazepines. Initial dose should not be more than 1.5 mg/day but can be increased at 0.5-1mg every three days in three divided doses until there is control of seizures.
4. **Topical anesthetics:** The use of these on the skin and mucous membrane reduces the systemic absorption and hence the side effects.
   (a) **Capsaicin:** It can be used as a topical cream and is a natural product extracted from chlillies, and is used topically to treat several pain conditions. When first applied, it causes neurogenic inflammation and results in burning sensation, followed by hyperalgesia. But after applying several times the burning and the hyperalgesia resolve.

Availability: 0.025%, 0.075%, 1%, 5% concentration, cream applied four 4 times a day – several weeks found to be effective.

5. **Topical NSAIDs:** Topical NSAIDs applications, which go directly onto the skin at the affected site using rub on creams, gels, patches, and plasters. At the same time, side effects tend to be localized to the site of application, such as itching and rashes.
   1. Diclofenac 1% gel: Voveron, Emulgel, relaxyl gel, diclonac gel, 2 – 3times a day.
   2. Ibuprofen 10 % gel; Ribufen gel, 2 – 3times a day.
   3. Naproxen 10% gel: Naprosyn gel, , 2 – 3times a day.
   4. Ketoprofen 2.5% gel Rhofenoid gel, 2 – 3times a day.
   5. Flurbiprofen 5% gel: Nimulid trans gel, zolandin gel, 2 – 3times a day.

Suggested reading:

1. Bells. Welden E, Orofacial pains classification, Diagnosis, Management third edition. Page 100-101.
2. E. Agostoni, R. Frigerio, P. Santoro, Atypical facial pain: clinical considerations and differential diagnosis, Neurological Sciences May 2005, Volume 26, Supplement 2, pp s71–s74.
3. Quail G, Atypical facial pain--a diagnostic challenge, Aust Fam Physician. 2005 Aug;34(8): 641-5.

Q 2) Define Pain. Give Classification Of Orofacial Pain. Describe Etiology, Clinical Features And Management Of Myofacial Pain Dysfunction Syndrome:

MUHS OCTOBER 2003 (10 Marks)

Definition:

Pain is an unpleasant sensory and emotional experience which is created by a noxious stimulus which is transmitted over a specialised neural network to central nervous system where it is interpreted as such.

Classification:

I. Somatic pain:

- A. Superficial somatic pain:
  1. Cutaneous pain
  2. Mucogingival pain
- B. Deep somatic pain
  1. Musculoskeletal pain
     - (a) Muscle pain
       1. Protective splintic pain
       2. Myofacial trigger point pain
       3. Muscle Spasm pain
       4. Muscle inflammation pain
     - (b) Temporomandibular joint pain
       1. Disc attachment pain
       2. Retrodiscal pain
       3. Capsular pain
       4. Arthritic pain
     - (c) Osseous and periosteal pain
     - (d) Soft connective tissue pain

2. Visceral pain:

- (a) Pulpal dental pain
- (b) Vascular pain
  1. Migrainous neuralgia
  2. Atypical odontalgia
  3. Common migraine
  4. Classic migraine
  5. Vascular inflammation pain
- (c) Visceral mucosa pain
- (d) Glandular, ocular, and auricular pain

(ii) Neuropathic pain:

A. Neuropathic pain

1. Traumatic neuroma pain

2. Paroxysmal neuralgia
   (a) Idiopathic neuralgia
   (b) Symptomatic neuralgia
3. Neuritic neuralgia
   (a) Peripheral neuritis
   (b) Herpes zoster
   (c) Postherpetic neuralgia

B. Deafferentation pain

1. Reflex sympathetic dystrophy (causalgia)
2. Anesthesia dolorosa
3. Atypical odontalgia / Phantom pain

(iii) Psychogenic pain:

A. Chronic Face pain
B. Psychoneurotic pain
   1. Conversion hysteria pain
   2. Delusional pain.

Etiology:

(i) Abnormal occlusion: Painful and damaging contacts lead to modifications in closure pathways and may result in muscle strain and spasm and abnormal pressure on temporo mandibular joint.

(ii) Occlusal abnormalities of teeth causing interference and incoordination and spasm of muscles of mastication.

(iii) Prosthetic problems like ill fitting partial dentures, increased vertical height in partial and complete dentures can lead to MPD syndrome.

(iv) Stress and emotional problems leading to clenching and grinding habits which result in muscle spasm, are thought to be major cause of MPD syndrome as suggested by Laskin in 1969 who then proposed the psychophysiological theory. According to this theory the psychophysiologically motivated oral habits is the most important cause of the painful muscle spasm, though mechanical factors that are related to occlusion can cause this condition by production of overextension or overcontraction of the muscles causing muscle fatigue.

Factors like improper dental restorations, loss of teeth leading to over contraction, dentures, either partial or complete, para-functional oral habits like clenching and grinding, and dental irritation caused by maloccluding restorations or overhanging margins of restoration all lead to this dysfunction syndrome.

(v) Temporomandibular joint problems like hypermobility due to laxity of ligaments and degenerative changes in the joint due to parafunctional habits, or overclosure of the joint due to bilateral loss of molars can ultimately lead to MPD syndrome.

According to Laskin the role played by stress along with

occlusal abnormalities leading to strain and spasm of muscles of mastication, the term myofacial pain dysfunction syndrome is more appropriate term than temporomandibular joint dysfunction syndrome.

NOXIOUS STIMULATION (DUE TO SUCH AS MECHANICAL, EMOTIONAL, INFECTIOUS, MEABOLIC, NUTRITIONAL, OR A COMBINATION OF THESE)

↓

DEVELOPMENT OF SPASM (PROTECTIVE MECHANISM)

↓

SHORTENING OF MUSCLES

↓

LOSE CAPACITY FOR VOLUNTARY RELAXATION AND EXHIBIT AN OVERACTIVE STRETCH REFLEX

↓

INVOLUNTARY SHORTENING OF ONE OR MORE MUSCLES

↓

ECCENTRIC POSITION OF CONDYLES

↓

DISORIENTATION OF JAW MOVEMENTS AND RESTRICTED OPENING OF THE MOUTH

↓

PAIN (DUE TO SPASM AND DECREASED RELAXATION OF MUSCLES)

↓

MORE SPASM OF MUSCLES

Fig. Figure showing the pathopysiology of myofacial pain dysfunction syndrome

Clinical features:

(i) Seen in middle aged group with predilection towards women.

(ii) The symptomatic episodes of pain can occur several times a day and between intervals patient is symptom free. The episodes increase during increased emotional strain and stress.
There is pain in a zone of reference which usually causes patient to seek treatment.

(iii) There is presence of trigger points in the muscles that cause pain on stimulation.

(iv) Taut muscle bands are present.

(v) Restricted jaw opening and associated symptoms.

(vi) No tenderness in the temporomandibular joint.

(vii) Ringing and pain in the ear and tooth ache are also manifestations of this condition.

(viii) Presence of bruxism, indentations on lateral border of tongue, ridging of buccal mucosa and excessive attrition of teeth are present.

Laskins diagnostic criterion:

(a) Unilateral dull aching pain in the ear or preauricular area or at the angle of mandible.
Pain is severe on arising in the morning.

(b) Muscle tenderness in the region of neck of the mandible and distal and superior to maxillary tuberosity.

(c) Clicking or popping noise in the TMJ.

(d) Limitation of jaw movement or deviation of mandible on opening.

Treatment:

(i) The treatment of this condition should be towards a total management rather than just a symptomatic treatment.

(ii) The patients need to be made to understand the reason of this condition and there should be no stress on the psychophysiological factors as the patient might not accept it. The initial information should be about the muscle fatigue and spasm and the explanation for the same.

(iii) Patients should be advised soft diet, and food to be taken as small cut pieces which can be easy to chew.

(iv) They should be educated to reduce the habits of clenching and grinding and also harmful habits like nail biting, lip biting should be advised to be avoided.

(v) Muscle relaxation exercises which include tongue, mouth opening and voluntary resistance exercises.

(vi) Moist heat should be applied for half an hour twice daily.

(vii) The affected area should be massaged with gentle kneading motion, which helps the return of venous blood, lymph and the catabolites that can help to reduce muscle spasm and pain.

(viii) Splint therapy especially if there is clenching and other forms of therapy are unsuccessful like-(i) Stabilization splint (ii) Relaxation splint (iii) Resilient splint (iv) Pivoting splint.

(ix) Physical therapies like ultrasound, high voltage electrogalvanic stimulation, cryotherapy, vapour coolant spray(ethyl chloride) applying over the involved muscle, ice pack application.

(x) Biofeedback which involves visual or auditory information about the contraction status of the muscle being monitored.

(xi) Tens therapy, acupuncture, diathermy, restorations, prosthodontic and orthodontic therapy are other modalities of treatment.

(xii) Pharmacotherapy includes analgesics like aspirin mostly, tranquilisers like benzothiazine derivatives, antidepressants like lithium carbonate, monoamine oxidase inhibitor, sedatives and hypnotics.

(xiii) Anesthetics like injection of local anesthesia in the trigger zones, intra articular anesthetic and hydrocortisone combination to be injected in the TMJ.

Suggested reading:

1. Anil Govindrao Ghom, Text book of Oral Medicine, Third Edition, page 632-636.
2. Ravi Patel, Himanshu Arora, Sarfaraz Memon, Usha Sharma, RamjeeLal Raigar Anant Raghav Sharma, Myofascial Pain - Dysfunction Syndrome: A Dilemma for the Clinicians: J Pre Clin Dent Res 2015; 2(5): 38-43 January-March.

Q 3) What is neuralgia? Describe different types of neuralgia of orofacial origin. Add a note on management of orofacial neuralgia.

TNMGRU

Neuralgia:

Paroxysmal or non-paroxysmal pain along the course of a nerve trunk.
Orofacial neuralgias:

1. Trigeminal neuralgia.
2. Glossopharyngeal neuralgia.
3. Geniculate neuralgia.
4. Occipital neuralgia.
5. Post Herpetic neuralgia.
6. Post-traumatic neuralgia.
7. Auriculotemporal neuralgia:

1. **Trigeminal neuralgia:** Most commonly involves maxillary, then mandibular and ophthalmic nerve.

The etiology includes vascular compression, focal demyelination, autoimmunity, hypersensitivity, and conditions like multiple sclerosis, direct injury to nerve, idiopathic or just aging process.

Clinical features:

- Sharp shooting, flashing, electric shock like, unbearable, moderate to very severe pain.
- One of the highest suicide rates.
- Known as suicide disease.
- Each single episode of pain lasts a few seconds to a maximum of two minutes.
- Pain may recur many times a day for weeks or months.
- periods of complete pain remission and there is no pain between attacks.
- Typical feature is the presence of trigger zones which are supraorbital foramina, infraorbital foramina, inner canthus of eye, lateral to the ala, mental foramen and intraoral areas.
- Triggering factors can be talking, chewing, washing face, shaving, brushing the teeth, wind blowing on face, or spontaneously.
- Relief is obtained by sleeping.

2. **Glossopharyngeal neuralgia:** It is a rare condition similar to trigeminal neuralgia but less intense pain.
   Neuralgia of the 9th nerve.

Etiology:

Most common cause is the intra or extra cranial tumours, and vascular abnormalities that compress the 9th nerve.

Clinical features:

- Trigger zones are present in the region of pharynx, tonsils, posterior tongue, ear, infra auricular and retro mandibular areas.
- Talking and swallowing can trigger the pain.
- It may be associated with a vasovagal reflex, which may cause syncope, hypotension or cardiac arrest.
- Application of topical anesthetic to the pharyngeal mucosa can eliminate pain and help in distinguishing from other neuralgias.

3. **Geniculate neuralgia:**

   Involvement of the sensory intermediate nerve root of the 7th cranial nerve.

   Etiology:

   It results from herpes zoster of the geniculate ganglion and the nervus intermedius of cranial nerve VII.

   Clinical features:

   - Pain is in front of and deep into the ear, anterior tongue and soft palate matching the distribution of the nerve. Pain is also in the deep musculature.
   - Location of pain matches the sensory distribution of the nerve that is in the external auditory canal, soft palate and posterior auricular region.
   - Trigger zone is within the ipsilateral distribution of the nerve.
   - Pain is not as sharp as trigeminal neuralgia and some degree of facial paralysis may occur indicating simultaneous involvement of motor root.

4. **Post herpetic neuralgia:** Pain of herpes zoster that continues for longer than a month is called post herpetic neuralgia.

   Etiology:

   Varicella–zoster virus injuries of the peripheral nerve by demyelination, wallerian degeneration, and sclerosis, and atrophy of dorsal horn cells in the spinal cord are the causes.

   Clinical features:

   - The condition occurs most commonly in individuals above 50 years of age.
   - The incidence is higher in women.
   - There is persistent pain, paresthesia, and hyperesthesia.
   - Pain is associated with sensory deficit.

5. **Occipital neuralgia:** It is a paroxysmal stabbing pain along the distribution of greater or lesser occipital nerves.

   Etiology:

   Trauma, myofacial pain of the neck muscles, neoplasms, infections and aneurysms.

Clinical features:
- Pain is in the occipital and neck regions.
- Palpation below the superior nuchal line may show extreme tender spot.

6. **Post-traumatic neuralgia:**

Etiology:

Trigeminal nerve injuries may result following facial trauma or traumatic surgical procedures like extraction of impacted third molars, placing of dental implants, removal of cysts and tumours of the jaws, genioplasties or osteotomies.

Clinical features:
- The pain is often of burning quality.
- There may be paresthesia, anesthesia and /or dysesthesia depending upon the nerve damage.
- Hyperalgesia may also be present.
- Pain may be persistent or occur on minor stimulation like touch.
- The pain may be diffuse and spread across dermatomes and is usually mild to moderate.

7. **Auriculotemporal neuralgia:** Is a neuralgia of the terminal branch of the mandibular nerve.

Is characterized by attacks of paroxysmal, moderate to severe pain on the preauricular area, often spreading to the ipsilateral temple. More prevalent in middle-aged females. Symptoms are excruciating pain attacks, especially in the temporal region.

Management:

I) Medical management:

It is almost similar for most of the neuralgias.

Carbamazepine:
- Drug of choice.
- Dosage 100-1200mg/Day
- Start With 200mg B.D. Then increase By 100mg, every 2 days to a Maximum of 1200 mg till pain disappears or side effects appear.

Oxcarbazepine:
- Preferred to carbamazepine as there are lesser side effects.
- Maximum dose is 2400-3000 mg/day.

Phenytoin:
- 2nd Drug of choice.
- Dosage 200-600 mg/day.
- Blood level 10-20 micro gm/Ml.
- Less effective than carbamazepine.
- Can be given intravenously for acute relapses of pain.

Baclofen:
- Less effective than carbamazepine.

- Least side effects.
- Dosage 10-80 mg/day.
- Can be combined with carbamazepine.
- It reduces spasticity in many neurological disorders like multiple sclerosis.

Gabapentin:

- Newer anti-epileptic drug.
- Dosage 100-5000 mg/day.
- Start with 300 mg O D.
- Then increase to 300-600 mg TDS.
- First line of drug for pain due to diabetic neuropathy & post herpetic neuralgia.

Valproic acid:

- Broad spectrum anticonvulsant
- Dosage 125-2500 mg/day.
- Blood level 50-100 microgm/ml.
- It increases brain concentration of gamma-aminobutyric acid (gaba).
- Affects sodium channels.

Lamotragine:

- Causes prolongation of na+ channel inactivation.
- Suppression of high frequency firing.
- Dosage 50-500mg/day.
- Blood level 2-5microgm/ml.
- Better tolerated than carbamazepine.

Clonazepam:

- Benzodiazepine.
- It potentiates gaba induced chloride influx to produce sedation.
- Dosage 0.5-8mg/day.
- Other treatments include capsaicin, lidocaine cream, pimozide, amytryptilline, lamotragine, proparacaine eye drops, misoprostol, laser treatment, TENS Therapy, NSAIDS, vitamins and minerals.

II) Surgical treatment:

- Peripheral injections of lidocaine, glycerol, absolute alcohol.
- Microvascular decompression of the involved nerve.
- Percutaneous radio frequency thermocoagulation, glycerol injections and compression of the ganglion by balloon microcompression.
- Rhizotomy, tractotomy of the involved nerve.
- Microsurgical rhizotomy.
- Gammaknife radiosurgery.
- Excision of the involved nerve.

Geniculate neuralgia:

A short course of high dose steroids are beneficial as is acyclovir therapy to reduce pain.

Post herpetic neuralgia:

Along with common modalities of treatment for other neuralgias, in this condition attenuated varicella-zoster virus vaccination is now-a days given as prevention.

Treatment with antiviral drugs at the onset of disease reduces the severity of this condition.

Post-traumatic neuralgias:

Apart from other common treatment modalities for orofacial neuralgias, in this type, systemic corticosteroids help to decrease the incidence and severity of traumatic neuropathies, especially when given in the first week after nerve injury.

Suggested reading:

1. Burket's, Oral Medicine Diagnosis and Treatment 10th edi. 279-282.

Q 4) Give the differential diagnosis of pain in and around the tooth:

RGUHS APRIL 2003 10 Marks

Pain:

Its an unpleasant emotional and sensory experience which is associated with actual or potential tissue damage, or described in terms of such damage.

- A "Toothache or tooth pain" is described as pain in and around the teeth or jaws basically due to dental conditions.
- The most common reasons attributed to tooth pain are dental caries, dental abscess, gingival diseases, tooth root irritations, fractured or cracked tooth syndrome, diseases of the TMJ, impacted teeth and eruption.

1. Pulpitis and dental abscess:

- Tooth ache is most commonly caused due to a cavity caused by dental caries.
- When the cavities are small and not deep, they go unnoticed.
- The cavities that are deeper can cause pain and collection of food debris. The pulp that is vital gets irritated by the bacterial toxins and the foods and liquids that are cold, hot or sour and sweet resulting in pain.
- Pulpitis can occur due to bacterial infection from caries or as a result of thermal and chemical insult following dental treatment as a result of inflammation.It could be reversible or irreversible.
- Severe injury to the pulp can lead to non-vitality of pulp tissue, resulting in periapical infection or apical alveolar abscess. A small gingival abscess also could be present near the tooth and cause pain.

- The pain associated with an abscess is described as throbbing or sudden aching which can last for hours and even days.
- A small and shallow cavity can be treated with dental filling and larger cavities could require a crown.
- However when the pulp is involved the treatment is generally a root canal or extraction of teeth in severe cases.

2. *Peridontal Diseases:*

- Periodontal lesions are the second most important reason for pain in teeth.
- It is caused by gingivitis and the abnormal loss of bone supporting the teeth and is caused by toxins that are secreted by the bacteria in the accumulated plaque.
- Pain is a symptom of more advanced gingival lesions, as the loss of the supporting structures leads to deep periodontal pockets. Bacteria in these pockets cause gingival infection, swelling and pain and results in further destruction of bone.
- Treatment consists of maintenance of oral hygiene and scaling and root planing so as to remove the calculus and plaque.

3. *Cracked tooth syndrome:*

- Its a dental pain that is caused by crack in the tooth and is not associated with caries or advanced periodontal lesions.
- When biting on the cracked tooth, it can lead to sharp shooting pain and this occurs usually on biting hard on hard food stuff and objects like pencils, nuts, bones etc.
- Treatment many a times is extraction but in some cases a full coverage crown could do the needful.

4. *Exposed dentine or cementum:*

- Attrition of tooth can cause exposure of dentine leading to hypersensitivity and pain of the affected tooth.
- Dentine underlying the enamel crown consists of minute tubules that are filled with fluid and connect directly with the nerve endings in the pulp. The dental pain that occurs is thought to be due to the osmolality theory, where in the fluids in the tubules evoke an action potential within the A delta and C fibres in the pulp, when they are mechanically stimulated.
- Gingival recession, recent scaling or erosions on teeth due to acidity can cause pain in teeth.

5. *Sensitivity of the tooth roots:*

- Exposed roots of teeth can also lead to painful tooth.
- The toxins from the bacteria affect the bone around the roots and cause the gingiva and the bone to recede, exposing the roots. This gingival recession can cause pain.
- The roots that are exposed can become very sensitive to the cold,

hot, and sour food and liquids as they are no longer protected by the supporting gingivae and bone.
- If the root exposure causes involvement of the pulp, a root canal may be required or extraction of tooth could be necessary.

6. ***Pericoronitis:***
   - Very common cause of dental pain can be due to teeth that are erupting or are impacted. Pain arises due to infection of the surrounding gingiva and mucosa of the erupting or impacted tooth. Acute pericoronitis most frequently affects the mandibular third molar. The upper molar tooth could impinge on the swollen flap of the soft tissue covering the lower molar and can aggravate the pain.
   - Pain may be continuous or intermittent and is aggravated on biting.
   - Impacted teeth can exert pressure on the adjacent teeth and especially if the other tooth is inflammed and infected it can result in severe dental pain. The treatment is usually analgesics, antibiotics and ultimately extraction of the impacted teeth.
7. ***Acute necrotising ulcerative gingivostomatitis:***
   - It is a fusospirochetal infection causing ulcerations in the interdental gingival.
   - Very often patients may feel pain in the teeth of affected area especially when chewing.
8. ***Post endodontic treatment:***
   - There can be severe aching pain in the teeth after endodontic treatment like root canal therapy or apicectomy.
   - The pain usually starts as sharp stabbing pain and then becomes dull and throbbing. Initially it can be created by a stimulus but later may continue without the stimulus.
   - This kind of tooth pain gets aggravated on lying down and can hinder the sleep of the patients. Heat application can increase and cold can reduce the pain.
9. ***Disorders of the TMJ:***
   - TMJ disorders can cause pain in and around the ears and the lower jaw and can be felt as tooth pain some times which cannot be pin-pointed to a particular tooth.
   - They are caused due to injury arthritis, muscle spasm and fatigue, and habitual clenching and grinding.
   - Teeth grinding can cause pain in the jaws, joints and teeth.
10. ***Muscle pain that is referred:***
    - Myofacial pain is a condition that is typically felt as dull, aching muscles with areas of localised tenderness.
    - These painful areas can refer the pain to other structures.
    - Pain of the muscles of the jaws can refer the pain to the teeth and can be felt as dental or intra-oral pain.

- Over use of the muscles can increase the pain.
- Treatment involves treating the muscles of mastication and reducing the factors that place strain on them.

11. *Trigeminal neuralgia:*

- Its a condition affecting the trigeminal nerve and the pain is described as sharp, shooting lancinating, unbearable pain even on harmless stimulation of the area such as brushing, shaving, washing face etc.
- This pain can some times be felt in the tooth as dental pain.
- When such a condition occurs, it could be difficult to diagnose as the pain has variable features. The presence of trigger zones and the absence of any dental decay can help in differentiating from actual dental pain.
- A proper neurological examination and the imaging of brain can help in diagnosis. Patient education, anticonvulsants and surgical treatment is required to treat this condition.

12. *Neuropathic pain:*

- Damage to the nerves that transmit sensation forms a group of conditions called neuropathic pain.
- The facial pain of neuropathic origin arises after injury to the face, teeth or the periodontal tissues.
- This condition can occur following extraction of teeth, trauma, surgery or in some cases routine dental procedures.
- The resultant effect is pain along with other symptoms like tingling, numbness, hypersensitivity which may persist even after the healing of the injury.

13. *Referral headache pain:*

- Changes in the nerves and blood vessels of the head region can result in migraines, cluster headaches etc.
- In some cases through referral of pain via the trigeminal nerve the headaches can be referred to the teeth and result in pain in teeth.
- The pain is severe throbbing and spontaneous and can have periods of remission.

14. *Cardiac toothache:*

- Problems of the heart such as angina or acute myocardial infarction cause the pain to be referred to the shoulders, arms and also the jaws.
- These conditions can refer pain to teeth also.
- A toothache with cardiac problems as the cause, the pain increases with exercise and reduces with medication for the cardiac conditions.

15. *Toothache associated with maxillary sinus and nasal mucosal conditions:*

- Sinusitis or rhinitis can some times result in pain especially in the maxillary teeth.

- The pain is dull and throbbing in nature and can be felt on several teeth.
- Thermal tests on teeth, chewing and percussion etc can increase the pain in tooth where sinus involvement is the cause.
- Infections of the upper respiratory tract, congestion of the nose or sinusitis or other conditions may lead to toothache.
- Visual examination of the nose, x-rays of the sinus or MRI can help in diagnosis.

16. *Malignancies in the head and neck region:*

- Some tumors, aneurisms and disorders of the intra-cranial region can lead to pain in teeth.
- Tumours of the nasopharynx and cerebellopontine angle tumours may cause referred pain to the teeth.
- The pain in tooth in such cases is associated with other symptoms like malfunctioning of nerve and other systemic symptoms like loss of weight, fatigue.
- When these symptoms occur it can help in deciding that more than a localised cause of tooth pain is present.
- Malignancies involving the oral cavity especially the carcinoma alveolus or central carcinomas and sarcomas of the jaws can cause pain in the teeth of the associated areas. The teeth may become mobile due to severe destruction of the bone.
- Proper radiography of the jaws, head and face region will be important for evaluation of these conditions.

17. *Dysfunction of the salivary glands:*

- Dysfunctions of the salivary glands can lead to referred pain to the teeth. The reason could also be the absence or reduction of salivary flow leading to compromise in the health of the teeth. Comprehensive evaluation of the salivary glands can help in diagnosis.

Suggested reading:

1. Tara Renton, Dental (Odontogenic) Pain Rev Pain. 2011 Mar; 5(1): 2–7.

CHAPTER 8

Gingival and Periodontal Diseases

Q 1) Enumerate the local and systemic causes of gingival enlargement. Describe the clinical and oral changes seen in leukemia and scurvy:

MUHS JUNE 2006 (10 Marks)

I) Local causes:

- Poor oral hygiene.
- Accumulation of plaque and calculus.
- Mouth breathing.
- Physical irritation of the gingiva due to faulty restorations and orthodontic appliances.
- Mal-alignment of teeth which may lead to difficulty in maintaining proper oral hygiene.
- Anterior deep bite.
- Cervical root resorption.
- Anomalies like enamel pearl and cemental tears.
- Root fractures and root perforations causing accumulation of plaque.

II) Systemic factors:

Conditioned enlargement.

- Pregnancy.
- Puberty.
- Deficiency of vitamin C.
- Pyogenic granuloma.

Gingival enlargement due to systemic diseases:

- Leukemia.
- Granulomatous diseases like sarcoidosis, orofacial granulomatosis.
- Neoplasms:
- Benign neoplasms like fibromas, papillomas, and giant cell granulomas.
- Malignant neoplasms like carcinomas and malignant melanoma.

- Gingival enlargements that are false as in cases where there is underlying bony or lesion associated with dental tissue.

Drug-induced enlargement:

Certain drugs such as anti-convulsants: phenytoin, phenobarbital, lamotragine, primidone, topiramate, vigabatrin.

Calcium channel blockers: Nifedipine, amlodipine and verapamil which are anti-hypertensives.

Immunosuppresant: Cyclosporin.

Leukemia:

Its a malignant condition which is progressive and increased number of immature and abnormal leucocytes are produced by the bone marrow and other blood forming organs that ultimately lead to anemia and other symptoms.

Classification:

- Acute:
  - (i) Acute lymphoblastic/ lymphocytic leukemia
  - (ii) Acute myelogenous / nonlymphocytic leukemia
- Chronic:
  - (i) Chronic lymphocytic leukemia
  - (ii) Chronic myelogenous leukemia

Clinical and Oral Manifestations of Leukemia:

- **Acute leukemia:** In acute leukemia there is a failure of maturation of leukocytes.

Clinical features:

- Age- most commonly children and young adults- 15-39 years.
- Sex- males more commonly affected than Females.
- Onset- Abrupt stormy onset with pyrexia and enlargement of spleen.
- Symptoms- Weakness, fever, headache, generalized swelling of lymph node, petechiae or hemorrhage in skin and mucous membrane, vomiting, nerve palsy.
- Signs- Due to anemia and thrombocytopenia – pallor, dyspnea, fatigue, petechiae, ecchymosis, epistaxis and melena. There is hepatosplenomegaly and cervical lymphadenopathy. Recurrent infections involving the lungs, urinary tract, skin, mouth, rectum, upper respiratory tract infection.
- Chloroma-localized tumor consisting of leukemic cells, surface of which turns into green when exposed to light due to presence of myeloperoxidase.
- Submental, cervical & pre and post auricular lymph nodes may be involved.

Oral Manifestations:

- Paresthesia of lower lip and chin and toothache.
- Oral mucous membrane shows pallor, ulcerations with necrosis, petechiae, ecchymosis, bleeding tendency.

- Gingival- Hypertrophy with cyanotic discoloration. It appears boggy, edematous, easily bleed.
- Teeth- mobility present.
- Lip- Crusting of lip may be seen.
- Infection- Oral infections like candidial, viral or bacterial infections are serious and potentially fatal complications in leukemic patients.
- Common complications of leukemia seen in the oral cavity are mucositis and infection induced by chemotherapy, also including herpes simplex ulcers and oral candidiasis.

Chronic leukemia:

It is characterised typically by the presence of large leukemic cells and differentiated WBCs in the bone marrow, peripheral blood and other tissues. It is associated with presence of a distinctive chromosomal abnormality i.e Philadelphia chromosome.

Clinical features:

- Most frequently in patients between the age of 35 and 60 years.
- No symptoms are noted by the patient during the first few years, and the disease may be discovered during a routine examination when splenomegaly or an elevated WBC count is noted.
- Early signs and symptoms are usually secondary to anemia or the packing of leukocytes into the spleen and bone marrow.
- The anemia causes weakness, fatigue, and dyspnoea on exertion, while bone pain or abdominal pain in the upper left quadrant results from the spleen and bone marrow changes.
- As the disease progresses, thrombocytopenia can cause petechiae, ecchymoses, and hemorrhage.

Oral manifestations:

- **Gingiva:** The most common oral finding is hypertrophy of gingiva associated with bleeding. There may be ulceration with necrosis and gangrenous degeneration with dark brown exudates and foul odor.
- Tongue is frequently swollen and dark.
- Regional lymphadenopathy is present.
- Rapid loosening of teeth due to necrosis of periodontal ligament has been reported.
- Destruction of alveolar bone is also seen.

Scurvy:

Deficiency of vitamin C for a prolonged time can result in scurvy.There is characteristic weakening of blood vessels and weak muscular support.

Clinical manifestations:

- **Infantile scurvy:** There is anorexia, lassitude, pain in the limbs, and enlargement of the costo-chondral junction.
- **Folliculosis:** There is rise of hair follicles above the skin and there

is perifollicular hemorrhages i.e tiny bleeding points around the hair follicle with piling up of keratin like material.

- Hemorrhage- in joints, in nerve sheath, under the nail or conjunctiva. Petechial hemorrhage in buttock, abdomen, legs, arm, ankle, nail bed. There may be bleeding from nose, anemia and wound healing could be delayed.
- Subperiosteal hemorrhage.
- Edema- on limb, face.
- Other features- premature aging, thyroid insufficiency.

Oral manifestations:

- Affects gingival and periodontal tissues.
- Scorbutic buds: Interdental and marginal gingiva swollen and bright red in colour, smooth and shiny surface producing appearance like scurvy bud. In later cases there is bogginess of the gingiva, ulcerations and easy bleeding.
- Gingiva appears violaceous red.
- Associated with fetid breath.
- Severe cases: Hemorrhage and swelling of periodontal ligament membrane, bone loss and loosening of teeth.

Suggested reading:

1. Anil Govindrao Ghom, textbook of oral medicine, 3rd edition, and 35, 340-344.
2. Burket's, Oral Medicine Diagnosis & Treatment, 10th edition, 443-448.
3. Newman MG, Takei HH, Klokkevold PR, Carranza FA (2012). Carranza's clinical periodontology (11th ed.). St. Louis, Mo.: Elsevier/Saunders. pp. 84–96.

CHAPTER 9

Diseases of Maxillary Sinus

Q 1) Enumerate the diseases of the maxillary sinus. write in detail about clinical features, radiographic features, differential diagnosis and management of the Squamous cell carcinoma of maxillary antrum.

MUHS MAY 2009 (10 Marks)

Diseases associated with the maxillary sinuses include both intrinsic diseases (originating primarily from within the sinus), and those that originate outside the sinus (most commonly odontogenic disease) that either impinge on or infiltrate the sinus.

1. **Traumatic:**
   - (a) Fracture of maxilla, tuberosity, nasal bone, zygoma and orbital floor.
   - (b) Blow out fracture.
   - (c) Isolated injury.
   - (d) Complex fracture.
   - (e) Hematoma due to traumatic injury.
   - (f) Foreign bodies displaced into the sinus- fractured tooth/ root.
   - (g) Oral antral fistula.
   - (h) Sinus contusion.
2. **Infection /Inflammatory conditions:**
   - (a) Non specific:
     - Acute and chronic sinusitis
     - Mucositis
     - Antral polyp
     - Empyema
     - Osteomyelitis
     - Osteoradionecrosis
   - (b) Specific
     - Actinomycosis
     - Aspergillosis
     - Blastomycosis
     - Histoplasmosis

- Leprosy
- Mucormycosis
- Leprosy
- Syphilis
- Sarcoidosis
- Tuberculosis
- Wegners granulomatosis
- Pseudo tumor

3. Cysts:

(a) Intrinsic:

- Mucus retention cyst(mucocele)
- Pseudo cyst
- Surgical ciliated cyst

(b) Extrinsic:

(i) Odontogenic

- Radicular
- Primordial
- Keratocyst
- Dentigerous

(ii) Non odontogenic

- Globullomaxillay
- Traumatic cyst
- Aneurismal bone cyst

4. Neoplasm:

(a) Benign:

(i) Odontogenic:

- Ameloblastoma
- Adenoameloblastoma
- Compound and complex composite odontome
- Calcified odontogenic epithelial tumor
- Cementoma

(ii) Non-odontogenic:

- Exostosis
- Enostosis
- Osteoma
- Chondroma
- Central haemangioma
- Antral polyp
- Antral papilloma
- Giant cell granuloma

(b) Malignant:

- Squamous cell carcinoma
- Midline lethal granuloma
- Multiple myeloma
- Metastatic carcinoma of the maxillary sinus

- Invasion by local malignant disease.

5. Metabolic and endocrinal:

1. Hyperparathyroidism
2. Fibrous dysplasia
3. Cherubism
4. Pagets disease
5. Langerhans cell histocytosis
6. Caffeys disease
7. Osteopetrosis
8. Cooleys anemia

6. Developemental

(a) Crouzon syndrome
(b) Treacher Collin's syndrome
(c) Binder syndrome

7. Calcification

(a) Anthroliths

Squamous cell carcinoma of the maxillary antrum:

Squamous cell carcinoma likely originates from metaplastic epithelium of the sinus mucosal lining.

Clinical Features:

- The most common symptoms of cancer in the maxillary sinus are facial pain or swelling, nasal obstruction, and a lesion in the oral cavity.
- The mean age of the patient is 60 years (range 25 to 89 years).
- Twice as many men as women are affected.
- Lymph nodes are involved in about 10% of cases, and the symptoms are present for about 5 months before diagnosis.
- Symptoms: Facial pain, swelling and nasal obstruction, unilateral nasal stiffness, intense pain or paresthesia of mid face.
- Sign: Ulceration or mass seen on the palate.
- Symptoms produced by neoplasms in the maxillary sinus depend on which wall(s) of the sinus is/are involved.
  (i) The medial wall is usually the first to become eroded, leading to such nasal signs and symptoms as obstruction, discharge, bleeding, and pain. These symptoms may appear trivial, and their significance may not be appreciated.
  (ii) Lesions that arise on the floor of the sinus may first produce dental signs and symptoms, including expansion of the alveolar process, unexplained pain and numbness of the teeth, loose teeth, and swelling of the palate or alveolar ridge and ill-fitting dentures. The neoplasm may erode the floor and penetrate into the oral cavity. Such oral manifestations appear in 25% to 35% of patients with cancer in the maxillary sinus.
  (iii) When the lesion penetrates the lateral wall, facial and

vestibular swelling becomes apparent and the patient may complain of pain and hyperesthesia of the maxillary teeth.

(iv) Involvement of the sinus roof and the floor of the orbit cause symptoms related to the eye: diplopia, proptosis, pain, and hyperesthesia or anesthesia and pain over the cheek and upper teeth.

(v) Invasion and penetration of the posterior wall lead to invasion of the muscles of mastication, causing painful trismus, obstruction of the eustachian tube causing a stuffy ear, and referred pain and hyperesthesia over the distribution of the second and third divisions of the fifth nerve.

Radiographic Features:

- In early stage radiographic features are non specific and thus difficult to differentiate between radiopacity due to sinusitis and polyp formation.
- As the lesion enlarges it may destroy sinus walls and leads to radiolucent areas in the surrounding bone. irregular widening of the periodontal ligament space.
- Medial wall may be thinned or destroyed and may extend into the nasal cavity.
- Destruction of the floor and the anterior and posterior walls may be detected.
    1. **Location:** Most carcinomas occur in the maxillary sinuses, but involvement of the frontal and sphenoid sinuses is also comparatively common.
    2. **Internal structure:** The internal aspect of the maxillary sinus has a soft tissue radiopaque appearance.
    3. **Effects on surrounding structures:** As the lesion enlarges, it may destroy sinus walls and in general, cause irregular radiolucent areas in the surrounding bone. A detailed examination of the adjacent alveolar process may reveal bone destruction around the teeth or irregular widening of the periodontal ligament space. Frequently the medial wall of the maxillary sinus is thinned or destroyed, although there may also be destruction of the floor and anterior or posterior walls that may be detected in the panoramic film. The medial wall of the maxillary sinus is best seen on the Caldwell and Waters projections. In addition to loss of the medial wall, it may extend into the nasal cavity.
- Differential diagnosis:
    - Sinusitis
    - Large retention pseudocysts
    - Odontogenic cysts.
    - Neoplasm should be suspected in any older patient in whom chronic sinusitis develops for the first time without obvious cause.

Treatment:

- Cytotoxic drug – local infusion of the cytotoxic drugs may be helpful for pain control.
- Radiotherapy – main mode of treatment, course of high voltage radiotherapy or gamma rays are given.
- If radiotherapy is ineffective then surgical excision of the maxilla is done.
- Reconstruction – after surgery, sophisticated prosthesis should be constructed.

References:

1. Anil Govindrao Ghom;' Textbook of Oral Medicine'; Edi-3, Chapter: 24;649-650.
2. Freny Karjodkar Essentials of Oral and Maxillofacial Radiology; Ch 26; Pg483.
3. Stuart C White, Michael J Pharoah, Oral Radiology Principles And Interpretation 5th edition, Chapter: 26; Page 587- 588.

CHAPTER 10

Immunologic Diseases

Q 1) Define autoimmune disease. Enumerate autoimmune diseases that have direct and indirect effect on oral cavity.

RGUHS OCTOBER 2005 (9 Marks)

Definition:

Its a disorder in which there is production of antibodies by the body that attack its own tissues, which leads to deterioration and in some cases to destruction of the tissues.

Autoimmune diseases (ADs) are characterized by an aberrant chronic activation of the immune system which causes tissue inflammation and damage in genetically predisposed individuals.

Autoimmune diseases occur in up to 3-5% of the general population. They are common in females for which, the reason is unknown.

Autoimmune diseases that have direct and indirect effect on oral cavity:

I) Hematological disorders:

Autoimmune Hemolytic Anemia (AIHA) is characterized by the presence of auto antibodies directed to antigens on the individuals own red cell membrane.

Oral manifestations include deposition of blood pigment in the enamel and dentin of the developing teeth, giving them a green, brown or blue hue. The stain is intrinsic and does not involve teeth or portions of teeth developing after cessation of hemolysis.

Immune Thrombocytopenic Purpura (ITP) is an autoimmune disorder characterized by a low platelet count and mucocutaneous bleeding.

Oral manifestations include gingival bleeding, petechiae, mucocutaneous bleeding and haemorrhage into tissues. Petechiae occur in the oral mucosa more commonly on the palate and appear as numerous tiny, grouped clusters of reddish spots only a millimeter or less in diameter.

II) Pernicious anemia:

Glossitis is the most common oral manifestation of pernicious anemia. Tongue is smooth and beefy red because of atrophic glossitis. Atrophy of papillae leads to bald tongue. Taste sensation also may be diminished.

III) Dermatologic diseases:

Pemphigus Vulgaris:

Pemphigus is a group of potentially life-threatening autoimmune mucocutaneous diseases characterized by supraepithelial bullae of the skin or the mucous membrane and the term is derived from Greek word Pemphix that means a bubble or blister.

Oral lesions typically run a chronic course, causing bullae, erosions, and ulcers.

Intact bullae are uncommon in the mouth.

Bullous Pemphigoid:

It is a subepidermal bullae forming disease affecting skin and mucous membrane characterized by dermal-epidermal junction separation, an inflammatory cell infiltration in the upper part of the dermis, and the autoanti-bodies that are targeted towards the hemidesmosomal proteins, BP230 and BP180.

Oral lesions begin as bullae, but they tend to rupture sooner, probably as a result of constant low-grade trauma to which the oral mucosa is subjected. Large, shallow ulcerations with smooth, distinct margins are present after the bullae rupture. Sometimes erosions are confined to the gingiva creating a picture of chronic desquamative gingivitis.

Cicatricial Pemphigoid (CP) or mucous membrane pemphigoid (MMP):

It is a rare chronic autoimmune disorder.

Oral mucosa is the most frequent site of involvement in patients with cicatricial pemphigoid and it is often the first site affected.

Lesions most commonly involve the gingiva, buccal mucosa, and palate.

The most frequent oral manifestation is desquamative gingivitis.

In severe disease, adhesions may develop between the buccal mucosa and the alveolar process, around the uvula and tonsillar fossae and between the tongue and floor of the mouth.

Psoriasis:

Its a chronic inflammatory disease of the skin with a strong genetic basis.

Oral psoriasis involves 2% of psoriatic patients.

They are commonly seen on lips, buccal mucosa, palate, gingiva and floor of the mouth.

The disease has typical patterns that range from white, raised, scaly lesions, commonly on the palate or the buccal mucosa, and also could be well demarcated, flattened, lesions that are erythematous with slightly raised, white, annular or serpiginous border.

Epidermolysis Bullosa Acquisita:

Is a chronic subepidermal blistering disease.

Oral lesions are rare and when involved will form large hemorrhagic bullae, most commonly on the buccal mucosa which heal with scar formation.

Oral Lichen Planus:

Oral lesions in lichen planus is present in 70-77% of dermatologically affected patients.

There are six recognized oral manifestations:

1. Reticular,
2. Papular,
3. Plaque,
4. Atrophic,
5. Erosive,
6. Bullous.

Reticular lichen planus is most common type affecting the oral cavity. Lesions consist of radiating white or gray, velvety, threadlike papules in a linear, annular or retiform arrangement forming typical lacy, reticular patches, rings and streaks over the buccal mucosa and to a lesser extent on the lips, tongue and palate.

Papular type is rare and present as small white raised papules of 0.5-1.5mm in diameter.

Plaque type appears as homogenous white patches which resemble leukoplakia.

Atrophic Lichen Planus presents as a diffuse red or erythroplakia type lesions.

In erosive lichen planus there are often extensive areas of erosion, which are irregular and affect mainly the buccal and the lingual mucosa and associated often with white lesions. Involvement of the gingiva produces desquamative gingivitis.

Bullous lichen planus is the least common type.

Erythema multiforme:

It is an acute, self-limiting disorder and is so called multiforme because it manifests variety of skin lesions.

Oral manifestations range from tender superficial erythematous and hyperkeratotic plaques to painful deep hemorrhagic bullae and erosions. The lips are commonly involved and may exhibit bloody crusty appearance. There is constant drooling of blood tinged saliva and eating and drinking process is hampered.

IV) Diabetes Mellitus Type I(IDDM):

Among various types of diabetes the insulin dependent type has an autoimmune basis.

In the oral cavity median rhomboid glossitis is considered as a specific pathognomonic oral manifestation associated with diabetes.Other features include gingivitis, periodontitis, oral candidiasis, burning tongue and delayed healing of tooth sockets after extraction.

V) Systemic autoimmune diseases:

Systemic lupus erythematosus(SLE):

Is a chronic, multi-systemic disease of unknown etiology.

Oral lesions of SLE develop in 5% to 25% of patients.

The lesions usually affect the palate, buccal mucosa and gingiva. Sometimes they appear as lichenoid areas, but they may also look nonspecific or even somewhat granulomatous. Varying degrees of ulceration, pain, erythema and hyperkeratosis may be present. Other oral complaints are xerostomia, stomatodynia, candidiasis, periodontal disease and dysgeusia.

Rheumatoid Arthritis:

Is a chronic systemic inflammatory disorder that may principally attack the joints.

The Temporomandibular joint (TMJ) is affected to some degree in more than 40% of persons with rheumatoid arthritis.

If TMJ is involved it is usually bilateral and occurs late in the disease.

The signs and symptoms include stiffness, crepitation, pain or ache, tenderness and limitation of mouth opening.

Sjogren syndrome:

SS is a chronic autoimmune disorder that has typical features of dry eyes, dry mouth, which is the result of destruction of the lacrimal and salivary gland that is immune mediated.

Subjective symptoms include mouth dryness, which is also called as xerostomia, which is a main feature of the SS. Severity of this dryness varies from patient to patient.

Other manifestations include, the increased need for liquid intake, difficulty in chewing, particularly dry foods, sensitivity to acids and alterations in the voice.

There is a feeling of burning and tingling sensation in the mouth and there is frequent hoarseness of the voice and a change in the sense of smell.

Objective oral manifestations consists of dryness of the oral cavity, reduction or inability to produce saliva, and difficulty in talking. There is dental caries in about 70% of the patients, and in 85% of cases, oral infections, especially candidiasis occurs.

Systemic sclerosis:

Is a chronic disease characterized by diffuse sclerosis of the skin, gastrointestinal tract, heart, muscle, lungs, and kidney.

The lips of a patient with scleroderma may appear to be pursed due to constriction of the mouth aperture, thus making it difficult to open the mouth.

Tongue becomes stiff and board like, causing difficulty in eating and speaking.

Gingival tissues are pale and firm.

The oral mucosa appears pale and feels rigid.

Reiter's Syndrome:

Is characterized by presentation of polyarthritis, ocular lesions and aseptic urethritis.

The oral lesions occur in less than 20% of patients with this disorder.

Lesions appear as painless, red, slightly elevated areas sometimes granular or even vesicular with a white circinate border on buccal mucosa, lips and gingiva.

Behcet's syndrome:

A disease of cause that is unknown, it is an inflammatory disorder which is characterised by recurrent oral aphthous ulcers, genital ulcers, uveitis and lesions of the skin.

The oral lesions are painful and very similar in appearance to recurrent aphthous ulcers. Ulcers are round, few mm to a cm in diameter having an erythematous border and covered by yellowish exudates occurring on soft palate and oropharynx.

Recurrent aphthous stomatitis is a disease that is common and is characterised by painful, recurrent, solitary or multiple ulcers of the oral mucosa. Based upon the clinical manifestations recurrent aphthous stomatitis has been classified into four categories: (1) Recurrent aphthous minor (2) Recurrent aphthous major (3) Recurrent herpetiform ulcerations and (4) Recurrent ulcers associated with Behcet's syndrome.

The minor aphthous begins as an ulcerative lesion having a well-circumscribed margin surrounded by an erythematous halo. The lesion is very painful and interferes with eating.

Recurrent aphthous major ulcers are large, oval, painful which may exceed 1cm in diameter and may approach upto 3cm, usually 1-10 in number occurring on the lips, cheeks, tongue, soft palate and fauces.

Recurrent herpetiform ulcers are characterized by crops of multiple small, shallow ulcers, often up to 100 in number, which may occur at any site in the oral cavity.

Suggested reading:

1. Mays JW, Sarmadi M, Moutsopoulos NMJ, Oral manifestations of systemic autoimmune and inflammatory diseases: diagnosis and clinical management, Evid Based Dent Pract. 2012 Sep;12(3 Suppl): 265-82.
2. Ravikiran Ongole, Textbook of oral medicine, oral diagnosis and oral radiology; 2nd edition.Chapter 20.Page no.-590-604.
3. Sridevi P, Munisekhar MS, Harika CH, Rama Krishna: Oral Manifestations of Autoimmune Diseases International Journal of Oral & Maxillofacial Pathology. 2012;3(4): 27-33

CHAPTER 11

Hematologic Diseases

Q 1) Enumerate the causes of cervical lymphadenopathy and clinical features of Hodgkins disease.

RUGHS APRIL 2005 9 Marks

Causes of cervical lymphadenopathy are as follows:

1. **Malignancies:**
   - Malignancies involving the oral cavity and areas of head and neck.
   - Lymphomas, Leukemias, Kaposi's sarcoma.
   - Langerhan's cell histiocytosis.
2. **Metastatic carcinoma to cervical nodes:** The cervical lymph nodes are more frequently the site of metastatic carcinomas than of primary tumors (lymphomas).
3. **Infections: Can lead to acute lymphadenitis:**
   - (a) **Bacterial:** Dental, Ear, Nose, Throat, Scalp, Cat-scratch disease, Mycobacterial lymphadenitis, Tuberculosis, Brucellosis, Syphillis, Leprosy, diphtheria.
   - (b) **Viral:** Upper respiratory tract infections, Oral, Infectious hepatitis, Herpes simplex, Measles, rubella, Infectious mononucleosis, Cytomegalovirus, HIV infection.
   - (c) **Fungal:** Histoplasmosis, Blastomycosis.
   - (d) **Chlamydial:** Lymphogranuloma venereum.
   - (e) **Parasitic:** Toxoplasmosis, Leishmaniasis.
4. **Autoimmune Disease:** Rheumatoid arthritis, systemic Lupus eryhthematosus, Sjogren's syndrome, Drug hypersensitivity.
5. **Miscellaneous and unusual conditions:** Castlemans' disease, Familial mediterranean fever, Sarcoidosis, kawasaki disease, Histiocytosis X.
6. **Iatrogenic causes:**
   - (a) Drugs: Allopurinol, Atenolol, Captopril, Carbamazepine, Gold, Penicillins, Phenytoin Primidone, Pyrimethamine, Quinidine.

(b) Serum sickness.

6. **Nontender lymphoid hyperplasia:** The majority of nontender benign enlargements of the cervical lymph nodes are lesions of nontender lymphoid hyperplasia.

Clinical features: Hodgkin's disease:

(i) It is characterized by age incidence that is bimodal, first peak in the young adults and the second peak in the 5th decade of life and affects males and females equally.

(ii) The onset is insidious, usually with painless enlargement of superficial nodes of one group. The cervical nodes are usually the first to be involved, but may also begin in the mediastinal abdominal, axillary, pelvic or inguinal nodes. The nodes of the neck that includes cervical and supraclavicular nodes. In about 80-90% of the cases the lymphnodes, cervical and supraclavicular nodes are involved. The chest lymph nodes are also affected often and can be so seen in the chest radiographs.

(iii) Cough, dyspnoea, and anorexia.

(iv) Itchy skin.

(v) Night sweats.

(vi) Unexplained weight loss.

(vii) Low grade fever.

(viii) Enlargement of the spleen occurs in about 40% of the patients with Hodgkin's lymphoma, however the enlargement is rarely massive and the size may fluctuate during the course of treatment.

(ix) Hepatomegaly: Increase in the size of the liver is present in about 5% of cases.

(x) Enlargement of the liver and spleen both can occur with the same disease.

(xi) Pain following alcohol consumption occurs in the involved nodes is common and its specificity is very high and can be regarded as pathognomonic of the Hodgkin's disease. The pain starts typically within just minutes after alcohol consumption. The pain could be sharp and stabbing or dull and aching.

(xii) Back pain that is non-specific and lower back commonly in Hodgkin's lymphoma has been reported in some cases.

(xiii) Due to low platelet count, red coloured patches on the skin, bleeding easily and petechiae are common.

(xiv) Very typical of this condition is very high fever that occurs in cyclical pattern and is called as Pel-Ebstein fever.

(xv) There is possibility of occurrence of nephrotic syndrome in cases of Hodgkin's lymphoma.

Oral manifestations:

- Lesions of the jaws as primary lesions are uncommon.
- Its effect secondarily can be seen in the oral cavity in the form of infections as a result of reduced host-immune response.

- Appearance: It may occur as an ulcer or a swelling or as an intrabony lesion, in which case it occurs as a hard swelling.
- Refer to short answer question.

Suggested reading:

1. Armitage JO (August 2010). "Early-stage Hodgkin's Lymphoma". N. Engl. J. Med. 363 (7): 653–62.
2. Parisi E, Glick M. Cervical lymphadenopathy in the dental patient: a review of clinical approach. Quintessence Int. 2005 Jun;36(6): 423-36.
3. Norman K wood, Paul.W.Goaz, Differential Diagnosis of Oral and Maxillofacial Lesions, 5th edition, 526-529.

Q 2) Define and classify Anemias. Discuss in detail about Iron Deficiency anemia:

RGUHS OCTOBER 2002 9 Marks

Definition: It is an abnormal reduction in the circulating blood cells number, the quantity of hemoglobin and the volume of packed red cells in a given unit of blood.

Classification:

1. Anemias with disturbed iron metabolism:
   - Iron deficiency anemia
   - Sideroblastic anemia
2. Megaloblastic anaemia:
   - Pernicious anemia.
   - Folic acid deficiency.
3. Anemia associated with chronic disorders:
   - Anemia of chronic infection.
   - Anemia of inflammatory connective tissue disorder.
   - Anemia associated with malignancy.
   - Secondary to chronic bleeding.
   - Myelophehisic anemia.
   - Anemia of uremia.
   - Anemia of endocrine failure.
   - Anemia of liver disease.
   - Hemolytic anemia
   - Extrinsic causes.
   - Splenomegaly.
   - Red cell antibodies.
   - Trauma in circulation.
   - Direct toxic effects.

- Membrane abnormalities.
  - Spur cell anemia
  - Paroxysmal nocturnal hemoglobinemia.
  - Hereditary spherocytosis.
  - Herediatary elliptocytosis.
- Disorders of interior of red cell:

- Defects in the embden myerhof pathway.
- Defects in hexose monophosphate shunt.

- Disorders of haemoglobin:
  - Sickle cell anemia.
  - Thalassemia.

Iron deficiency anemia:

Iron is essential for synthesis of 'heme' portion of haemoglobin.

Iron deficiency anemia is caused by imbalance between iron intake and loss or inadequate utilization.

Iron deficiency is the single most prevalent nutritional deficiency worldwide.

Risk factors:

- As women loose blood during menstruation, they are at greater risk for developing iron deficiency anemia.
- Infants and children especially with low birth weight and born prematurely and those who fail to get sufficient iron from breast milk or formula are prone to develop this condition.
- People who are vegetarians, don't eat meat and if they dont eat other iron rich foods can develop this condition.
- People routinely donating blood can suffer from depleted stores of iron and are at higher risk of developing this kind of anemia.

Etiology:

- **Inadequate intake:** inadequate intake or insufficient iron in diet may lead to deficiency. Foods that are rich in iron include meat, eggs, green leafy vegetables and foods fortified with iron.
- **Malabsorption:** malabsorption of iron due to hypochlorhydria and diarrhea may lead to deficiency. Intestinal disorders like the celiac disease may affect the efficiency of the intestines to absorb nutrients from food leading to iron deficiency anemia and also if part of the small intestine has been removed surgically, it can affect the absorption of iron and other nutrients.
- In pregnancy iron supplements if not given can lead to this kind of anemia because their iron stores need to serve their increased volume of blood and also have to provide the source of hemoglobin for the growing fetus.
- **Increased requirement:** increase requirement of iron in a growing child.
- Increase loss of iron due to injury, recurrent epistaxis, peptic ulcer. Chronic blood loss due to menstrual or menopausal bleeding. Bleeding from the GIT can occur due to over use of the over-the counter pain killers and aspirin.
- **Gastrotomy:** Sub total or complete gastrotomy may cause iron deficiency anemia.

Stages of iron deficiency anemia:

- Prelatent iron deficiency- body storage of iron are depleted but circulating hemoglobin and serum iron remain normal.
- Latent iron deficiency- in it body storage of iron are exhausted and serum iron is reduced.
- Early anemia- in which hemoglobin concentration is reduced. Serum iron is low.
- Marked anemia – Hemoglobin concentration is below 10 gm/ 100 ml of blood.

Clinical features:

- It occurs chiefly in women in 4th and 5th decades of life.
- The patient experiences tiredness, headache paraesthesia, lack of concentration.
- Nails becomes brittle, flattened and spoon shaped and is termed as koilonychia.
- Neuropathy: Tingling and pins and needle sensation in extremities.
- Dysphagia- patients developing pharyngeal mucosal web formation.
- Gastrointestinal symptoms- liver and spleen may be palpable.
- Patient may get Knuckle pigmentation.
- Sideropenic anemia- iron gets accumulated in mitochondria and appears as a ring of granules round the nucleus. These are called ring sideroblasts.

Oral manifestations:

1. Pallor of mucosa- in iron deficiency anemia pallor of oral mucosa and gingiva is the most common sign. The normal pink color is lost due to lack of oxygenated blood in capillary bed in lamina propria and is associated with lowered levels of haemoglobin.
2. Atrophy of oral mucosa on tongue and buccal mucosa.
3. Redness, soreness or burning of tongue. Filiform papillae of the anterior two third of the tongue are the first to undergo atrophy, and later the fungiform papillae may also be involved leading to smooth, bald tongue.
4. Cracking and fissuring at corner of mouth causing angular cheilitis.
5. Softening of epithelium which leads to linear ulceration of skin upto and beyond mucocutaneous junction. Recurrent aphthous ulceration and candidiasis can also occur in iron deficiency anemia.
6. Slow healing: after oral surgical procedures.
7. Gingival enlargement can occur in some cases.

Diagnosis:

Clinical:

Koilonychias, Neuropathy, Angular cheilitis, Depapillation of tongue may help in diagnosis.

Laboratory and other diagnostic aids:

1. Anemia is microcytic and hypochromic and peripheral smear show abnormal forms of RBC's.
2. Reduced hemoglobin level as low as 4gm/100 ml.
3. Normal or slightly reduced RBC count.
4. MCV, MCH, MCHC are all reduced.
5. Ferritin: This protein is responsible for storing iron in the body and low levels of this can indicate low levels of iron in the body.
6. Endoscopy: Its done to check bleeding from hiatus hernia or an ulcer present in the stomach.
7. Colonoscopy: Its recommended to rule out bleeding from the lower intestinal sources.
8. Ultrasound: This procedure is carried in pelvic area of women to find out the causes of excess menstrual bleeding like the fibroids.

Management:

- The etiology of iron deficiency should be established and the underlying cause can be treated.
- Oral contraceptives can be given to reduce the menstrual blood flow.
- For treatment of peptic ulcers antibiotics and other medicines can be given.
- Surgery can be performed to remove a polyp that could be bleeding, tumours or fibroids.

Supplememt of iron:

The ferrous iron supplements that are generally prescribed are, ferrous fumarate, ferrous gluconate and ferrous sulphate.

Almost all patients can be treated by oral supplements of iron by giving ferrous fumerate or ferrous sulphate. It is given in dose of 300mg three to four times a day for a period of 6 months.

The daily dose that is recommended are 150mg/day-180mg/day of elemental iron that is given in divided doses twice or thrice/day.

The parenteral route of administration is suitable for few patients who are unable to take iron by mouth or who are unable to or absorb iron by mouth.

Iron intravenously or non-viable red cells give about 80-160mg of iron/day.

The recommended single dose of iron sorbitol is 1.5mg of iron per kg of body weight, given daily.

Suggested reading:

1. Anil Govindrao Ghom, textbook of oral medicine 3rd edition, 858-859.
2. Terri D. Johnson-Wimbley, David Y. Graham Diagnosis and management of iron deficiency anemia in the 21st century Therapy, Adv Gastroenterol. 2011 May; 4(3): 177–184.

CHAPTER 12

Miscellaneous

Q 1) Discuss in details the different conditions producing chronic sinuses in angle of mandible.

TNMUGRU FEBRUARY 2009 (10 Marks

A sinus (hollow, bay, or curve) is the tract of a lesion that has one opening.

Classification for different condition producing chronic sinuses in angle of mandible:

Inflammatory Conditions:

- Chronic dentoalveolar / periodontal abscess
- Chronic osteomyelitis
- Osteoradionecrosis
- Infected Cysts
- Suppurative infection of the parotid and submandibular salivary gland
- Pustule
- Infected lymphnodes
- Space infection

Infectious Diseases:

- Actinomycosis
- Tuberculosis of jaw
- Syphilis

Malignancy:

- Oral carcinoma / malignancy
- Salivary gland malignancy

Other Conditions:

- Sinus secondary to trauma /injury
- Postsurgical pit / sinuses

Developmental Defects:

- Second branchial sinus

- Congenital aural sinuses

A) Inflammatory Conditions:

1. **Chronic Dentoalveolar and Periodontal Abscess:**
   - The dentoalveolar abscess is a common lesion that is a pyogenic infection of the periodontal ligament and bones and frequently occurs as a draining sinus.
   - Most dentoalveolar abscesses result from a direct extension of an acute pulpitis or an acute nonsuppurative periodontitis or from an acute exacerbation of a periapical granuloma, cyst, or chronic abscess.
   - Less commonly the dentoalveolar abscess arises from an infection of the alveolar socket after surgical removal of a tooth.
   - Sinuses at angle of mandible usually associated with the infection from the mandibular molar roots, particularly of the third molars.
2. **Chronic Osteomyelitis:**
   - Osteomyelitis is an inflammation of the bone caused by pathogenic microorganisms.
   - The sinus extends from the medullary bone through the cortical plate to the mucous membrane or skin.
   - The sinus opening may be close to or distant from the offending infection.
   - The mandible is more frequently involved than the maxilla.
   - The osteomyelitis in posterior body of mandible and ramus of mandible can lead to the sinus formation at the angle of mandible.
3. **Osteoradionecrosis:**
   - Osteoradionecrosis (ORN) is a disease condition of hard and soft tissue after irradiation of the region.
   - When ulceration of the surface mucosa or skin occurs, it forms extraoral sinuses.
   - Osteoradionecrosis involving the retromolar trigone and the alveolus associated with mandibular molar region can form the sinus opening at the angle of mandible.
4. **Cysts:**
   - Infected, Inflammatory cysts associated with mandibular molars, Dentigerous cysts involving impacted mandibular third molar and Odontogenic keratocysts in mandibular ramus / body region can produce sinus at the angle of mandible.
   - The common soft tissue cysts that occur in the mandibular angle region are sebaceous, epidermoid, dermoid, thyroglossal, preauricular and branchial. Secondary infections from this cyst can form sinus at the angle of mandible.
5. **Salivary Gland Diseases:**
   - Malignancies like pleomorphic adenoma, mucoepidermoid

carcinoma, adenoid cystic carcinoma and suppurative infections like bacterial sialadenitis of parotid or the submandibular salivary gland can form the sinus over the skin near to the angle of mandible.

6. **Pustule:**
   - A pustule is a small, superficial elevation of the skin or mucous membrane; it is filled with pus and generally are the result of psoriasis, impetigo, acrodermatitis continua, or superficial bacterial diseases.
   - Pustules become draining lesions for a short time after they rupture and may occur at the angle of mandible region.
7. **Infected Lymphnodes:**
   - Infected submandibular group of lymphnodes can form a draining sinus at or near the angle of mandible.
   - Lymph nodes can be infected secondary to inflammation or infections of dental or periodontal origin from posterior mandibular molars or metastasis of cancer.
8. **Space infection:**
   - Space infections like submandibular or buccal or masseteric space infections can drain as sinus at the angle of mandible.
   - Submandibular space infection is caused due to dental/ periodontal infection by mandibular molars. And if the perforation is below the mylohyoid line it causes the sinus over the skin at the angle of mandible.

B) Infectious Diseases:

1. **Actinomycosis:**
   - It is a chronic granulomatous suppurative disease caused by anaerobic bacteria commonly Actinomyces israeli.
   - The cervicofacial type of Actinomycosis forms the sinus at the angle of mandible.
   - Submandibular region is the most frequent site of infection. Cheek/ masseter region and parotid gland may also be involved.
   - Sinus formation is common in this disease, through which the pus drains.
   - Skin surrounding the sinus is purplish.
2. **Tuberculosis:**
   - Tuberculosis (TB) is a chronic bacterial infection, caused by Mycobacterium tuberculosis that leads to the formation of granulomas in the infected tissues.
   - The bacteria can infect oral tissues and lymph nodes (scrofula) and if the submandibular nodes are involved may form a sinus at the angle of mandible.
   - The lesions involving oral cavity occur in the soft tissue and supporting bone of mandible and in extraction sites of posterior mandibular molars can lead to sinus formation at the angle of mandible.

3. **Syphilis:**
    - Syphilis is a venereal disease caused by spirochetes, Treponema Pallidum.
    - Secondary Syphilis- The ulcers if secondarily infected especially the buccal mucosal lesions near the angle of mandible may penetrate the mucosa over the skin and form a sinus opening.
    - Tertiary Syphilis- Gumma, typical feature of this stage may rapidly progress to large zone of necrosis with denudation of bone. If it is in mandibular posterior alveolus it may perforate to form a sinus at angle of mandible, but it is rare.
4. **Cancrum oris:**
    - It is rarely seen in developed countries, may produce an orocutaneous sinus at the angle of mandible.

C) Malignancy:

1. **Oral carcinoma/Sarcoma:**
    - 90% of Malignancies occurring in the oral cavity are squamous cell carcinoma.
    - Malignancies involving the osseous structures of mandible i.e ramus, retromolar trigone, posterior alveolus of mandible, gingiva of posterior mandibular molars can lead to sinus at angle of mandible.
    - Neoplastic sinus may be the result of disease that has progressed through soft tissue or bone, can perforate to form a sinus. Secondary infections in these carcinomatous lesions can cause draining sinus at the angle of mandible.
    - Sarcoma involving the mandible can get secondarily infected and cause sinus at the angle.
2. **Salivary gland malignancy:**
    - Malignancy like pleomorphic adenoma, mucoepidermoid carcinoma, adenoid cystic carcinoma of parotid gland directly forms the sinus over the skin near to the angle of mandible, because the gland lies superficial over the masseter muscle.
    - The sinuses from submandibular gland infection are formed at the lower border of mandible on lateral side of neck near the angle of mandible.

D) Other Conditions:

1. **Orocutaneous Sinuses Secondary to trauma /injury:**
    - Orocutaneous fistula/sinus is a troublesome defect which may occur rarely at the angle of mandible.
2. **Postsurgical Pit:**
    - The postsurgical pit is the result of wound breakdown secondary to infection or failure to obliterate dead space in wound or improper and inadequate wound closure.
    - The postsurgical pit forms at the angle of mandible after the surgical management of the diseases involving ramus / body of

mandible and soft tissue at the angle of mandible.

E) Developmental Defects:

1. **Second Branchial Sinus (Lateral Cervical Sinus):**
   - A sinus or fistula of the second branchial cleft or pouch is somewhat common in the lateral neck.
   - They sometimes occur in a more superior location along the anterior border of the sternocleidomastoid muscle or near the angle of mandible.
2. **Congenital Aural Sinuses:**
   - Congenital aural sinuses (auricular fistulae, preauricular fistulae, preauricular pits) occur in approximately 1% of the population.
   - Very few or rarely may occur near the angle of mandible.

Suggested reading:

1. Stuart C White, Michael J Pharoah, Oral Radiology, Principles and Interpretation first South Asia edition, pg.no.315-28.
2. Norman K. Wood and Paul. W. Goaz, Differential Diagnosis Of Oral And Maxillofacial Lesions, 5th Edition, chapter 13, page no. 209-230.

Q 2) Describe the papillae of tongue. Enumerate & describe the conditions in which there are atrophic changes in the papillae:

MUHS MAY 2002 (10 Marks)

The tongue surface has fleshy bump like structures called the papillae. The Papillae of the tongue are the projections of the mucous membrane or corium which gives the anterior two-thirds of the tongue its characteristic roughness. They are present on the dorsal surface of the tongue and are absent on the lingual surface. There are 5 types of papillae present on the tongue surface and are

1. Circumvallate papillae.
2. Fungiform papillae.
3. Filiform papillae.
4. Foliate papillae.
5. Papillae simplices.

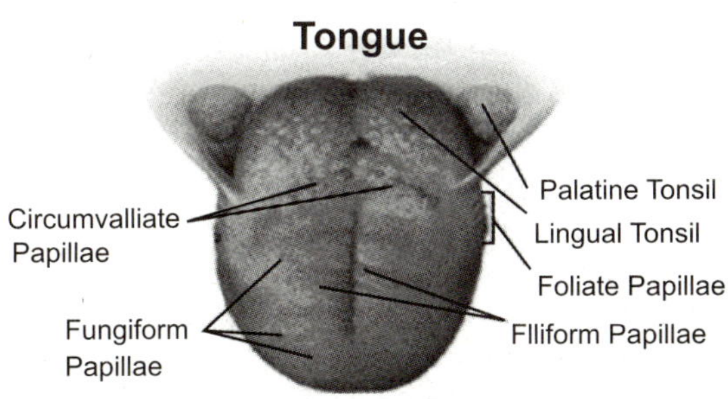

Fig. Different papillae of tongue

1. **Circumvallete papillae:** They are usually 8 to 12 in numbers, 1to 3 mm in diameter, and are the largest of the papillae. They are usually situated in front of sulcus terminalis. Each papillae is a cylindrical projection surrounded by a circular sulcus, flattened with a circular depression and are surrounded by a moat like trough.
2. **The fungiform papillae:**
   - These are numerous papillae present near the tip and margins of the tongue and some are distributed over the dorsum surface of the tongue being most numerous in the anterior part.
   - They are round & mushroom – shaped, consists of a narrow pedicle & large rounded neck & is distinguished from the filliform papillae by their larger size & bright red color.
   - Their number is about $100/cm^2$ on the tip & $50/cm^2$ in the middle.
   - Contain terminal epithelial differentiation products such as K1 / K10 keratins & Filaggrin.
   - They are richly innervated, well vascularised & carry taste buds.
3. **Filliform papillae:**
   - These are smallest, numerous papillae that are evenly distributed over the dorsum of tongue arranged in rows in the presulcal area parallel to the sulcus terminalis except for the tip, where they run transverse & gives tongue a characteristic velvety appearance.
   - They are conical, broadest at the base & whitish due to marked degree of keratinisation.
   - They are $500/cm^2$ and are heavily concentrated in centre of dorsum of tongue.
4. **Foliate papillae:**
   - They are vertical folds of the mucosa located at the margins of the tongue, anterior to the palatoglossal arch.
   - They have cornified surface with numerous taste buds along lateral walls in the early life.
   - Atrophy of these papillae are seen in older age.
5. **Papillae simplices:**
   - These are the connective tissue papillae which are similar to the connective tissue papillae of the dermis of the skin. These are present beneath the entire tongue surface.

The conditions in which there are atrophic changes or depapillation of the tongue occurs are classified as:

(a) Local disease:

1. Benign migratory glossitis
2. Eosinophillic granuloma
3. Traumatic injuries
4. Lesions due to automutilation
5. Allergic stomatitis
6. Facial hemiatrophy

7. Cranial arteritis
8. Chronic candidiasis.

(b) Systemic disease:

1. Iron deficiency anemia
2. Plummer –Vinson's syndrome
3. Pernicious anemia
4. Niacin deficiency
5. Folic acid deficiency
6. Peripheral vascular disease
7. Dermatomyositis
8. Diabetes
9. Syphilis
10. Zoster infection
11. Tuberculosis

(c) Neurological diseases:

1. Glossodynia
2. Dyskinesia
3. Paralysis
4. Oropharyngeal dysphagia

1. **Benign migratory glossitis:** Synonyms: 'geographic tongue', 'wandering rash', 'glossitis areata exfoliativa'& 'erythema migrans'. These are irregularly shaped reddish areas of depapillation & shows thinning of dorsal tongue epithelium which is surrounded by narrow zone of regenerating papillae that are whiter than the surrounding tongue surface.
2. **Eosinophillic granuloma:** Synonyms: 'ulcerated granuloma', 'traumatic granuloma'.
   It is not related to eosinophillic granuloma of bone & the cause is not known, and which is characterised by a proliferative ulceration that is well demarcated and is covered by thick fibrin and detritus.
   Occurs at any age, no sex predilection and usually the dorsum of the tongue is involved, and may involve the margins and inferior surface of the same.
   Lesions are ulcerative, not indurated and well circumscribed with putrid odour.
3. **Traumatic injuries:** Mechanical or chemical trauma such as jagged tooth, rough margins of the restoration involuntary contact of the tongue with certain dental medications such as phenol and eugenol.
   There is an area of localised depapillation with papillary regeneration present.
   Yellowish, non indurated well circumscribed ulcer at the border of the tongue is usually due to sharp edge.
4. **Allergic stomatitis:**
   - Its a condition in which there is edematous changes in part or

the entire oral mucosa because of hypersensitivity reaction.

- Certain drugs can also cause this condition such as antibiotics cancer chemotherapeutic agent & anticholinergic agents.
- Allergens such as monomer of the dentures, mouth washes and chewing gum and lipstick.
- Swelling of the tongue that is edematous & depapillation of tongue is seen.

5. **Facial hemiatrophy:** There is atrophy of the half of the tongue.
6. **Cranial arteritis:**
   - An inflammatory condition of large and medium sized arteries in elderly persons are rheumatic polymyalgia and temporal arteritis.
   - Ulcerations & gangrene of tongue, pain in tongue and intermittent blanching is also seen in some cases.
7. **Acute atrophic candidiasis:** Also known as antibiotic sore mouth Causes depapillation of tongue.

(b) Systemic diseases:

1. **Iron deficiency anemia:**
   - Atrophic changes first appears on the dorsum surface of the tongue, especially at the tip & lateral borders with loss of filliform papillae.
   - In severe cases entire dorsum becomes smooth, glazed, pale or fiery red & is painful.
2. **Plummer-vinson-syndrome:**
   - Sideropenic anemia includes atrophic glossitis, angular cheilitis, generalized atrophy of the oral mucosa, ulcerations and secondary candidiasis.
   - The tongue is red or pale, painful & fissured.
3. **Pernicious anemia:**
   - Paresthesia & atrophy of filliform & fungiform papillae.
   - In severe cases there is complete atrophy of the tongue and it becomes smooth and fiery red.
4. **Niacin deficiency:**
   - Niacin deficiency results in 'pellagra' which is characterized by fiery red tongue devoid of papillae.
   - Filliform papillae are most sensitive & disappears first and fungiform papillae are enlarged.
   - In advanced cases all the papillae are lost.
5. **Deficiency of folic acid:**
   - The glossitis is severe and the tongue appears fiery red with atrophy of fungiform & filliform papillae.
   - Tongue is swollen with cracks seen on the dorsum surface.
6. **Peripheral vascular disease:**

   (a) **Oral submucous fibrosis:**
   - This also thought to be a premalignant condition, with collagens deposition in the lamina propria of the oral

mucosa. The tongue appears depapillated with limitation in the movement.

(b) **Scleroderma:**
- Tongue appears scarred, shrunken & atrophic due to fibrosis of sub mucosal tissues which is secondary to small vessels obliteration due to an autoimmune process.
- There occurs shrinking of tongue, loss of its mobility, change in pattern of papilla and vivid red appearance due to disturbances of circulation.

(c) **Lupus erythematosus:** In this condition there is atrophy and ulceration that is caused by arteritis.

7. **Dermatomyositis:**
   - In early stage tongue appears swollen and in later stages, becomes harder and in the late phase it appears atrophic.
8. **Diabetes:**
   - Atrophic glossitis in diabetic patients results due to vascular changes.
   - Central papillary atrophy of the dorsum is characteristic.
9. **Syphilis:**
   - Depapillation of the tongue usually seen in secondary & tertiary syphilis.
   - Atrophy of filliform & fungiform papillae.
10. **Zoster infection:** Its caused by herpes zoster virus and is, characterized by numerous vesicle formation on the ventral surface of the tongue.
11. **Tuberculosis:** Can cause atrophy and ulcers on the tongue.

c. Neurological diseases:

1. **Glossodynia:** Also known as painful tongue, is associated with atrophy of the tongue.
2. **Paralysis:** Also called as glossoplegia, is associated with paralysis & atrophy of the muscles of one- half of the tongue and atrophy of sides of tongue.

Suggested reading:

1. Anil Govindrao Ghom; Textbook of Oral Medicine, 3rd edition, 506-517.
2. B D Chaurasia's Human anatomy; Edi: 5 th; Ch: 17; pg: 250.

Q 3) Oral manifestations of systemic diseases:

TNMGRU FEBRUARY 2011 (20 Marks)

The mouth is a mirror of health or disease, a early warning system. Oral manifestations can occur in many systemic disorders.The lesions in such cases occur in the oral mucosa, gingiva, tongue, teeth, periodontal tissues, salivary glands, skeleton of the face, extra-oral skin and other related structures.

1. **Nutritional Disorders:** Vitamins- Vitamins are essential micronutrients of diet.

Oral manifestations:

(a) Vitamin A:

- There is retardation of the rate of eruption and alveolar bone formation.
- The gingiva becomes hyperplastic, Impaired healing & tissue regeneration, increased risk of candidiasis, periodontal diseases and microabscess formation.
- Decreased taste sensitivity, xerostomia, disturbed or arrested enamel development, increased caries risk.

Oral manifestations of hypervitaminosis A:

- It is characterized by dry and fissured lips.

(b) Vitamin D:

Rickets (vitamin D deficiency)

- Delayed eruption, malalignment, enamel hypoplasia, mottled enamel.
- Pulp chamber is high, delayed closure of root apices, pitting surface of enamel which is more prone to caries.
- Radiographically thinning of cortical structures and narrowing of PDL space.
- In Vitamin D resistant rickets there are multiple periapical infections with poorly defined or complete loss of lamina dura.

(c) Vitamin E (tocopherol):

Deficiency leads to atrophic degenerative changes in the enamel and loss of pigmentation.

(d) Vitamin K (phylloquinone):

- Deficiency can result in gingival bleeding.

(e) Vitamin B-complex:

These are water soluble vitamins. It includes Vitamin B1, Vitamin B2, Vitamin B3, vitamin B6, vitamin B9, vitamin B12.

The most common oral manifestations of deficiency of vitamin B include:

- Oral mucosa- entire mucosa of the oral cavity becomes painful and fiery red.
- Profuse salivation.
- Glossitis- In the initial stages there is glossitis involving the tip and/or the lateral borders of the tongue. In later cases the tongue becomes so swollen that indentation from teeth are found on the lateral borders of tongue.
- Stomatitis- The mouth is sore and shows angular stomatitis or cheilitis. Tenderness, pain and ulceration seen at the interdental papilla & spreads rapidly.

(f) Vitamin C (Ascorbic acid):

Deficiency can lead to scurvy which may manifest as:

- Interdental and marginal gingiva is bright red, swollen, smooth, shiny surface producing appearance like scurvy bud. In later cases there is bogginess of the gingiva, ulcerations and bleeding and in severe cases- hemorrhage and swelling of periodontal ligament membrane, bone loss and loosening of teeth.
- Breath- Fetid breath.

2. Metabolic Disorders:

(a) **Disorders of protein metabolism:**

(i) **Amyloidosis:**

- Difficulty in chewing, swallowing, or talking.
- Macroglossia, decreased mobility of tongue, yellowish nodules on the lateral border, indentations of teeth. Gingiva is hypertrophied, Xerostomia present.

(ii) **Kwashiorkor and marasmus:**

- There is loss of papillae of the tongue and there is bright red colour development, bilateral angular cheilosis.
- Fissuring of lips, loss of circum oral pigmentation, xerostomia.
- Epithelium readily becoming detached from the underlying tissues, leaving a raw, bleeding surface.
- Decreased Overall growth of the jaws and delayed Eruption and retarded incisor and molar growth and hypoplasia of the deciduous teeth.

(iii) **Porphyria:**

Oral manifestations:

1. The permanent and deciduous teeth can show a red or brownish discoloration which under ultraviolet light, exhibit red fluorescence.
2. Bullous erosive lesions of oral mucosa may be present, atrophic cheilitis and advanced periodontal diseases.

(b) **Disorders of carbohydrate metabolism:** The caries index becomes significantly low.

(c) **Disorders of lipid metabolism:**

A. Langerhans cell histiocytosis: It is a inflammatory reticuloendothelioma condition in which there is pathological accumulation of histiocytes & eosinophillic leukocytes. It is also called as histiocytosis X. It is of three types-

(a) **Hand- schuller-christian disease:**

- sore mouth, halitosis, unpleasant taste, poor wound healing, gingival inflammation.

(b) **Letterer-siwe disease:**

- gingival hyperplasia, ulcerations, loosening and premature loss of teeth.

(c) **Eosinophilic granuloma:**
- juvenile periodontitis
- sockets fail to heal normally

3. **Endocrine Disorders:**

(a) Hypopituitarism:
- There is delayed eruption and shedding of the teeth.
- The teeth tend to have shorter roots than normal, and the supporting structures are retarded in growth.
- Hypopituitarism in the adults:
- Decreased salivary flow due to hypofunctioning of salivary glands thus increased caries activity and periodontal disease.

(b) Hyperpituitarism:

Oral Manifestations of Gigantism:
- Skeletal changes include frontal bossing and prognathic mandible.
- Patient may develop class III malocclusion with interdental spacing.
- Hypercementosis is a common finding in the intra oral radiographs.
- The teeth in gigantism are proportional in comparison to the jaw size and the rest of the body. The roots can be longer than normal.

Oral Manifestations of Acromegaly:
- Accelerated condylar growth thus large mandible.
- Resulting prognathism may be extreme, giving the head a typical acromegalic appearance.
- As a result of the enlarged tongue the teeth in the mandible can be tilted buccally or labially.
- Microscopically, the surface epithelium and the connective tissues are hyper plastic.

(c) **Pancreatic Hormones:** Diabetes occurs due to disorder of pancreatic hormone.
- Xerostomia is present which can act as a predisposing factor in the causation of oral infections.
- There can be associated bilateral enlargement of the parotids that are diffuse, and non-tender and is called diabetic sialadenosis.
- In cases of poorly controlled diabetes, there is alteration in taste and burning mouth syndrome.The dryness of the mucosa which is also damaged, gets predisposed to development of candidiasis.
- There is atrophy of the papillae on the dorsal surface of the tongue. Loss of alveolar bone, Loosening of teeth.

(d) **Parathyroid Hormone:**

Hypoparathyroidism:

If in the early stages of life, hypothyroidism develops when the teeth are in developmental stage, enamel hypoplasia of the pitting type and failure in eruption of tooth can occur.

Hyperparathyroidism:

Brown's tumours may affect the mandible or maxilla along with other bones.

(e) **Hypoadrenocorticisim:**

- Orofacial manifestations consist of hyperpigmentation which is bronze in colour of the skin which is exposed to the sun and the pressure points occurs.
- The oral mucosa melanosis often preceeds the skin changes. The buccal mucosa shows diffuse brown macular pigmentation.

4. **Renal Diseases:**

(i) Renal failure: Various etiological factors for renal failure are – Glomerulonephritis, pyelonephritis, hemolytic uremic condition etc.

Oral manifestation of renal failure includes:

- Ammonic and metallic taste, Xerostomia.
- Erythematopultaceous form- acute rise in Blood Urea Nitrogen level may cause uremic stomatitis, characterized by red mucosa covered with thick exudates and pseudomembrane.
- Ulcerative form- frank ulcerations present.
- Low caries activity, Enamel hypoplasia.

(ii) **Uremic Stomatitis:** In this condition, the buccal mucosa, floor or the tongue dorsum shows presence of painful plaques and crusts.

(iii) **Kidney transplantation:**

- Oral mucosa- pale with diminished colour demarcation between the alveolar mucosa and the attached gingiva.
- Salivary glands enlarged and xerostomia seen, and odor of urea and metallic taste also present.
- Gingiva- low grade gingival inflammation and bleeding.
- Candidal infection of tongue and petechiae, ecchymosis, erosive glossitis, burning present.

5. **Gastrointestinal Diseases:**

(i) Crohn's disease:

- The patients with this condition exhibit swelling that is diffuse involving one or both lips and there can be angular cheilitis and cobblestone appearance of the buccal mucous with hyperplastic mucosa that is rigid.
- Linear ulcerations are seen in the buccal vestibule which are painful, midline of the lower lip may show fissuring, and the gingiva can be erythematous and edematous.

(ii) **Ulcerative Colitis:**

- Ulcers similar to aphthous ulcers may develop in the oral cavity.

(iii) **Gastro-esophageal reflux disease:** Regurgitation of gastric content will reduce the pH of oral cavity and may lead to erosion of enamel.

6. **Hematologic Disorders:** It includes disorders of RBC, WBC and platelets.
   (a) Disorders of RBC:
   (i) Iron deficiency anemia:
   Oral manifestations include:
   - Pallor of mucosa and gingiva- It is due to lack of oxygenated blood in the capillary bed in the lamina propria and is associated with lowered levels of hemoglobin.
   - There is generalised atrophy of the buccal mucosa and tongue.
   - Atrophy of the filliform papillae of the anterior 2/3rds of the tongue, angular cheilitis, and soreness and burning of the tongue is present.
   - When the condition is severe even the fungiform papillae get affected and the tongue is left devoid of paillae and becomes smooth and glistening.
   - There can be occurrence of recurrent aphthous ulcers and candida lesions.
   - There is tendency to slow healing and gingival enlargement may also be seen.
   - In plummer-vinson syndrome there is typical dysphagia, iron deficiency anemia, koilonychia and glossitis which is seen in severe form in middle aged women. There is also presence of angular cheilitis, soreness and fissuring of the tongue.

   (ii) **Erythroblastosis fetalis:** It is a type of isoimmune hemolytic anemia, also called as 'hereditary disease of newborn' and occurs because of Rh incompatibility that results from destruction of fetal blood brought about by a reaction between the maternal and fetal blood factors.

   Oral manifestations include:
   - Teeth- It may manifest in teeth by blood pigment deposition in the enamel and dentin and gives a green, brown or blue hue.
   - Enamel hypoplasia is also seen. Mainly affects upper anteriors, deciduous cuspid and first molar crown.
   - Rh hump-A ring like defect is called as Rh hump. It is caused by enamel hypoplasia on tooth crown.
   - Radiographically there is increase in the thickness of cranial bone which includes maxilla and mandible due to increased thickness of diploe. Radiating spicule may also be seen.

   (iii) **Sickle cell anemia:** It is a chronic hemolytic disorder that is characterised by hemoglobin that is abnormal and which under low tension of oxygen, causes sickling of cell.

Oral manifestations include:

- Oral mucosa shows pallor.
- Teeth- There may be delayed eruption and hypoplasia of the dentition.
- Osteomyelitis- Patients are more prone to develop osteomyelitis due to hypovascularity of bone marrow secondary to thrombosis.
- Nerves- Paresthesia of mental nerve.
- Jaw Bones- Mongoloid Facies with high cheek bone and bimaxillary prognathism.

(iv) **Thalassemia:**

- The oral mucosa is pale and shows lemon yellow tint because of chronic jaundice.
- Rodent and chipmunk facies may be seen.

(b) **WBC disorders:**

(i) **Leukemia:**

- **Acute leukemia:**
- Paresthesia of lower lip and chin.
- Oral mucous membrane shows pallor, ulcerations with necrosis, petechiae, ecchymosis, bleeding tendency.
- Gingival hypertrophy with cyanotic discoloration. It appears boggy, edematous, easily bleed and teeth mobility and toothache present.
- Infection- Oral infections like candidial, viral or bacterial infections are serious and potentially fatal complications in leukemic patients.
- **Chronic leukemia:**
- Gingiva: The most common oral finding is hypertrophy of gingiva associated with bleeding. There may be ulceration with necrosis and gangrenous degeneration with dark brown exudates and foul odor.
- Tongue is frequently swollen and dark.
- Regional lymphadenopathy is present.
- Rapid loosening of teeth due to necrosis of periodontal ligament has been reported.
- Destruction of alveolar bone is also seen.

(ii) **Multiple Myeloma:**

- **Oral manifestations:** There can be swelling, numbness and pain in the jaws, formation of epulis, and there could be unexplained mobility of teeth.
- The swellings that are intra-oral tend to be ulcerated, roundish and bluish red. The swelling is tender on palpation and crackling like egg shell may be present.
- Macroglossia can occur due to amyloid deposit.

(c) **Platelet Disorders:**
Oral manifestations of:

(i) **Thrombocytopenic purpura:**

- Submucous petechiae and ecchymosis commonly occur especially at the junction of hard and soft palate. And in some cases may be seen on tongue.
- Excessive bleeding after tooth extraction.
- Extensive spontaneous gingival bleeding can be seen.
- Hemorrhagic bullae can also occur intraorally due to collection of blood.

(ii) **Von Willebrand disease:**

- Gingival bleeding and post extraction bleeding are the most common oral manifestations.

(d) **Hemorrhagic Disorder:**

1. Hemophilia:
   - Persistent bleeding from frenum of lip and tongue.
   - There is prolonged bleeding after tooth extraction.
   - Gingival hemorrhage and hematoma of floor of mouth can be seen.

7. **Granulomatous Disorders:** Granulomatous diseases are a heterogeneous group of disorders that are characterized by a specific pattern of chronic inflammation called Granulomatous inflammation, in which granulomas are formed.

1. **Tuberculosis:** Caused by acid fast bacillus M. tuberculosis.
Oral manifestations of:

(i) **Tuberculosis:**

- Primary oral tuberculosis involves gingiva which can show diffuse, hyperemic, papillary or nodular proliferation.
- Tongue is the most commonly affected in secondary tuberculosis, followed by palate, lip, buccal mucosa, gingiva and frenula.
- There can be presence of ulcer that is irregular, deep or superficial and that grows slowly in size.

(ii) **Leprosy:** Also called as Hansen's Disease, a chronic non-fatal infectious disease affecting mainly cooler parts of the body such as the skin, mouth, respiratory tract, eyes, peripheral nerves, superficial lymph nodes and testis caused by Mycobacterium Leprae.

Oral manifestations of leprosy:

- If the trigeminal nerve is involved hyperesthesia or parasthesia of the face, lips, tongue, palate, cheeks or gingiva may occur.
- Small tumor like masses called lepromas, which develop on the tongue, lips and hard palate. These nodules show tendency to break down and ulcerate.
- Dental deformity of lepromatous leprosy includes pink

discoloration of the upper incisors due to invasion of the pulp by infected granulomatous tissue that can produce pulpitis and pulp death.

(iii) **Syphillis:** Syphilis is a venereal disease caused by spirochetes, Treponema Pallidum.

Oral manifestations:

- **Primary Syphilis-** A chancre of lip is the most common extra genital lesion. Other affected sites are tongue, gingiva and tonsillar area. Enlarged lymphnodes in the submaxillary, submental and cervical regions.
- **Secondary Syphilis-** Slightly raised, greyish white patches called mucous patches on the tongue, soft palate, tonsil or cheek. The ulcers coalesce to give the characteristic snail tracks appearance.
- **Tertiary Syphilis-** The representative lesion is gumma which begins as a small, pale, raised area of the mucosa that ulcerates and rapidly progresses to large zone of necrosis with denudation of bone. In palate may perforate to nasal cavity.

(iv) **Wegener's Granulomatosis:** The gingiva presents with a florid and granular hyperplasia. It is swollen, reddened, with multiple short bulbous projections that are hemorrhagic and friable, and exhibit a red bumpy surface giving the strawberry-like appearance.

(v) **Sarcoidosis:**

- Multiple nodules as well as painless ulcerations of the tongue, gingiva, buccal mucosa, labial mucosa, and palate.
- The lesions have a granularity, may be hyperkeratotic, and present as brown-red or purple in color.

8. **Oral manifestations of skin diseases:**

(i) Lichen planus: Lesions consist of whitish, gray, velvety, papules that are thread like arranged in linear, annular or retiform arrangement which form typical lacy, reticular patches, rings or streaks.

Wickham's striae: tiny white elevated dot at intersection of white lines.

On gingiva it presents as desquamative gingivitis.

(ii) **Pemphigus:** Its an autoimmune vesiculobullous disorder.

Oral manifestations:

Bullous lesions occur on oral mucosa which break down easily and form ulcers.

(iii) **Pemphigoid:** Subepithelial bulla are formed in oral cavity.

(iv) **Psoriasis:**

Oral manifestations:

Grey or yellow/white plaque, white lesions that are silvery, having erythematous base, small papillary lesion with scaly surface.

(v) **Systemic lupus erythematosus:**

Oral manifestations:

Caused by vasculitis and appear as frank ulcerations or mucosal inflammation.

Sites–buccal mucosa, palate, gingiva.

There is involvement of vermillion zone of lower lip(lupus cheilitis).

vi) **Discoid lupus erythematosus:**

Oral manifestations:

It begins as erythematous areas, more often depressed, without induration, with white spots.

Margins may show formation of narrow zone of keratinisation.

Fine white striae radiate from margins.

(vii) **Scleroderma:**

Oral manifestations:

Microstomia, lips rigid, oral aperture narrow.

Mask like appearance, purse string appearance.

Tongue is hard and rigid.

Telangiectasia on hard palate, lips.

(viii) **Erythema multiforme:**

Oral manifestations:

Can occur anywhere in oral cavity but gingiva and hard palate are relatively spared.

Lesions begin as erythematous patches that undergo epithelial necrosis and evolve into large shallow erosions and ulcerations with irregular borders.

Oral lesions merge quickly and are uncomfortable and painful. Bloody crusty appearance of lips with drooling of saliva is seen.

(ix) **Warty dyskeratosis:**

Oral manifestations:

Pink/white papule on keratinised mucosa (hard palate, alveolar ridge).

(x) **Hereditary benign intra epithelial dyskeratosis:**

Oral manifestations:

Appears as white spongy macerated lesion of buccal mucosa with or without folds.

Milder cases exhibit opalescent appearance of leukoedema.

It frequently involves corners of mouth and appear as soft plaques with pin point elevations when mucosa is stretched.

(xi) **Acanthosis nigricans:**

Oral manifestations:

Tongue, lips, buccal mucosa, gingiva are involved.

Hypertrophy of filiform papillae producing shaggy,

papillomatous surface of dorsal tongue.
Buccal mucosa shows velvety white appearance.
Gingival enlargement also seen.

(xii) **Pachyonichia congenita:**

Leukokeratosis of tongue, buccal mucosa.
Scalloped edges of tongue.
Angular cheilitis.
Enamel hypoplasia, neonatal teeth, hypodontia, severe caries.

(xiii) **Dyskeratosis congenita:**

Oral manifestations:

Diffusely distributed vesicles & ulcers followed by white patches of necrotic epithelium.

(xiv) **Epidermolysis bullosa:**

Oral manifestations:

The palate, peri-oral areas and perinasal areas show hemorrhagic bullae.
The mouth shows diminished opening due to scarring around it.

Suggested reading:

1. Angela C. Chi, Brad W. Neville, Joe W. Krayer, Wanda C. Gonsalves, oral manifestations of systemic diseases, American Family Physician, Volume 82, Number 11, December 1, 2010, 1381-1387.

Q 4) Enumerate the various causes of Cervico-Facial Lymphadenopathy. Write the differential diagnosis of cervical lymphadenopathy:

RGUHS OCTOBER 2000 (10 Marks)

Causes of cervico-facial lymphadenopathy:

I) **Infectious diseases:**
- (a) **Viral:** Infectious hepatitis, infectious mononucleosis, herpes simplex, rubella, adenovirus and HIV.
- (b) **Bacterial:** Staphylococci, streptococci, cat-scratch disease, tuberculosis, tularemia, diphtheria, primary and secondary syphilis and leprosy.
- (c) **Fungal infections:** coccidiomycosis, histoplasmosis and paracoccidiomycosis.
- (e) **Parasitic:** Leishmaniasis, toxoplasmosis, filariasis.
- (f) **Rickettsial:** Rickettsialpox, scrub typhosis.

II) **Immunologic diseases:**
- (a) Rheumatoid arthritis:
- (b) Mixed connective tissue disease.
- (c) Systemic lupus erythematosus.
- (d) Dermatomyositis.

(e) Sjogren's syndrome.
(f) Serum sickness.
(g) Hypersesnsitivity to drugs.
(h) Primary biliary cirrhosis.
(i) Graft-versus-host disease.

III) Malignant lesions:

(a) **Hematologic:** All, Cll, multiple myeloma, hodgkin's lymphoma, non-hodgkin's lymphoma.

IV) Gaucher's, Niemann-pick.

V) Endocrine diseases: Thyroiditis, hyperthyroidism, adrenal insufficiency.

(a) Castleman's disease.
(b) Sarcoidosis.
(c) Dermatopathic lymhadenitis.
(d) Lymhomatoid granulomatosis.
(e) Kikuchi's disease.
(f) Kawasaki's disease.
(g) Histiocytosis X.
(h) Hypertriglyceridemia.

Differential diagnosis:

1. **Infections:** Upper respiratory tract that is infected by viruses and bacteria in adults and children lead to acute bilateral cervical lymphadenopathy.

   The symptoms consist of cough, congestion of the sinus, rhinorrhoea, and there could be occasional fever and malaise. Bilateral lymph node swelling of the cervical nodes which can be painful and tender and can persist for several weeks even after the symptoms have resolved.

   The typical symptoms will help in diagnosis.

2. **Local infections:** Localised infections commonly lead to cervical lymhadenopathy. Bacterial infections of the head and neck region result in cervical lymphadenopathy in case where the nodes draining that area respond to the infection or when the infection gets localised in the nodes themselves.

   Local infection can reveal an offending tooth or sialadenitis of the major salivary glands or periodontal infections.Maxillary sinusitis also can be the cause.

   The bacterial infections result in acute enlargement of the nodes which are tender, warm and erythematous.In more than 50% of the cases the submandibular nodes involvement is present. The enlarged tender nodes can eventually become fluctuant. The cervical lymphadenopathy can also occur due to viruses like the herpes simplex and the coxackie virus. These viruses cause primary herpetic gingivostomatitis and herpangina respectively. There are vesicles and ulcerations of the oral cavity, palate and the oro-pharynx and there could be fever and malaise.

In children the most common manifestation of non-tuberculous mycobacterium, chronic lymphadenopathy is the most common presentation.

3. **Systemic infection:** Cervical lymphadenopathy is a common manifestation of several viral infections.Viral infections that are systemic can cause many conditions like the hand-foot-mouth disease, chicken pox, measles and rubella.

   Viruses like the epstein barr virus, HIV, cytomegalovirus, HHV-6 cause infections that can involve the oral mucosa and along with rashes, fever, malaise can cause bilateral cervical nodes involvement of both anterior and posterior nodes. The lymphnodes in these conditions are firm, erythematous. Infectious mononucleosis often leads to involvement of anterior and posterior cervical lymphadenopathy. Other infections causing this condition could be bacterial and protozoal in nature.
4. **Other infectious agents:** Cervical lymphadenopathy can be caused by a broad array of infective organisms. Syphillis caused by T.pallidum results in this condition. In Lyme disease there can be apart from cervical lymhadenopathy, fever, malaise, and multiple system findings. In rubella there is typical lymphadenopathy of the posterior cervical triangle. It can also be seen in the sero conversion stage of HIV infection.
5. **Cat-scratch disease:** Subacute cervical lymphadenopathy is a typical feature in this disease. The causative organism is the Bartonella species. At the site of inoculation pustular lesions occur along with cervical lymphadenopathy.Biopsy of the lypmh nodes can show the cat-scratch bacilli with special staining techniques.
6. **Tuberculosis:** Mostly caused by M.tuberculosis and the symptoms and signs are loss of weight, sweating at nights, fever, malaise and anorexia. Typical feature is the persistent cough and hemoptysis and non-purulent sputum may help in diagnosis. Tuberculous cervical lymphadenitis or scrofula is the most common extra-pulmonary manifestation of the disease.

   Koch's test and x-ray chest will help confirming diagnosis.
7. **Toxoplasmosis:** Its caused by a parasite, toxoplasmosis gondii and the most common manifestation is the cervical lymphadenopathy with warm, tender enlargement of the nodes. The diagnosis is based on clinical findings and by the rising anti-body titres of IgG which are typically high in the acute phase of the infection and low titres persist for life.
8. **Mailgnancy:** In malignant conditions of the head and neck regions enlarged palpable nodes are present. Several metastatic tumours may persist as cervical lymphadenopathy. Typical findings of malignancy are present involving enlarged lymph nodes. The duration of lymphadenopathy in these cases is of longer time and is associated with gradual enlargement. The nodes could be involved

unilaterally and multiple or bilateral.

9. **Autoimmune diseases:** Several autoimmune disorders can result in local or disseminated lymphadenopathy for several reasons.

   Rheumatoid arthritis:

   Its a condition in which there is chronic inflammation of the synovium and affects the small joints of the upper and lower extremities.

   Rheumatoid arthritis involving the TMJ may lead to cervical lymphadenitis. Lymph nodes excised from the individuals with rheumatoid arthritis will show a severe reactive follicular hyperplasia and interfollicular plasmacytosis.

   Systemic lupus erythematosus:

   Its a chronic multisystem disorder and involves systems of renal, cardiac, muco-cutaneous and CNS. Other symptoms include arthralgia or arthritis, rashes, edema of the ankle or periorbital edema, neurologic complaints, fatigue and fever. Initial clinical manifestation in 2% of cases has been reported to be cervical lymphadenopathy. Biopsy of the lymphnodes will reveal a diffuse hyperplasia and small lymphocytes, plasma cells and prominent immunoblasts. The lymphadenopathy responds well to corticosteroids.

   Sjogren's syndrome:

   Its a chronic autoimmune disorder that has characteristic xerostomia, xerophthalmia and exocrine gland involvement.There can be cervical lymphadenopathy in about 20% of the cases. The biopsy of the nodes will show paracortical hyperplasia and prominent proliferation of the vessels and several lymphoid follicles and germinal centers.

10. **Other causes:** kikuchi's disease runs a benign, self-limiting course and is a rare disease that affects the young adults and is commonly seen in Asians.

    There is typical presence of cervical lymphadenopathy that is tender and associated with fever and night sweating. The diagnosis is made after biopsy of the lymphnodes and immunoperoxidase stains may be used for final diagnosis.

11. **Reactions of drugs:** Several drugs cause signs involving the systems and it includes lymphadenopathy. Anticonvulsants and sulphonamides are notorious in causing lymphadenopathy. It could be related to a hypersensitivity reaction. There could be muco-cutaneous eruptions, fever, hematologic abnormalities, hepatitis, interstitial nephritis and lymphadenopathy.

Suggested reading:

1. Ernesta Parisi, Cervical Lymphadenopathy in the Dental Patient: A Review of Clinical Approach, Quintessence International Volume 36 • Number 6 • June 2005 425-431.

ORAL AND MAXILLOFACIAL RADIOLOGY

LONG ANSWERS QUESTIONS

CHAPTER 1

Radiation Biology

Q 1) Enumerate hazards of radiation. Discuss effects of radiation on oral tissues:

RGUHS APRIL 2000 (10 Marks)

Radiation hazards can be classified as:

1. Deterministic.	1) Direct.	1) Acute.	1) Somatic effect.
2. Stochastic.	2) Indirect.	2) Chronic.	2) Genetic effects.

A) Somatic Effects:

(i) **Somatic Stochastic Effect:** These are the effects in which probability of the occurrence of a change increases, rather than its severity.

Eg: Radiation induced cancer is a stochastic effect because greater the exposure of a person or population to radiation, increases the probability of cancer and not its severity.

(ii) **Somatic Deterministic effects:** Also called as non-stochastic effects. These are the effects which have increased probability of occurrence, increase with increase in dose and have dose threshold, below which the response cannot be seen. It results from specifically high doses of radiation.

For example during Radiotherapy. Examples include ulceration and desquamation of skin, damage to connective tissue, cataract formation.

B) Genetic Effects: This kind of damage is not seen in the person who is irradiated but is seen in their offsprings. Genetic damage follows non-threshold type of response, that is small amounts of radiation has the potential to produce lesser number of mutations in chromosomes.

C) Acute Effects: It occurs when a large amount of radiation is given in short period, for example in atomic bomb explosions and nuclear accidents. A single whole body dose of 500 rads can cause death.

Immediate effects due to large amounts of radiation:

- Skin-excessive exposure can cause dermatitis.
- Finger-fingernails may become brittle or crumble.
- Hair-Epilation can occur due to excessive radiation.
- Blood forming tissues: Excessive radiation can cause leucopenia.
- Eyes-Very high radiation doses can cause cataract and retinal detachment can occur.

D) **Chronic effects:** This occurs due to small amounts of radiation absorbed over long periods of time.

- Carcinoma: cancer of skin is an example of chronic radiation hazard.
- Leukemia: This can occur due to primary and secondary radiation. Radiographers hence are susceptible to develop this disorder.
- Retardation of bone and teeth growth are some effects of chronic radiation.

Radiation Effects on the Oral Cavity

The oral cavity has effects of radiation mainly during irradiation for the treatment of radiosensitive oral malignant tumors, usually squamous cell carcinomas. About 5000 Rads is administered during the course of the treatment. The effects of this treatment on the oral cavity is as follows:

(i) **Oral Mucous Membrane:** At the end of the second week of radiotherapy, the mucous membranes begin to show areas of redness and inflammation (mucositis).

As the therapy continues, the irradiated mucous membrane begins to break down, with the formation of a white to yellow pseudomembrane (the desquamated epithelial layer)

At the end of therapy the mucositis is usually most severe, discomfort is at a maximum, and food intake is difficult.

Good oral hygiene minimizes infection. Topical anesthetics may be required at mealtimes.

Secondary yeast infection by Candida albicans is a common complication and may require treatment.

After irradiation is completed, the mucosa begins to heal rapidly.

Healing is usually complete by about 2 months. At later intervals (months to years) the mucous membrane tends to become atrophic, thin, and relatively avascular.

This long-term atrophy results from progressive obliteration of the fine vasculature and fibrosis of the underlying connective tissue.

These atrophic changes complicate denture wearing because they may cause oral ulcerations of the compromised tissue. Ulcers can result from a denture sore, radiation necrosis, or tumor recurrence. A biopsy may be required to make the differentiation.

(ii) **Taste Buds:** Taste buds are sensitive to radiation. Doses in the therapeutic range cause extensive degeneration of the normal

histologic architecture of taste buds.
Patients often notice a loss of taste acuity during the second or third week of radiotherapy.
Bitter and acid flavors are more severely affected when the posterior two thirds of the tongue is irradiated, and salt and sweet when the anterior third of the tongue is irradiated.
Taste acuity usually decreases by a factor of 1, 000 to 10, 000 during the course of radiotherapy.
Alterations in the saliva may account partly for this reduction, which may proceed to a state of virtual insensitivity, with recovery to near normal levels some 60 to 120 days after irradiation.

(iii) Salivary Glands: The major salivary glands are at times unavoidably exposed to 20 to 30 Gy during radiotherapy for cancer in the oral cavity or oropharynx.
The parenchymal component of the salivary glands is rather radiosensitive (parotid glands more so than submandibular or sublingual glands).
A marked and progressive loss of salivary secretion is usually seen in the first few weeks after initiation of radiotherapy, the extent of reduced flow is dose-dependent and reaches essentially zero at 60 Gy.
The mouth becomes dry (xerostomia) and tender, and swallowing is difficult and painful because the residual saliva also loses its normal lubricating properties.
Patients with irradiation of both parotid glands are more likely to complain of dry mouth than are those with unilateral irradiation.
The small volume of viscous saliva that is secreted usually has a pH value 1 unit below normal. This pH is low enough to initiate decalcification of normal enamel.
In addition, the buffering capacity of saliva falls as much as 44% during radiation therapy.
If some portions of the major salivary glands have been spared, dryness of the mouth usually subsides in 6 to 12 months because of compensatory hypertrophy of residual salivary gland tissue.
Reduced salivary flow that persists beyond a year is unlikely to show significant recovery.
In the months after irradiation the inflammatory response becomes more chronic and the glands demonstrate progressive fibrosis, adiposis, loss of fine vasculature, and concomitant parenchymal degeneration, thus accounting for the xerostomia.
Salivary changes have a profound influence on the oral microflora and secondarily on the dentition, often leading to radiation caries.
After radiotherapy that includes the major salivary glands, the microflora undergo a pronounced change, rendering them acidogenic in the saliva and plaque.
Patients receiving radiation therapy to oral structures have increases

in Streptococcus mutans, Lactobacillus and Candida. Because of their small volume of thick, viscous, acidic saliva, such patients are quite prone to radiation caries.

IV) Teeth: During development of the teeth radiation in therapeutic doses causes retardation of their growth.

If it precedes calcification then the radiotherapy can destroy the tooth bud. After the calcification has begun, irradiation can inhibit differentiation of cells which can lead to malformation and arrest of general growth.

Children receiving radiation therapy to the jaws may show defects in the dentition that is permanent like retardation in development of roots, dwarfed teeth, or there could be failure to form one or more teeth.

The teeth that undergo radiation during development can complete the calcification and erupt prematurely.

The severity of the damage is dependent on the dose.

Irradiation of teeth may cause retardation of the root formation, and the eruptive process is relatively resistant to radiation. Even if the root formation is altered the teeth will erupt.

The teeth in adults are quite resistant to the effects of radiation.

Tissue of the pulp that consists mainly of reverting and fixed postmitotic cells, show long term fibro atrophy after irradiation.

The crystalline structures of the enamel dentin and cementum show no major effects of radiation, and radiation does not increase their solubility.

(iv) Radiation Caries: Radiation caries is a rampant form of dental decay that may occur in individuals who receive a course of radio therapy that includes exposure of the salivary glands.

Clinically, three types of radiation caries exist. The most common is widespread superficial lesions attacking buccal, occlusal, incisal, and palatal surfaces.

Another type involves primarily the cementum and dentin in the cervical region. These lesions may progress around the teeth circumferentially and result in loss of the crown. A final type appears as a dark pigmentation of the entire crown.

The incisal edges may be markedly worn. Some patients develop combinations of all these lesions.

The histologic features of the lesions are similar to those of typical carious lesions.

It is the rapid course and widespread attack that distinguish radiation caries.

The best method of reducing radiation caries is daily application for 5 minutes of a viscous topical 1 % neutral sodium fluoride gel in custom-made applicator trays.

Use of topical fluoride causes a 6-month delay in the irradiation-induced elevation of Streptococcus mutans.

Avoidance of dietary sucrose, in addition to the use of a topical fluoride, further reduces the concentrations of S. mutans and Lactobacillus.

The best result is achieved from a combination of restorative dental procedures, excellent oral hygiene, and topical applications of sodium fluoride. Patient cooperation in maintaining oral hygiene is extremely important.

Teeth with gross caries or periodontal involvement are often extracted before irradiation.

V. Bone: Treatment of cancers in the oral region often includes irradiation of the mandible. The primary damage to mature bone results from radiation-induced damage to the vasculature of the periosteum and cortical bone, which are normally already sparse.

Radiation also acts by destroying osteoblasts and, to a lesser extent, osteoclasts.

Subsequent to irradiation, normal marrow may be replaced with fatty marrow and fibrous connective tissue.

The marrow tissue becomes hypovascular, hypoxic, and hypocellular. In addition, the endosteum becomes atrophic, showing a lack of osteoblastic and osteoclastic activity, and some lacunae of the compact bone are empty, an indication of necrosis.

The degree of mineralization may be reduced, leading to brittleness, or little altered from normal bone. When these changes are so severe that bone death results, the condition is termed osteoradionecrosis.

Osteoradionecrosis is the most serious clinical complication that occurs in bone after irradiation.

The decreased vascularity of the mandible renders it easily infected by microorganisms from the oral cavity.

This bone infection may result from radiation-induced breakdown of the oral mucous membrane, by mechanical damage to the weakened oral mucous membrane such as from a denture sore or tooth extraction, through a periodontal lesion, or from radiation caries.

This infection may cause a non-healing wound in irradiated bone that is difficult to treat.

It is more common in the mandible than in the maxilla, probably because of the richer vascular supply to the maxilla and the fact that the mandible is more frequently irradiated.

The higher the radiation dose absorbed by the bone, the greater the risk for osteoradionecrosis.

Patients must be referred for dental care before undergoing a course of radiation therapy to reduce the severity of or prevent radiation caries and osteoradionecrosis.

Radiation caries can be minimized by restoring all carious lesions before radiation therapy and initiating preventive techniques of good oral hygiene and daily topical fluoride.

The risk for osteoradionecrosis and infection can be minimized by removing all poorly supported teeth, allowing sufficient time for the extraction wounds to heal before beginning radiation therapy, and adjusting dentures to minimize the risk for denture sores.

When teeth must be removed from irradiated jaws, the dentist should use a traumatic surgical technique to avoid elevating the periosteum, provide antibiotic coverage, and use low concentration epinephrine-containing local anesthetics that do not contain lidocaine.

Often patients require a radiographic examination to supplement the clinical examination.

These radiographs are especially important because untreated caries leading to periapical infection can be quite severe with the compromised vascular supply to bone.

The amount of added radiation is negligible compared with the amount received during therapy and should not serve as a reason to defer radiographs.

Whenever possible, however, it is desirable to avoid taking radiographs during the first 6 months after completion of radiotherapy to allow time for the mucosal membrane to heal.

Suggested reading:

1. Stuart C White, Michael J Pharoah, Oral Radiology, Principles and Interpretation 5th Edition, page no. 25-37.

CHAPTER 2

Radiation Protection

Q 1) Discuss radiation protection:

MUHS MAY 2007 10 Marks

The principle of radiation protection is to do those things that will minimize exposure of patient and dental personnel and still provide benefits for the patient from use of diagnostic radiography.

The means of protection can be divide into:

1. Protection for the operator.
2. Protection for the patient.
3. Protection for the environment.

1. **Protection for the operator:** The two most important sources of X-rays to which the operator is exposed to are:
   (a) The primary X-ray beam .
   (b) Scattered radiation originating from the irradiated tissues of the patient.
   (c) Other sources include:
      - Leakage radiation through the tube head housing.
      - Scattered X-ray from filters, cones.
      - Scattered radiation coming from object other than the patient, such as walls and furniture that the primary beam may strike.

   (a) **Protection against primary beam:**
      - The operator can leave the room or take a suitable position behind a barrier or wall during exposure.
      - Dental operatory should be designed and constructed to meet the minimum shielding requirements.
      - Position distance rule: which states that the operator should stand at least six feet away from the source of radiation or the operator should be at an angle of 90°, 135°, with respect to the direction of the central ray.
      - If there is no shield or barrier the operator should use a lead apron.
      - The film should never be held by operator. Ideally film holding devices should be used.

- There should be no use of fluorescent mirrors in the oral cavity at the time of exposure.
- Avoid holding the X-ray tube head of the machine. The suspension arm should be adequately maintained to prevent housing movement and drift.

(b) **Protection from secondary and scattered radiation:**
- Use of high speed film.
- Replace the short plastic cone with an open ended lead lined cone.
- Adequate filtration of the primary beam.
- Use of collimator, to reduce the diameter of beam.
- Use of film badge/ TLD badge/ pocket dosimeter, for personnel radiation monitoring, to avoid accumulated over exposure.

(c) **Protection against leakage radiation:**
- Neither the tube housing nor the cone should be hand held during exposure.
- The machine should be periodically checked for leakage.

2. **Protection for the patient:** Patient dose is usually reported as the amount of radiation received by target organs. One of the most common measurements is the skin or surface exposure. Other target organ commonly reported include the bone marrow, thyroid glands and gonads.
   - **Mean active bone marrow dose:** The dose derived as specific dose relevant to a particular stochastic effect, e.g. leukemia.
   - **Thyroid dose:** Thyroid glands are highly susceptible to radiation induced cancer.

   Thus, due to proximity of thyroid gland to the X-ray beam is crucially important in determining the magnitude of dose received.
   - **Gonad dose:** radiograph that involve the abdomen result in highest dose to the gonads.
   - Becoming aware of the potential risk associated with use of ionizing radiation is the first step towards exposure and dose reduction in diagnostic radiography.
   - **Prescription of radiographs:** Patients should be carefully evaluated and the dentist should make a proper judgement as to the need of a radiograph. The decision about the type number and frequency of radiographs should be taken with utmost care. The principle of As Low As Reasonably Achievable (ALARA)should be followed.
   - **Patient selection:** A refferal criteria including the clinical findings that identify the patient and radiographic examination that will provide more information that affect treatment and prognosis.
   - **Conduct of the examination:** when the decision is made that

a radiographic examination is justified, the way in which the examination is conducted greatly influences patient exposure to radiation. It is divided into:

- **Selection of image receptor:** use of high speed films, which help to reduce exposure time. Although the image quality may be compromised, E speed film should be used routinely which doesnot lead to loss of diagnostic information.
- **Screen films:** The use of intensifying screen also helps to reduce exposure time to the patient, but the diagnostic result of nonscreen films are far superior.
- **Intensifying screens:** use of intensifying screens lead to a compromise on image quality, in order to reduce exposure to the patient.
- **Focal spot film distance:** as X-rays are less divergent at a longer distance, there is a decrease in the volume of the patient exposed.
- **Source skin distance:** as the source skin distance is increased, the collimation must be correspondingly increased to reduced the beam size, thereby reducing the volume of tissue irradiated, thus reducing the patient dose.
  - Equipment operating below 50 kvp should have a minimum target-film distance of 10 inches.
  - Equipment operating above 50 kvp should have a minimum target film distance of 18 inches.
- **Collimation of the beam:** collimation helps to control the size and shape of the x-ray beam, allowing only the primary radiation beam to emerge. Collimation decreases the risk of radiation, minimizes scattered radiation and decreases the fog, with sharper image and better contrast.
- **Filtration:** filtration preferentially absorbs low energy photons which are undesirable as they add to the patients skin dose but do not have enough energy to penetrate the tissue and bring about image formation.
  - The amount of filtration should be in accordance with the machine's operating range:
    Below 50kvp: 0.3-0.5mm of half value aluminum layer.
    50-70kvp: 1.2-1.5mm of aluminum.
    Above 70 kvp: 2.1-4.1 mm of aluminum.
- **Use of high kvp:** higher kvp is used to keep the incident skin doses acceptable. The equipment should be capable of operating at a kilo voltage of 60 kvp or higher.
- **Use of positioning indicating devices:** These help to minimize the volume of tissue irradiated in intraoral radiography, it is necessary to increase the object film distance by using longer position indicating devices to direct the x-ray beam. One of the commonly used PID is the long open ended cylinder.

- **Film holding devices:** these offer protection to the patient, because:
    - Their use often reduces frequency of retakes, as the film can be positioned more accurately in the patient's mouth.
    - They also provide an external guide to indicate the film position.
    - The possibility of misaligning the x-ray tube and cone cut, is also reduced.
    - Some of the holders also collimate the beam to the size of the film being used, which further reduces patient exposure.
    - The exposure to the patient's fingers is also reduced, as the patient does not have to hold the film.
- **Timers:** the x-ray timer should be accurate and reproducible.
- **Use of protective barrier:**
    - Leaded apron should be used to protect the patient, especially in case of children, individuals of reproductive age and pregnant women.
    - Use of gonadal shields.
    - Use of leaded thyroid shield, this is recommended specially when cephalometric examination are carried out on children because of greater sensitivity of thyroid in young people. The thickness of lead used should be 0.2mm.
- **Use of proper technique:** the use of proper technique for the imaging of the particular anatomy of the patient.
- **Processing the image:** if the film are not processed properly, retakes are required, increasing the patient exposure and cost.
- **Interpretation of image:** the radiograph should be viewed under proper conditions with an illuminated viewer. Proper interpretation precludes the necessity of retaking the images and subjecting the patient to additional exposure.

3. **Protection for the environment:**
    - Primary beam should never be directed at any one other than the patient.
    - Patient should be positioned such that the X-ray beam is aimed at the wall of the room and not through the door or other opening where people may be located.
    - Wall made of 3″ of concrete, 3″ x 16″ of steel or 1mm of lead will suffice to protect adjacent rooms, even if the work load in the radiology department is high.
    - It is necessary for the operator to see the patient as he is being irradiated, so a window is provided.
    - Continuing education: practitioners should stay informed of new information on radiation safety issue as well as developments

in equipment, material and techniques and adopt appropriate items to improve radiographic practice.

- Regular radiation surveys, should be performed at regular interval as the amount of exposure is dependant upon many factors, such as:
  - The machine's kilovoltage
  - The work load of x-ray machine
  - The x-ray absorbing ability of the walls
  - The amount of time the adjacent areas are occupied by people.
- Radiation monitoring is measuring of the x-ray exposure of operators or associated personnel as a protective measure. There are various monitoring devices available:
  - *Electrical*
    Ionization chamber
    Thimble chamber
    Proportional counter
    Geiger counter
  - *Chemical*
    Film
    Chemical dosimeter
  - *Light*
    Scintillation counter
    Gerenkov counter
  - *Thermoluminescence*
    Thermoluminescent dosimeter.
  - *Heat*
    Calorimeter.

Suggested reading:

1. Freny R Karjodkar, Essentials of oral and maxillofacial radiology. Edi. 1, Chapter 6, page no. 35-42.

CHAPTER 3

Processing of X-Ray Films

Q 1) Discuss the requirements of an ideal dark room and details of dark room chemistry.

MUHS NOVEMBER 2011 10 Marks

Ideal Dark Room:

- The main function of the darkroom is to create a totally dark environment where the exposed x rays can be manipulated, handled and processed to obtain an image that is diagnostic in an efficient, precise and standardized manner.
- As processing operations are carried out in total darkness, every piece of equipment must be in a specific place.
- Ideal darkroom should have following characteristics;

1. **Dimensions:**
   - The darkroom should be convenient to the x-ray machines and dental operatories and should be at least 4 × 5 feet (1.2 × 1.5m).
   - The darkroom should have sufficient space to accommodate the processing tanks or automatic processors.
2. **Lightproofing:**
   - One of the most important requirements is that it be lightproof.
   - To accomplish this, a light-tight door or doorless maze (if space permits) is used.
   - The door should have a lock to prevent accidental opening, which might allow an unexpected flood of light that can ruin opened films.
3. **Ventilation:**
   - The room must be well ventilated for the comfort of those working in the area and to exhaust the heat from the dryer and moisture from the drying films.
   - A comfortable room temperature helps to maintain the optimal conditions for the development, fixation and washing solutions.
   - If supplies / unexposed x-ray film are to be stored in the darkroom, ventilation is doubly important because temperatures of 90° F

or higher can cause a generalized increase in density (film fog) on the film.

4. **Safe-lighting:**
   - The processing room should have both white illumination and safe-lighting.
   - Safe-lighting is low-intensity illumination of relatively long wavelength (red) that does not rapidly affect open film but permits one to see well enough to work in the area.
   - It is best to place one safelight above the work area on the wall behind the processing tanks and somewhat to the right of the fixing tank.

Intensity of illumination:

- To minimize the fogging effect of prolonged exposure, the safelight should have a 7.5 to 15-watt bulb and should be mounted at least 4 feet above the surface where opened films are handled.
- Arrangement of safe light filters should be such that three zones of illumination i.e. Dimmest zone, Medium zone and Bright zone.

Types of filters:

- X-ray films are very sensitive to the blue-green region of the spectrum and less sensitive to yellow and red wavelengths.
- The red GBX-2 filter is recommended as a safelight in darkrooms where either intraoral or extraoral films are handled, because this filter transmits light only at the red end of the spectrum.
- The older Moralite / ML-2 filters (yellow light) are not appropriate for fast intraoral dental film or extraoral panoramic or cephalometric film.
- Film handling under a safelight must be only for 5 minutes as the emulsion of the film has some sensitivity to light from a safelight with prolonged exposure.
- Written filter (cannot be used for screen films).

Test for checking unsafe illumination:

- Coin test / penny test: Coin is placed on unexposed film under the safe light. Develop the film. If the developed film showing outline of the coin, it indicates that the safe light intensity is too great and not safe. This test is to evaluate for fogging caused by inappropriate safe lighting conditions.
- Careful observation for light leakages.

Dark Room Chemistry:

After a radiograph is taken it is processed in the dark room to convert the latent image into visible image.

This is done by manual processing with the help of two main chemical solutions that are the developer solution and a fixer solution.

These solutions are contained in a metal tank.

There are three tanks present. On the left is present the developer solution in which the film is immersed first.

The second tank contains water which is used to rinse the film after developing.

The third tank contains the fixer solution in which the film is placed for fixing.

1. Film Processing Solutions (Chemical composition):

- **Developer Solution:**

  The developing solution contains four components: (1) developer, (2) activator, (3)preservative, and (4) restrainer.

  Developer:

  - Two developing agents used are; a pyrazolidone-type compound, usually Phenidone (1-phenyl-3-pyrazolidone), and hydroquinone (paradihydroxy benzene).
  - Phenidone serves as the first electron donor that converts silver ions to metallic silver at the latent image site.
  - This electron transfer causes the oxidation of Phenidone.
  - Hydroquinone provides an electron to reduce the oxidized Phenidone back to its original active state so that it can continue to reduce the silver halide grains to metallic silver.

  Activator:

  - Sodium or potassium hydrozide are activator in developing solution.
  - The developers are active only at alkaline pH values, usually around 10. This is achieved with the addition of alkali compounds (activators).
  - The activators also cause the gelatin to swell so that the developing agents are able to diffuse in a speedy manner in to the emulsion and reach the suspended silver bromide crystals.

  Preservative:

  - The developing solution contains an antioxidant or preservative, usually sodium sulfite.
  - The preservative protects the developers from oxidation by atmospheric oxygen and thus extends their useful life.
  - The preservative also combines with the brown oxidized developer to produce a colorless soluble compound. If not removed, they stain the film.

  Restrainer:

  - Bromide, which is usually potassium bromide, and benzotriazole are used as restrainers in developing solution.
  - They help in restraining the development of unexposed silver halide crystals.
  - Although bromide and benzotriazole depress the

reduction of both exposed and unexposed crystals, they are much more effective in depressing the reduction of unexposed crystals.

- The restrainers act as anti-fog agents and increase contrast.

- **Fixing Solution:**

  The primary function of fixing solution is to dissolve and remove the undeveloped silver halide crystals from the emulsion.

  Clearing Agent:

  - An aqueous solution of ammonium thiosulphate ("hypo") dissolves the silver halide grains.

  Preservative:

  - Ammonium sulfite is the preservative in the fixing solution.
  - It prevents oxidation of the thiosulfate clearing agent, which is unstable in the acid environment of the fixing solution.
  - It also binds with any colored oxidized developer carried over into the fixing solution and effectively removes it from the solution, which prevents staining of the film.

  Acidifier:

  - Acetic acid buffer system helps to keep the fixer pH constant. This pH is required to promote good diffusion of the thiosulphate in to the emulsion.

  Hardener:

  - Aluminum sulphate is most commonly used as a hardening agent.
  - Aluminum complexes with the gelatin during fixing and prevents damage to the gelatin during subsequent handling.
  - The hardeners also help in the reduction of swelling of the emulsion when the films are washed finally and hence lessen the mechanical damage to the emulsion and shorten the drying time.

- **Replenishing solutions:**

  Developer and fixer replenishing solutions are a part of darkroom chemistry and are important to maintain the proper strength of the solutions used for processing of films.

Suggested reading:

1. Freny. R. Karzodkar, Essentials of Oral and Maxillofacial Radiology, 2nd edition . pg no.133-143.
2. Stuart C White, Michael J Pharoah, Oral Radiology, Principles and Interpretation.6th edition Page no. 94-110.

Q 2) Discuss in detail processing of Radiographs and formation of latent image:

BFU MAY 2006 1(5 Marks)

Processing is the name given to series of procedures that are carried out in the dark room, that results in chemical changes in the radiographic film that is exposed to x-rays, and make the invisible latent image that is present in the sensitised emulsion of the film into a permanent visible radiographic image.

Processing of radiographs can be classified as:

I) **Manual:** There are three types:
   (i) Time temperature.
   (ii) Modified time-temperature.
   (iii) Visual.

II) **Automatic processing.**

III) **Daylight processing.**

IV) **Self developing films.**

Processing of films includes the following procedures:

1. Immerse exposed film in developer.
2. The developer is rinsed off in the water bath.
3. Immerse film in fixer.
4. Washing the film in the water bath to remove the fixer.
5. Drying of the film and mounting it for viewing.

After the film is exposed to the x-rays, the grains of silver halide in film emulsion consists of silver atoms that are neutral at the sites of latent image. These areas of latent image make the crystal sensitive to the developing solution and ultimately the image formation.

The function of the developer is to convert the silver bromide crystals with silver atoms that are neutral that are deposited at the latent image sites, in to black solid metallic silver grains. The function of the fixer is to remove the unexposed silver halide crystals that are undeveloped on the film in unexposed areas.

The radiographic image hence consists of light areas (radiopaque)in which very few x-ray photons have reached and dark or radiolucent areas where the film has been struck with several x-ray photons.

Developing solution:

The developing solution contains four basic components all dissolved in water.

Reducing agents	Phenidone serves as the first electron donor that converts silver ions to metallic silver at latent image site.
Phenidone	
Hydroquinone	
Metol or elon	
Phenidone is used in automatic processing	Hydroquinone provides an electron to reduce the oxidized phenidone back to its original active state so that it can continue to reduce silver halide grains to metallic silver.

	Metol or elon helps develop the shadow areas or shades of gray on the film and brings out the details. It does not produce a high contrast. It is less sensitive to temperature changes.
Activator Sodium hydroxide Potassium hydroxide Potassium carbonate/ sodium carbonate.	Developers are active only at pH values around 10; and this pH is achieved only by addition of activators and they are also called the accelerator. The activators also cause the gelatin to swell so that the developing agents can diffuse more rapidly into emulsion to reach silver bromide crystals
Preservative Sodium sulfite	It extends the useful life of solution. Preservative combines with oxidized developer to produce a compound that subsequently stains images brown if not washed out.
Restrainer Potassium bromide or benzotriazole	Prevents excessive fogging of film and increases the contrast
Hardener Glutaraldehyde	This is added to automatic processing to prevent the emulsion from softening and sticking to rollers.
Fungicide	To prevent bacterial growth

Rinsing:

After the developing of the film, the emulsion on the film swells and gets saturated with the developer. At this time, the films are rinsed in water for about 30 seconds with gentle, agitation and continously and then put in the fixer.

Rinsing of the film helps to dilute the developer and slows down the developing process. It also helps to remove the alkaline activator so as to prevent neutralisation of the acid fixer. This process is typically done in the manual processing but not with most automatic processors.

Fixing solution:

This solution contains four components and are dissolved in water.

Clearning agent Ammonium thiosulfate or sodium thiosulfate	It removes the unsensitized silver halide crystals. It forms stable water soluble complexes with silver ions, which diffuse from the emulsion.
Acidifier Acetic acid	It contains an acetic acid buffer system (pH 4 to 4.5) to keep the fixer pH constant and the acid fixing solution also inactivates residual developing agents in the film emulsion

Preservative Ammonium sulfate	Prevents oxidation of thiosulfate clearing agent.
Hardener Aluminum sulfate	It complexes with gelatin during fixing and prevents damage to gelatine.

Washing:

Once the fixing is done the film is washed in water so as to remove all the thiosulfate ions and complexes of silver thiosulfate. The efficiency of washing gets declined when the temperature of water falls below 60 degrees F.

Formation of latent image:

1. When the x-ray photons fall on the film, they react with the silver halide crystals chemically and form a invisible image at the site of interaction which is called as latent image. By the process of developing and fixing this latent image is converted to visible image.
2. The sulfur compounds play an important part in the formation of image and so does the physical irrgularities in the crystals that are produced by the iodide ions. Sulfur compounds create sensitivity site, the sites in the crystal that are sensitive to radiation.
3. When exposed to radiation, the photosensitive crystals of silver halide get altered chemically and produce the latent image
4. When the silver halide crystals are irradiated photons of x-ray primarily interact with the ions of bromide by compton and photoelectric interactions.
5. Because of these interactions, there is removal of an electron from the bromide ion and they are converted to neutral bromine atom. These free electrons keep moving in the crystal, till they reach the site of sensitivity where they get trapped and handover the negative charge to the site.
6. These sensitivity sites which is now negatively charged attracts interstitial silver ions that are free and positively charged. Then the silver ions reach these negatively charged sites of sensitivity and are reduced to form a neutral atom of metallic silver. The sites in which these neutral silver atoms are present are called the latent image sites.
7. This process occurs for numerous times within the crystal. The overall distribution of the crystals with the sites of latent image in the film after the exposure to the x-rays constitutes the latent image. Then when the films are processed with the developer and fixer, this latent image is converted to visible image.

Suggested reading:

1. Stuart C White, Michael J Pharoah, Oral Radiology, Principles and Interpretation 5th Edition, 94-104.

Q 3) What is the composition of radiographic film? Describe the mechanism of image formation. Add a note on the composition of developing and fixing solution and their functions.

RGUHS APRIL 2006 (9 Marks)

Composition:

The films of x-rays have two components:

1. **Base:** The base functions mainly as support to the emulsion.
   It should possess flexibility enough, so that easy handling of the film is possible and is 0.18mm in thickness and is made up of polyethylene pterephthalate.
   The base is translucent uniformly and doesnot cast any pattern on the radiograph.
   According to some the base should have a slight blue tint and it will help in improving the viewing of diagnostic detail.
   The base of the film should have properties to withstand exposure to processing solutions with out becoming distorted.
2. **Emulsion:** It consists of two important components, the first is the grains of silver halide which are sensitive to visible light and x-rays and the gelatin matrix in which the grains are suspended.
   The grains of silver halide are composed of mainly the crystals of silver bromide. Iodide which has larger size than the bromine is added to the ultra-speed films to disrupt the regular size of the silver bromide crystals and thus increases the sensitivity to x-rays. Trace amounts of sulphur containing compounds control the photosensitivity of the silver halide crystals. Sometimes trace amounts of gold is also added to increase the sensitivity.
   When the film is being manufactured, the crystals of silver halide are suspended in the gelatin matrix and applied to both sides of the film base.
   The medium in which the crystals are suspended are made up of gelatinous or non-gelatinous material which helps to disperse the silver halide grains evenly. A thin layer of adhesive is applied to the base of the film so as to ensure proper adhesion of the emulsion to the base.
   During the processing of the films the gelatinous matrix absorbs the solutions used in processing and helps the chemicals to reach and react with the silver halide crystals.

Supercoat:

It is a protective, transparent, non-abrasive layer over the emulsion.

This is an additional layer of gelatin which is applied to the surface to serve as a protective coat and prevents damage to the film during mechanical handling.

This additional layer of gelatin acts as a barrier and prevents the film from scratching or damaging and contamination and also prevents pressure from the rollers in automatic film processors.

The films are made as double emulsion films by coating the emulsion on each side of the base.

When the emulsion consists of a double layer, less amount of radiation can be used to produce an image.

One corner of each dental film has a small, raised dot that is used for film orientation.

When the film is placed in the patient's mouth, the side of the film with the raised dot is always positioned facing the x-ray tube.

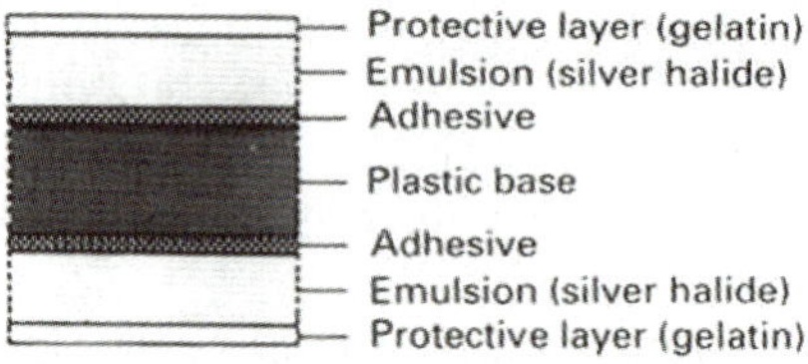

Fig. Composition of x-ray film

Mechanism of image formation:

Image formation consists of two stages:

1. Latent image formation.
2. Visible image formation.

Latent image:

The silver halide crystals present on the film are sensitised chemically by the addition of trace amounts of sulphur compounds that bind to the crystals on the surface. The sulphur compounds play a crucial role in image formation.

There are several sensitivity sites on the crystals, and the process of formation of image begins by trapping of the electrons which are generated when there is irradiation of the emulsion.

When the photosensitive silver halide crystals are exposed to radiation it alters them chemically and there is production of latent image.

After exposure to radiation of the silver halide crystals the x-ray photons primarily interact with the bromide ions by the compton and photoelectric effect. This results in removal of an electron from the bromide ions.

The bromide ion as a result of loss of an electron gets converted to a neutral atom of bromine. The electrons that are liberated move in the crystal and reach the sensitivity site, where after getting trapped they donate a negative charge to the site. This site that is now negatively charged attracts the positively charged free interstitial silver ions. By this interaction the there is reduction of the silver ion and there is formation of neutral atom of metallic silver. The sites thus, which consist of the neutral silver atoms become the site for latent image.

Visible image:

When the films are taken through a processing method this latent image gets converted to visible image.

In the latent image site the neutral silver atoms sensitise the crystals so that there can be development and formation of image . Larger the aggregation of the neutral silver atoms, more is the sensitivity of the crystal to the effects of the developer.

In a film that is optimally exposed to radiation have, the latent image sites that are capable of being developed have at least four or five silver atoms. The function of the developer is to convert the silver bromide crystals with neutral silver atoms at the sites of the latent image, in to solid metallic grains of silver. The function of the fixer is to remove the silver bromide crystals that are unexposed and undeveloped and leave the film clear in the unexposed areas.

Hence the final radiographic image consists of light area where only few photons have reached the film and dark areas of the film that were bombarded by many photons.

Composition of developing and fixing solutions and their functions:

Developing solution contains the following chemicals:

1. **Developer:** The function of the developer mainly is to convert the exposed silver halide crystals in to grains of metallic silver.
   There are two types of developing agents used in dental radiology:
   (a) **Pyrazilodone type compound usually Phenidone:** At the latent image sites, phenidone acts as the first electron donor that converts the silver ions to metallic silver. This transfer of electrons forms the iodised form of phenidone.
   (b) **Hydroquinone:** The function of hydroquinone is to provide an electron to reduce the phenidone that is oxidised back to its original state of activeness so that it can continue to reduce the silver halide grains to metallic silver.
2. **Activator:** As the developers are active at an alkaline pH of 10, it is achieved by the addition of alkali compounds that are activators such as sodium or potassium hydroxide. Buffers like sodium carbonate are added to maintain this condition. The gelatin also swells due to action of activator because of which the developing agents can diffuse more speedily and effectively within the emulsion and reach the sites of suspended silver bromide crystals. Sodium hydroxide in conjunction with sodium carbonate may be used to give higher contrast.
3. **Preservative:** Sodium sulphite which is an anti-oxidant and preservative is usually contained in the developer. Its function is to protect the developer from getting oxidised by the atmospheric oxygen and helps to extend the useful life of the developer. It also combines with the oxidised brown developer to produce a colourless soluble compound. If the oxidation products are not removed they interfere with action of developing and will stain the film.
4. **Restrainer:** Potassium bromide and benzotriazole are added to the developer so as to control the development of silver halide crystals

that are unexposed .The restrainers help to increase the contrast and act as anti fog agents. Though the bromide and the benzotriazoles help in depressing the exposed and unexposed crystals of silver halide more effectiveness is with unexposed crystals of silver halide reduction of both the exposed and unexposed silver halide crystals, they are more effective with unexposed silver halide crystals.

5. **Replenisher:** The phenidone and hydroquinone get consumed in the normal course of processing of films and the bromide ions and other by-products get released in the solution. There is inactivation of the developer by exposure to atmospheric oxygen. Due to these actions a seasoned solution is produced and the speed of the film and the contrast stabilise. There is need to replenish the developing solutions of both manual and automatic processing, with fresh solution each morning so as to prolong the life of the developer.
6. **Hardener:** Glutaraldehyde is added especially in automatic processing to prevent the emulsion from softening and sticking to the roller.
7. **Fungicide:** To prevent bacterial growth.
8. **Buffer:** To maintain pH (+7).Sodium bicarbonate is usually used.
9. **Solvent:** Water is used as solvent of the chemicals and as a medium in which they react with the silver bromide of the film emulsion.

Fixer Solution:

The fixer solution contains the following components:

Clearning agent:

Ammonium thiosulfate or sodium thiosulfate: It removes the unsensitized silver halide crystals. It forms stable water soluble complexes with silver ions, which diffuse from the emulsion.

Acidifier:

Acetic acid: The contents are a buffer system of acetic acid with pH of 4-4.5 so as to keep the fixer pH constant. The acid fixing solution also inactivates the residual developing agents in the film emulsion.

Preservative:

Ammonium sulphate: Prevents oxidation of thiosulfate clearing agent.

Hardener:

Aluminum sulphate: A complex is formed with gelatin during the process of fixing and there is prevention of damage to gelatine.

Suggested reading:

1. Freny R Karjodkar, Essentials Of Oral and Maxillofacial radiology, chapter 10, pg no.131-132.
2.) Stuart C White, Michael J Pharaoh, Oral Radiology, Principles And Interpretation, 5th edition, 72-73, 94 , 96-97.

CHAPTER 4

Intraoral Radiographic Examinations

Q 1) Enumerate intraoral radiographic technique. Describe the procedure of localizing an impacted left maxillary canine:

RGUHS APRIL 1999 (10 Marks)

There are following intraoral radiographic techniques:

1. Periapical radiography:
   - (a) Paralleling technique
   - (b) Bisecting angle technique
2. Bite Wing radiography:
3. Occlusal radiography:

Radiographic Assessment:

There are various radiographic methods that can be used for localization of impacted maxillary left canine.

There can be:

1. Right angle technique:
   - Intraoral.
   - Extraoral.
2. Clarks technique/tube shift/SLOB rule.
3. True occlusal view.
4. Panoramic radiography.
5. Computerised Tomography and Cone Beam Computerised Tomography.
6. Rapid prototyping.

1. **Right Angle Technique/ Millers technique:**
   - In the right angle technique, two radiographs that are at right angles to each other are taken.
   - In intraoral radiography, the use of combination of a intraoral periapical radiograph with a occlusal radiograph for localization of impacted canine.
   - In extra oral radiography a lateral cephalogram and a PA Skull is taken.

(a) **Intraoral technique:**

(i) Intra-oral periapical radiography(IOPA):
- ❖ Procedure:
- ❖ The patient is positioned erect in the chair with the ala-tragus line parallel to the floor.
- ❖ The film is placed against the palate in left maxillary canine region, with the long axis of the tooth superimposed on the central long axis of the film.
- ❖ The projection of central ray through the ala of nose of left side and perpendicular to the plane bisecting the angle between the long axis of the film and the root of the tooth at an angle of $+40^\circ$ to $+45^\circ$ is made.
- ❖ The periapical radiograph shows left impacted canine lying apical to roots of lateral incisor and first premolar.

(ii) Maxillary anterior occlusal radiograph:
- ❖ The film is placed cross wise into the mouth and gently pushed back until it contact the anterior border of both the ramus.
- ❖ The central ray directed at a vertical angulation of $+45^\circ$ and horizontal angulation of 0° towards the middle of the film through the tip of nose.
- ❖ The maxillary anterior occlusal radiograph shows that the left maxillary canine lies palatal to the roots of the lateral incisor and first premolar.

(b) **Extraoral technique:**

(i) Postero-Anterior Views:

Procedure:
- ❖ For the localization of impacted left maxillary canine in PA skull, the cassette is placed in vertical position. The left and right side of the patient should be marked on the cassette.
- ❖ Position of the patient is done by adjusting the sagittal plane perpendicular to the film and the patient's head is tipped downwards so that the forehead and nose touch the film. The radiographic baseline is horizontal and perpendicular to the film. The film is adjusted so that lips is centered on the film.
- ❖ The central ray is directed at right angles to the film through the midsagittal plane through the occiput.
- ❖ Postero-anterior radiography is helpful for evaluating the medio-lateral position of the impacted canines in respect to a line that connects the inferior border of the orbits.
- ❖ By evaluation of the angle that is formed by the long axis of the tooth and the transorbital line, this is possible.
- ❖ There is a decrease in prognosis and increase in the difficulty of treatment as the angle between the long axis of the tooth and the transorbital line decreases.

(ii) **Lateral Cephalogram:** The height of the impacted tooth and the antero-posterior position of the cuspid with respect to the apices of the incisors can be established by this technique.

Procedure:

- The cassette is placed perpendicular to the floor with its long axis placed vertically.
- The side of the patient's head is positioned against the casette. The mid saggital plane is perpendicular to the floor and parallel to the film/ cassette. The patient's head is stabilized with the help of ear rods, nasion positioner and the orbital rod. The patient is asked to keep the teeth in occlusion.
- The central ray is directed perpendicular to the cassette through the porion. The distance between x-ray source and midsagittal plane of the patient is 60 inches.
- This will indicate the position of impacted canine in an antero-posterior dimension.
- This may thus help to establish whether the impacted tooth is positioned palatally or labially.

2. **Clark's rule/parallax method/tube shift technique:**
   - The apparent displacement of an image in relation to the image of an object of reference is called parallax and its caused due to an actual change in the x-ray beam angulation.
   - Change in the position of the x-ray tube causes the change in angulation of the beam. The object of reference is usually the root of an adjacent tooth.
   - Two radiographs of the impacted left maxillary canine is taken. With proper technique and angulation the first radiograph is obtained. By keeping all the parameters constant and equivalent of the first radiograph, a second radiograph is taken and only the direction of the central ray in relation to horizontal or vertical angulation is changed.
   - If the angulation is given more distal to the first radiograph, and the impacted canine moves more distally then it is situated palatally. If the horizontal angulation is given more distally and the canine moves mesially, it is located buccally. (SLOB-same lingual opposite buccal)
3. **True occlusal view:** In this technique a cassette with intensifying screen is used. The cassette is placed inside the mouth as for standard occlusal view and the patient is asked to bite on the cassette. The central ray is entered through the vertex perpendicular to the centre of the film. The occlusal surface of the teeth appear in cross section, button shaped and the lingual and cortical borders are clearly defined. This technique can give idea about the location

of the left impacted maxillary canine whether located palatally or buccally.

4. **Panoramic Radiographs:** Ericson and Kurolin in 1988 described number of sectors to denote different types of impactions.
   (i) **Sector I:** If the tip of the cusp of the canine is between the inter-incisor median line and the long axis of the central incisor.
   (ii) **Sector II:** If the peak of the cusp of the canine is between the major axis of the lateral and central incisor.
   (iii) **Sector III:** In this case the peak of the cusp of the canine is placed between the major axis of the lateral incisor and the first premolar.
   - Angle a was used to denote the angle formed between the inter-incisor midline and the long axis of the canine and d was used to denote the perpendicular distance of the peak of the cusp of the impacted canine in respect to the plane of occlusion.
   - Localisation of the impacted canines by means of the sector methods have more prognostic than the diagnostic value. The resorption of the root of the lateral incisor is at risk and increases by 50% if the cusp of the canine belongs to the sector I and II and if the angle a is greater than 25 degrees.
   - In case the canine is in the sector I then the treatment duration is longer and it is shorter if found in sector III, with respect to sector II. As this angle increases the treatment necessity and the degree of difficulty of the treatment increases.

5. **3-D Techniques:** Computerised Tomography and Cone Beam Computerised Tomography:

   In conventional radiography, due to superimposition of the structures on the areas of interest, it becomes difficult to discern the details which are important for proper diagnosis and treatment planning.
   - The tissue contrast is excellent in computed tomography(CT) and there is elimination of blurring and overlapping of the adjacent teeth and help in exact localization of the teeth. However the cost, risk, access and expertise in reading has limited its use.
   - Cone beam Computed Tomography is a latest trend of volumetric image acquisition which can give a three dimensional view of an object. The view of impacted left maxillary canine can be taken and the 3-D view can help to accurately locate the canine and also the lingual or buccal placement of it.

6. **Rapid prototyping:**
   - In this technique there is use of various technologies to use the data from a computer-aided design files and the production of physical models and devices by a material addition process.
   - Exact position of the canine to be known is important in the

treatment of impacted maxillary canines. It can be a challenge for the oral surgeons and the orthodontists. In this newer technique use of computed tomography with rapid prototyping is used to diagnose and plan the proper treatment for the impacted left maxillary canines. In a patient with maxillary left canine impaction, the computed tomography image files of the same can be edited to produce by the use of rapid prototyping, an anatomic model of the maxillary teeth and the use of a single attachment model which is used later to fabricate a attachment that is of metal to be bonded to the tooth that is impacted. This model can be used to denote the precise anatomic relationship between the tooth that is impacted and the other teeth. The metal attachment that is formed from the prototype can be bonded to the maxillary canine during surgery.

- In the evaluation of the impacted maxillary canines the rapid prototyping can become the diagnostic procedure of choice.

Suggested reading:

1. Freny R. Karjodkar, Essentials Of Oral and Maxillofacial Radiology, First Edition, Chapter 11, 12, page no. 97-155.
2. Surubhi Kumar, Praveen Mehrotra, Jitendra Bhagchandani, Ashish Singh, Aarti Garg, Snehi Kumar, Ashish Sharma, Harsh Yadav, Localization of Impacted Canines. Journal of Clinical and Diagnostic Research. 2015 Jan, Vol-9(1): ZE11-ZE14

CHAPTER 5

Panoramic Imaging

Q 1) Discuss the principles, technique, advantages and disadvantages of panoramic imaging:

TNMGRU AUGUST 2013 10 Marks

Principle:

Panoramic radiography is a form of rotational tomography.

Panorama: Can be defined as an unobstructed view of a region in every direction.

Tomography: It is a technique in which the image of a section of the object is obtained which is sharply defined by deliberately blurring the images of objects that are above, below, in front of or behind it.

A conventional radiograph is a two dimensional image of a three dimensional object and there is unavoidable superimposition of anatomic structures that are not of interest.

In tomography there is controlled movement of both the tube and film through out the exposure. This movement is so arranged that in a predetermined plane there is no relative movement of the tube and the film. In this layer the image is sharpest.

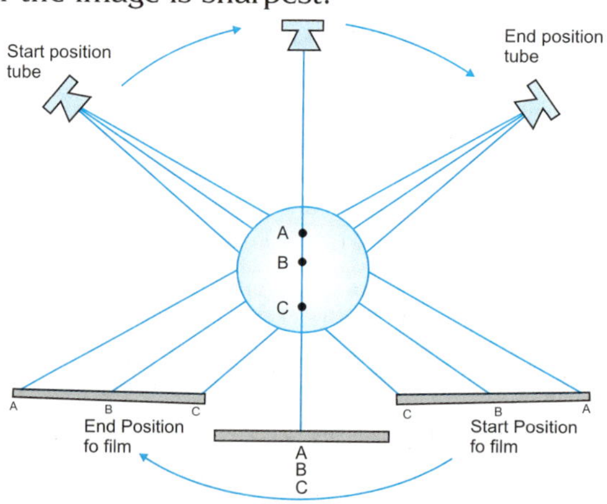

Fig. The position of B remains constant where as those of A and C change and hence the slice B is seen clearly

In panoramic radiography the x-ray tube is linked mechanically to the film holder by a rigid metal bar and there is a pivot around which they can swing freely.

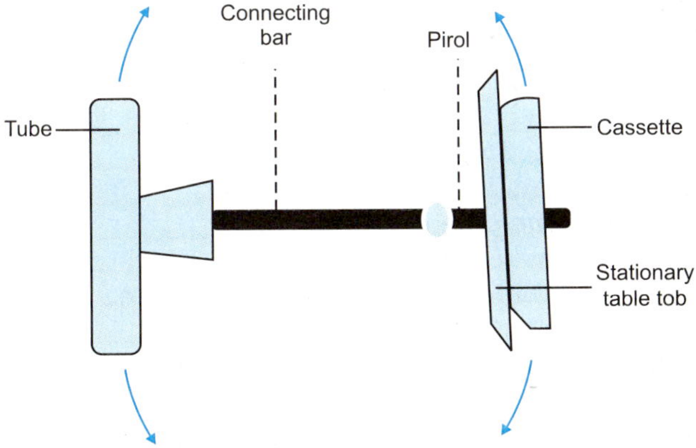

Fig. Set up of panoramic radiography with film and x-ray tube connected with rigid metal bar with a pivot for free swing

This helps to obtain a curved tomographic cut which is as near as possible to the shape of the dental arch.

A narrow beam of x-rays(slit)is used by placing two metal plates across the x-ray window.

As the x-ray source and the film rotate at equal speed the beam exposes only a part of the film at one time as the exposed and the unexposed part of the film is covered by a protective shield and has a slit like opening to coincide with the slit opening on the x-ray tube. This prevents scattered radiation and prevents darkening of film and film fogging.

Since only a small portion of the film is exposed at any one time there is no superimposition of layers and will be seen as one continuous tomograpic layer.

The thickness of the tomographic layer is decided by the angle of swing of the film and x-ray tube assembly. Larger the swing, thinner the tomographic cut.

Different machines have different modes of movement. Some have continuous movement and others have three axi of rotation, two for posterior segment and one for the anterior segment.

In the beginning the tube is on the right side of the patient and it images the left side posterior segment. Then the axis changes to image the anterior segment and lastly it changes to image the right side posterior segment.

Focal trough: It is a three dimensional imaginary zone. the objects when placed in the centre are most sharply defined.

Different machines have different shapes and size of focal trough.

Technique:

- The machine is adjusted on panoramic mode.
- The patient is asked to remove glasses and other metallic items

from the head and the neck, like necklaces, neck chain, napkins, zippers, hairpins etc.

- Patient either stands or can sit erect with back straight so as to prevent superimposition of cervical spine in the anterior region.
- Neck is extended so as to prevent large opaque artifacts in the midline.
- The Patient's head should be tilted downward so that the ala-tragus line is 5 degrees down and forward.
- Align the mid sagittal plane of the patient 's head with the vertical central line of the chin rest.
- The patient is asked to bring mandible forward so as to bring the maxillary and mandibular incisors to the same plane and bite into a notched positioning device.
- It has to be ensured that the mandible is not shifted to any one side.
- Patient closes the lips and places the tongue against the roof of the mouth.
- Patient is explained how the machine works.
- The exposure is then made with preset timing and KVp adjusted according to need.

Advantages:

- Positioning is simple and minimal expertise is required.
- Convenient for the patient.
- Useful visual aid in patient education and case presentation.
- Minimal requirement of patient co-operation.
- Can be used with comfort in patients with severe trauma and inablility to open their mouth .
- Broad coverage of the facial bones & teeth.
- The anatomical structures are most identifiable and the teeth are oriented in their correct relationship to the adjacent structures and to each other.
- Useful for mass screening.
- Multiple lesions can be seen on one film.
- The overall view of the jaws helps in rapid assessment of any underlying possibility of unsuspected disease.
- Easy assessment of single or multiple fractures on one film. Especially helpful to visualize bilateral condylar fractures.
- The maxillary antrum of both sides, their floor, anterior and posterior walls can be seen and compared on one film.
- The initial evaluation of periodontal status can be done.
- The mixed dentition phase can be easily assessed especially prior to orthodontic treatment.
- Multiple impacted supernumerary and other teeth can be visualized on one film.
- The exposure time is less and radiation dose is minimal especially when compared to full mouth radiography.

Disadvantages:

- The movement of x-ray tube and film assembly and the larger target –object distance causes magnification and image unsharpness.
- The amount of horizontal and vertical distortion varies from one part of the film to another. This results in uneven magnification of the image & structure and spaces may be seen larger than the actual size.
- Unable to display the fine anatomic details available on intra oral radiographs.
- Is not as useful as periapical radiography for detecting small carious lesions, fine structure of the marginal periodontium, periapical disease, and exact extent of cysts and tumours .
- Have tendency to produce overlapping of teeth images, most particularly in premolar area.
- Cervical spine may superimpose and the anterior teeth may not be clearly visualized.
- Some patients jaw sizes may not conform to the shape of the focal trough of a particular machine and hence structures may appear blurred.
- Ghost images of anatomic and non-anatomic structures may interfere with the diagnostability of the radiograph.
- Not very suitable for children and handicapped patients because of the length of exposure time.
- Equipment is expensive and requires high maintenance.

Suggested reading:

1. Freny R Karjodkar, Textbook Of Dental And Maxillofacial Radiography, 2nd edition, 236-255.

CHAPTER **6**

Periodontal Diseases

Q 1) Discuss The Role Of Radiography In The Diagnosis And Management Of Periodontal Disease:

TNMGRU Sept. 2002 (15 Marks)

Introduction:

- Radiographs are an integral component of a periodontal assessment for those with clinical evidence of periodontal destruction.
- For the diagnosis of periodontal diseases both radiographic and clinical data is essential.
- The bone amount that is present.
- The condition of the alveolar crests.
- Loss of bone in the areas of furcation.
- The width of the periodontal ligament space.
- Local factors causing or intensifying the periodontal disease.
- Presence of calculus.
- Restorations that are not properly contoured and overhanging restorations.
- Caries
- Morphology and length of the roots.
- Ratio of crown to root.
- Inflammatory lesions of the apex.
- Resorption of roots.

Clinical assessment of the need for radiographic examination in periodontal patients:

- In clinical examination of periodontitis, probing pocket depths and/or recession provides information about the condition.
- Radiographic examination gives some information on: evident bone levels; evident patterns of bone loss, even or angular; tooth-root lengths, morphologies and topographies; and importantly length of tooth-root radiographically surrounded by alveolar bone.
- Clinical attachment loss is the diagnostic tool for periodontitis and also the calculating tool for determining clinical severity of

periodontitis.

- But remaining tooth-root support is the major complementary estimation provided only by radiographic imaging, which while not diagnostic, is of prime importance in treatment planning decisions, in prognosis estimation, and, in contributing to the eventual outcome, the retention of periodontitis affected teeth in acceptable function for life.

Radiography in the diagnosis of periodontal diseases:

- There is inflammatory lesions of the marginal bone in periodontal diseases.
- Bone activity shows osteoblastic as well as osteoclastic activities.
- Changes in the morphology of the crestal bone will occur due to osteoclastic activity.
- Destruction of bone is the initial response.
- Osteosclerosis will be seen in chronic lesions.

1. **Mild marginal periodontitis:**
   - Erosions that are localised of the marginal bone is seen and there is thinning of the crestal lamina dura.
   - The lamina dura loses the sharp borders in the adjacent teeth and there is loss of spiking in the anterior region.
   - The bone height is slightly reduced about less than 1/3rd .
   - Bitewing and periapical radiographs are useful to detect the bone loss.
2. **Moderate marginal periodontitis:**
   - There is generalised horizontal bone loss.
   - There is vertical loss of bone and loss of buccal and lingual cortices seen as localised defects.
   - Radiographically it is difficult to view the buccal and lingual defects and can be seen as areas of decreased density over the surface of the roots.
   - Conventionally bitewing radiographs are helpful.
   - To visualise the buccal and lingual cortical changes cone beam computed tomography can be very useful.
3. **Chronic periodontitis:**

   In some clinical situations restorations may impede the accessibility of the periodontal probe into a pocket and/or may obscure the cement-enamel junction, and so compromise the clinical assessment of the presence and severity of chronic periodontitis. In such a situation radiographic evidence of alveolar bone loss may be helpful. Similarly, subgingival calculus or root surface topographies or malformations may impede the passage of the periodontal probe. In these situations radiographic evidence of alveolar bone loss may be helpful as it may direct the attention of the examining clinician to probe carefully sites or teeth with evident radiographic bone loss.

   Conventional radiographs such as IOPA or bitewing radiographs can be misleading as the condition could have been treated and actual assessment should be by clinical evaluation. However digital intra-oral radiography and CBCT could help in assessing the condition.

4. **Severe Periodontitis:**
   - Extensive horizontal bone loss or extensive vertical osseous defects may be present.
   - As with moderate bone loss, the lesions seen during surgery usually are more extensive than is suggested by the radiographs alone.
   - Panoramic and bitewing radiographs will help in diagnosis .
5. **Buccal Or Lingual Cortical Plate Loss:**
   - The buccal or lingual cortical plate adjacent to the teeth may resorb.
   - This type of loss is indicated by an increase in the radiolucency of the root of the tooth near the alveolar crest.
   - The shape seen usually is a semicircular shadow with the apex of the radiolucency directed apically in relation to the tooth.
   - In such case bitewing and cone beam tomography will help to diagnose the condition.
6. **Horizontal loss of bone:**
   - In cases of horizontal bone loss, the crest of the buccal and lingual cortical plates and the intervening interdental bone is resorbed.
   - In this case periapical and bitewing radiographs are useful.
7. **Vertical Osseous Defects:**
   - With these defects the crest of the remaining alveolar bone displays an oblique angulation to the line of the CEJs in the area of involved teeth.
   - Bitewing and periapical radiographs are useful in such case.
8. **Osseous Deformities in the Furcations of Multi Rooted Teeth:**
   - Progressive periodontal disease and its associated bone loss have the tendency to extend in to the areas of furcation of teeth that have multiple roots.
   - Widening of the periodontal ligament space at the apex of the interradicular bony crest of the furcation is shows that the periodontal disease process involves the furcation.
   - The bony defect may involve either the buccal or lingual cortical plate and extend under the roof of the furcation.
   - Bitewing and cone beam tomography are useful to see the bone loss.
9. **Periodontal abscess:**
   - In periodontal abscess, a radiolucent region appears, superimposed over the root of a tooth.
   - A bridge of bone may be present over the coronal aspect of the lesion, separating it from the crest of the alveolar ridge.
   - Periapical and bitewing radiographs are helpful.

10. **Aggressive periodontitis:**
    - The radiographic appearance of the bone loss in the localized aggressive periodontitis is vertical.
    - The generalized form of aggressive periodontitis can involve several teeth or all the dentition.
    - Rapid bone loss may be of the vertical or angular or horizontal pattern.
    - There could be vertical or horizontal bone loss in patients.
    - The level of bone is in the apical 1/3rd of the root.
    - The localized form may present with a very characteristic "mirror image" pattern of bone destruction which can be seen in radiographs.
    - IOPA, bitewing and Panoramic radiographs can be useful along with clinical assessment to study the bone loss.
    - Digital panoramic and CBCT can help in diagnosing the generalised bone loss.
11. **Localised juvenile periodontitis:**
    - Primarily seen the second decade.
    - Most commonly the first molars and central incisors are involved.
    - The bone loss is very rapid.
    - Plaque amounts are minimal.
    - Progressively over time other teeth are involved.
    - Preiapical and bitewing radiographs are useful in evaluating the periodontal status.
12. **Periodontitis As A Manifestation Of Systemic Disease:**
    - Periodontitis as a manifestation of a disease process can be diagnosed and characterized on the basis of the findings from a clinical examination without the need for radiographs.
13. **Necrotizing Periodontal Diseases:**
    - Necrotizing ulcerative periodontitis in which there is not only necrosis of gingival tissues but also necrosis of periodontal ligament, and alveolar bone.
    - Both of these diagnoses are established on the basis of the symptoms and the clinical signs, and radiographs are not required.
14. **Periodontitis Associated With Endodontic Lesions:**
    - For diagnosing periapical periodontitis, usually periapical radiographs, are required, and if periodontal pathology is evident clinically a long-cone paralleling technique is preferred for the taking of the periapical radiographs.

With the advent of recent advances in radiology like digital intraoral radiography(Radio visio graphy), digital panoramic radiography, digital subtraction radiography, CBCT and CT scanning, the bone loss and bony defects, whether lingual, buccal, mesial or distal can be minutely observed by zooming in on the defects and can be accurately measured by soft ware. It thus helps in diagnosis and treatment planning in a more accurate way.

Conventional and digital radiographic views to assist periodontal treatment planning:

I) Conventional Radiographs:

- **Intraoral Periapical Radiographs:**
  - Full-mouth surveys of paralleling periapical radiographs have been considered to be a "gold standard" for periodontal diagnosis and treatment planning.
- **Conventional Bitewing Radiographs:**
  - They are not so useful in informing periodontal treatment and treatment planning if bone loss is advanced.
  - Vertical bitewing radiographs can be helpful if clinically there is nothing suggestive of any previous endodontic therapy or current periapical periodontitis alone or in combination with periodontal destruction.
- **Panoramic Radiographs:**
  - Panoramic radiographs are helpful in the investigation of patients with periodontal diseases, because of time efficiency, greater patient tolerance, and often a lower radiation exposure.
  - Panoramic radiographs may not reveal alveolar bony defects as accurately as periapical radiographs.

II) Digital Radiographs:

Digital intra-oral radiography:

Dental image analyser tool can reliably replace conventional measuring on intra-oral film radiographs for measuring bone in periodontitis patients. Such image analyser tools may well become more of mainstream devices for quantifying bone loss, and also post-periodontal therapy bone gain or bone level stability.

Digital Panoramic Radiographs:

- The ability to manipulate the panoramic images, such as zooming in and changing contrast, is very useful feature in assessment of bony defects and root morphologies.
- Open (access) flap debridement surgeries have confirmed an impression of a greater ability in anticipating the shape, depth and extent of bony defects by digital panoramic radiographs compared to viewing conventional panoramic oral radiographs.
- The ability to zoom in and magnify defects and to adjust the contrast and brightness allows for vastly improved "visualization" of bone levels and intra-bony defects.
- Periapical periodontitis was more scoreable on screen from digital panoramic radiographs than on printed digital panoramic radiographs, supporting the advantages gained from manipulating

the digital panoramic oral images in assessing bony lesions rather than interpreting only one static panoramic oral image.

Digital Subtraction Radiography:

- Digital subtraction radiography in periodontology allows the detection of small changes in alveolar bone, which might otherwise go undetected.
- For achieving this serial radiographs need to be taken with the best possible reproducible projection geometry and using standardized image processing.

CBCT:

- CBCT may provide detailed information about furcation involvements in patients with chronic periodontitis and so may influence treatment planning decisions.
- The horizontal and vertical location bars can be adjusted to centre on the defect of interest. Zoomed-in images of the periodontal defects centred in, can show the three-dimensional appreciation of the defect and the tooth-roots can be elaborated. Operators can adjust the position of the image, power of zoom-in and zoom-out and contrast of the images in order to assess a particular region of interest. The thickness of the slices across an area of interest can also be adjusted down to an interval of 0.2 mm.
- It allows for the three-dimensional nature of defects to be built up, for the root morphologies and topographies to be studied, for buccal and lingual bony landmarks to be discerned, which is not possible in conventional radiography.

Suggested reading:

1. EF Corbet et al, Radiographs in periodontal disease diagnosis and management, Australian Dental Journal 2009; 54: (1 Suppl): S27–S43.
2. Stuart C White, Michael J Pharoah, Oral Radiology, Principles and Interpretation 5th Edition, 299.

CHAPTER 7

Inflammatory Lesions of Jaws

Q 1) Classify radiolucent lesions of the jaw .Write in detail about osteomyelitis etiology, C/F, D/D & management .

TNMGRU OCTOBER 2003 (15 Marks)

Radiolucent lesions of the jaw:

They are classified into:

(i) Unilocular/ Solitary Radiolucencies:

(a) Well defined radiolucencies:

- Periapical Radiolucencies:
  - (a) Pulpoperiapical Radiolucencies:
    - Chronic and acute dentoalveolar abscesses
    - Periapical granuloma
    - Radicular cyst
    - Scar
    - Surgical defect
    - Osteomyelitis
    - Pulpoperiapical disease and hyperplasia of maxillary sinus lining
  - (b) Dentigerous Cyst
  - (c) Periapical Cementoosseous Dysplasia (Periapical Cementoma)
  - (d) Periodontal Disease
  - (e) Traumatic Bone Cyst
  - (f) Nonradicular Cysts
  - (g) Malignant Tumors
- **Pericoronal Radiolucencies:**
  - (a) Pericoronal or Follicular Space
  - (b) Dentigerous Cyst
  - (c) Unicystic (Mural)Ameloblastoma

(d) Ameloblastoma
(e) Adenomatoid Odontogenic Tumor
(f) Calcifying Odontogenic Cyst or Tumor
(g) Ameloblastic Fibroma

✪ **Radiolucencies not contacting tooth:**

(a) Postextraction Socket
(b) Residual Cyst
(c) Traumatic Bone Cyst
(d) Lingual Mandibular Bone Defect
(e) Odontogenic Keratocyst
(f) Primordial Cyst
(g) Ameloblastoma-Unicystic
(h) Focal Osteoporotic Defect of The Jaws
(i) Surgical Defect
(j) Giant Cell Granuloma
(k) Giant Cell Lesion (Hyperparathyroidism)
(l) Focal Cementoosseous Dysplasia
(m) Incisive Canal Cyst
(n) Midpalatine Cyst
(o) Cementifying And Ossifying Fibroma (Early Stage)
(p) Benign Nonodontogenic Tumors

(b) Solitary Ragged & poorly defined border radiolucencies:

(a) Chronic Osteitis
(b) Chronic Osteomyelitis
(c) Hematopoietic Bone Marrow Defect
(d) Squamous Cell Carcinoma
(e) Fibrous Dysplasia-Early Lesion
(f) Metastatic Tumors of the Jaws
(g) Malignant Minor Salivary Gland tumors
(h) Osteogenic Sarcoma-Osteolytic type
(i) Chondrosarcoma

(ii) Multilocular Radiolucencies:

(a) Multilocular Cyst
(b) Ameloblastoma
(c) Central Giant Cell Granuloma
(d) Giant Cell Lesion of Hyperparathyroidism
(e) Cherubism
(f) Odontogenic Myxoma
(g) Odontogenic Keratocyst
(h) Aneurysmal Bone Cyst
(i) Metastatic Tumors of The Jaws
(j) Vascular Malformations and Central Hemangioma Of Bone

(iii) Multiple Separate, Well-Defined Radiolucencies:

(a) Multiple Cysts Or Granulomas

- (b) Basal Cell Nevus Syndrome
- (c) Multiple Myeloma
- (d) Metastatic Carcinoma
- (e) Langerhans' Cell Disease (Idiopathic Histiocytosis)

(iv) Generalized Rarefactions Of The Jawbones:

1. Hyperparathyroidism:
   - (a) Primary
   - (b) Secondary
   - (c) Tertiary
2. Osteoporosis:
   - (a) Postmenopausal and senile osteoporosis
   - (b) Drug-induced osteoporosis
   - (c) Osteoporosis of Cushing's syndrome
   - (d) Osteoporosis of malnutritional states
   - (e) Thyrotoxic osteoporosis
3. Osteomalacia
4. Hereditary hemolytic anemia
   - (a) Thalassemia
   - (b) Sickle cell anemia
5. Leukemia
6. Langerhans' cell disease (idiopathic histiocytosis)
7. Paget's disease (early stage)
8. Multiple myeloma (late stage)

Osteomyelitis:

In Greek osteon means bone, myelos means marrow, and it means inflammation.

Osteomyelitis may be defined as an inflammatory condition of bone, that begins as an infection of medullary cavity, rapidly involving the haversian systems and eventually involving the periosteum of the infected areas.

Predisposing Factors:

1. **Conditions that alter host defenses:** Such as chronic debilitating systemic diseases like diabetes mellitus, agranulocytosis, leukemia, severe anemia, malnutrition, drug abuse, chronic alcoholism, sickle cell disease and febrile illness such as typhoid.
2. **Conditions that alter vascularity of bone:** It include therapeutic irradiation osteoporosis, paget's disease, fibrous dysplasia, bone malignancy, metastasis etc, affects the cellularity of the jaw.
3. **Virulence of organisms:** Some organisms precipitate thrombi formation by virtue of their destructive lysosomal enzymes.

Etiology:

- ✪ Odontogenic infections:
  Such as periapical, periodontal, pericoronal and infection from the infected dental cysts.

- Compound fractures of the bone.
- Local traumatic injuries to the gingiva leads to periostitis, which leads to osteomyelitis if the patients resistance is low to infection.
- Middle ear infection & respiratory infection: via hematogenous route.
- Furunculosis of chin (spread through lymphatic channel via infected lymph nodes).
- Peritonsillar abscess.
- Microorganism responsible for osteomyelitis are:

Staph. Aureus, Staph. Albus & Klebsiella, pseudomonas, protease, β-hemolytic streptococci, and to a lesser extent gram –ve rods and anaerobes may cause acute infections.

Classification of Osteomyelitis:

- According to duration & severity
  1. Acute
  2. Chronic
- Depending on the presence & absence of suppuration.
  1. Suppurative:
     - (a) Acute suppurative osteomyelitis
     - (b) Chronic suppurative osteomyelitis
     - (c) Infantile osteomyelitis
  2. Non-suppurative type
     - (a) Chronic non suppurative
       - Diffuse sclerosing
       - Focal sclerosing
     - (b) Osteoradionecrosis.
     - (c) Garre's sclerosing osteomyelitis
     - (d) Osteomyelitis due to specific infection
       - Actinomycosis
       - Tuberculosis
       - Syphilis

1. **Acute Suppurative Osteomyelitis Or Acute Pyogenic Osteomyelitis:** It is the sequelae of periapical infection which spreads diffusely through the medullary spaces, with subsequent necrosis of bone.

   Clinical features:

   Occurs in adults, more common in mandible and involves alveolar process, angle of mandible, posterior part of ramus and coronoid process. In maxilla it is fairly well localized, where as in mandible it tends to be more diffuse and wide spread.

   Early cases are characterized by-
   - Symptoms such as deep seated boring pain, continuous pain associated with high grade fever, malaise vomiting & anorexia.
   - Paresthesia or anesthesia of lip and regional lymphadenopathy.
   - Teeth involved may become loose and sore.

- Trismus may be present.
- There are no sinus tracts, but there is pus exudation from the infected extraction socket.
- In children, it is severe, fulminating and usually involves maxilla than mandible. It causes necrosis of the developing tooth bud and long term involvement leads to TMJ ankylosis & affects the growth & development of facial structures,

2. **Sub Acute Phase (10-14 Days Later):**
   - Deep pain, fever and malaise, anorexia.
   - Pus exudation from the sulcus & fetid odor.
   - Fistulas may be present.
   - Firm cellulites, that is tender.
   - Bone expansion may be present.
3. **Chronic Osteomyelitis:**
   1. **Primary:** Relatively less virulent organisms cause this type.
   2. **Secondary:** It occurs after the acute phase in cases where the treatment could not eliminate the infection. The time limit that differentiates the acute from chronic form is about one month.
      - There is presence of pain that is dull and aching and tenderness is minimal.
      - There is induration of soft tissue and wounds of the bone and overlying soft tissues are non-healing.
      - Draining fistulas of the intra oral or extraoral sites are present.
      - Exposed bone with sloughing and pus.
      - The deposition of the subperiosteal new bone causes enlargement of the bone and thickening or wooden character of bone.
      - May cause pathological fractures.
      - Brodie's abscess which is sterile, is common in long bones but rare in jaws.
      - Loose and sensitive teeth.
      - Commonly seen are anesthesia and paresthesia.
4. **Chronic Diffuse Sclerosing Osteomyelitis:**
   - Occurs only in the mandible and in older individuals (3rd decade).
   - Bone is mildly expanded and tender.
   - Recurrent episodes of pain, sometimes excruciating and swelling.
   - Nerve, paresthesia may also be present.
5. **Garre's Periostitis (Chronic non suppurative sclerosing osteomyelitis):** It is a non-suppurative inflammatory process, where there is peripheral subperiosteal bone deposition caused by mild irritation and infection.
   - Occurs in children and young adults.

- Unilateral swelling involving the lateral and inferior aspects of the mandible.
- Absence of pain or tenderness over the expanded bone.
- It varies from 1-2 cm to the involvement of the entire length of the affected side.
- Causes discomfort when secondarily infected.
- Lymphadenopathy, hyperpyrexia & lymphocytosis.

6. **Focal Sclerosing Osteomyelitis:**
   - Incidental radiological finding during the investigation for the offending tooth.
   - Mild pain may be present.
7. **Infantile Osteomyelitis:**
   - Seen few weeks after birth.
   - Rare type seen in infants maxilla especially molar region.
   - May be caused due to prenatal trauma, or due to contaminated nipples or finger in mouth, it is also believed to occur by hematogenous route (streptococcus).
   - May have sudden onset with high fever, rapid pulse, vomiting, delirium.
   - Facial cellulitis involving orbit leading to closure and proptosls.
   - Subperiosteal abscesses in the alveolar region, buccal mucosa and palatal region.
8. **Radiation Osteomyelitis /Osteoradionecrosis:**
   It is the infection of the irradiated bone following the exposure to intense radiation i.e. 40 80 GY. There is marked decrease in the vascularity, leading to degenerative changes in the osteocytes and bone marrow, making it more susceptible to trauma & infection. Decrease or absence of inflammatory response.
   C/F:
   - Occurs due to triad of radiation, trauma & infection.
   - Common in mandible.
   - Intense pain with inflammation, swelling &drainage develops.
   - Facial fistulas develop from the subperiosteal tissue.
   - Positive vitality test of the involved tooth.
   - Exposed bone, trismus, fetid odour, pyrexia.
   - Pathological fractures.
9. **Syphilitic Osteomyelitis:** Caused by T. Palladium and is seen in secondary and tertiary stages and congenital form.
10. **Tubercular Osteomyelitis:**
    - When the blood borne bacilli lodge in the cancellous bone the spread is usually hematogenous.
    - Direct inoculation of the bacilli into the oral mucosa because of an ulcer or through a tooth socket can lead to spread to the bone.
    - There is formation of cold abscess where there no typical

reddening and increase in temperature locally.
- When the lesion is located centrally and there is only swelling present in the absence of draining sinus, it mimics parotid swelling and is called lumpy jaw.

11. **Actinomycotic Osteomyelitis:**
    - Caused by Actinomyces Israeli.
    - In cervicofacial type jaws are involved especially the mandible.
    - On the skin clinically can be seen soft or firm masses of tissue which are dark red, purplish and oily with zones of fluctuation that are small.
    - There is spontaneous serous fluid drainage containing yellowish granular material called 'sulphur granules' which represent colonies of bacteria.
    - It produces dense bone & scarring of soft tissues & has been described as lumpy jaw.
    - Caused by Actinomyces Israeli.
    - Jaws are involved in cervicofacial type, especially mandible.
    - Clinically soft or firm tissue masses on the skin, which are purplish, dark red, oily with small zones of fluctuations.
    - Spontaneous drainage of serous fluid containing yellowish granular material called 'sulphur granules' which represent colonies of bacteria.
    - It produces dense bone & scarring of soft tissues & has been described as lumpy jaw.

Differential diagnosis:

1. **Fibrous dysplasia:** the new bone formed in osteomyelitis is laid down by the periosteum & is on the outside of the outer cortical plate. Where as in fibrous dysplasia the bone is formed on the inside of the mandible.
2. **Squamous cell carcinoma:** Malignant tumors invading the bone & superimposed with secondary infection via an ulcer is difficult to differentiate from the acute phase of osteomyelitis. If the destruction of periosteal bone is present then the probability of malignant lesion is more.
3. **Langerhans cell histocytosis:** Sclerotic bone reaction is seen in osteomyelitis which is not seen in langerhans cell histocytosis.
4. **Leukemia & lymphoma:** They simulate similar periosteal reaction. A complete hemogram can help in distinguishing from osteomyelitis.
5. **Osteosarcoma:** Bone destruction with characteristic spiculated periosteal response i.e. sun ray appearance. The lesions are very fast growing and destructive.
6. **Eosinophillic granuloma:** Bone lesions radiographically are better defined & show no evidence of sclerosis.
7. **Ewings sarcoma:** sun ray appearance (osteophytes), facial

neuralgia & lip paresthesia are the frequent complications.

8. **Caffeys disease:** seen in early age before 2 year, in the angle or ramus of the mandible & involves clavicle.
9. Peripheral osteomas, exostosis, tori should be clinically distinguished.
10. **Ossifying subperiosteal hematoma:** History of trauma to the area may establish the diagnosis.

Management:

1. Incision & drainage–drainage of fluctuant area under antibiotic cover.
2. Irrigation & debridement of necrotic area followed by irrigation with hydrogen peroxide & saline.
3. **Empiric therapy:**
   Regime i:
   - Aqueous penicillin 2 million units. IV, 4 hourly
   - Oxacillin1g, IV, 4 hourly.

   Regime ii: if patient is asymptomatic after 48 to 72 hours, then penicillin V500mg, 6 hourly & dicloxacilin 250 mg orally 4 hourly for an additional 2- 4 weeks.
4. **Definitive therapy:**
   Culture & sensitivity testing is performed and the antibiotic therapy is then modified accordingly.
   - Initial therapy with gram stain result:
     - Initial course of oxacillin 1g IV after every 4 hours.
     - Followed by orally dicloxacillin250mg after every 4 hours.
     - An oral antibiotic like penicillin v may be started after 48 hours.
   - If patient is allergic to penicillin the following antibiotics are prescribed
     1. Clindamycin: 300-600mg orally 6 hourly.
     2. Cephalosporin: 250- 500 mg orally 6 hourly
     3. Cefazolin: 500mg orally IV/IM after every 8 hourly
     4. Cephalexin: 500 mg every 6 hourly
     5. Erythromycin: 2g IV after every 6 hourly.

     followed by 500mg orally, every 6hourly.
5. **Other modalities:**
   - Intra Arterial Antibiotics.
   - Local Implantation of Antibiotics.
   - Prostaglandin Inhibiting Salicylates Therapy To Diminish Osteolytic Destruction In Osteomyelitis Model.
6. **Extraction:** Extraction of carious tooth to remove the source of infection.
7. **Supportive therapy:**
   Adequate rehydration in the forms of fluids.
   Rich nutritional diet.

Multivitamin supplement.

8. **Sequestrectomy:** It is removal of sequestra which takes at least two weeks to form after which they persist. If not removed it will get chronically infected &infect the surrounding tissues& will lead to further sequestration & bone loss.
9. **Saucerization:** Saucerisation is the unroofing of the cortex for thorough debridement of the medullary cavity. It results in better visualization of sequestra & excision of the margins of the infected bone.
10. 2 polyethylene chain tubes which are 3-4 mm in diameter and about 6-10 inches in length are placed through separate incision after sequestrectomy or decortication.
    - To allow drainage of pus one tube is attached to a low pressure suction.
    - The second tube is used for irrigation and administration of antibiotics.
    - Everyday saline irrigation is done first which is followed by instillation of antibiotics that is done till–ve culture are obtained.
11. **Decortication:** Decortication refers to the removal of the lateral and the inferior border of the mandible for upto 2cm beyond the affected area and the mandible is stabilised with plates if the removal is extensive and a risk of fracture is feared.
12. **Hyperbaric Oxygen Therapy:** HBO therapy consists of breathing 100% oxygen at 2.4 absolute atmosphere pressure for 90 minute sessions or Dives for as many as 5 days a week, totaling 30 or more dives often followed by another 10 or more dives.
13. Resection of jaw.
14. Trephination.
15. Immediate or delayed reconstruction with bone graft.

Suggested reading:

1. Freny R Karjodkar, Essentials of oral & maxillofacial radiology, Ch: 20; pg no: 283-290.
2. Neelima Anil Malik; textbook of oral &maxillofacial surgery. Edi: 2 nd ch: 41 pg no 640-647.
3. Norman K. Wood, Paul W. Goaz; Differential diagnosis of oral & maxillofacial lesions, Edition: 5 th pg no: 252- 393.

CHAPTER 8

Cysts of Jaws

Q 1) Define cyst, classify cyst of the jaws. Describe clinical features, causes of recurrence, radiographic appearance, d/d and treatment plan of odontogenic keratocyst.

MUHS MAY 2011 (10 Marks)

Definition:

Cyst is a pathological cavity which is filled with fluid, semifluid or gaseous content but not always lined by epithelium which is not formed due to pus accumulation.

-1974 kramer

A cyst is a sac lined by epithelium, which may contain fluid, semisolid or gasseous material. The epithelial cells proliferate first and then undergo degeneration and liquefaction during the formation of a cyst. There is exertion of equal pressure by the liquefied material on the walls of the cyst from within.

Classification of Cysts of jaws:

A) Epithelial cysts:

(a) **Odontogenic:**

Developmental:

- Primordial cyst
- Keratocyst
- Gingival cyst of infants
- Gingival cyst of adults
- Lateral periodontal cysts
- Dentigerous cyst
- Eruption cyst
- Calcifying collateralodontogenic cyst
- Botryoid cyst

Inflammatory:

Periodontal cyst

1. Radicular Cyst
2. Lateral Cyst
3. Residual Cyst

Paradental cyst (inflammatory collateral cyst, mandibular infected buccal cyst)

(b) Non-odontogenic cysts:

- Nasopalatine (incisive canal cyst)
- Median cyst
- Median alveolar cyst
- Median mandibular cyst
- Globulomaxillary cyst
- Nasolabial cyst
- Palatal cyst of infants

(c) Cyst associated with maxillary antrum:

Benign mucosal cyst of the maxillary sinus

1. mucocele
2. serous cyst
3. cyst of McGregor (mesothelial cyst)
4. lymphangiectatic cyst
5. Surgical ciliated cyst of the maxilla

(d) Cyst of the soft tissues of the face and neck:

- Dermoid cyst
- Epidermoid cyst
- Branchial cyst
- Thyroglossal duct cyst
- Anterior median lingual cyst
- Gastromucosal cyst
- Cystic hygroma
- Paracytic cyst (Hyatid cyst)
- Cyst of salivary gland-mucocele and ranula

B) Non-epithelial cysts:

Pseudocysts:

- Aneurysmal bone cyst
- Traumatic (Simple) Bone cyst)
- Static bone cyst (Stafne's Bone Defect)
- Focal osteoporotic bone marrow defect

The term 'odontogenic keratocyst' was introduced by Philipsen (1956) The odontogenic keratocyst (OKC) is now designated by the WHO as a keratocystic odontogenic tumour (KCOT).

Definition:

Odontogenic keratocyst can be defined as a benign unicystic or multicystic, intaosseous tumour that is of odontogenic origin, which has characteristic lining of parakeratinised stratified squamous epithelium and has the potential for aggressive and infiltrative behavior.

Clinical Features:

1. More common in young adults.
2. Shows male predilection.
3. Pronounced in blacks than whites.
4. KCOTs are twice more frequent in the mandible than in the maxilla.
5. More common in the posterior body of mandible & ramus region, especially angle of mandible and in maxilla in canine region.
6. In mandibular canine & molar region involvement of an impacted tooth has been reported in 25 to 40% of cases .
7. Symptomless unless infected, causes pain, soft tissue swelling & drainage, paresthesia of lower lip, if there is pathological fracture.
8. Aspiration reveals a thick, yellow, cheesy, odourless, creamy or caseous material(keratin).
9. Teeth may be displaced, if it expands through cancellous bone & body of mandible.
10. Multiple KCOT's are found in the syndromes such as:
    (a) Gorlin goltz syndrome
    (b) Marfans syndrome
    (c) Ehlers – danlos syndrome
    (d) Noonan's syndrome

Causes of Recurrence: Reccurence of OKC is very high. Striking tendency for recurrence-25-30%-with most recurrences developing during the first 5-7 yrs after the therapy .

In 1976, Brannon, proposed 3 mechanisms for KCOT recurrence:

1. Satellite cyst–occurrence of satellite cyst, which is a bud-like projection of basal cell layer into the connective tissue .Cystic lining can be allowed to remain during the procedure of enucleation -incomplete removal of the cyst lining.
2. Growth of a new KCOT from satellite cysts.
3. Development of a new KCOT in an adjacent area that is interpreted as a recurrence.
4. Intrinsic growth potential that may be responsible for recurrence.
5. Proliferation of basal cell: May arise from proliferation of the basal cells of the oral mucosa particularly in the 3 rd molar region and the ascending region of the ramus of mandible.

Radiographic features:

1. Varies from 5 cm or more in diameter. Shape is usually ovoid and has tendency to extend along the body of the mandible with little medio lateral expansion. Margins are hyperostotic. Relatively late expansion of odontogenic keratocyst contributes to late detection.
2. 90% of the OKCs occur in the posterior part of the body of the mandibe that is posterior to canines and in the ramus about 50% cases.

3. The location of the epicenter is superior to the inferior alveolar nerve canal. This cyst some times has the same position pericoronally and is almost difficult to differentiate from a dentigerous cyst.
4. As with other cysts, the OKCs almost always have a cortical border unless it is infected secondarily. It generally has a smooth, round and oval that is similar to that of other cysts and may have scalloping at the borders.
5. Internally the cyst is almost radiolucent, and the presence of keratin may just give a hazy appearance but doesnot cause radiopacity. In some cases curved septa may be present internally and the lesion could exhibit a multilocular appearance.
6. Roots of adjacent teeth may be displaced but usually the cyst extend around the roots and size-varies from, .5 cm or more in diameter. Shape is usually oval and there is antero-posterior growth, with very little medio-lateral expansion. Margins are hyperostotic. This cyst when involves the maxilla can occupy the entire maxillary sinus.

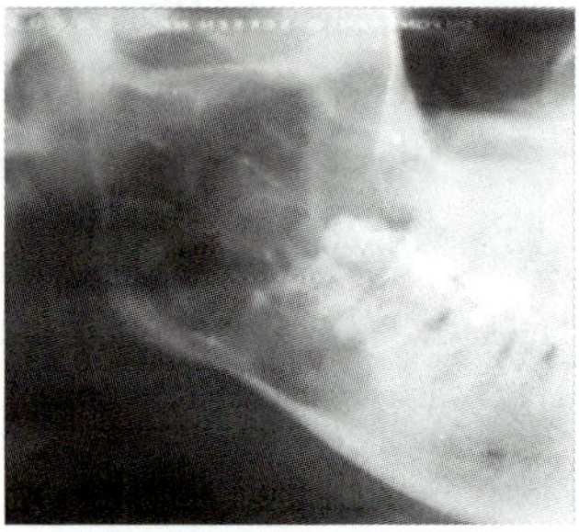

Fig. OKC involving the mandible, body as well as the ramus

Radiological types of KCOT:

1. Envelopmental type, this embraces an adjacent unerupted tooth.
2. Replacement type, this form in place of normal teeth.
3. Extraneous type, these are in the ascending ramus away from the teeth.
4. Collateral type, those adjacent to the roots of teeth.

Differential diagnosis:

1. **Dentigerous cyst:** Always associated with a tooth. The cystic lining is attached at the cementoenamel junction typically which is not so with the OKC.
2. **Ameloblastoma:** Occurs in older age, causes expansion of the jaws buccolingually and usually involves the horizontal and the vertical component of mandible.
3. **Primordial cyst:** absence of tooth without a history of extraction favors primordial cyst.
4. **Residual cyst:** history of extraction of tooth, amber coloured fluid and flask shaped residual radiolucency.
5. **Traumatic cyst:** characteristic radiographic feature is scalloped margins, straw coloured fluid on aspiration and typically involving the interdental bone.
6. **Giant cell granuloma:** usually found in the anterior region of the jaw.

7. **Odontogenic myxoma:** It is rare but must be considered if the tooth has failed to develop and may appear as a cyst like radiolucency. Has a typical tennis racket like appearance.

Suggested reading:

1. Stuart C White, Michael J Pharoah, Oral Radiology, Principles and Interpretation 5th Edition, Page no. 393-397.

Q 2) Classify cysts of the jaws. Describe the clinical and radiographic features of Dental Cysts:

TNMGRU NOVEMBER 2001 (15 Marks)

Classification of Cysts of jaws:

A) Epithelial cysts:

(a) Odontogenic:

Developmental:

- Primordial cyst
- Keratocyst
- Gingival cyst of infants
- Gingival cyst of adults
- Lateral periodontal cyst
- Dentigerous cyst
- Eruption cyst
- Calcifying collateral odontogenic cyst
- Botryoid cyst

Inflammatory:

- Periodontal cyst
  1. Radicular Cyst
  2. Lateral Cyst
  3. Residual Cyst
- Paradental cyst (inflammatory collateral cyst, mandibular infected buccal cyst)

(b) Nonodontogenic cysts:

- Nasopalatine (incisive canal cyst)
- Median cyst
- Median alveolar cyst
- Median mandibular cyst
- Globulomaxillary cyst
- Nasolabial cyst
- Palatal cyst of infants

(c) Cyst associated with maxillary antrum:

- Benign mucosal cyst of maxillary sinus
  1. mucocele
  2. serous cyst
  3. cyst of McGregor (mesothelial cyst)
  4. lymphangiectatic cyst

- Surgical ciliated cyst of the maxilla

(d) Cyst of the soft tissues of the face and neck:

- Dermoid cyst
- Epidermoid cyst
- Branchial cyst
- Thyroglossal duct cyst
- Anterior median lingual cyst
- Gastromucosal cyst
- Cystic hygroma
- Paracytic cyst (Hydatid cyst)
- Cyst of salivary gland- mucocele and ranula

B) Non-epithelial cysts:

Pseudocysts:

- Aneurysmal bone cyst
- Traumatic (Simple) Bone Cyst
- Static Bone Cyst (Stafne's Bone Defect),
- Focal Osteoporotic Bone Marrow Defect

Clinical and radiographic features of dental cysts:

Developmental Dental Cysts:

1. **Gingival cysts of infants:** Gingival cyst of newborn is also called as dental lamina cyst and as its lined by epithelium, its a true cyst. Its lumen is usually filled with keratin that is desquamated and contains ocassionally inflammatory cells.

   Clinical features:

   - Can manifest as few or many, white to yellowish, round to oval, nodes in the maxillary and/or mandibular gingiva and alveolar ridge of newborns. These nodes generally measure 2 to 3 millimeters in their largest dimension.
   - Their location is typically on the alveolar ridges of the new born and infants.
   - They generally donot cause any discomfort to the infants and are usually asymptomatic.
   - In some cases they may become large enough and be noticeable clinically and appear as discrete white swellings on the ridges. They degenerate on their own or rupture by the end of 2 weeks to 5 months of post natal life.
   - When these cysts are located in the midline of the palate in the raphe region, they are referred to as palatine cysts and when on the buccal, lingual or crest of the ridge, then called as alveolar or gingival cysts.

   Radiographic features:

   As it doesnot involve alveolar bone, no radiographic changes are seen.

2. **Odontogenic keratocysts:**

   Clinical features:

- Its origin is from the dental lamina.
- The mandibular 3rd molar region is most commonly involved and the ratio of mandible to maxilla is 2: 1.
- Can also involve the canine region of the maxilla and mandible.
- Ramus of the mandible is also often involved.
- The OKC has an estimated recurrence rate of about 60%.
- They can occur singly and some times multiple lesions can be present and in such cases is a part of the basal cell nevoid carcinoma syndrome(Gorlin syndrome).
- Though can occur at any age, most commonly is found in the 3rd-4th decades .
- There can be complaints of pain, swelling or discharge from the lesion.
- There can be displacement of the teeth as the cyst enlarges.

Radiographic features:

- OKCs are unilocular presenting a well defined peripheral rim.
- They generally grow mesiodistally following path of least resistance due to very thin epithelial lining.
- Scalloping of the borders can be seen.
- It often has a cloudy appearance due to presence of keratin.
- Multilocular radiolucent OKC is also observed, generally representing a central cavity having satellite cysts.
- When it is multilocular and especially if located in the third mandibular molar area, it may be confused radiographically with an ameloblastoma.
- Occasionally OKC may mimic a dentigerous cyst and contain the crown of a retained tooth within its lumen.

3. **Dentigerous cyst:** Its an odontogenic cyst that surround the crown of an impacted tooth. It is caused by accumulation of the fluid between the crown of the tooth and the reduced enamel epithelium. The crown thus projects into the lumen of the cyst and the roots remain outside.

Clinical features:

- Asymptomatic, occassionally pain or swelling.
- Usually not clinically visible without radiographs.
- Firm hard mass.
- Appears in place of missing tooth.
- Usually involve unerupted mandibular third molars, other frequent sites include canines of the maxilla and the third molars and mandibular second premolars.
- This cyst most often involves individuals in the age group of 20-40 years.

Radiographic features:

- Well circumscribed radiolucency around crown of tooth.

- Surrounding bone corticated due to slow growth.
- Unilocular .
- There are three types: Central, lateral and radicular:
- There is a greater chance of resorption of roots of the adjacent teeth in dentigerous cysts than any other cyst.

4. **Eruption cysts:** It is a type of odontogenic cyst having similar histologic features as that of the dentigerous cyst, and it surrounds the crown of a tooth which has erupted through the bone but has yet to erupt through the soft tissues and appears clinically as soft fluctuant swelling on the ridges of the alveolus.

   Clinical features:

   - It is a variation of the dentigerous cyst and part of it occurs in the soft tissue.
   - Common particularly with premature eruption of teeth any erupting tooth, molar and canines most frequently.
   - The eruption cyst can hinder the eruption of the affected tooth through the soft tissues overlying the bone.
   - Well demarcated directly over the crown on an erupting tooth.
   - This cyst tends to produce a swelling that is soft and fluctuant and smooth over the tooth that is erupting and the colour could be of the normal gingiva or pale bluish.
   - Unless it is secondarily infected, its painless.

   Radiographic features:

   There is little bone involvement except the dilated and open crypt of the tooth surrounding the unerupted crown and can be seen in the radiograph, apart from that it may show soft tissue shadow pericoronally.

5. **Gingival cyst of adults:** Its a odontogenic cyst which is small in size and developmental, derived from the rests of dental lamina and consists of a lining of the embryonic epithelium of cells that are cuboidal and have distinct focal thickenings like the lateral periodontal cyst.

   Clinical features:

   - Common in 5th and 6th decades of life.
   - Uncommon cyst.
   - Usually asymptomatic.
   - Firm, compressible.
   - Dome-like swelling often bluish or blue-gray filled with fluid.
   - Occurs commonly on facial gingiva or alveolar mucosa.
   - Mandibular canine-premolar area.
     Radiographic changes not seen.

6. **Calcifying epithelial odontogenic cysts:** The origin of these cysts is from the developmental odontogenic epithelial tissues.

   - It shows several features of the odontogenic cysts and

tumours.

- It affects females below the age of 40 and males above the age of 40 years.
- It is commonly associated with an un-erupted tooth.
- The intra-bony lesions can lead to expansion of the bone and could be quite extensive.

Radiographic features:

- It appears as a unilocular or multilocular well defined cystic lesion.
- In the beginning it appears as a non-specific cyst as there are no calcifications within the cyst. Small areas of calcification may start appearing in later stages, and may appear as small irregular opaque bodies within the radiolucent lumen and later may appear in substantial amounts and could occupy major part of the lesion. This is the only cyst showing calcifications and hence opacities.

7. **Lateral periodontal cysts:** Its a developmental odontogenic cyst which is non-expansile, and is slow growing, derived from the rests of dental lamina and consists of an epithelial lining of embryonic cells that are cuboidal and 1-3 cells in thickness and distinct focal thickenings.

Clinical features:

- Caucasian male predilection.
- Slow growing most often in mandibular lateral incisor, canine and the pre-molar areas.
- Non-expansile .
- Most often asymptomatic.
- Common in young adults.

Radiographic features:

- Shows a well-defined, unilocular, round or ovoid or tear drop shaped radiolucent area.
- The position of the cyst is somewhere between the apex of the tooth and the cervical margin of the vital teeth.
- Their size can vary from very small, about 1mm to involving the entire length of the root.

8. **Botryoid odontogenic cyst:**

Clinical features:

- Its a rare multilocular variant of the lateral periodontal cyst that is developmental and odontogenic cyst.
- It occurs intra-osseously and has typical multilocular pattern which can resemble a bunch of grapes.
- Commonly seen in mandible followed by maxilla and seen mostly in anterior region.
- Occurs in middle age and slight predominance in females.

Radiographic features:

- Seen as unilocular or multilocular lesions.

- Though less aggressive they have high recurrence rates similar to OKCs.

9. **Glandular odontogenic cyst:**

   Clinical features:
   - Also known as the "sialo-odontogenic cyst".
   - This cyst arises in the tooth bearing areas of the jaws and has typical epithelial lining of cuboidal or columnar cells which are both at the surface and crypt linings or they appear as cyst-like spaces within the epithelial thickness.
   - Has a high recurrence rate.
   - It displays an aggressive growth potential.
   - Though this lesion has been recently recognized, adequate number of cases have been reported.

   Radiological features:
   - It presents as multilocular expansile lesion in the anterior quadrants of mandible followed by maxilla. They should be differentiated from central giant cell granuloma and aggressive ameloblastoma.
   - Some lesions may involve extragnathic structures, such as the sinuses, floor of the nose or the orbital floor.

Inflammatory Dental Cysts:

1. **Radicular cyst:** A cyst of inflammatory origin, its a odontogenic cyst which is preceded by a periapical granuloma and forms due to stimulation of the epithelial rests of malassez that are present in the periodontal membrane.

   Clinical features:
   - Its the most common cystic lesion affecting the jaws.
   - Usually seen in adults between 2nd and 5th decade of life.
   - They can also occur as a result of trauma and in such cases, no caries will be seen.
   - The radicular cyst is usually devoid of symptoms and some times can become very large by the time its discovered.
   - These cysts can result in expansion of the areas affected.
   - Radicular cysts that involve the lateral incisor of the maxilla can cause expansion of the palatal bone and the mucosa.

   Radiographic features:
   - It appears as a well defined unilocular radiolucency at the apex of the involved tooth.
   - It is usually 1.5-3 cms in size.
   - It can expand and cause displacement of the structures in the neighbouring areas. It can especially cause displacement of the maxillary sinus and in the mandible can displace the mandibular canal.
   - Resorption of roots can be seen ocassionally.
   - It generally has well corticated margins but in case of infections there can be loss of the well corticated margins.

- Globulomaxillary cyst like radiolucency if occurring in the apical region of a lateral anterior maxilla incisor tooth.

2. **Residual cyst:**

   Clinical features:
   - It is a cyst that remains after the causative tooth is removed.
   - Residual cyst occurs due to incomplete surgical removal of a radicular or other inflammatory cyst.
   - The histological and clinical features of the radicular cyst are very similar to those of the residual cyst except for the site of the extracted teeth.

   Radiographic features:
   - It is a well-defined unilocular radiolucent structure of varying size at the edentulous area of a previous extracted tooth site.
   - As the tooth is not present it looks like a flask shaped radiolucent lesion.

3. **Paradental cyst:**
   - Clinical features:
   - They are associated with the lateral part of the partially erupted vital teeth of the mandibular molars.
   - These cysts usually involve the older individuals and the tooth affected is generally the mandibular third molars. The infected buccal cyst of the mandibular region involving the first or second molar is seen in children or young adults.

   Radiological features:
   - It can be seen as a well defined radiolucency distal and buccal to a tooth that is partially erupted.
   - A true occlusal view will show its placement more buccally than distally.

4. **Inflammatory collateral cyst:**

   Clinical features:

   These are generally associated with the lateral aspects of the tooth roots of non-vital teeth.

   Radiographic features:

   The radiographic features are quite similar to the lateral periodontal cyst but the associated tooth will be clinically non-vital.

Suggested reading:

1. Aman Moda, Gingival Cyst of Newborn, Int J Clin Pediatr Dent. 2011 Jan-Apr; 4(1): 83–84.
2. D S MacDonald-Jankowski, Glandular odontogenic cyst: systematic review, Dentomaxillofac Radiol. 2010 Mar; 39(3): 127–139.
3. Mervyn Shear, Paul m. Speight, Text Book Of Cysts Of The Oral And Maxillofacial Regions, 4th edition, 1-2.
4. Vitor H Farina, Adriana AH Brandão, Janete D Almeida, and Luiz AG Cabral, Clinical and histologic features of botryoid odontogenic cyst: a case report, J Med Case Reports. 2010; 4: 260.

CHAPTER 9

Benign Tumours of Jaws

Q 1) Classify benign odontogenic tumors of the jaws. Differentiate between benign and malignant tumors. Describe clinical, radiographic, features and radiographic differential diagnosis for ameloblastoma.

MUHS MAY 2009 (10 Marks)

A tumor is defined as a lesion that occurs due to abnormal growth of cells which persists after the initial stimulus has been removed. This occurs when the cell growth defies the normal mechanism of regulation.

The benign odontogenic tumors are neoplasms that arise from the dental lamina or any of its derivatives.

Benign Odontogenic Tumors:

I) Tumours arising from Odontogenic Epithelium without Odontogenic Ectomesenchyme:
   1. Ameloblastoma.
   2. Pinborg's tumour or calcifying epithelial odontogenic tumour(CEOT)
   3. Clear cell odontogenic tumor.
   4. Squamous odontogenic tumor.

II) Odontogenic epithelium with odontogenic ectomesenchyme, with or without dental hard tissue formation:
   1. Ameloblastic fibroma.
   2. Ameloblastic fibrodentinoma (dentinoma).
   3. Odontoameloblastoma.
   4. Adenomatoid odontogenic tumor (AOT).
   5. Complex odontome.
   6. Compound odontome.

III) Odontogenic ectomesenchyme with or without included odontogenic epithelium:
   1. Odontogenic fibroma.

2. Myxoma (odontogenic myxoma, myxofibroma).
3. Benign cementoblastoma (true cementoma).

Waldron included AOT as epithelial odontogenic tumor but according to WHO's classification (1992 the AOT is included in the mixed Odontogenic tumor.)

Difference Between Benign and Malignant Tumors:

Sr no	Benign Tumors	Malignant Tumors
1	Mobile mass.	Fixed or ulcerating mass.
2	Smooth and round with a surrounding fibrous capsule.	Irregular shaped with no capsule.
3	Cells multiply slowly.	Cells multiply rapidly.
4	Tumor grows by expanding and pushing against the surrounding tissue.	Tumor grows by invading and destroying surrounding tissue.
5	Mass is mobile. Not attached to surrounding tissue.	Mass is fixed. It is attached to the underlying tissue.
6	Never spread to other sites (metastasize).	It always spreads to the surrounding tissues if not removed.
7	Easier to remove and does not recur after excision.	Difficult to remove and recurs after excision.

Ameloblastoma:

Ameloblastoma was described as "adamantinoma" by Brocca and Malassez in late eighteenth century. The term 'ameloblastome' was coined by Ivy and Churchill in the year 1934.

Definition:

Ameloblastoma is defined as, locally-invasive epithelial benign odontogenic tumor with a tendency to recur. Tumor consists of proliferative odontogenic epithelium in a fibrous connective tissue stroma. It is considered as locally malignant.

Robinson described ameloblastoma as unicentric, non-functional, with growth that is intermittent, anatomically benign, and persistent clinically.

The origin of ameloblastoma is as follows:

1. Late and secondary development sources.
2. Early embryonic origin.
3. Basal cells of the surface epithelium of oral mucosa.
4. The heterotrophic epithelium from other parts of the body, especially the pituitary gland.

The probable etiological factors are: chronic irritation, infection with history of traumatic injury or extraction and dietary deficiencies.

Clinical Features:

- Accounts for 1% of all tumors and 11% of all odontogenic tumors.

- More common in males among the age group of 20-50 years and sometimes in the 7th decade.
- The male is slightly more affected than females.
- The lesion may involve either of the jaws but the mandible is affected more than maxilla, the ratio being 5: 1. In mandible, it involves the posterior part and ramus and in case of maxilla in the 3rd molar region is usually involved. Right side mandible is more commonly affected than the left side.
- It is a central lesion of bone, slow-growing, and of long duration, initially symptomless, gradually increasing in size.
- There is expansion of the buccal and the lingual cortical plates, lingual expansion more than buccal. Produces marked enlargement and deformity of the cortex of the jaw, but rarely causes destruction.
- The teeth in that area may be vital or may show resorption of roots.
- There is gradual facial asymmetry, with mobility and displacement of the involved teeth.
- If the nerve is compressed and there is secondary infection pain and paresthesia may develop.
- Maxillary involvement is more dangerous as the lesions can spread easily to the adjacent structures such as paranasal air sinuses, orbit or the nasopharynx.
- In later stage, lesions become hard, non tender and show oval shaped or fusiform enlargement .
- Fluctuation and crackling like egg shell can be elicited due to thinning of the surrounding bone.

Radiographic features:

- Radiodensity: In early stages, there is area of bone destruction which is well defined and surrounded by hyperostotic borders.
- Margins: Outline is smooth, scalloped, well defined and corticated.
- Internal structure: Usually multilocular but could be unilocular, and coarse or fine trabeculae may be present within the tumor.
- Appearance: 5 types of radiological appearances are seen:
  1. Presence of septa and its arrangement may give rise to numerous small compartments causing a honey comb appearance.
  2. soap bubble appearance is named when the compartments are larger.
  3. Unilocular dental cyst like especially when it occurs at the root apex.
  4. Radiating trabeculae originating from center of the lesion giving spider nevus like appearance.
  5. Unicystic variety: In case of mural ameloblastoma, the radiological appearance is like single cyst.
- Subclinical lesion: subclinical lesion usually presents as many small rounded cavities in the bone with well defined corticated borders.
- Effect on surrounding structures: it causes extensive root

resorption and root displacement and apical displacement of the tooth. Expansion and thinning of cortical plate leads to crackling of eggshell of bone.

- Perforation of bone or window formation occurs when the periosteum cannot keep up the pace with the expanding, lesion and is a feature seen in the later stages.

Radiographic investigation:

CT: Helps to confirm the diagnosis and also demonstrate the accurate extent of the tumor, detects perforation of the outer cortex and invasion into the soft tissues.

MRI: Detects the nature and extent of invasion in the soft tissue.

CBCT is also a good radiographic technique to depict the exact extent of the lesion.

Lateral oblique radiographs of body and ramus of mandible also show extension of the lesion.

Digital panoramic radiographs can depict the lesions clearly but the extent cannot be defined properly due to inherent magnification in these views but may be helpful in the absence of sophisticated and high cost radiological techniques like computed tomography or MRI.

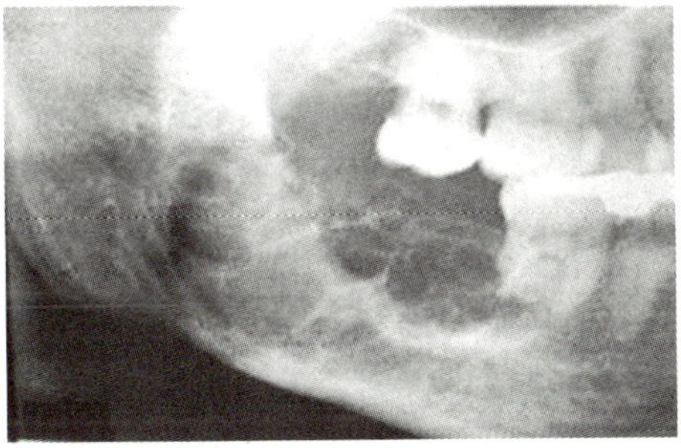

Fig. Ameloblastoma with a Honey comb pattern

Radiographic differential diagnosis for ameloblastoma:

- Small and unilocular ameloblastoma:
- **Dentigerous cyst:** When they are located around the crown of an unerupted tooth, its difficult to differentiate from dentigerous cyst.
- **Residual cyst:** There is history of extraction of the affected tooth and has typical flask shaped appearance.
- **Lateral periodontal cyst:** Its commonly associated with the incisors, canine and the premolars in the maxilla and ameloblastoma has more affinity for the mandible.
- **Traumatic bone cyst:** occurs in mid –twenties and ameloblastoma in 3 rd and 4 th decade. This cyst also can be seen extending into the inter –radicular areas which is not seen in ameloblastoma.
- **Primordial cyst:** Occurs in place of tooth, or associated super-numerary tooth, and other features similar to traumatic bone cyst.
- Multilocular ameloblastoma:

- **Odontogenic keratocysts:** contains curved septa, but tends to grow mesiodistally than bucco-lingually hence causing less expansion of bone and it also shows hazy opacity due to presence of keratin.
- **Odontogenic myxoma:** history of missing tooth, presence of one or two thin, sharp, straight septa, with typical tennis racket or step ladder like appearance, non expansile and tending to grow along the bone.
- **Odontogenic fibroma:** septa are usually wide, granular and ill-defined, with small irregular trabeculae present.

Suggested reading:

1. Freny R Karjodkar, Essentials of oral and maxillofacial radiology, first edition 2014, 345-350.
2. Norman K Wood, Paul W. Goaz, Differential Diagnosis of Oral and Maxillofacial Lesions. 5th ed. St. Louis: Mosby, 1997. 342-43.

Q 2) Describe in detail the radiographic appearance of various odontomes and give the differential diagnosis.

TNMGRU APRIL 1996, (16 Marks)

- Odontoma is a hamartoma which is odontogenic in origin and in which there is complete differentiation of the both the epithelial and the mesenchymal cells and enamel, dentin and cementum is laid down in abnormal positions.
- Broca in 1866 was the first to name it as such and he describes it as a tumour due to over growth of all the dental tissues.

Classification:

(a) **Ectodermal origin:** Enameloma(enamel pearl, enamel nodule)

(b) **Mesodermal origin:**

   (i) Dentinoma

   (ii) Cementoma

(c) **Mixed:**

   1. Complex composite odontoma: These are non-descrete masses of dental tissue.
   2. Compound composite odontoma: There are multiple well formed teeth.
   3. Compound complex odontoma: These contain multiple teeth like structures and along with it calcified masses of dental tissue that are placed in a random manner.
   4. Geminated odontoma.
   5. Dilated odontoma.
   6. Dens in dente.

(a) Odontomes of ectodermal origin:

   (i) **Enameloma:**

   - Also known as Enamel pearl.

- It is a small globule of enamel 1.3 mm in diameter and occurs on the roots of molars.

Radiographic features:

- It appears smooth round and comparable in radiopacity to the enamel covering the crown. It appears as a radiopaque shadow.
- Shape is hemispherical.
- Appears as a well circumscribed rounded, density in association with a root.
- The dentine casts a small radiolucent shadow in the centre of the radiopaque sphere of enamel.
- It seen best when present on the mesial and distal side of the root.

Differential Diagnosis:

- **Calculus:** Isolated piece of calculus, can be clinically verified and it will not be rounded.
- **Pulp stone:** an increase in vertical angulations will move the image of enamel pearls away from the pulp chamber.
- When the distal portion of the mesial root is projected over the mesial part of the distal root, an area of radiodensity similar to enamel pearl will be seen. However a radiograph so taken that the rays pass through the contiguous part of the roots will help to differentiate.

(b) Odontomas of mesodermal origin:

(i) **Dentinoma:** Its a rare tumour of odontogenic origin which is composed of odontogenic epithelium, immature connective tissue and dysplastic dentin placed in irregular manner.

Radiographic features:

- It appears as radiopaque mass or several masses associated with the crown of an unerupted tooth usually surrounded by a radiolucent area.
- It can lead to destruction of local bone.

(ii) **Cementoma:** Its fibro-osseous lesion that is reactive and is derived from the odontogenic cells present in the periodontal ligament usually located at the apex of the tooth.

Radiographic features:

Stage I–Radiolucent:

- The lesion appears as a circumscribed radiolucency associated with localised destruction of bone.
- The margins of the lesion vary from well defined but not corticated, poorly defined or partly ill defined.
- Loss of lamina dura around involved tooth.

Stage II–Mixed stage:

- Radiopaque tissue 'cementicles' having round, oval or irregular shape appear in the radiolucent structure.

Stage III–Radiopaque:

- Complete opacification of lesion occurs.
- It is a well defined radiopacity which is surrounded by a radiolucent capsule causing its separation from the adjacent bone.
- The margins vary from well defined to poorly defined.
- Loss of lamina dura, no root resportion.
- If large enough, this tumor can cause expansion of the mandible but with an intact outer cortex.

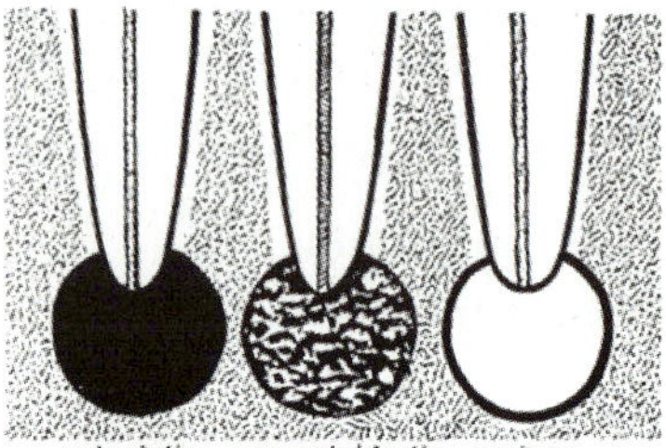

Fig. Three different stages of cementoma.

Differential diagnosis:

In early (radiolucent) stage:

Periapical rarefying osteitis: Associated with pulpal disease and the associated tooth is sensitive to percussion.

In mixed stage:

(a) **Benign Cementoblastoma:**

- Rare lesion and is usually associated at the apex of mandibular molars.
- Tumour has attachment to the root surface, and the root may be resorbed partly.
- Radiating pattern of internal structure.
- Expansion is more concentric & less undulating than cementoma.

(b) **Odontomes of mixed origin:**

(i) Odontoma:

- It is located above the crown of the unerupted tooth, and is sometimes between the teeth but is rarely seen at the apex.
- Organizations of the internal aspect into tooth like structure helps in diagnosis.

(c) **Cemento-ossifying fibroma: It shows aggressive growth pattern:**

In stage III:

- Dense bone island: radiolucent periphery indicate cementoma.

1. **Complex and compound odontoma:** The WHO in 2005 classified the odontomas based on the histopathologic findings:
   - Complex odontomas, in which the tissues of the teeth are formed well but are amorphous and arranged in a disorderly arrangement.
   - Compound odontomas, in which the tissues of the teeth are normal and are arranged in an orderly manner but their size and conformation is altered, and results in small multiple teeth like elements which are called denticles or odontoid.

   Radiographic features:

   1. **Compound composite odontome:**
      - Appears as number of tooth like structures in the region of canine.
      - Internal structures: Shows number of small shapeless dense masses of solid tissue which have equal or more density. In some cases there may be two or more tooth like mass present with conical enamel capped crowns and there could be fusion of the root portion.
      - If only few teeth are present, a pericoronal and periodontal characteristics of unerupted teeth can be seen on each individual tooth. In case of presence of large number of teeth then it is surrounded by thin radiolucent line which represents the follicular space of the unerupted teeth.
      - Margin is well defined. It may be smooth or irregular and can show sclerotic borders.

2. **Complex composite odontome:**
   - The appearance is that of dense radiopaque object, which is seen sometimes lying in clear space. Density is greater than bone and more than or equal to the teeth.
   - Internally, it shows an area of well defined radiolucency which contains masses of calcified tissue that are irregular which is associated with unerupted teeth.

   Differential diagnosis:
   - Cemento ossifying fibroma: There is a difference between the complex odontomas and the cemento-ossifying fibroma by their tendency to associate with unerupted molar teeth and more radiopaque than cemento-ossifying fibroma.
   - Periapicalcemental dysplasia: They are generally multiple and are centered on the periapical region of the teeth periphery, has wider uneven sclerotic border. Odontomes have well defined sclerotic borders and the soft tissue capsule surrounding it is uniform and well defined than cemental dysplasia.
   - Dense bone island: They lack the soft tissue capsule seen in the odontomas.

- Hypercementosis: It is attached to the root part and is separated from the surrounding bone by the periodontal ligament space that is radiolucent and which surrounds the entire root.
- The condensing osteitis should be ruled out as it involves the peri-apex of the teeth which are usually non-vital and lacks the radiolucent rim.
- Osteosclerosis which is periapical is quite irregular in shape and there is absence of the radiolucent border.

3. Geminated Odontome:

- Geminated odontomes: It shows two or more, quite well developed teeth that are fused to each other.

Radiographic features:

- Radiograph reveals altered shape of hard tissue and pulp chamber of geminated tooth.

Differential diagnosis:

- Geminated odontome can be differentiated from fusion of teeth, as there is missing teeth in fusion.

4. Dilated odontoma:

- Its a developmental anomaly that is rare and there is dilation of the root and crown because of a deep invagination that is lined with enamel.
- It is considered to be a severe form of dens invaginatus.

Radiographic features:

A tooth associated with a dilated odontome has a round or oval shaped radiopacity with a radiolucent interior.

Suggested reading:

1. Freny R. Karjodkar, Essentials Of Oral And Maxillofacial Radiology, Chapter 26, Pg No 538-596.
2. Morawala Abdul: Compound Composite Odontoma and Its Management, Hindawi Publishing Corporation, Case Reports in Dentistry, Volume 2014.
3. Stuart C White, Michael J Pharoah, Oral Radiology, Principles and Interpretation 5th edition, chapter 22, pg no.366-404.

CHAPTER 10

Fibro-Osseous Lesions

Q 1) Classify Fibro-osseous lesions of the jaws. Discuss the clinical and radiographic features of Fibrous Dysplasia:

TNMGRU FEBRUARY 2012 (10 Marks)

Definition:

Fibrous dysplasia is a fibrosseous condition involving one or more bones of the cranial and extra cranial skeleton, consisting of nonencapsulated lesions which have undergone change that is localised in the normal metabolism of bone, and shows replacement of the normal cancellous bone by cellular fibrous tissues containing islands of metastatic bone.

Classification:

Medullary bone origin:

1. Fibrous dysplasia
2. Cherubism
3. Paget's disease
4. Juvenile ossifying fibroma
5. Gaint cell tumor
6. Aneurysmal bone cyst
7. Jaw lesions in hyperparathyroidism
8. Fibro-osteoma

Periodontal membrane origin:

9. Periapical cemental dysplasia
10. Florid osseous dysplasia
11. Cementossifying fibroma
12. Cementifying fibroma
13. Ossifying fibroma

Clinical types:

1. Monostotic fibrous dysplasia: In this case there is involvement of

only one bone.

2. Polyostotic fibrosis dysplasia: More than one bone is involved.
   (a) **Jaffe type:** In this type there is fibrous dysplasia that involves several bones and there are pigmented lesions of the skin, especially the cafe au lait spots.
   (b) **McCune- Albright syndrome:** It is a more severe form of fibrous dysplasia where almost all bones of the body are involved and there is presence of skin pigmentations along with endocrinal disturbances of various types.
   (c) **A craniofacial form:** lesions are confined to bones of the craniofacial complex.
   (d) **Monomelic:** where there is involvement of only one extremity. This is very rare.
   (e) **Subclinical fibrous dysplasia:** sometimes an unsuspected lesion of fibrous dysplasia may be discovered on routine radiographic examination, without any clinical evidence of the suspected disease, these may be termed as subclinical fibrosis dysplasia.

Clinical features:

1. **Monostotic type:**
   - This accounts for 70% of all cases, involving one bone and quite often involve the jaws. Most common bones in order of affectation are the ribs, femur, tibia, maxilla and the mandible.
   - Maxilla is more commonly involved than the mandible and more common in premolar molar region.
   - Older age group with no sex predilection.
   - Lesions become static after skeletal growth stops but may become active in pregnant females or with use of oral contraceptives.
   - Often discovered as an incidental radiographic findings.
   - Patient may complain of swelling on one side of the face or enlargement of the alveolar processes, involving the buccal and labial cortical plates.
   - The involved teeth may be malaligned, tipped or displaced. Presence of supernumerary teeth has been reported which are commonly found in midline of maxilla and mandibular premolar region. These teeth may affect eruption of normal teeth.
   - The presence of pain and pathologic fractures are not usually present. In case the craniofacial lesions are extensive and have impinged on various foramen, then neurologic symptoms like anosmia, blindness or deafness may occur.
2. **Polyostotic type:**
   (a) **Jaffe type:**
      - Involvement of multiple bones along with the presence

of pigmented lesions of the skin, that is cafe-au-lait spots.

- Age of occurrence is less than 10 years of age.
- Lesions become static after skeletal growth stops.
- There may be expansion and deformity of jaws.
- Disturbances in normal eruption pattern.
- Facial asymmetry which can lead to pathologic fractures. In case of extensive involvement of the cranio-facial bones, the lesions can impinge on the foramina and lead to anosmia, blindness or deafness.
- Serum alkaline phosphates level is normal but sometimes elevated.

(b) **Mc Cune Albright syndrome:**

- Most commonly occurs in females.
- Associated with endocrine disturbances like precocious puberty, goiter, hyperthyroidism, cushing syndrome and acromegaly.
- Development of secondary sexual character like pubic hair, axillary hair, development of breast at 5 years of age.
- Bone and skin lesions are unilateral mostly long bone affected.
- There may be expansion and deformity of jaws.
- Disturbances in normal eruption pattern.
- Facial asymmetry which can lead to ballooning of jaws.

(c) **Craniofacial type:**

- Most commonly involves maxillary antrum, zygomatic process, orbital floor, base of skull.
- There is severe facial deformity with malocclusion.
- Craniofacial lesions causes impingment on nerve foramina producing symptoms such as anosmia, blindness and deafness.

Radiographic features:

1. **Location:** it involves the maxilla twice common as that of mandible and most frequently in the posterior aspect of premolar molar region. Lesions more commonly are unilateral or in rare cases extensive lesion may be bilateral.
2. **Periphery:** lesions are most commonly ill defined and there is gradual blending of the normal trabecular bone with the abnormal. Some times however, the boundary between the normal and abnormal bone can be sharp and even corticated specially in early lesions.
3. **Internal structure:**

   (a) **Early lesion:** it is radiolucent with ill defined borders.

Surrounding the radiolucency there is wider band of increased density giving granular appearance. It can be unilocular or presence of bony septa can lead to the appearance of multilocularity.

(b) **Intermediate lesion:** lesion is mixed radiolucent and radiopaque depending on stage of maturity. New bone appears as small radiopacity of poor density. Lesions in the mandible are more pronounced and are homogenous in the maxilla and base of skull.

(c) **Mature lesions:** lesions appear as radiopaque where the bone is prominent. Abnormal trabeculae are thinner and shorter, with irregular shape and more in numbers than the normal trabeculae.

Obisesan et al classification of radiographic appearance of fibrous dysplasia:

(i) **Ground glass appearance:** This resembles the shattered glass of a wind shield.

(ii) **Peau de orange/ orange peel appearance:** Areas of alternating granular density and radiolucency gives the orange peel appearance.

(iii) **Whorled plaque like type:** Plaques of amorphous material having intermediate radiodensity.

(iv) **Diffuse sclerotic type:** homogeneous dense areas are present which merge to normal bone.

(v) **Cyst like type:** lesions are radiolucent giving unilocular or multilocular appearance well defined margins.

(vi) **Pagetoid type:** affected areas of bone expands and shows areas of radiopacity and radiolucency seen in pagets disease.

(vii) **Chalky type:** lesions are well circumscribed with amorphous dense radiopaque material.

4. **Effect on surrounding structures:** In case the lesions are small, they may not affect the surrounding structures. The effect on the bone involved will include expansion, with maintenance of a thinned outer cortex. Lesion may expand into antrum consequently and occupy most of the maxillary antrum. Loss of lamina dura of involved teeth. Displaced teeth interfere with normal eruption. Root resorption or destruction of tooth bud may occur. Inferior alveolar canal is displaced superiorly.

Suggested reading:

1. Freny R karzodkar, Essentials of Oral and Maxillofacial Radiology, 2nd ed, pg no. 419-29.
2. Stuart C White, Michael J Pharoah, Oral Radiology, Principles and Interpretation, 6 th ed, pg no. 428- 32.

CHAPTER 11

Diagnostic Imaging of Temporomandibular Joint

Q 1) Describe radiographic techniques to diagnose TMJ diseases and disorders:

TNMGRU OCTOBER 1997 (18 Marks)

Temporomandibular joint is a unique complex joint which executes both hinge and sliding movements. It is also called as the ginglymo-di-arthroidal type of joint. There are number of imaging modalities for imaging temporomandibular joint. But, for majority of cases diagnostic imaging has not proven to be a valuable test for directing treatment or for predicting outcome and long term course.

Conventional radiographic projections:

1. Transcranial Projection
2. Transpharyngeal Projection
3. Transorbital Projection
4. Corrected Submentovertex Projection
5. Panoramic radiography
6. Reverse Towne's projection
7. Conventional Tomography
8. Other investigations:
    (a) Arthrography.
    (b) Computed tomography (CT).
    (c) Cone beam computed tomography(CBCT)

I. Transcranial Projection:

Technique:

1. The patient is positioned in a dental chair. The film cassette is placed on the side to be imaged. The x-ray beam is directed downward from the opposite side, through the cranium and above the petrous ridge of the temporal bone.
2. The tube head of the x-ray is placed with the central ray aimed downwards at 25° to the horizontal, across the cranium, centering

through the TMJ of interest.

3. The horizontal direction of the beam may be individually corrected for the condylar long axis, an average 20-degree anterior angle may be used.

The main clinical indications include:

1. For investigation of joint diseases like rheumatoid and osteoarthritis.
2. Investigation of conditions that are pathological involving the head of the condyle like fractures, cysts or tumour from the lateral aspect only.
3. To assess the position of the condylar head in the fossa.
4. Agenesis of condyle, Condylar hypoplasia/ hyperplasia, ankylosis.

(ii) Transpharyngeal Projection:

Technique:

1. The patient is asked to hold the cassette against the side of the face on the TMJ of interest. The film and the sagittal plane of the head are parallel.
2. The x-ray beam is directed superiorly at -5 degrees through the sigmoid notch of the opposite side and 7 to 8 degrees from the anterior.
3. The patient opens the mouth maximally to avoid superimposition of the condyle on the temporal component. Because of the negative beam angulation, this view depicts the medial aspect of the condyle.

The main indications include:

1. Investigation of the existence of diseases of the joints like osteo and rheumatoid arthritis.
2. Investigation of pathological conditions of the condylar head which includes fractures, cysts or tumour.
3. The condylar head shape and the condition of the articular surface of medial pole of the condyle like condylar hypoplasia (unilateral or bilateral), condylar hyperplasia (unilateral or bilateral), bifid condyle .
4. Effective for visualizing erosive changes of the condyle rather than more subtle changes.
5. Defects associated with specific diseases or syndromes.

(iii) Transorbital Projection:

Technique:

- The transorbital projection provide an anterior view of the TMJ.
- In this view, patient's head is tilted downward 10 degrees so that the canthomeatal line is horizontal.
- The x-ray beam is directed from the front of the patient through the ipsilateral orbit on the TMJ of interest.

- The film is placed behind the head of the patient, perpendicular to the beam of x-ray.
- The patient opens maximally or, as an alternative, protrudes the mandible, thereby positioning the condyle at the summit of the articular eminence and avoiding superimposition of skull base on the condyle.

The main indications include:

1. Entire mediolateral dimension of the articular eminence, condylar head, and condylar neck is visible, which makes this view particularly useful for visualizing condylar neck fractures.
2. The morphology of the convex surface of the condylar head can be evaluated like condylar hypoplasia, hyperplasia.
3. In assessing the degenerative changes or other anomalies.

(iv) Corrected Submentovertex (Basal) Projection:

- The submentovertex (SMV) projection provides a view of the base of the skull and the condyles that are superimposed on the necks of the condyle and rami of the mandible.
- For this reason the SMV projection often is used to determine the angulations of the long axis of the condylar head for corrected tomography.

Technique:

- The film is positioned parallel to transverse plane of the patient and perpendicular to the midsagittal and coronal planes. To achieve this, the patient's neck is extended as far backwards as possible, with the canthomeatal line forming a 10-degree angle with the image receptor.
- The central beam is perpendicular to the image receptor, directed from below the mandible towards the vertex of the skull (hence the name submentovertex or SMV), and centered about 2 cm anterior to a line connecting the right and left condyles.

The main indications include:

This view may be used as an adjunct to views depicting the TMJs in the lateral plane and is particularly useful for evaluating facial asymmetries, condylar displacement, or rotation of the mandible in the horizontal plane associated with trauma or orthognathic surgery.

V. Panoramic radiography:

Technique:

- Panoramic radiography is a procedure that produces a single tomographic image of the structures of the face including both maxilla and mandible and surrounding structures.
- The chin of the patient and the plane of occlusion should be properly positioned so that a line from the tragus of the ear to

the outer canthus of the eye that is the 'canthomeatal line' is parallel with the floor. Canthomeatal line forms 10 degrees with the Frankfort horizontal plane.

- There is a movement of the source of x-ray and the film which is reciprocal around a central point which is called as the image layer, within which the object of interest is placed. The objects that are placed in front of or behind this layer of image are not clearly captured because of their relative movement to the center of rotation of the film and the source of x-ray.
- In this condyles of both sides can be visualized simultaneously which roughly give some idea about the anatomic structure or the pathology. But it is not a primary imaging modality for TMJ radiography.

The main indications are:

1. TMJ pain dysfunction syndrome.
2. Investigations of the pathological conditions that affect the head of the condyles.
3. Fractures of the condylar heads or necks.
4. Ankylosis.
5. Agenesis of condyle.
6. Condylar hypo/hyperplasia.

VI. Reverse towne's Projection:

Technique:

The patient is positioned facing the film with the head tipped forwards in the forehead-nose position, the mouth is open, and the X-ray tube head is aimed upwards at 30° from behind.

The main clinical indications are:

1. Fractures of the condylar heads and necks.
2. Condylar hypo/hyperplasia.
3. Developmental anomalies.

VII. Conventional Tomography:

Techniques:

- This technique can provide multiple image slice at right angle to the joint. it is superior to the transcranial view in depicting true condylar position and revealing osseous changes.
- Tomography usually involves imaging several different sections of the area under investigation. Enables visualization of a section of the patient's anatomy by blurring regions of the patient's anatomy above and below the section of interest.

Main indications are:

1. Complete assessment of the entire joint so as to determine the presence and the location of bony disease and abnormality.

2. Assessment of the head of the condyle and articular fossa in case when the patient is unable to open the mouth.
3. To assess the fractures of the articular fossa and intracapsular fractures.
4. An alteration in the position of the head of the condyle, implying an abnormality in disc position.

VIII. Other investigations:

(a) Arthrography:

Technique:

1. 0.5- 1 ml of non-ionic aqueous contrast medium is injected carefully into the lower joint space using fluoroscopy to aid the accurate positioning of the needle. Most commonly used contrast media are iodine compounds.
2. A series of radiographs are taken following joint space opacification with the jaw's closed and opening movements.
3. The disc appears as a radiolucent void between two opaque areas of contrast medium.
4. The perforation is detected by the flow of contrast agent into the superior joint space from the lower space, and adhesions are detected by the manner in which contrast agent fills the joint space.
5. It is indicated when information on disk position, function, morphology, and the integrity of discal attachments is required or when persistent history of locking is present. When there is limited opening of unknown etiology this technique is indicated.

Main indications are:

- Displacement of the disc anteriorly or antero-medially.
- Presence of any perforations is main indication of this technique.

b. Computed tomography:

Technique:

- CT scanner consists of a radiographic tube that emits a finely collimated x-ray beam that is fan shaped and directed to a series of detectors that are scintillating or ionisation chambers.
- CT produces digital image slices. Multiple image slices are made in both the axial and coronal plane.
- The advantages of CT are that they can produce the hard and soft tissue images of the joint, which includes the disc, in different planes.
- Main indications are:
- These are useful for assessing osseous deformities of the jaws or surrounding structures.
- Presence and extent of ankylosis and neoplasms and the extent of bone involvement in some arthritides.

- Imaging complex fractures.
- Evaluating complications from the use of polytetrafluoroethylene or silicon sheet implants such as erosions into the middle cranial fossa and heterotrophic bone growth.
- Severe juvenile rheumatoid arthritis.
- Trauma, particularly condylar head fractures and birth injury, and bleeding into the joint.
- Ely's cyst, tumors:

c. CBCT:

- Cone beam computed tomography is a more complex and accurate imaging with 3 dimensional visualization as compared to routinely used analog and digital radiographs.
- Its a technique in which x-ray beam that is cone shaped is centered on a two dimensional detector that produces a series of 2D images.
- Modified Feldkamp algorithm is applied for reconstruction of these images in a 3D data set. The data hence can be reformatted in a volume rather than a slice thus giving 3 D information.

Main indications are:

- It is imaging technique of choice in assessing bony changes of the TMJ like erosions.
- Presence and extent of ankylosis and neoplasms and the extent of bone involvement in some arthritides.
- Imaging complex fractures.
- Arthritis.
- Trauma, particularly condylar head fractures and birth injury, and bleeding into the joint.
- Ely's cyst, tumors.

Suggested reading:

1. Eric whaites, Essential of Dental Radiography and Radiology, 3rd ed, pg no 385-402.
2. Pramod Kumar, Nitin Upadhyay. Recent advances in Temporomandibular Joint Imaging: An Upadate. Journal of Dental Sciences & Oral Rehabilitation. 2013; Oct-Dec: 15-19.
3. Stuart C White, Michael J Pharoah, Oral Radiology, Principles and Interpretation 5th Edition, 538-575.

CHAPTER 12

Trauma to Teeth and Facial Structures

Q 1) Enumerate the various radiographic techniques for the diagnosis of fractures of mandible:

RGUHS APRIL 2000 (10 Marks)

Fracture of mandible according to the frequency of occurrence are as follows:

(i) Body of mandible.
(ii) Sub condylar area fractures.
(iii) Angle of mandible.
(iv) Dentoalveolar fractures.
(v) Ramus region.
(vi) Symphyseal fractures.
(vii) Coronoid fractures.

Radiography for fractures of mandible can be classified into:

- Intra-oral.
- Extra-oral.
    (i) Conventional.
    (ii) Computerised Tomography/ Cone Beam Computerised tomography.

1. **Intra-oral radiography:**
    - **Intra-oral periapical radiographs:** They can reveal:
        - Association of tooth to line of fracture.
        - Existing pathology related to tooth in line of fracture.
        - Fracture of tooth in line of fracture.
    - **Occlusal radiographs:** They can reveal:
        - **Anterior:** Assessment of fracture in anterior teeth and alveolar bone and assessment of displacement fractures of the anterior mandible in the vertical plane.
        - **Cross sectional:** Assessment of displacement fractures of the anterior body of the mandible in the horizontal plane.

- Lateral occlusal views can depict the fractures of mandible and depending upon the region apt occlusal radiographs can be taken.
- True occlusal radiographs can show details of whether the buccal or lingual cortical plates are involved.

2. Extra-oral radiography:

I) Conventional:

1 (Lateral oblique(Right and left)

(i) **Body of mandible:** Head is tilted towards the side being examined and the mandible is protruded .
Film is centered over the first molar, parallel and 2 cms below the inferior border of the mandible.
Central ray is directed toward the molar-premolar region from a point 2cm below the angle of the opposite side of the mandible.

(ii) **Ramus of mandible:** Head is tilted towards the side being examined such that the condyle of the area of interest and the contra lateral angle of the mandible form horizontal line. To prevent superimposition of cervical spine on ramus protrude the mandible.
Film is placed over the ramus and far enough posteriorly to include the condyle.
Central ray is directed towards the center of the imaged ramus, from 2cm below the inferior border of the opposite side of the mandibular at the area of the first molar.
These radiographs can reveal:

- Fracture of body of mandible proximal to the canine region.
- Fractures of angle, ramus and condylar region.

2. Postero-anterior view of mandible:

- Fractures of posterior thirds of the body of the mandible, angles, rami, and lower condylar necks.
- Can reveal displacement of fractures in the ramus, angle and body region.
  - Film is placed in a cassette holder with the long axis vertically.
  - Patient is positioned with saggital plane perpendicular to the film.
  - Head is tipped down wards so that the forehead and nose touch the film.
  - The radiographic base line is horizontal and perpendicular to the film.
  - The film is adjusted so that the lips are on the centre of the film.
  - Central ray is directed at right angles to the film at the level of the angle of the mandible.

3. Rotated postero-anterior view:

- Can depict fractures between symphysis and canine region.

4. Reverse Towne's view:

The patient is positioned facing the film with the head tipped forwards in the forehead-nose position, the mouth is open, and the X-ray tube head is aimed upwards at 30° from behind.

- It is ideal for showing lateral or medial displacement of condyle.

5. Towne's view:

- It is primarily used to visualise the condyles and hence can depict condylar fracture.

6. Water's view/Basal view:

- In P.A views the symphyseal region can be obscured by the cervical spine. In such cases the Water's view and basal views can be taken to evaluate the symphyseal region by negating superimposition of the spine.

7. Conventional T.M.J views:

(i) **Transpharyngeal projection:** The patient holds the cassette against the side of the face over the TMJ of interest. The film and the sagittal plane of the head are parallel.

(ii) The x-ray beam is directed superiorly at -5 degrees through the sigmoid notch of the opposite side and 7 to 8 degrees from the anterior .

- This technique can reveal fracture of the neck and condyle of the mandible.

(ii) **Transorbital projection:**

- In the transorbital view, patient's head is tilted downward 10 degrees so that the canthomeatal line is horizontal.
- The film is located behind the head of the patient and perpendicular to the beam of x-ray.
- The x-ray beam is directed from the front of the patient through the ipsilateral orbit on TMJ of interest.
- Its an antero-posterior view which can depict medial displacement of fractured condyle.
- It can also show fracture of the neck of condyle.

8. Panoramic radiography:

Panoramic radiography is a procedure that produces a single tomographic image of facial structures including both maxilla and mandible and surrounding structures.

The patient's chin and occlusal plane must be properly positioned so that a line from the tragus of the ear to the outer canthus of the eye that is the 'canthomeatal line' is parallel with the floor. Canthomeatal line forms 10 degrees with the Frankfurt horizontal plane.

There is a reciprocal movement of an x-ray source and an image receptor around a central point, called the image layer, in which the object of interest is located. Objects in front of or behind this image layer are not clearly captured because of their relative movement to the center of rotation of the receptor and x-ray source.

- It can show multiple mandibular fractures in one radiograph.
- Bilateral condylar fractures can be seen at one time.
- Bony detail of alveolar-ridge, tooth root, fractures can be evaluated very well.

II) Computerised Tomography:

1. **Cone Beam Computerised Tomography:**
   - It has been found in studies that as compared to panoramic radiography, the CBCT is superior because the fractures of the condyle and the coronoid processes and the anterior mandibular area are difficult to assess due to superimpositions.
   - As compared to the conventional radiographs the CBCT is superior to detect the fractures of patients in cases of maxillo-facial trauma and provides more detailed information about subtle dentoalveolar fracture.
   - Can depict additional information like displaced fragments and multiple fragments.
   - Can demonstrate fractures not visible on conventional radiographs.
   - In patients with suspected mandibular fracture CBCT increases diagnostic certainty to about 90.5% according to some studies.
2. **Computed Tomography Scan:**
   - With sagittal and coronal reconstructions, CT scans can depict all the portions of the mandible in 3 planes, but direct coronal views are always preferred. Besides identifying the fracture, it is easier to determine the degree of fragment displacement with CT scanning than with plain radiography.
   - CT scanning is the best method for detecting subtle or fractures that are questionable. CT scanning can also better show hard-to-see fractures through the thin cortex of a pathologic lesion.

Suggested reading:

1. Seth A. Reiner, David L. Schwartz, Keith F. Clark, N. Robert Markowitz, Accurate Radiographic Evaluation of Mandibular Fractures Arch Otolaryngol Head Neck Surg. 1989;115(9): 1083-1085.

CHAPTER 13

Salivary Gland Radiology

Q 1) Describe Sialography In Detail & Write Briefly On Significance In Various Salivary Gland Disorders.

RGUHS APRIL 2005 (9 Marks)

Sialography:

(a) Sialography is the radiographic visualization of the salivary gland following retrograde instillation of soluble contrast material into the ducts.

(b) It is one of the oldest procedures for imaging and was first mentioned by Carpy in 1902.

(c) Is a specialized radiographic procedure performed for detection of disorders of major salivary glands (usually submandibular and parotid).

(d) The technique is employed for both parenchymal (acinar) and ductal abnormalities.

(e) It involves cannulation and filling with a radio-opaque/contrast agent to make them visible on the radiograph.

Techniques For Sialography:

The three main techniques available for introducing the contrast medium into the ductal system after cannulating the relevant duct orifice are as follows:

1. **Simple injection technique:** Water based or oil based contrast medium is introduced by use of gentle pressure of the hands till the patient experiences a feeling of tightness or discomfort in the glands, and 0.7 ml for the parotid gland, 0.5 ml for the submandibular gland is used.

   Advantages:

   1. Simple.
   2. Inexpensive.

Disadvantages:

1. The pressure that is used arbitrarily can cause damage to the gland.

2. **Hydrostatic technique:** The water based contrast medium is allowed to freely flow in to the gland under the gravitational force till the patient feels discomfort.

   Advantages:

   1. The introduction of the contrast medium in a controlled manner less likely causes damage and doesnot give artefactual picture.
   2. Simple
   3. Inexpensive.

   Disadvantages:

   1. Reliant on the patient's responses.
   2. The patients have to lie down during the procedure and hence need to be positioned in advance for the filling phase radiographs.

3. **Continous infusion pressure-monitored technique:** A water based medium is used and a constant rate of flow is adopted and pressure on the ducts is monitored through out.

   Advantages:

   1. There is less likelyhood of damage due to controlled introduction of the contrast medium under known pressure.
   2. Does not cause overfilling of the gland.
   3. Does not rely on the patient's responses.

   Disadvantages:

   1. Complex equipment is required.
   2. Time consuming.

Procedure for sialography:

(a) Armamentarium: 5 or 10cc syringe, Lacrimal dilators, Contrast media, Cotton 4 x 4 Gauze pads, IV extension tube, Cannulae - varying sizes & designs, Sterile gloves, Topical anesthetic, Sialagogue, like 5 lemon slices / lemon extract / chewing gum.

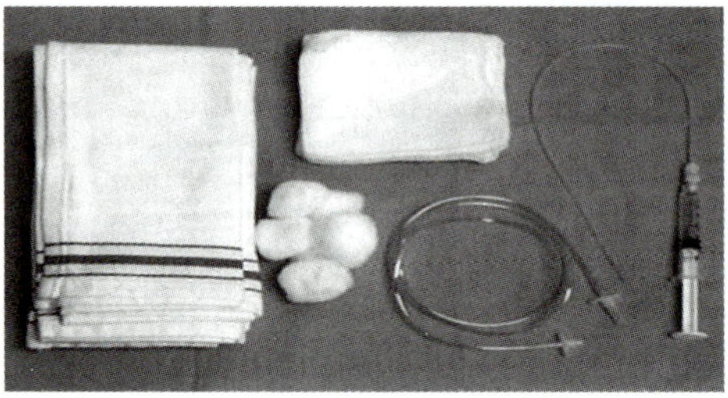

Fig. Armamentarium for sialography

B. Procedure:

Step 1: preliminary plain film evaluation.

Step 2: Injection / filling phase.

Step 3: Evacuation phase.

(a) Parotid gland:

- A radiograph is taken before infusion of contrast media into the gland.
- Salivary gland orifice is located and it is dried with small sponge.
- Ductal orifice is explored with lacrimal probe.

(b) Submandibular duct:

- It is located as small papilla at the side of lingual frenum.
- Probe should pass through the length of floor of the mouth to the level of posterior border of the mylohyoid muscle.
- Probe is moistened with patient's saliva, then it is directed into the orifice and slowly advanced down the duct for about 4 to 5 cm.
- 5-ml of contrast media is injected, loaded with Renographin 40 or Hypaque which is slowly infused.
- Radiographic exposure is made immediately.
- After the procedure cannula is removed, patient is instructed to massage gland and suck on lemon drops to promote flow of saliva and contrast media out of gland.
- Radiographs are taken after 1hour after procedure, if contrast media remains follow up visits should be done.

Radiographs to be taken:

1. **Mandibular occlusal view:** it is used for submandibular gland. Sialolith are better visualized.
2. **Lateral oblique:** duct pattern is not distorted.
3. Anteroposterior view and puffed cheek AP views of both glands demonstrate medial & lateral gland structures.
   For Parotid gland: patient is asked to keep mouth open.
4. **Panoramic projection:** Erosion of bone / destruction of mandible in case of salivary tumors.

Significance in various salivary gland disorders:

1. **Sialographic appearance of calculi:** Sialoliths or calculus in the ductal architecture may be evident as radioopaque or radiolucent appearance commonly seen in submandibular gland. Radio-opaque sialoliths may appear as filling defect in the main duct. They may be single or multiple long cigar shape / oval/ round shape with smooth borders ranging from little more than pin head to a length of inch / more upto 5mm.
2. **Sialographic appearance of sialodochitis:** Sialodochitis is an inflammation of the ductal system of the salivary glands. Most commonly occurs in submandibular gland and parotid gland. There is dilation of the ductal system. If interstitial fibrosis develops it is apparent in sialograms as a sausage string appearance.
3. **Sialographic appearance of sialadenitis include:** Contrast media appears as blobs or dots of the contrast medium in the

glands, known as sialectasis, which is due to the inflammation of the tissues of the glands resulting in production of saccular dilation of the acini.

4. **Sialographic appearance of sjogren's syndrome:** The early stages of the disease are witness to the initiation of punctuate (less than 1mm) and globular (1 to 2 mm) spherical collections of contrast agent evenly distributed throughout the gland. These collection are referred to as sialectasis. Main duct is normal. Wide spread blobs or dots of the contrast medium in the gland known as "punctate sialectasis/ and snowstorm appearance".Typical appearance is also called as cherry blossom appearance.
5. **Sialographic appearance of intrinsic tumours:** Sialography may suggest a space occupying mass when the ducts are compressed or smoothly displaced around the lesion giving 'ball in hand appearance'. Most common presentation of parotid gland.

Suggested reading:

1. Freny R Karjodkar, Essentials Of Oral and Maxillofacial Radiology, first Edition, Pg no.856-859
2. Eric whaites, Essentials of dental radiography and radiology, third edition, pg 407.
3. Stuart C White, Michael J Pharoah, Oral Radiology, Principles and Interpretation 5th Edition, pg 660-676.

CHAPTER 14

Periapical Radiolucencies and Opacities

Q 1) Describe periapical radiolucencies and radiopacities:

RGUHS OCTOBER 2000 (10 Marks)

1. Periapical radiolucencies:

(i) **Periapical granuloma:** The periapical granuloma by far represents the most common type of pathologic radiolucency. It represents a successful attempt to neutralise the irritating toxic products coming out of root canal.

On radiographic examination the lesion is a well-circumscribed radiolucency somewhat rounded and surrounding the apex of the tooth.

It may have a thin radiopaque border.

Radiographs of the involved tooth may reveal deep restorations, extensive caries.

(ii) **Radicular cyst:** The radicular cyst is the second most common pulpoperiapical lesion.

It is the most common of all odontogenic cysts.

Most radicular cysts involve the apices of the permanent teeth.

About 60% involve the lateral incisors.

These cysts involve deciduous teeth, most commonly the molars.

Radiolucency is at least 1.6 cm in diameter.

(iii) **Periapical scar:** The periapical scar is composed of dense fibrous tissue and is situated at the periapex of a pulpless tooth in which usually the root canals have been successfully filled.

It is a well-circumscribed radiolucency that is more or less round and on radiographic examination resembles the periapical granuloma and cyst.

The periapical scar occurs most often in the anterior maxillary teeth.

(iv) **Chronic and acute dentoalveolar abscesses:** Abscesses make up about 2% of all pathologic periapical radiolucencies.

The primary abscess develops in a periapical region that is normal on radiographic examination.

The secondary abscess may be of the chronic or the acute type.

A periapical radiolucency is a feature of the secondary abscess.

The radiolucency may vary from small to quite large to involve much of the jaw.

The initial periapical lesion may even cause an expansion of the cortical plate.

In later stages the margins of the radiolucency may vary from well defined with a hyperostotic border to poorly defined in chronic cases.

(v) **Surgical defect:** A surgical defect in bone is an area that fails to fill in with osseous tissue after surgery.

The periapical radiolucency is usually rounded in appearance, is smoothly contoured, and has well-defined borders.

It usually does not measure more than 1 cms in diameter.

The radiolucent shadow may be projected directly over the apex or a few millimeters beyond the apex of the resected root of the endodontically treated tooth.

(vi) **Osteomyelitis:** Defined as an infection of bone that involves all three components: periosteum, cortex, and marrow.

Acute osteomyelitis is seen as rounded periapical radiolucency that resembles the image seen in a periapical cyst, granuloma, or abscess.

Chronic osteomyelitis may demonstrate four distinct radiographic pictures:

Completely radiolucent, mixed radiolucent and radiopaque, completely radiopaque, and proliferative periostitis.

If a sequestrum is present and large enough, it shows as a radiopacity within a radiolucency.

(vii) **Pulpoperiapical disease and hyperplasia of maxillary sinus lining:** Pulpoperiapical inflammation or infection and periodontal conditions frequently produce local inflammatory hyperplasia of the adjacent antral soft tissue floor.

These appear as gray shadows that may be dome shaped in the maxillary sinus floor or a gray radiopacity that appears as a cap over the adjacent troublesome root.

(viii) **Dentigerous cyst:** Although a dentigerous cyst forms adjacent to the crown of an unerupted tooth, sometimes the position of the crown of the involved tooth and the extension of the cyst is such that the pericoronal radiolucency is projected over the apex of a neighboring tooth.

(ix) **Periapical Cemental Dysplasia:** It is the lesion previously known as periapical cementoma.

The early stage is radiolucent and the lesions are usually somewhat rounded, have well-defined borders, and are associated with teeth having vital pulps.

(x) **Periodontal Disease:** It causes a relatively common periapical radiolucency.

Such a radiolucency is usually caused by advanced periodontal bone loss involving one tooth more severely than the teeth immediately adjacent.

(xi) **Traumatic Bone Cyst:** Its a pseudocyst more commonly involving the mandible. On radiographic examination a traumatic bone cyst is a well-defined (cystlike) radiolucency above the mandibular canal, is predominantly round to oval, and may be positioned somewhat symmetrically about the periapex of a root.

It usually extends superiorly between the premolar and molar roots, producing a scalloped appearance.

The lateral and inferior borders of the elongated variety have smooth, regular contours.

(xii) **Nonradicular Cysts:** On occasion, nonradicular cysts may be projected over the apices of teeth.

The most common offenders are the incisive canal cyst, midpalatine cyst, median mandibular cyst, traumatic bone cyst and primordial cyst.

(xiii) **Malignant Tumors:** Malignant tumors may produce the following images:

(I) a well-defined periapical radiolucency; (2) a poorly defined periapical radiolucency; or (3) a large, ragged, well-defined radiolucent tumor that has destroyed a large segment of the surface bone and has involved the apex of a tooth.

I) True periapical radiopacities:

(i) **Condensing Or Sclerosing Osteitis:** Condensing or sclerosing osteitis is a sclerosis of bone induced by an inflammation or infection that most often occurs as a pulpoperiapical lesion.

The condensing osteitis occurs chiefly at the apex of a pulpless tooth or a tooth with an infected pulp.

The radiographic image varies greatly in size, shape, contour, and discreteness of margins.

(ii) **Periapical Idiopathic Osteosclerosis:** Also known as enostosis is a relatively common finding on full-mouth radiographs of dentulous patients over 12years of age. Size may vary from a few millimeters to 2 cm in diameter. Its shape may range from generally round to very irregular, and sometimes a triangular configuration.

The degree of density may vary from a slight accentuation of the trabecular pattern to a dense homogeneous radiopaque mass.

Borders may be well defined or vague and well contoured or ragged.

(iii) **Mature Periapical cemental dysplasia:** On radiographs the completely mature periapical cemental dysplasia appears as round or oval with smoothly contoured borders. It varies in diameter from 0.5 to 2 cm.

This mature lesion is uniformly dense, is devoid of trabecular pattern, and may have a thin radiolucent border.

(iv) **Unerupted Succedaneous Teeth:** When the permanent crowns of succedaneous teeth are completely formed and the resorption of the root ends of the corresponding deciduous teeth is initiated, the images of the permanent tooth crowns represent periapical radiopacities.

(v) **Foreign Bodies:** Radiopaque foreign bodies in the periapex are usually root canal-filling materials.

The images are produced by extruded gutta percha, silver points, sealer, or retrograde amalgam restoration, and the filled root canal.

(vi) **Hypercementosis:** Hypercementosis is excessive formation of cementum on the surface of the root of the tooth.

On radiographs the altered shape of the root is apparent if there has been a reasonable amount of cemental hyperplasia and the root is surrounded by a normal periodontal ligament space and lamina dura. On anterior teeth may appear as a spherical mass of cementum attached to the root end.

II) False Periapical Radiopacities:

(i) **Anatomic Structures:** Anterior nasal spine, ala of the nose, malar process of the maxilla, external oblique ridge, mylohyoid ridge, mental protuberance, and hyoid bone may project over apices of teeth.

(ii) **Impacted Teeth, Supernumerary Teeth, And Compound Odontomas:** May be projected over the apices of teeth and are false radopacities.

(iii) **Tori, Exostoses, And Peripheral Osteomas:** May appear on radiographs as single or multiple, smoothly contoured, somewhat rounded, dense radiopaque masses.

These radiopaque images are not circumscribed by a periodontal ligament space and lamina dura.

(iv) **Retained Root Tips:** Retained root tips, especially in the molar regions may be situated so that their radiopaque shadows are projected over the apex of an adjacent tooth.

(v) **Foreign Bodies:** Objects such as metal fragments, buttons, zippers, hooks, other metal dress accessories, jewellery, and various dental materials and fragments of instruments that may project over the root apices.

(vi) **Mucosal Cyst Of The Maxillary Sinus:** On radiographs the cyst usually appears as a relatively dense, dome-shaped mass with its base on the floor of the maxillary sinus.

The apices of the maxillary first and second molars may appear to be within the opaque image of the cyst.

(vii) **Ectopic Calcifications:** Ectopic calcifications in the soft tissues surrounding the jaw may be projected on radiographs at the apices of teeth as radiopacities.

- **Sialoliths:** If they are not expelled from the duct, however, they eventually become large enough to be visible as radiopacities. Those of the submandibular salivary glands would be projected at the mandibular teeth apices and those in the parotid duct will be projected on maxillary molar teeth.
- **Rhinoliths and Antroliths:** Their images may be cast over the apices of adjacent maxillary teeth on periapical radiographs. They may appear as a dense, homogeneous radiopacity or may show concentric rings of radiopaque material.
- **Calcified Lymph Nodes:** Calcified lymph nodes occur in the cervical and submaxillary Regions.
  On radiographs a single round, oval, or linear calcified radiopaque mass may be seen as periapical radiopacities.
- **Phleboliths:** Phleboliths (angioliths) are calcified thrombi occurring in venules, veins, or sinusoidal vessels of hemangiomas.
  They may occur singly or as multiple calcifications, are usually small radiopacities, may be round or oval, and may show concentric light and dark rings and may be projected over teeth apices.
- **Arterial Calcifications:** Sometimes when the facial artery is involved these may be seen as periapical radiopacities.

Suggested reading:

1. Norman K Wood, Paul W. Goaz, Differential Diagnosis Of Oral And Maxillofacial Lesions, 5th edition, 457-475. 259-276.

CHAPTER 15

Miscellaneous

Q 1) Define ideal radiograph. Describe the technique for intraoral periapical radiograph in detail with merits and demerits.

MUHS DECEMBER 2005 (10 marks)

Ideal Radiograph:

Can be defined as a radiograph with desired density or overall darkness, optimum details to make the details fully apparent, and which shows the part completely with minimum distortion and maximum details.

There are two techniques used to take periapical radiographs:

(a) The paralleling or long cone or right angle technique.
(b) Short cone or bisecting angle technique.

(a) The Paralleling technique:

- It is a method that is preferred for taking IOPA radiographs. It is so named because the film is placed parallel to the long axis of the tooth and it minimises image distortion.
- To make the tooth and the film parallel, the radiographer has to place the film many a times in the center of the oral cavity away from the teeth.
- This method results in the teeth being parallel to the film, but as the distance between them is more it can result in magnification and loss of definition due to increased unsharpness.
- To minimise magnification, the focal spot to film distance is increased by using a long cone.
- The essence of this technique is that the x ray film is supported parallel to the long axis of the tooth and the central ray of the x-ray beam is directed perpendicular to both the tooth and the film.
- Rules to be followed in paralleling technique:
- Placement of film: It should be so placed so that the area of the teeth to be examined should be covered completely.
- Film position: The film has to be placed parallel to the long axis of the tooth. The film is placed away from the tooth and

the holder has to be placed in the midline of the oral cavity to achieve this.

- The rotation of holder is so done, that the teeth to be examined should touch the block. The patient is instructed to gently bite together so that the film holder is stabilised in proper position.
- The focal spot to film distance is determined correctly as the long cone is aligned with the locator ring.
- Then the exposure is made.

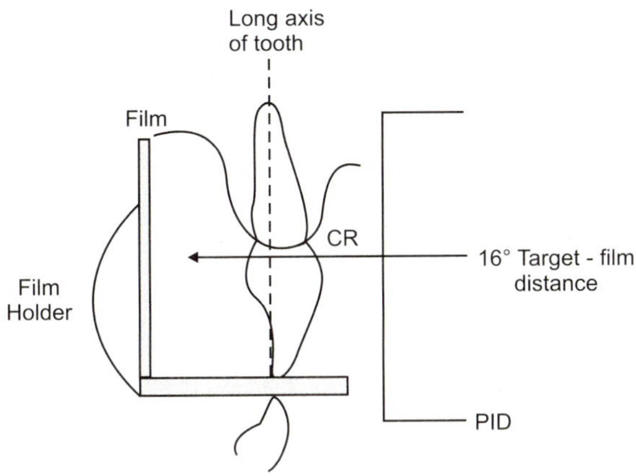

Fig. Positioning of film holder and direction of central ray in long cone technique

Advantages of Paralleling Technique:

- **Accuracy:** the paralleling technique produces an image that has dimensional accuracy which is due to: Increased source film distance, Object and film are parallel, Though the object film distance is increased it is compensated by increased source film distance and therefore there is decreased enlargement.
- **Simplicity:** Technique is simple, easy to use.
- **Duplication:** This technique is easy to standardize and can be accurately duplicated or repeated.
- Decreased secondary radiation.
- The radiograph produced give: An excellent bone level assessment.

No elongation or foreshortening seen in periapical region.

Inter proximal caries can be seen clearly.

- The shadow of the zygomatic bone is projected above the molar teeth apices.
- Periodontal bone level can be seen clearly.
- Periapical tissues can be seen clearly with minimum elongation and foreshortening.
- Useful in handicapped and compromised patients.

Disadvantages Of Paralleling Technique:

- Film Placement: The film holding device is difficult to use in children and the patients having reduced mouth opening.

- Positioning the film holders within the oral cavity can be difficult for operators who lack experience.
- Film holders can cause discomfort and gagging.
- Increase in exposure time.
- Holders need to be autoclavable.

b. Bisecting angle technique:

- It is based on the simple geometrical principle known as "the rule of isometry" or "ciesenzky's rule of isometry" which states the triangles having two angles that are equal and which share a common side are equal.
- In this technique the film is placed in close apposition to the tooth along the lingual surface and the point where the tooth and film come in contact, an angle is formed between the plane of the film and the long axis of the tooth.
- Operator must visualize a plane that divides a plane which divides in half or bisects the angle formed by the long axis of the tooth and the film. This plane is known as "imaginary bisector".
- Because of this bisector, two equal angles are created and also provides a common side for the two imaginary triangles.
- The hypotenuse of one imaginary triangle is represented by the long axis of the tooth and the other by the plane of the film.
- Nevertheless, by directing the central ray perpendicular to a plane that is imaginary and bisects the angle formed by the tooth and the film, the practitioner can make the length of the tooth's image on the film correspond to the actual length of the tooth. This angle between a tooth and the film is especially apparent when teeth are radiographed in the maxilla or anterior mandible.
- Even though the projected length of a tooth is correct, the image is still distorted because the film and object are not parallel and the beam of x-ray is not at right angles to both of them. This distortion tends to increase along the image toward the apex.

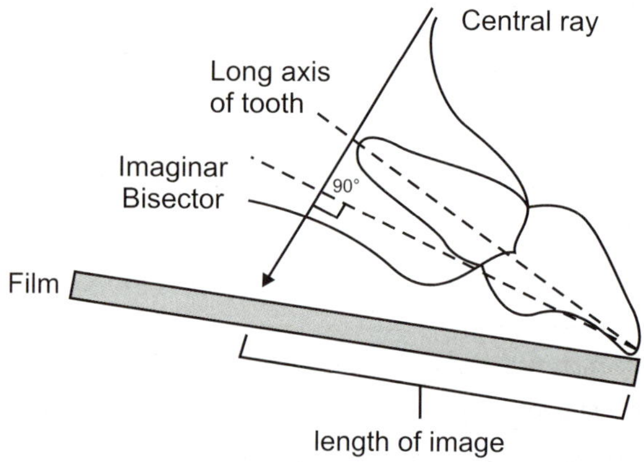

Fig. Position of film and direction of central ray in short cone technique

Advantages of Bisecting Angle Technique:

- Can Be Used Without Film Holder.
- Positioning Is simple, comfortable And quick.
- Decreased exposure time.
- No sterilization of the holder is required.

Disadvantages of Bisecting Angle Technique:

- Image distortion is more commonly seen.
- Angulation problems can lead to more chances of elongation and shortening.
- In finger holding technique, the patient may shift the position of film.
- Coning off can occur when the central ray is not directed at the center of the film.
- Periodontal bone levels and proximal caries are poorly represented.
- Buccal roots of premolars and molars are foreshortened.

Suggested reading:

1. Freny R Karjodkar, Essentials of Oral and Maxillofacial Radiology, chapter 11, pg no.99-115.

Q 2) Enumerate multilocular lesions of the oral cavity. Write in detail about clinical features, radiographic appearance & differential diagnosis of the central haemangioma:

MUHS WINTER 2012 (10 Marks)

Compartments in the bone that are pathologic, multiple, adjacent and often coalescing cause radiolucencies that are multilocular. Though they can be seen in the maxilla they are more commonly in the mandible.

The terms soap bubble, honeycomb, and tennis racket are frequently used to describe the various radiographic images of multilocular lesions.

Soap bubble - lesions consisting of several circular compartments that vary in size and appear to some what overlap.

Honeycomb - lesions whose compartments are small and tend to be uniform in size.

Tennis racket - lesions composed of angular rather than rounded compartments that result from the development of more or less straight septa. Therefore these compartments tend to be triangular, rectangular, or square.

Multilocular radiolucent lesions of the oral cavity include the following:

1. Multilocular cyst
2. Ameloblastoma
3. Central giant cell granuloma
4. Giant cell lesion of Hyperparathyroidism

5. Cherubism
6. Odontogenic myxoma
7. Odontogenic keratocyst
8. Aneurysmal bone cyst
9. Metastatic tumors to the jaws
10. Vascular malformations
11. Central hemangioma of bone

Rarities:

1. Ameloblastic variants
2. Arteriovenous malformations
3. Burkitt's lymphoma
4. Calcifying epithelial odontogenic tumor
5. Cementoossifying fibroma.

Proliferation of blood vessels that create a mass that resembles a neoplasm, though in many cases, a hamartoma is called hemangioma. They can affect any part of the body but are most common on the skin and subcutaneous tissues. The intraosseous (central type) is most commonly seen in the vertebrae and skull. It rarely occurs in the jaws, and is more common in mandible than maxilla. The lesions could be developmental or traumatic in origin.

Central haemangioma:

1. Cavernous hemangioma: consists of dilated blood containing spaces, lined by endothelium.
2. Arterial or plexiform haemangioma: arises from the arteries.

Clinical features:

- Central hemangioma lesion is developmental or traumatic in origin. It arises either from the periosteum & resorbs the underlying bone or occurs within the bone as an anomaly of blood vessels within the marrow spaces.
- Hemangiomas are more prevalent in females than males, the ratio being 2:1.
- The occurrence is most commonly in the first decade but may occur later in life.
- Enlargement is slow, producing a non tender expansion of the jaw that occurs over several months or years.
- The swelling may or may not be painful, is not tender. and usually is bony hard.
- Pain, if present, probably is the throbbing type.
- In some cases the tumours can be compressible and pulsatile and on auscultation bruit may be detected.
- Anesthesia of the skin supplied by the mental nerve may occur.
- In the area affected there can be loosening and migration of the teeth.

- Gingival bleeding from around the necks of the affected teeth can occur,
- The teeth can show a rebound mobility; that is, when depressed into their sockets, they rebound to their original position within several minutes because of the pressure of the vascular network around the tooth. This is also called as the pumping tooth syndrome.
- Aspiration with a syringe produces arterial blood that may be under considerable pressure.
- Kasabach-Merritt syndrome: it is associated with extensive hemangioma in infants, thrombocytopenia & haemorrhage due to entrapment of platelet within the tumor.

Radiographic features:

- affect the mandible about twice as often as the maxilla.
- In the mandible the most common site is the posterior border and the ramus region and also within the inferior alveolar canal.
- In some instances the periphery is well defined and corticated, and in other cases it may be ill defined and even simulate the appearance of a malignant tumor.
- Linear spicules of bone can form that emanate from the surface of the bone in a sunray-like appearance can occur in case when the hemangioma breaks through the outer cortex and causes displacement of the periosteum.
- When there is trapping of the residual bone around the blood vessels, it can cause a multilocular appearance.
- Small radiolucent locules may resemble enlarged marrow spaces surrounded by coarse, dense, and well-defined trabeculae.
- These internal trabeculae may produce a honeycomb pattern composed of small circular radiolucent spaces that represent blood vessels oriented in the same direction of the x-ray beam.
- Some lesions reveal coarse, linear trabeculae that appear to radiate from an approximate centre of the lesion giving spokes of a wheel or cart wheel appearance.
- When the inferior alveolar canal is involved, the whole canal is increased in width and often the normal path of the canal is altered into a serpiginous shape sometimes creating a multilocular appearance.
- Some lesions may be totally radiolucent.
- The roots of teeth in the region of the vascular lesion often are resorbed or displaced.
- When the lesion involves the inferior alveolar nerve canal, the canal can be enlarged along its entire length and its shape may be changed to a serpiginous path.
- The mandibular and mental foramen may be enlarged.

- Hemangiomas can influence the growth of bone and teeth.
- The involved bone may be enlarged and have coarse, internal trabeculae.
- Also, developing teeth may be larger and erupt earlier when in an intimate relationship with a hemangioma.

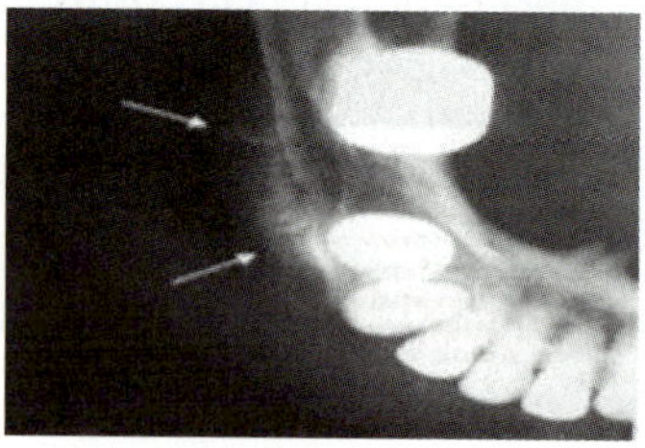

Fig. Sun-ray appearance of haemangioma

Differential Diagnosis:

1. **Central giant cell granuloma:** Central giant cell granuloma crosses the midline where as central hemangioma does not.
2. **Giant cell lesions of hyperparathyroidism:** Biochemical investigations to be carried out to will rule out hyperparathyroidism.
3. **Aneurysmal bone cyst:** Hemangioma will show profuse haemmorhage on aspiration.
4. **Ameloblastic fibroma:** In hemangioma, honeycomb appearance, local gingival bleeding with pumping action of tooth is seen.
5. **Odontogenic myxoma:** Tennis racket pattern seen in myxoma.
6. **Ameloblastoma:** It occurs in old age.
7. **Metastatic tumor:** H/O of primary tumor is present.
8. **Cherubism:** Usually bilateral with typical facial appearance.
9. **Traumatic bone cysts:** Well defined entity with better defined borders.
10. **Central giant cell granuloma:** Central giant cell granuloma crosses the midline where as central hemangioma does not.
11. **Giant cell lesions of hyperparathyroidism:** Biochemical investigations to be carried out to rule out hyperparathyroidism.

Vascular malformations, including the Central Hemangioma, are dangerous lesions of the jaw because rapid exsanguination often follows tooth extraction and jaw fracture. Because of this lethal potential, when a bony radiolucent lesion is encountered in the jaws, a Central Hemangioma or arteriovenous aneurysm must always be considered, especially since such a tumor often demonstrates a variety of radiographic appearances.

Specifically the clinician should form a strong impression of Central Hemangioma when encountering:

- a pumping tooth.
- localized gingival bleeding around a loose tooth coupled with radiographic evidence of bony change in the region.
- large quantities of blood are easily aspirated from the area.

Treatment:

Central hemangiomas must be treated without causing delay because trauma that causes disruption of the integrity of the jaws that are affected and may result in exsanguinations that are lethal.

Specifically, embolization (introduction of inert materials into the lesion by a vascular route), surgery (en bloc resection with ligation of the external carotid artery), and sclerosing techniques have been used singly or together.

Suggested reading:

1. Burket's, Oral Medicine Diagnosis and Treatment 10th edi. 445-449.
2. Norman K wood, Paul. W. Goaz, Differential Diagnosis of Oral and Maxillofacial Lesions, 5th edition. 333-356.

Q 3) Discuss the differential diagnosis of radiolucencies on coronal part of teeth.

RUGHS OCTOBER 1999 (10 Marks)

Pericoronal radiolucencies comprise those lesions which cause radiolucency in the coronal region of the tooth or teeth. The teeth are usually not erupted or may be clinically covered by the cystic fluid under the overlying mucosa.

✪ Lesions which produce pericoronal radiolucencies are as follows:

Most common	Rarities
• Pericoronal Or Follicular Space • Dentigerous Cyst • Unicystic (Mural)Ameloblastoma • Ameloblastoma • Adenomatoid Odontogenic Tumor • Calcifying Odontogenic Cyst Or Tumor • Ameloblastic Fibroma	• Ameloblastic variants • Calcifying epithelial odontogenic tumor • Envelopmental primordial cyst • Ewing's sarcoma • Extrafollicular dentigerous cyst • Follicular primordial cyst • Langerhans' cell disease • Malignant teratoma • Odontogenic carcinoma • Odontogenic fibroma • Odontogenic keratocyst • Odontogenic myxoma • Odontoma in pericoronal location (premineralized stage) • Ossifying fibroma • Other radiolucencies projected onto images • of impacted tooth crowns • Paradental cyst

- Pseudotumor of hemophilia
- Salivary gland tumors (central)
- Squamous cell carcinoma
- Squamous odontogenic tumor

(a) Pericoronal Or Follicular Space:

- The crowns of teeth that are unerupted are generally surrounded by a dental follicle which is a soft tissue remnant of the enamel organ known as the reduced enamel epithelium.
- Radiographically, it appears as a homogenous radiolucent halo having thin radiopaque border which is continuous with lamina dura.
- Radiolucent halo merge with PDL space.

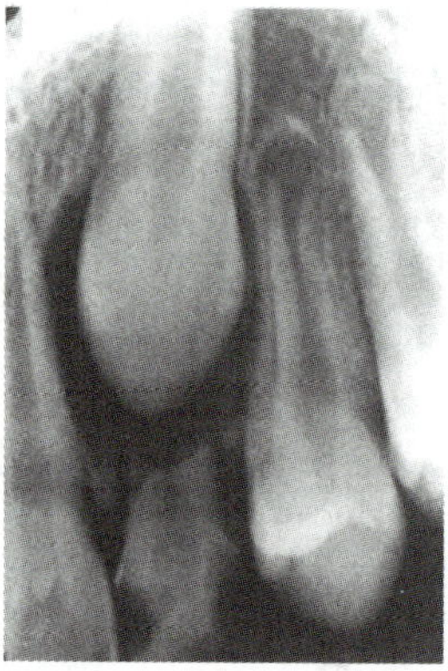

Fig. Follicular spaces surrounding maxillary canines

(b) Dentigerous cyst:

- It is the most common pathologic pericoronal radiolucency.
- The cyst is always associated with the crown of an impacted, embedded or a tooth that is unerupted.
- It has a lumen lined with epithelium derived from the enamel organ or from other remnants of the dental lamina.
- Most frequently involved teeth are the mandibular third molars and premolars, maxillary canines and the third molars.,
- Epicenter is located above the crown of the involved tooth.
- An important diagnostic point is that this cyst attaches at the cementoenamel junction.
- Dentigerous cysts have a typical well defined cortical border and has curved or circular outline. If infection is present, the cortex may be missing.
- The internal structure of the cyst is radiolucent completely except for the crown of the involved tooth.
- A dentigerous cyst has the tendency to displace and cause resorption of the adjacent teeth.
- One of the most difficult differential diagnoses to make is

between a small dentigerous cyst and a hyperplastic follicle. A cyst should be considered when tooth displacement or considerable expansion of the involved bone is present. The size of the normal follicular space is 2-3 mm. If the follicular space exceeds 5 mm, a dentigerous cyst is more likely present.

(c) Unicystic (Mural) Ameloblastoma

- The unicystic ameloblastoma that forms in the wall of a existing dentigerous cyst occurs second in number to the dentigerous cyst as the most commonly pathologic pericoronal radiolucency.
- The unicystic (mural) ameloblastoma is asymptomatic and remains undetected until the pericoronal radiolucency is observed on a routine radiograph.
- When the lesion enlarges gradually, a swelling that is non-tender can be seen on clinical examination. This swelling occurs because of the expansion of the buccal and lingual cortical plates of the jaws and can be felt on palpation as a hard and bony swelling.
- Radiographically a localized thinning and haziness of the hyperostotic radiopaque rim of the pericoronal radiolucency must make the clinician to suspect that there could be penetration by mural ameloblastoma in the fibrous capsule of a dentigerous cyst that has occurred and is initiating the invasion of bone between trabeculae.

Ameloblastoma:

- It grows slowly and silently without clinical signs in early stages & later it causes migration, mobility, tipping.
- Radiographically these multilocular lesions may appear as soap bubble, honey comb or tennis racket pattern.
- Cortices are spared & expanded & in some cases they can be destructed.
- Common finding is the resorption of roots.

(d) Adenomatoid Odontogenic Tumor (Adenoameloblastoma):

- The AOT is a benign and uncommon tumour and is not invasive.
- The origin is thought to be from residual odontogenic epithelium.
- It is a tumour that grows slowly and does not cause bone infiltration. They however tend to displace teeth and donot usually cause root resorption.
- Most of them occur in association with teeth that are unerupted or in the dentigerous cyst walls, and some AOTs are not associated with teeth, and a few are extraosseous.
- More frequent in the maxilla than in the mandible.
- Unerupted teeth frequently associated with this tumor (in order of frequency) are the maxillary canine, lateral incisor, and mandibular premolar.

- Lesion is completely radiolucent and mimics a dentigerous cyst in growth pattern and appearance.
- Continued growth which is rather slow may cause expansion of the cortical plates and may result in swelling that is clinically visible and can cause asymmetry, but invasion of the soft tissue does not occur.

(e) Calcifying Odontogenic Cyst or Tumor:

- It is a mixed radiolucent – radiopaque lesion but in early stages it appears as a completely radiolucent cyst like lesion.

(f) Ameloblastic fibroma:

- Its a true odontogenic tumour that is mixed, containing nests and strands of odontogenic and ameloblastic epithelium in a primitive, dental papilla like connective tissue.
- The ameloblastic fibroma unlike the AOT is not usually associated with an unerupted tooth but occur in the similar age group of below 20 years.
- The ameloblastic fibroma does not demonstrate a predilection for either gender.
- Although this tumor may arise in either jaw, the majority occur in the mandibular premolar and molar regions .
- This mixed odontogenic tumor grows slowly by expansion of the cortex and usually does not invade bone.
- On radiographic examination the ameloblastic fibroma is usually seen as a pericoronal radiolucency but may appear unilocular or multilocular.
- It can show cortical expansion & may spread the roots of adjacent Teeth.

Suggested reading:

1. Norman K .Wood, Paul W. Goaz, Differential Diagnosis Of Oral And Maxillofacial Lesions, 5th Edition, Chapter 17, Pg No.279.
2. Stuart C White, Michael J Pharoah, Oral Radiology, Principles and Interpretation 5th edition, chapter 20, pg no 384-408.

Q 3) Discuss the causes of distortion of images in the radiographs:

FEBRUARY 2006 (15 Marks)

Distortion can be defined as magnification that is unequal of different parts of the same object.

Distortion is defined as a misrepresentation of the shape or size of an object that is being examined.

It is of two types:

1. Image size distortion.
2. Image shape distortion.

Image size distortion:

It is also called as magnification and is increase in size of the image on the final x-ray as compared to the actual size of the object.

Image size distortion results from the relative distances of the focal spot-to-film and object to film.

When there is divergence of the path of the x-ray photons of an x-ray beam, there is an enlargement of the image of the object on the radiograph.

Factors that influence magnification are:

(a) Target-film distance:

This is determined in the intra-oral machines by the length of the position indicating device.

- Longer the position indicating device more parallel are the x-rays that strike the object from the middle of the beam instead of the more diverging rays from the periphery of the beam. This reduces magnification.
- Shorter the position indicating device length, less parallel x-rays from the middle of the beam strike the object, and more diverging x-rays from the periphery hit the object, resulting in greater magnification.

(b) Object-film distance:

- Lesser the object–film distance, lesser is the magnification.
- Increasing the object-film distance increases the magnification.

(c) Use of intensifying screens:

The use of these increases the film-object distance, which produces some amount of magnification.

The formulas for magnification are:

The percentage of magnification of an object at any source to film distance and object to film distance can be determined by:

$$\frac{\text{Source - Film - Distance}}{\text{SFD - OFD}} - \text{OFD} \cdot 100\% = \text{Percentage of magnification}$$

The rule for magnification: The actual size of the object is proportional to the size of the projected radiographic image of the object, as the source-object distance is to the source-film distance.

S1(size of the object)/S2(size of the image)=Source-Object distance/ Source-Film distance.

Formula to calculate size distortion is:

Image width/object width=focal spot to film distance(FFD)/film to object distance (FOD).

Accordingly with an increase in the focal spot-film distance and a decrease in the object-film distance the magnification can be minimised.

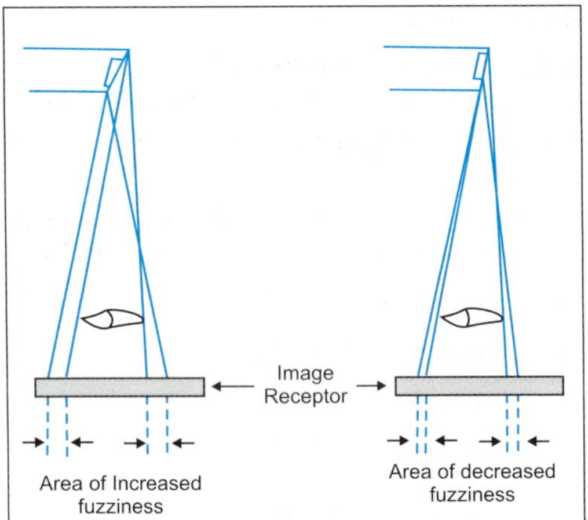

Increasing the distance between the focal spot & object nesults in an image with increased sharpness & less magnification

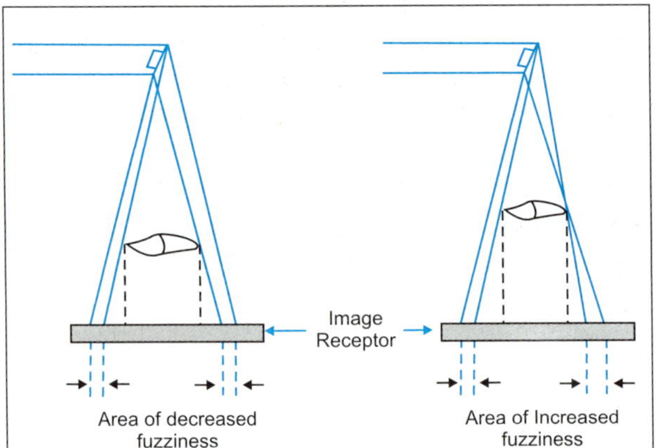

Decreasing the distance between the object & film increases the sharpness and results in less magnification of object

Fig.

The use of long cones in periapical radiography as a aiming device can reduce the magnification.

Furthermore, as mentioned above, this technique also improves image clarity by increasing focal spot-object distance.

Image shape distortion:

Image shape distortion occurs because of unequal magnification of the different portions of the same object. This usually results when all parts of the object of interest are not at the same focal spot-object distance.

Dimensional distortion of a radiographic image is the variation in the actual shape and size of the structure that is being radiographed. A distorted image occurs as a result of magnification that is unequal of different portions of the same object.

The physical shape of the object may often prevent its optimal orientation, resulting in some shape distortion.

The factors that cause image shape distortion are:

(a) Alignment of the object and the film: The object of interest and the film should be parallel to each other, because if they are not, and there is an angular relationship between them, it can produce variation of distance between the object and the film, resulting in distortion.

The distorted image may be too long or too short, that is elongated or shortened.

(b) X-ray beam angulation: To minimise distortion of dimension the beam of x--ray should be perpendicular to the tooth and the film as well, so as to record the tooth and their adjacent structures in their actual relationship.

- If the vertical angulation is increased then there will be shortening of the image.
- If the horizontal angulation is decreased, there will be elongation of the image.
- If the horizontal angulation is increased or decreased there will be overlapping of the structures.

Thus:

When the central ray of the x-ray is perpendicular to the film but the object of interest is not parallel to the film causes the resultant image to be distorted because of the unequal distances of the various parts of the object from the film. This type of shape distortion is called foreshortening because it causes the radiographic image to be shorter than the object.

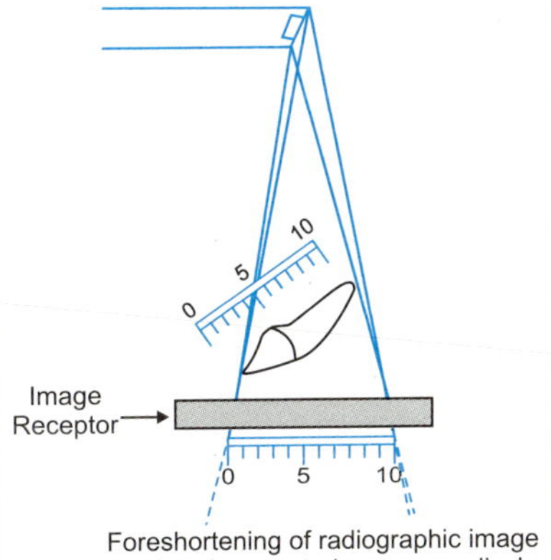

Foreshortening of radiographic image results when central ray perpendicular to film but object is not parallel to film

Fig. Central ray perpendicular to the film, but the object is not parallel to the film resulting in foreshortening

Sometimes the x-ray beam is oriented at right angles to the object but not to the film. This results in elongation, with the object appearing longer on the film than its actual length.

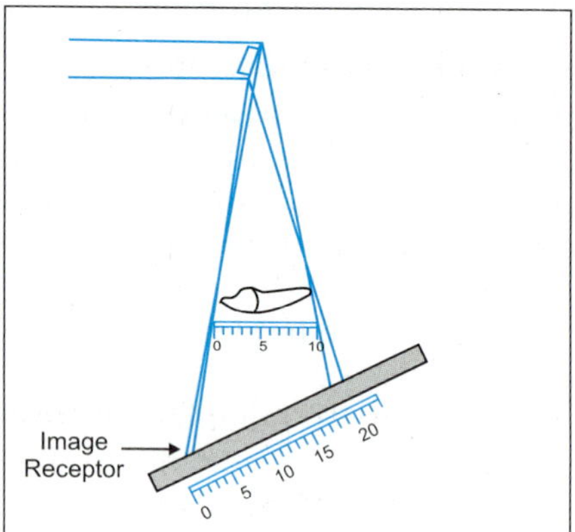

Fig. Central x-ray beam perpendicular to the object but not the film causing elongation of image

This is most evident on maxillary molar projections:

When the central ray is given an excess of vertical angulation there is disproportionately longer appearance of the palatal roots of the molars than the buccal roots.

Reduction of distortion:

The teeth and the alveolar processes are units of facial bone and are fixed components of the skull.

If the head position is stabilised the position of teeth and the surrounding structures is automatically stabilised.

Care should be taken so that:

- The plane of occlusion should be parallel to the floor.
- The sagittal plane should be perpendicular to the floor.

This can reduce the errors associated with angulation of the beam.

If the height of the palatal arch is more, the vertical angulation should be decreased.

(c) The film should never be bent in the direction of the long axis of the tooth and the holder of the film should be used to prevent the movement of film during exposure.

Causes of distortion in panoramic radiographs:

(i) **Patient positioned too far back from the focal trough:** Results in narrowing of images of the dental arches.

(ii) **Patients head twisted to one side:** Results in unequal size of the dental arches.

(iii) **Chin is tipped too low:** Causes vertical narrowed images of the arches.

(iv) **Chin is tipped too high:** Results in widened magnified images of the arches.

(v) **Chin is not on the rest:** Results in narrow arches but wide magnification.

(vi) Patient is not standing straight.

(vii) When lips are open and the tongue is not touching the palate.

- Patient movement in same direction as the beam leads to prolonged exposure of the same area increasing horizontal dimension of the image.
- Movement of patient in opposite direction as that of the beam leads to decrease in horizontal dimension of the image.
- Sudden jerky movement of the patient in the same direction as the beam, the area is projected twice.
- Sudden movements that are jerky of the patient in the opposite direction as the beam, leads to a part of object missing in the image.
- In case of the up and down movement of the patient during exposure leads to indentation in the lower border of the mandible, blurring and unsharpness.

Suggested reading:

1. Freny. R. Karjodkar, Essentials of oral and maxillofacial radiology, 1st edition, 89-91.
2. Stuart C White, Michael J Pharoah, Oral Radiology, Principles and Interpretation 5th Edition, 87-89.

Q 4) What is an Ideal radiograph? Enumerate the various factors influencing the quality of radiographs. Describe in detail the role of processing procedures on the quality of radiographs.

TNMGRU AUGUST 2004 (16 Marks)

Ideal radiograph:

- An ideal radiograph is that which has the desired density and overall blackness and that which shows the area of interest completely, without distortion and with maximum details and has the right amount of contrast to make the details completely apparent.
- An ideal radiograph is that which has optimum density, maximum detail and contrast sufficient to make the details apparent. The image should be sharp, centered and should have the same size and shape as that of the object of interest.

Characteristics of an ideal radiograph:

(a) Visual characteristic:

  (i) Density

  (ii) Contrast

(b) Geometric characteristics:

(iii) Sharpness or detail
(iv) Resolution or definition
(v) Magnification
(vi) Distortion

(c) Anatomical accuracy of the radiographic images.

D. Adequate coverage of the anatomical region of interest.

Various factors influencing the quality of radiographs:

1. Factors related to the x-ray beam:
   (a) Exposure time.
   (b) Milliamperage.
   (c) kilovoltage peak.
   (d) Tube-film distance.
   (e) Focal spot size.
   (f) Collimation.
   (g) Filtration.
   (h) Equipment efficiency.
2. Factors related to the object:
   (a) Object thickness.
   (b) Object density.
3. Factors related to the technique:
   (a) Position of patients head.
   (b) Placement and position of film.
   (c) Angulation of the x-ray beam.
4. Factors related to recording of the x-ray image of an object:
   (a) Reduction in secondary radiation.
   (b) Films and film storage.
   (c) Intensifying screens.
   (d) Film processing.

Role of processing procedures on the quality of radiographs:

1. **Storage of films:** Films should be stored in cool dry place away from ionising radiation, chemical fumes including mercury and mercury containing compounds. If proper care is not taken the resultant image may not be ideal.
   Fumes or smoking in the room can cause film fog.
2. **Dark Room:** Processing is carried out in a darkroom and hence the ideal conditions should be:
   - Location of the darkroom must be near the area where the x-ray unit is installed.
   - The size of the darkroom and the, working space should be adequate and there should be no contamination with the processing chemicals, water, dust and debris.
   - Adequate storage space for processing chemicals and films.
   - General cleanliness especially of work surfaces and hangers.
   - Light tightness of the room has to be perfect. Standing in the darkroom in total darkness with the doors close and safe lights

switched off, visual inspection of light leakage is compulsory.

- General room lighting requires incandescent light to perform tasks such as cleaning, stocking materials and mixing chemicals, and though not directly involves processing it ultimately helps to get ideal radiographs.
- Safelights should be in good condition and following checks are required:
  - (i) Type of filter: This should be compatible with the colour sensitivity of the film used, eg. blue, green, or ultraviolet.
  - (ii) The filters should not be scratched as it can affect the final image.
  - (iii) The bulb wattage should not be more than 15 watts, otherwise it can lead to darkening of the film.
  - (iv) To ensure no light leakage and proper safe ligting, simple coin test should be done.
  - (v) They should be mounted at least four feet above the working table.
  - (vi) Temperature and humidity of the darkroom should be maintained at 70 degrees farenheit. If above 90 degrees then film fog can result.
  - (vii) Humidity of the dark room should be between 50-70%. When it is very high, the film emulsion will not dry and if it is too low, can result in static electricity.
  - (viii) Plumbing of darkroom should have hot and cold running water to get correct water temperature in the processing tank.
  - (ix) Hangars should be present and the clips should be clean otherwise chemical deposits on clips can result in streaking of films.

3. **Processing of films:** Requires two solutions, that is developer and fixer. Following care should be taken:
   - The solutions should be made up to the manufactures's specification.
   - Special care should be taken to avoid slightest contamination of the developer solution by the fixer. Hence the fixer tank should be filled first because, the splashes from the fixing solution in to the developing tank can be washed away before putting the developer.
   - Any kind of contamination of the solutions with oil or other impurities should be avoided as it can result in deposits on the film.
   - Temperature should be maintained at optimum that is 65-75 degrees farenheit.
   - The solutions must be regularly replenished, ideally every 2 weeks and records should be maintained.
   - Solutions should be monitored for deterioration. This can

be done using radiographs of a step-edge phantom.

4. **Cassettes:**
   - Intensifying screens should be regularly cleaned with a proprietary cleaner. The films and intensifying screens should be dust and dirt free or can lead to white spots or lines on the film.
   - Light tightness of the cassettes should be checked by loading the cassette with an unexposed film and kept on a window sill in daylight for a few minutes. Any ingress of light will result in film fog on developing.
   - Regular checking of the screen-film contact should be done. The cassette is loaded with a film and same sized piece of graph paper. The film is exposed with a very short exposure time. After the film is processed, any areas of poor film/screen contact will be demonstrated by loss of definition of the image of the graph paper.
   - For digital phosphor storage plates, regular cleaning and visual checks for scratches or other defects should be done.
5. **Processing methods:**
   (I) Manual: There are three types:
      (i) Time temperature.
      (ii) Modified time-temperature.
      (iii) Visual.
   (II) Automatic processing.
   (III) Daylight processing.
   (IV) Self developing films.
   (V) Manual processing and its effect on quality of radiograph:

General procedure:

In the time-temperature, visual and modified temperature methods the process begins by:

- The levels of developer and fixer solutions should be checked. If the solution level is low fresh solution has to be added.
  This can ensure that the strength of solutions is good and even the film can be completely immersed in the solutions so that proper image can be formed.
  Water should not be added to increase the levels as it weakens the strength of the solution.
  If the developer is weak it can result in light radiographs and if it is more than required it can lead to film fog.
  The developer should not be contaminated, exhausted or diluted because this can lead to light radiographs.
  Exhausted developer can cause yellow or brown stains on films.
  If the fixer is not replenished it can result in reticulation on the film.

The fixer acidity needs to controlled. Excessive acidity can cause brittleness and blisters on the film.
Weak fixer solution can cause orange peel appearance on films.

- The solution should be stirred with rod or paddle.
  This ensures equalisation of the temperature of the solution. Unbalanced temperature of the solutions can result in blistering of the film.
- The temperature of the developing solution should be between 65-75 degree farenheit.
  If not, it should be regularised. Optimum temperature is 68 degree farenheit, below 60 degrees the development will be too slow and can result in light radiographs.
  If temperature is above 80 degrees it can develop too rapidly and can cause film fog.
  Very hot developing solutions can cause frilling of the film.
  Warm solution can cause grainy appearance of the films.
  Sudden extreme changes in temperature can cause orange peel appearance of films.
- The darkroom is closed and the white light is turned off and safe light is turned on. It should be checked for light leakage, which will cause fim fog.
- The film is removed from the cassette gently with dry hands .
  The films should be handled with dry hands to prevent the black wrapping paper from sticking to the films which can cause black spots on the film.
  Handling should be gentle or can result in nail marks, bent films, peeled emulsions, tears. Excessive bending of films can produce white lines or spots on the film.
  Rapid removal of film can cause static electricity artifacts.
- The white light if turned on accidentally before putting the film in developer can cause dark radiograph.
- The film should be held only at the edges to prevent fingerprints mark.
  The film is clipped to the film hanger carefully. The clips of hangers should be clean otherwise chemical deposits on clips can result in streaking of films.
- In time temperature method according to the temperature of the solution the timer is set.
- The hanger with the film is immersed in the developing solution.
- Care is taken that the developer doesn't splash the film before it is put in developer as it can lead to black spots on films.
  The film should not touch one another or the developing tank as it can result in partial image.
  The films should be handled with care as rough handling can cause tear of the emulsion.
- The timer is set. The chances of over or under developing

leading to dark or light radiographs is minimised.

- The film hanger is agitated up and down for several times so as to prevent air bubble from clinging to the film.
  Failure to agitate the film can result in streaks and blisters on the film. However if very vigourously agitated then dark flow marks can result on the film.
  The films should not be touched during developing as it can cause black spots.
- In visual method the film is dipped in developer solution for ten seconds and observed under safe light. Too much exposure to safe light can lead to fogging of the film.
- When the timer goes off the hanger is removed and is placed in the circulating water of the rinsing tank.
  The water should be clean as dirty or contaminated water can cause streaks on films.
  Very rigorous washing can lead to peeling of emulsion from the film.
- Then the film is put in the fixer solution and gently agitated for 5 seconds after every 30 seconds so as to eliminate the bubbles and bringing the fixer in close contact with the film.
  Finger contamination with fixer and spot of fixer on film before processing can cause white spots, lines on films.
  Fixing time is about twice that of developing time. If excessively fixed, can cause light radiographs and inadequate fixing can cause dark radiographs and also streaks on the film.
  Excessive fixation can also cause faded image on the film.
- After fixing, the excess fixer is shaken off and the film is placed under running water for 10 minutes. It is necessary to remove all the chemicals from the film to improve the radiographic quality.
  Inadequate washing or dirty and contaminated water can lead to streaks on the film.
  Insufficient final wash can lead to fading of the film.
- Drying: Can be done in a dryer or at room temperature in a dust free area. It helps improve the image quality and helps in proper viewing.
  Excessive drying temperature should be avoided as it can lead to brittleness of the finished radiograph.

- **Automatic processing:**
  Consists of:
  - Processor housing.
  - Film speed slot.
  - Roller film transporter to move the film speedily through the developer, fixer, water and the compartments for drying.
  - The temperature and replenishing of the solutions same as in manual methods are necessary to get ideal radiographs.

- The rollers should be cleaned to remove heavy deposits of developer solution and other foreign bodies and dust or roughness of the rollers can cause defects that can prevent the formation of ideal radiographic film.
- Choosing the correct type of film for the time cycle of the developer should be done.
- **Daylight processing:**
  It involves stripping the film in a light proof pouch and eliminates the use of darkroom.
- **Self developing films:**
  The x-ray film is contained in a sachet containing the developer and fixer. After exposure the developer tab is pulled and milked down to towards the film to develop the film and then the fixer tab is pulled and film is fixed. Then the film is rinsed under running water for 10 minutes. No darkroom facility is required but the overall image quality is poor and the image deteriorates rapidly.

6. **Reduction:** An overexposed and overly developed film will be too dark and may affect the diagnostic value. A photographic reducer containing an oxidising agent, potassium ferricyanide which oxidises the silver to silver ferrocyanide, which then is dissolved by the sodium thiosulphate solution, can be used to reduce the darkness, instead of repeating the radiographs. This is called as Farmer's solution.
7. **Chemical intensification of radiographs:**
   - Sometimes the radiographs may be too light and instead of repeating, chemical intensification can be done. These act by converting the silver which forms the image into a compound which is more opaque, and more coloured or of a different physical form.
   - A number of coloured intensifying solutions are available:
     - In-chromium intensifier.
     - In-5 silver intensifier.
     - Copper -iodide intensifying solution.
     - XR-10 intensifying solution.
     - Line-toner solution..

The processed radiograph of low density is immersed in the intensifying solutions for a time of 3-8 minutes which depends on the density that is required.

Suggested reading:

1. Langland Olaf E., Langlais Robert P., Preece John W. Principles of Dental Imaging; 2002: 2nd edition,
2. White S.C., Pharoah M.C. Oral Radiology, Principles and Interpretation; 2011, 6th edition.